Games, Sports, and Exercises
FOR THE PHYSICALLY DISABLED

Games, Sports, and Exercises
FOR THE PHYSICALLY DISABLED

RONALD C. ADAMS

Director of Therapeutic Recreation and Adapted
Physical Education, Kluge Children's Rehabilitation Center and Research Institute,
University of Virginia Medical Center,
Charlottesville, Virginia

JEFFREY A. MC CUBBIN, Ph.D.

Department of Exercise and Sport Science,
Oregon State University,
Corvallis, Oregon

FOURTH EDITION

Lea & Febiger Philadelphia
London

1991

Lea & Febiger
200 Chester Field Parkway
Malvern, Pennsylvania   19355-9725
U.S.A.
(215) 251-2230
1-800-444-1785

Lea & Febiger (UK) Ltd.
145a Croydon Road
Beckenham, Kent BR3 3RB
U.K.

First Edition, 1972
   Reprinted, 1974
Translation:
   Spanish Edition by Editorial PAIDOS, Buenos Aires, Argentina, 1978
Second Edition, 1975
   Reprinted, 1978
   Reprinted, 1979
Third Edition, 1982
Fourth Edition, 1991

Library of Congress Cataloging-in-Publication Data

Games, sports, and exercises for the physically disabled /
   Ronald C. Adams . . . [et al.].—4th ed.
      p.   cm.
   Includes bibliographical references.
   ISBN 0-8121-1180-X
   1. Recreation therapy. 2. Physically handicapped—Recreation.
3. Exercise therapy. 4. Sports for the physically handicapped.
5. Physically handicapped—Rehabilitation. I. Adams, Ronald C.
   RM736.7.G35   1990
615.8'24—dc20   90-31284
                                                 CIP

Reprints of chapters may be purchased from Lea & Febiger in quantities of 100 or more.

PRINTED IN THE UNITED STATES OF AMERICA

Print number: 5   4   3   2   1

Preface

Considerable changes have been made in the Fourth edition of Games, Sports, and Exercises for the Physically Disabled. The new edition includes major revisions to most of the chapters. The authors have considerable experience in working with the physically disabled population in comprehensive clinical situations. Their strategies, intervention, and research have inspired further efforts to survey an expanded list of disability groups, including methods of delivering services. The text contains current thinking and state-of-the-art information on physical activity guidelines and intervention strategies, all of which have been tested and found practical by the authors. Useful ideas for practical application are featured throughout the text.

Both authors have extensive background knowledge in transferring medical information into practical procedures in school physical education programs. This is the most complete text on the market that emphasizes the similarities of therapeutic recreation and adapted physical education, and draws experiences from both disciplines to formulate applications for approved intervention. Clinical and nonclinical approaches are discussed thoroughly to give the reader a balanced approach to therapeutic and adapted service programs.

Updated and expanded material includes current issues pertinent to competitive sports for the disabled. Clearly, the competitive aspects of involvement in sports and games are basic to human nature. However, the purpose of this book is to analyze all aspects of physical activity and to further enhance a comprehensive programs' study of recreational, therapeutic, and competitive programs. The concepts underlying the use of gross motor sports, games, and therapeutic exercises are emphasized not only in theoretical form, but also in practice to indicate that pleasurable experiences can be engendered for the physically disabled.

It is not the intent of this book to overplay the use of adapted or innovative equipment in physical activity programs. Many physically disabled individuals do not have the physical attributes to participate fully in meaningful activity. The use of adapted equipment to compensate enhances their capacity for independent mobility, and in turn improves their effectiveness and efficiency in overcoming physical challenges. The rationale is to provide greater attention to the progress of involvement and less to the device or product as the disabled person engages in meaningful activity.

This edition addresses common concerns for the prospective therapist or instructor who will be confronted with assessing and programming for physically disabled individuals. The text broadens both the education of undergraduate and graduate students and the methods used to deliver services in both therapeutic recreation and adapted physical education. Direct care providers should also find this text to be of interest, as the wealth of material stresses the effects of physical activity on primary treatment outcomes. The suggested games, sports, and physical activities offer an exciting alternative for the disabled and nondisabled alike.

Charlottesville, Virginia Ronald Adams
Corvallis, Oregon Jeffrey A. McCubbin

Acknowledgments

The authors express gratitude to the many contributors to this book, including those who supplied material from numerous sports organizations, equipment suppliers, and manufacturers. Special thanks are also forwarded to the many health professionals at the University of Virginia Medical Center who contributed their knowledge and insight into the preparation of this book.

Unique contributions were made by David Burton, Recreational Therapy Supervisor at the Kluge Children's Rehabilitation Center, for his section on Hydrotherapy, and by Dr. Marion Alexander from the University of Manitoba, Canada, for her information on Marathon Racing. We extend our grateful appreciation for their efforts.

Deepest thanks are also extended to Ms. Laura Pretorious from the Kluge Children's Rehabilitation Center for her excellent photographic contributions, and to the many parents of patients at the Center who gave permission for their children to be photographed.

R.C.A.
J.A.McC.

Contents

1 *Understanding and Assessing Persons with Physical Disabilities*

Everyone has a handicap, a basic limitation that prevents normal functioning or the ability to be self-sufficient in one area or another. "Handicap" is used in the context of this book to assist in describing a basic congenital or acquired mental or physical defect. It can be assumed that a disability can be a hindrance to completing certain tasks. To this degree, an individual is restricted and under such circumstances the term handicapped will be used. However, many disabled persons have overcome enormous obstacles and physical challenges in life. As a rule, they prefer to be called disabled and not handicapped since the latter term only suggests a more pronounced need for assistance.

Moreover, when environmental changes are made to accommodate the needs of a person with a disability, and when that person has also undergone necessary adaptations, then even someone with a severe disability may be only minimally handicapped. A person who is blind may not be handicapped in work that does not require visual orientation. A person in a wheelchair may be no more frustrated in a barrier-free job situation than the person who takes it for granted that one has to ride the bus to work every morning.[1]

How many persons are physically disabled? Although the exact number is not really known, available medical records indicate that there are approximately 170,000 children born with defects each year in the United States. Add to this the number of persons disabled, paralyzed, or otherwise incapacitated by injury or disease; thousands more are mentally retarded or socially and culturally deprived; clearly there are staggering numbers of people who need remedial, compensatory, and rehabilitative programs.

UNDERSTANDING PERSONS WITH PHYSICAL DISABILITIES

Humans, in their efforts to better understand that most complex and sophisticated of all living creatures, themselves, have employed all sorts of experiments, tests, descriptions, and surveys in their continuing search for self-knowledge. Society has trained and prepared them, dissected and probed them, but an understanding of the mechanism of acceptance—acceptance of self and acceptance of others—still eludes us. It is quite obvious that individuals function satisfactorily within their environment almost in direct relationship to their ability to accept others, to others' capacity to accept them, and to their tolerance and acceptance of themselves. The need is the same for persons with physical limitations, only the approach is altered. If society remains unyielding and inflexible, demanding the same attainments from this group as from the so-called average, or normal, human, there seem little likelihood of resolving the problems. The psychologic and social effects accompanying some handicaps may create greater problems than the actual physical impairment.

The primary focus in dealing with the disabled population should be directed toward those qualities most similar to those of the average person. Focusing on the aberrant condition serves only to alienate this group further and to diminish the possibility of their leading nearly normal lives. The fundamental drives for success, recognition, and approval are desired by everyone, regardless of their physical appearance. Physically disabled humans are no exception. They especially need opportunities for self-exploration and achievement; they need to become involved and accepted. Their disability need not prevent them from attaining success and winning recognition and approval. Society has an especial obligation and challenge to consider the needs of disabled humans and to meet their needs in the way most likely to preserve their moral integrity and dignity.

It is generally recognized that the achievement of vocational success involves varying and progressive levels of attainment. Succinctly stated, the levels of maturation that lead to successful careers include: (1) acceptance; (2) success; (3) progression; and (4) competence.

It is obvious that before any program is initiated, the task of gaining participant involvement is of primary importance. This problem is relatively insignificant for most groups, since the participants are accustomed to becoming involved and are quite readily accepted into a group. Physically disabled individuals, however, have often been isolated from peer group relationships, as well as from community and school activities. As a result, they have experienced little social interaction, and not infrequently, they are fearful of participation in a group other than their own family. It is relatively easy to understand their problem, since throughout their life, usually as a direct consequence of being handicapped, they typically have had little opportunity to become involved. As a result, those social skills that make involvement possible have never been fully developed.

Often the physical appearance of the disabled persons is notably different, even bizarre on occasion, further removing them from the mainstream of life and interaction with unimpaired members of their age group. Many have severe locomotor deficiencies and/or physical deformities. The more unusual their appearance, the greater the possibility that they find themselves an oddity—something to be stared at or ridiculed—an attitude which serves to foster and perpetuate a morbid awareness of their differences. Major tasks of a therapeutic recreation specialist or an adapted physical education teacher are to promote self acceptance and to instill confidence that will permit physically disabled people to develop skills and talents that compensate for their limitations. They must be persuaded that any attempts at involvement will be in some measure successful with a minimum of frustration. It is important to point out that a major obstacle to successful goal setting is lack of confidence.

The successful program leader is able to convince individuals that group rules and regulations can be modified and that concern for their potential ability in the home, school, and community is the major objective. Other peer group members must realistically recognize their physical limitations, but at the same time, accept them as a real participant.

Success, the second level in the maturation process of vocational fulfillment, not only is vital, but also must be repeated often. Unless some level of success is attained and recognized in the various tasks attempted, virtually no further gains are realized. We all thrive on success, particularly on recognized success, and disabled individuals need their successes, however minimal, recognized even more than the normal person. Their contributions quite frequently require unusual exertion of effort considerably beyond that imagined by the ordinary individual. It needs to be recognized not only for its individual integrity but also for its contribution to the total group effort.

As physically challenged people experience success, they will usually seek more difficult tasks requiring greater efforts. These efforts can be measured quantitatively, as well as qualitatively, through the progression of acquired skills, thereby factually demonstrating an improvement in level of competence. Once they are accepted into a group where their success is evident, they will feel confident in their ability to pursue further tasks. They will normally remain involved and make further contributions to the success of the group.

The final level of vocational maturation is competence. As physically disabled persons continue making meaningful contributions to the welfare of the group, other members typically place more and more trust in their ability. Essentially they win recognition and approval from their peers at the same time that they satisfy their own curiosity about their ability to succeed. The result is a whole individual, in terms of their place in a peer group, since they utilize their potential to maximum advantage despite disability.

The Program of Adapted Sports, Games, and Exercises

Seventy years ago, physical education was a program primarily concerned with the development of strong bodies and minds. Beginning in about 1920, more and more emphasis was placed on programs that incorporated modern educational theory into the activities of the playing field and the gymnasium. Exercise, games, and sports for the physically disabled as an integral part of medical practice have won greater prominence with each succeeding year since World War II. The impetus came partially from the needs of the armed forces to keep fighting men in top physical and mental condition and partially from rehabilitation programs for wounded servicemen.

Today, physical education is an important part of the program of general education. Physical activities and sports of all kinds are designed to improve posture, physical development, general fitness, and health, as well as to provide fun and recreation. Annarino states,

The weighting of objectives is determined by a number of factors: namely, the growth and developmental stages of the students, teaching styles, teacher competencies, and teacher values. Other criteria for weighting value would be the uniqueness of the objective to the physical education discipline and the degree of objective measureability.[2]

Based on these criteria, the uniqueness of the organic, neuromuscular, and interpretive objectives would be allotted more weighting value and the social and emotional objectives, less value.

To show these factors in graphic form may help to point up their significance. Table 1–1 places the content and experiences of physical education under 5 traditional objectives and gives clues for the selection of curriculum and the techniques of measurement.

The developmental objectives of physical education for the physically disabled are the same, and only the rules, regulations, organization, and procedures for each particular activity require minimal adjustment to provide a flexible, but rewarding, opportunity for leisure-time activities.

A program of sports, games, and exercises for the physically disabled includes a wide variety of activities. Some may be conducted in a nursing home, some in a neuropsychiatric hospital, others in a general or surgical hospital, and still others in a school, college, or institutional setting. Those who work in this field in educational institutions are commonly referred to as adapted physical educators, and those employed in treatment centers and hospitals are known as therapeutic recreators (as identified in this text), or recreational therapists.

Therapeutic recreation as defined by the National Therapeutic Recreation Society is

Table 1–1.
Developmental Objectives of Physical Education

ORGANIC

Proper functioning of the body systems so that the individual may adequately meet the demands placed upon him by his environment. A foundation for skill development.

Muscle Strength
The maximum amount of force exerted by a muscle or muscle group.

Muscle Endurance
The ability of a muscle or muscle group to sustain effort for a prolonged period of time.

Cardiovascular Endurance
The capacity of an individual to persist in strenuous activity for periods of some duration. This is dependent upon the combined efficiency of the blood vessels, heart and lungs.

Flexibility
The range of motion in joints needed to produce efficient movement and minimize injury.

NEUROMUSCULAR

A harmonious functioning of the nervous and muscular systems to produce desired movements.

Locomotor Skills
Walking	Skipping	Sliding	Leaping	Pushing
Running	Galloping	Hopping	Rolling	Pulling

Nonlocomotor Skills
Swaying	Twisting	Shaking	Stretching
Bending	Handing	Stooping	

Game Type Fundamental Skills
Striking	Catching	Kicking	Stopping
Throwing	Batting	Starting	Changing direction

Motor Factors
Accuracy	Rhythm	Kinesthetic awareness	Agility
Power	Balance	Reaction time	

Sport Skills
Soccer	Softball	Football	Baseball
Track & Field	Archery	Speedball	Hockey
Basketball	Golf	Bowling	Tennis
Fencing	Volleyball	Wrestling	

Recreational Skills
Shuffleboard	Croquet	Deck tennis	Hiking
Table tennis	Swimming	Horseshoes	Boating

INTERPRETIVE

The ability to explore, to discover, to understand, to acquire knowledge, and to make value judgments.

A knowledge of game rules, safety measures, and etiquette.

The use of strategies and techniques involved in organized activities.

A knowledge of how the body functions and its relationship to physical activity.

A development of appreciation for personal performance. The use of judgment related to distance, time, space, force, speed, and direction in the use of activity implements, balls, and self.

An understanding of growth and developmental factors affected by movement.

The ability to solve developmental problems through movement.

SOCIAL

An adjustment to both self and others by an integration of the individual to society and his environment.

The ability to make judgments in a group situation.

Learning to communicate with others.

The ability to exchange and evaluate ideas within a group.

The development of the social phases of personality, attitudes, and values in order to become a functioning member of society.

The development of a sense of belonging and acceptance by society.

The development of positive personality traits.

Learning for constructive use of leisure time.

A development of attitude that reflects good moral character.

EMOTIONAL

A healthy response to physical activity through a fulfillment of basic needs.

The development of positive reactions in spectatorship and participation through either success or failure.

The release of tension through suitable physical activities.

An outlet for self-expression and creativity.

An appreciation of the aesthetic experiences derived from correlated activities.

The ability to have fun.

From Annarino, A.: The five traditional objectives of physical education. JOHPER, *41:* June, 1970.

a special service within the broad area of recreation services. It is a process which utilizes recreation services for purposive intervention in some physical, emotional, and/or social behavior to bring about a desired change in that behavior and to promote the growth and development of the individual.

This definition reflects broadening realms of therapeutic recreational service that apply to recreational services for special groups in the community and in other types of agencies, as well as in hospitals and other medically oriented facilities.

Recreational programs encompass a gamut of activities such as arts and crafts, music, dramatics, camping, physical activities, community service, collections, and hobbies (Table 1–2). Physical education focuses on activities involving physical fitness, motor skills, movement, and physical prowess (Table 1–3).

The ultimate goal through either physical education or therapeutic recreation is self-actualizing behavior in which an individual functions as independently as possible (some may prefer as dependently

Table 1-2.
Differentiated Characteristics in Therapeutic Recreational Service

Type & Level of Service	Basic Goals of the Service & Participation	Relationship of TR Specialist with Client or Patient
Therapeutic recreation service	**Therapeutic Goals** Contribution to treatment Contribution to rehabilitation Behavior change Social adjustment Therapeutic reaction procedures	**Intensive** One-to-one Small group
Recreation for ill and handicapped	**Participation Goals** Sheltered opportunity Adaptation Remedial teaching Counseling	**Concentrated** Small group Large group
Standard recreation program	**General Recreation Goals** Physical conditioning Mental well-being Personal growth and development Creative fulfillment Individual expression	**Active** Large group Mass participation

Leisure activity	**Individual Goals**
	Amusement
	Diversion
	Relaxation
		Implied
		Residual role through
		  attitudes, skills, habits
		  imparted to clients

From Nesbitt, J.A.: The mission of therapeutic recreation specialists: to help and to champion the handicapped. Therapeutic Recreation Journal, 4:43, 1970.

independent or as independently dependent as possible) and to as large a degree as possible, integrated with his nonimpaired, nondisabled, and nonhandicapped contemporaries.

Physical education by and large is a means to an end. Recreation often is considered an end in itself. While some skill teaching takes place in recreation programs, skill teaching is the hallmark of physical education. Conversely, preparing an individual to use

his leisure time in more constructive and wholesome ways is a basic goal of all physical education.

In this text, the terms instructor and program leader refer to a physical or occupational therapist, a therapeutic recreation specialist or a physical education instructor. In some instances, the terms are used interchangeably, and in such cases, our remarks apply to either a hospital/treatment center or a school. The term client is frequently used to identify anyone who

Table 1-3.
Differentiated Characteristics of Physical Education Services

Type & Level of Service	Desired Outcomes
REGULAR SERVICES	
Extraschool activities Interschool activities Regular physical education activities	Totally integrated program of physical activities
HALFWAY SERVICES	
Partially integrated school programs Developmental activities Modified sports and games Specialized exercise programs	Maximum physical, mental function Physical movement skill Social adjustment Emotional adaptability
SPECIAL SERVICES	

Segregated school programs
Clinical programs
Hospital programs
Institutional programs
	Physical, social, and emotional changes through:
	  Counseling
	  Treatment, corrective, and therapeutic approaches
	  Diagnostic/prescriptive procedures

From: A clarification of terms, JOHPER, 42:1971.

is receiving special recreational services. In this text it is used interchangeably with the term patient in a treatment setting. The terms recreationist and therapeutic recreation specialist are used interchangeably and refer to a professionally skilled program leader who develops activities for established needs.

ASSESSING THE PERSON WITH A PHYSICAL DISABILITY

Written records and reports assessing the goals of leisure and therapeutic recreation are an integral part of the total treatment process.

Goal Directed Leisure Recreation Assessment

Assessment records and reports written for patients participating in such leisure recreation as municipal, summer camp, or institutional programs evaluate various aspects of patients' skills and attitudes toward leisure. In most cases, the reports require a minimum amount of writing, often accomplished through checklists. A written profile on each individual should include his past leisure experiences and his interest in learning new leisure skills. The therapist or instructor should record the level of individuals' skills when they enter a program and make notes on their progress periodically.

Goal-Directed Therapeutic Recreation Assessment In a Treatment Setting

Written assessment records and reports enhance the effectiveness of therapeutic recreation. Obviously, effective programs must be centered around the client and intended to improve his physical, social, mental, and/or emotional behavior. In addition, the program leader must demonstrate and document a client's progress, particularly if the client was referred to the therapist or treatment center for therapeutic recreation services. The type of assessment framework or report obviously depends on a number of factors, including the philosophy behind and reason for the goals, the type of treatment program (leisure recreation or therapeutic recreation), the size of the treatment facility, and the number of clients it serves. Ongoing monitoring and documenting of information is especially important in an interdisciplinary setting in which various disciplines, each complementing another, provide the structure for a unified treatment plan.

Individualized Program Planning

In an effort to identify specific therapeutic objectives, the therapeutic recreation specialists at the Kluge Children's Rehabilitation Center at the University of Virginia Medical Center designed a system termed Patient Therapy Plan (PTP) which helps determine goals and objectives for each patient. The information recorded for the PTP is designed to provide a baseline of data that will help in the identifi-

cation of developmental objectives (see Table 1–1). Specifically, the PTP provides a recording system that guides the referring agent (physician) in noting initial assessment data and progress. In addition, the PTP is an operating plan for the practicing instructor who is responsible for selecting specific therapeutic activities. The format of the PTP is based on one to three components depending on the individual case. The PTP can include one, two or all three of the following intervention plans:

1. Supportive plan. This relates primarily to psycho-social stimulation. It includes providing guidelines and encouraging the patient while he is adjusting to his treatment plan and making the transition to a hospital/rehabilitation center environment. The objective, of course, is to provide recreational services with the expressed purpose of riveting people's attention and concerns away from their illness or disability to more pleasurable aspects of play and leisure activities. If patients are tolerating their treatment with no undue emotional effects and have adjusted well to the therapy environment, then the supportive intervention plan need not be utilized. However, this plan is used quite frequently, because changes in the client's attitude and acceptance of limitations are usually desired.

2. Observation plan. This plan involves the use of directive (structured) or nondirective (unstructured) recreational activities to obtain baseline data regarding the patient's personality, compliance to treatment, and motor skills. In some situations, this means using standardized testing instruments to evaluate the patient's physical performance. This plan is used primarily for patients whose treatment outcomes are anticipated, for it contributes to an interdisciplinary evaluation of the outcome of treatment. However, the observation intervention plan is not used for every patient. The information gained from it is used most often to make recommendations to other professional agencies, for school placement, or for behavioral management. The assessment information is also used for parent education.

3. Habilitation/Rehabilitation plan. This plan is designed to achieve maximum possible physical and psychologic fitness. Habilitation is designed to help patients who have been handicapped since birth make use of their abilities to the limits of their capabilities. Rehabilitation is designed to teach or restore function after an illness or injury. The objective is to introduce activities that promote independent functioning and mobility. The intervention plan is often used to complement such other disciplines as occupational or physical therapy, and its expressed purpose is to increase muscle strength, endurance, and the

range of motion of specific extremities. A habilitation/rehabilitation plan is generally designed for long-term patients who are undergoing vigorous treatment for the development of self-sufficient habits and attitudes.

After the intervention plan(s) is established, the developmental objectives are identified. The client's needs are determined by referring to a system such as that shown in Table 1–1. It is important to point out, however, that the objectives cannot be documented until after the program leader engages his client in a few activity sessions.

The developmental objectives should be considered and circled on the PTP form in order of preference. All high-priority or major objectives should be circled one, and all low-priority or minor objectives circled 2 or in sequence (2, 3, 4, or 5) depending upon the individual case and the weight of specific concerns. The 1 to 5 scale is designed to identify those objectives that have a high priority, although in some cases, all 5 developmental objectives demand equal consideration. Generally, if the objectives are clear and specific, the therapy plan will have both major and minor objectives. A short statement should be made after each major objective to clarify the program plans in detail (Figs. 1–1 and 1–2).

The next phase of the PTP is the Observation (O) Report. The program leader should note the client's performance and participation in therapy and his response to the major objectives outlined previously. If possible, the observation report should be concise—no longer than one paragraph. This length may vary, however, if the instructor needs to describe in detail the assessment criteria from a standardized test.

The last part of the PTP is the Plan (P). This information should include a brief statement regarding the prescriptive plan, possibly including both short-term and long-term goals. The instructor should specify program content, intervention tools, and whether therapy sessions are group or individualized situations. A short-term plan concerns the immediate action to be taken by a program leader while the patient is undergoing active treatment as an inpatient. A long-term plan concerns the follow-up procedures taken after the patient leaves the treatment facility. If there is no follow-up, the long-term plan can obviously be omitted from the PTP.

In physical rehabilitation, treatment services are designed to improve social, emotional, cognitive, and physical functioning behaviors. A basic inventory assessment of the client's recreational interests is useful in coordinating leisure/social involvement during the hospitalization period. The PTP should reflect information on patient interests relative to recreational activities. However, programming is often based upon activity analysis concepts, judged accordingly by the practicing therapist. It is not unusual for the therapist to choose a particular activity for reasons which are specific to rehabilitation goals. It is often useful early in a treatment program, and as the patient progresses, the process of rehabilitation progresses from prescriptive to elective programming.

The PTP also includes information on identified needs and measurable goals. Needs can focus on the objectives that are defined in the PTP. Measurable goals may be subjective where there is interpretation of certain behavioral outcomes or objective if various testing instruments or measurements are used during the assessment or treatment process. Due to a short term hospitalization course, it might be impossible to target improvement in any one particular area. This might be the case, for example, with a postoperative patient who is following a 48-hour nursing care plan and then is discharged for home convalescence. With more frequent contacts (long-term patients who are hospitalized longer than 2 weeks) it is easier to measure desired changes.

Frequency and duration documentation should include number of daily sessions and total length of therapy time during each session. In addition, a flow sheet (not illustrated) should be added to document frequency, duration, and date of service with the therapist's signature or initials. This is a requirement by many third party insurance carriers. The treatment modality should also be identified. A modality is a procedure or tool used to accomplish an objective. In Therapeutic Recreation objectives are accomplished through providing activities and through the person who provides the activities. Each activity has identifiable unique qualities. Being able to identify the unique qualities allows a therapist to select activities which have the greatest chance for goal attainment. This is the reason why the procedure should be described in the PTP.

The PTP may change as the patient improves or as changes occur in his physical, social, mental, and/or emotional behavior. To update information, a statement recorded under the observation section (O) is sufficient. The date should be recorded as well as the circumstances surrounding the change in status. This information may be recorded daily, weekly, or over an extended period of time, depending on the individual case (Fig. 1–3). Biweekly reports are recommended.

The SOAP Assessment and Evaluation System

Another popular documentation system is referred to as SOAP notes (subjective and objective data, assessment, and plan). Often used by nurses and clinical therapists, it has been adopted for usage by recreationists as well. In this system, the therapist interprets the statement made by the client, for example, "Please leave me alone, I need my privacy!" The follow-up procedure is for the therapist to document objective analysis, either observational or testing, followed by assessment of the client's condition, and plan or intervention strategy.

PATIENT THERAPY PLAN

Name of Patient *Alissa Grimes*

Recreational Interests: *Reading*

Age: *13*

History NO. *63 5802*

Diagnosis: *S/P Multiple Trauma + Closed Head Injury secondary to Motor Vehicle Accident*

Referring Physician:
Dr. C. Y. Futgory

Reason for Admission or Referral for Therapy:
Rehabilitation + gait training

Identified Needs and measurable goals: *Have patient assume independent aligned posture. Refer to below for needs. Observe effects of standing and record length of time for each session (maximum 20-30 minutes as per Physical Therapy)*

THERAPEUTIC INTERVENTION PLAN: Check and describe the plan (s) of choice.

1. _____ Supportive _____

2. _____ Observation _____

3. _✓_ Habilitation or Rehabilitation *Improve functional skills and independent habits*   Modality: *Dual games. Hydrotherapy*

Frequency and Duration:
Daily - ½ hr. in gym, ½ hr. of hydrotherapy

PROGRAM OBJECTIVES: List in order of preference by circling the number opposite the objective.   In some cases, equal emphasis should be place on various objectives.   In some situations, circle no. 1 more than one time.   This information is by no means a point to an end, but provides information regarding program guidelines and therapeutic objectives.   Circle No. 1 for all major objectives.

1. Organic................(1),2,3,4,5   *Organic - Promote active exercise to ↑ range of motion in the right upper-extremity. Improve standing balance + tolerance during recreational exercise.*

2. Neuromuscular.........1,(2),3,4,5

3. Interpretive..........(1),2,3,4,5   *Interpretive - Facilitate understanding of how to adapt to physical limitations.*

4. Social................1,2,(3),4,5

5. Emotional.............1,2,(3),4,5

List a statement that describes each major objective (s)

O: *Alissa is an outgoing adolescent who is making good progress. Her attitude is excellent, + is adjusting extremely well to the therapy plan. There is improvement in strength + functional usage of the right upper-extremity. Also, she is tolerating 20 minute periods of standing with no discomfort. In hydrotherapy, she is using the elementary backstroke to ↑ range of motion in the right upper-extremity. She is also walking in the shallow area of the pool to improve endurance + balance reactions.*

P: *Continue individual therapy sessions. Attempt to increase length of standing time in R.T.*

DATE: *March 15, 1988*   THERAPIST *Ellen Thompson, C.T.R.S.*

Fig. 1–1.   Patient therapy plan.

PATIENT THERAPY PLAN

Name of Patient *Regina Daniels*

Age: *15*

Diagnosis: *Hodgkins Disease (stage II B)*

Recreational Interests: *Music*

History NO. *63-8764*

Referring Physician: *Dr. Cary*

Reason for Admission or Referral for Therapy: *Admitted for radiation therapy. Intervention for adolescent adjustment reaction.*

Identified Needs and measurable goals: *Refer to intervention plan. Subjectively analyze & document emotional changes, if any, to malignant disease & treatment protocol.*

THERAPEUTIC INTERVENTION PLAN: Check and describe the plan (s) of choice.

1. __✓__ Supportive *Psycho-social stimulation*

2. __✓__ Observation *Document behavioral issues and attitudinal changes.*

3. _____ Habilitation or Rehabilitation _____

Frequency and Duration: *Daily - 2 ½ hr. sessions*

Modality: *Social games / Special events*

PROGRAM OBJECTIVES: List in order of preference by circling the number opposite the objective. In some cases, equal emphasis should be place on various objectives. In some situations, circle no. 1 more than one time. This information is by no means a point to an end, but provides information regarding program guidelines and therapeutic objectives. Circle No. 1 for all major objectives.

1. Organic.....................1,2,③,4,5
2. Neuromuscular................1,2,③,4,5
3. Interpretive................1,②,3,4,5
4. Social......................①,2,3,4,5
5. Emotional...................①,2,3,4,5

Social - Adjustment to both self & others by an integration to society & her environment. Encourage constructive use of leisure time.
Emotional - Provide outlet for self-expression. Support acceptance of illness, treatment & possible limitations and/or effects.

List a statement that describes each major objective (s)

O: *Regina is a shy, somewhat depressed adolescent. She responds to questions, but demonstrates minimal spontaneous conversation. To this point, she has chosen to stay in her room and prefers a quiet environment. I feel she is slowly developing a sense of security through efforts to be more responsive to suggestions. At this stage, Regina is basically interested in playing passive table games.*
P.

Continue to visit patient in her room, to explore personal feelings & engage in quiet recreational outlets. Encourage peer interaction & involvement whenever possible.
Assess adjustment to treatment issues.

DATE: *4-25-88*   THERAPIST *Karen Overbay, CTRS*

Fig. 1–2. Patient therapy plan.

UNIVERSITY OF VIRGINIA HOSPITAL

PROGRESS RECORD

Alissa Grimes
#63 5802

P
R
O
G
R
E
S
S

R
E
C
O
R
D

Therapeutic Recreation 4-1-88

O: Alissa continues to remain a highly motivated patient. Due to her rapidly increasing interest in aquatics, Alissa has expressed a desire to learn an assortment of swim strokes. For this reason, her therapy plan will also focus on neuromuscular objectives for the purpose of skill attainment in this particular medium.

P: The parents have expressed a desire to enroll Alissa in a YWCA swim program upon discharge. Continue to follow PTP as documented on March 15th, but add neuromuscular objective to list of proposed intervention areas.

Ellen Thompson, CTRS

HS 82 8

Fig. 1–3.   Progress note.

Model Assessments

The aim of many therapeutic recreation and adapted physical education programs is to provide through competent leadership a diverse program of developmental activities, games, sports, and rhythms suited to the interests and/or physical capacities of disabled patients or students.

Elaborate assessment methods are not necessary for the acquisition of baseline data regarding physical performance levels. However, it is important for every therapist or instructor to follow a few guiding principles regarding assessment before he enlists a patient or student in a physical activity program. The specificity of the disability and the potential performance level of each individual must be assessed before an accurate decision can be made regarding involvement in selected forms of athletics and recreational exercise. Consideration must be given, in general, to: (1) movement characteristics of the person, (2) social and emotional needs, and (3) program goals and objectives. In effect, assessment is a prerequisite to determining specific measureable outcomes of a program.

Sample Assessment for a Crutch-User

Evaluate Medical History, Condition Of Crutches, Crutch Stance And Tripod Position, Standing Balance And Tolerance, And Crutch Gait (Partial Or Non-Weight Bearing). Every instructor should evaluate the medical history of a student or patient who is using crutches in a physical education or recreational exercise program. Some individuals will be on programs of intermittent walking and sitting (spending a portion of time in a wheelchair with the alternate periods of time spent using crutches). Under such circumstances, activity can include forms of exercise to develop the muscle groups needed to manage crutches and/or to improve balance and tolerance for standing. Crutches are used by persons who have both temporary and permanent limitations. It is essential that the program leader know the approximate length of the time for which a student or patient will be using crutches if the problem is only temporary. Consultation with a physical therapist is recommended.

The instructor should observe the student or patient who is using crutches. Improper use can deter effective motor responses and patterns. Particular attention should be paid to 3 basic concerns: (1) condition of the crutches, (2) crutch stance, and (3) type of crutch gait (Appendix D).

The axillary, or underarm, crutch (Fig. 1–4) can be adjusted to meet the needs of the student or patient. The support screws of the extension shafts and hand bars should be secured tightly. Each shoulder piece should have a rubber cover over it to lessen the pressure of the hard wood in the axillary spaces. A rubber tip always covers the base of each crutch to prevent it from slipping.

In the crutch stance, or relaxed standing position, the head is up straight and the pelvis is positioned

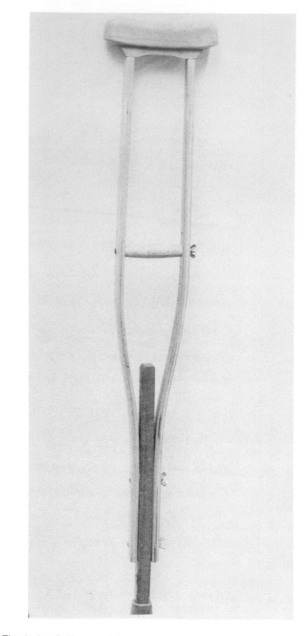

Fig. 1–4. Axillary crutch.

over the feet. The crutches are approximately 6 to 8 inches in front of and to the side of the feet. The elbows are bent at a 25 to 30 degree angle; the shoulders are down but not hunched; and the elbows should not be extended. It should be possible to place about 2 fingers between the tops of the crutches and the armpits. The weight is borne by the arms and hands so that weight is never borne by the apexes of the axillae (Fig. 1–5).

For individuals who have powerless or weak abdominal, back or hip-joint muscles (as persons using long leg-braces often have), the tripod position is necessary. In this position, the crutches are placed 8 to 10 inches in front of and to the side of the feet. The

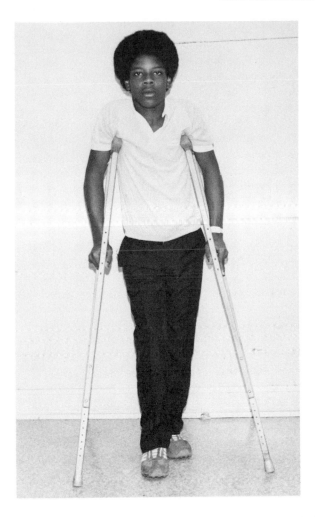

Fig. 1–5. Crutch stance. Postoperative patient after removal of Knowles pins that were used to correct a displaced fracture of his right femur. The patient was placed on a guarded weight-bearing program, using a 3-point gait, for 3 months.

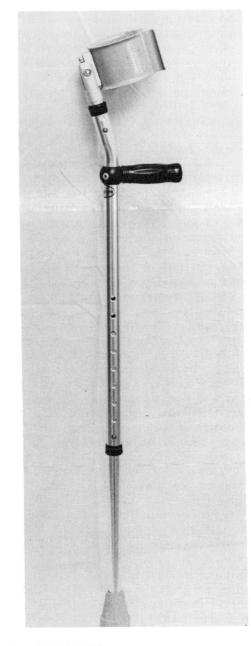

Fig. 1–6. Lofstrand crutch.

pelvis is tilted forward so that the slanted crutches provide anterior support. In this position, the individual can assume a position for bimanual activities and summation of forces, e.g., the catching of balls by freeing both upper limbs and transferring the weight of the crutches to the apexes of the axillae. It must be remembered, however, that this position can become tiring and that activity must be controlled so that proper balance is maintained at all times. The tripod position is used most frequently by individuals using a swing-to-gait, a swing-through-gait, or a drag-to-gait.

Another popular crutch is the Lofstrand crutch, which consists of a single tube of aluminum with a metal cuff at the top that fits around the forearm (Fig. 1–6). To use this crutch, however, the student must have good control of his trunk, pelvis, and upper extremities.

In walking with Lofstrand crutches, the body weight is transferred to the hand bars, and the crutch gait patterns are the same as those used with axillary crutches (also see Appendix D). One advantage that the Lofstrand crutch has over the axillary crutch is the fact that, because of the stability of the metal cuff around the forearm, the student or patient can release his hold on the hand bar without dropping the crutch.

Before the student or patient using crutches is asked to participate in physical activity programs, several exercise drills can be utilized to develop his confidence and skill. By standing against the wall with shoulders and heels touching the wall, the patient can sway on the crutches from side-to-side to accustom his hands and arms to bearing weight. A simple balance exercise can involve lifting one crutch to the count of 5 while support is maintained by the other crutch and the lower limb(s). The exercise can be repeated for the opposite side. After this, if the user demonstrates no problems he can pick one crutch up about 6 inches from the floor and then place it down. This can be repeated with the other crutch. After crutch-balancing exercises performed against the wall are mastered, crutch-balancing away from the wall is practiced. Obviously, depending on the functional ability of each individual, not all crutch-users will be able to perform all of the aforementioned exercises.

Assess Effects Of Using Crutches In Specific Activities, Including Crutch-Balancing Exercises, And Negotiation Of Steps And Platforms. Evaluate Importance Of Using Crutches As Balance Aids On One Side Of Body In Order To Free The Dominant Side For Upper Limb Movements Such As Throwing And Catching. Determine If Positional Changes (Prone, Sitting) Should Be Used To Compensate For Lack Of Proficiency In A Particular Activity. Assess The Use Of The Crutch As A Striking Implement From Standing Position. The student or patient should be taught how to use a crutch as an aid to balance during physical activities. Some individuals who have good trunk control can balance themselves with both feet and one crutch. When the other crutch is placed on the floor, the dominant limb becomes free for throwing or other game-type movements. The student or patient can lean into the support crutch, but he can also learn to shift weight smoothly to the feet and maintain balance while doing so (Fig. 1–7). The one-crutch balance support stance can be used by individuals using a 2-point, 3-point or 4-point gait.

Some individuals with good balance skills can use a crutch as a striking implement to hit balls from a stationary position that are placed on the floor. Support is maintained by one or both feet and one crutch, while the dominant limb controls the other crutch and strikes objects with it. Obviously, the student or patient should have sufficient trunk balance and upper extremity strength if he performs this advanced skill.

Depending on the nature of the activity, the program leader must determine if the student or patient should perform from a position other than standing. For example, the sitting or prone positions would be more suitable than the standing position for air-riflery. Different positions can also be assumed by individuals who have precarious balance skills, particularly those wearing long leg-braces. In general, the sitting or prone positions may be utilized to compensate for poor standing tolerance and balance.

Determine If A Standing Appliance, i.e., Standing Platform Or Supportive Device, Can Be Used To Facilitate Upper Trunk Movement And/Or Improve Standing Balance And Tolerance Without Crutches. The standing platform (Fig. 1–8) or a similar appliance can be used by individuals who are using crutches for mobility. In rehabilitation, for example, a standing

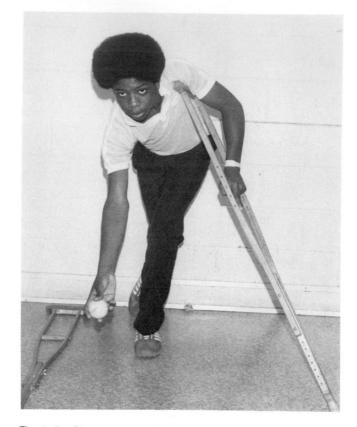

Fig. 1–7.   Patient using one axillary crutch for balance support. This patient was encouraged to use his crutches during physical activities, but not to place full weight on the affected leg.

appliance allows crutchless standing and can be used by disabled persons to develop the muscle groups needed for crutch management. Standing balance and tolerance can be improved while, at the same time, upper trunk mobility is provided.

The standing platform provides opportunities for lateral and rotational flexibility. Eliminating the physical constraints of crutches allows the upper extremities to control objects in space with complete freedom of movement. The platform can be used successfully with individuals who are on partial or full weight-bearing programs, including those using long leg-braces.

Sample Assessment for a Wheelchair-User. It is important to point out that the lightweight or sport wheelchair is gaining in popularity because of the many optional features that can be customized for the user. These include antitip tubes, adjustable axle positions, quick release wheels, etc. Various growth options such as adjustable seat width are even available for those using a junior/pediatric wheelchair. Depending upon the individual, each person will demonstrate a wide variety of needs. The following information is based on concerns for the standard wheelchair user. However, certain assessment issues will apply to both the standard and sports chair user.

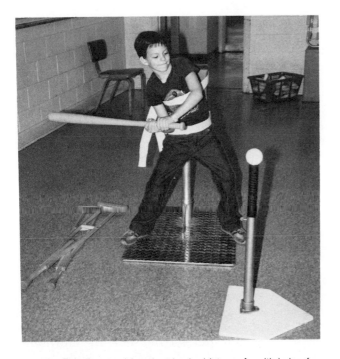

Fig. 1–8. This 7-year-old patient had a history of multiple leg fractures secondary to a bicycle accident. After cast removal, he began a rehabilitation program that included ambulation training with the aid of crutches. The standing platform was used in a therapeutic recreation class to offer him an outlet for emotional release through physical activity and an opportunity for crutchless standing. The standing platform also complemented the patient's physical therapy by increasing his standing tolerance for gait training.

Evaluate Medical History, Movement Potential, And Motor Function Of User, i.e., Functional Significance Of His Spinal Cord Lesion, His Trunk Balance, Positioning Of His Lower and Upper Extremity Segments, His Ability To Do Independent Transfers, And Importance Of Pressure Relief Schedules For Those Who Are Prone To Skin Breakdown. It is imperative that the program leader carefully examine a patient's medical records to determine any specific concerns that may need close attention. In a public school, the physical education teacher may retrieve some of this information from consulting with the parents. A history of current problems should be identified. For example, an individual may be taking medication, or segments of his body may require specific positioning. This kind of information plays an important role in the identification of precautions and the planning of programs. Additional information retrieved from medical records should include important facts about social, emotional and general intellectual functioning.

Obviously, the potential for movement and the motor function of each individual must be assessed. For example, a quadriplegic whose fifth cervical segment is unaffected will have some shoulder function, but little function in the extremities. The presence of more unaffected levels will add critical function. A C-8 quadriplegic is significantly more functional because he has the ability to extend his elbows, grasp with his fingers, and use his thumb appreciably. In effect, the management and potential functioning abilities of a patient or student vary depending on the level of spinal cord lesion and degree of muscle power. Consideration for use of adapted or assistive aid also depends on these factors.

The program leader must be cognizant of individuals who are prone to contracture deformities (e.g., muscular dystrophy) and spasticity (e.g., cerebral palsy). Proper positioning in a wheelchair is crucial to maintain proper segmental alignment, avoid exaggerating an existing deformity and eliminate the possibility of increasing excess muscle tone. Strapping techniques for persons with cerebral palsy can be used to maintain alignment of body parts, control spastic patterns or athetoid movements. This is done to enhance performance skills in competitive or recreational sports. The program leader should work jointly with an Occupational or Physical Therapist to assure proper guidance in this area (refer to section on Cerebral Palsy). Additional concerns may include decubiti (pressure sores), urinary infections, gallstones, and incontinence. The patient or student will be able to fully utilize his remaining muscle power only if these complications can be minimized or resolved.

It is important to know whether an individual can transfer from a wheelchair to an armless chair or a mat (refer to section on transfers). If not, trunk balance becomes a factor of concern in program planning. The instructor should observe the person and notice how he propels the wheelchair over a natural-grade surface. If the patient or student leans forward or uses compensatory shoulder movements for propulsion, then his trunk balance generally is not adequate for certain activities in which speedy movement is required (e.g., basketball, dashes). The ability to compensate quickly and accurately when trunk balance is upset increases the quality of performance in athletic or recreational exercise activities. Trunk weakness may be compensated for by using a semi-reclining back or by adding height to the back of the chair. In most cases, individuals who can transfer independently can perform activities in a sitting position from a mat with their backs resting against a wall.

It is also extremely important to know about pressure relief schedules for individuals with poor or no skin sensation. The patient or student who has a spinal cord injury with sensory loss needs at least an 8-cm. seat cushion. Because many persons with myelomeningocele and spinal cord injuries lack sensation, decubitus ulcers occur frequently. For preventive reasons, the person is taught to elevate his trunk every 10 to 15 minutes (Fig. 1–9). If he cannot assume the "push-up" position, then it is frequently necessary for him to lean sideways until the pressure is relieved from one ischial tuberosity. Manual assistance is required in some instances.

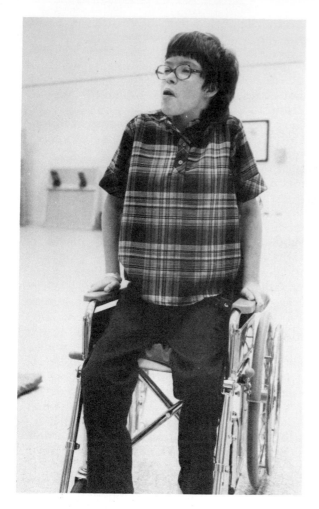

Fig. 1–9. Wheelchair push-up.

Occasionally, a child who is using a wheelchair may have the ability to stand for brief periods of time. Frequently, individuals who wear leg braces to protect and support weakened segments or joints (e.g., those people with muscular dystrophy or stroke hemiplegia) are encouraged to maintain a standing position for brief periods during the day. It is conceivable that standing time can be incorporated into a period of physical activity with the aid of a standing appliance (e.g., a standing table or a standing platform).

Evaluate Functional Capacity Of Wheelchair, i.e., Condition Of Braking System, Heel Cups, Foot Rests, And Arm Rests. Successful participation in physical activities depends upon a wheelchair that is safe and in good condition. For safety reasons, brakes should be required on all standard chairs. Wheelchairs should also be checked for anterior-posterior stability according to the user's weight distribution. Unfortunately, many wheelchairs have defective brakes which interfere with the individual's motor performance. Under such circumstances, sand bags can be placed behind the front casters and the tires to stabilize the chair during activities that involve trunk

extension and rotation. Also, an able-bodied assistant can provide stability by holding onto the push handles. Removable arm rests are especially helpful in certain activities, for example, in the sports of archery and bowling, because performance skills are improved by increased range of motion and elimination of structural wheelchair barriers. Ideally, all standard features of a wheelchair should be operating effectively to guarantee a foundation for efficient movement patterns (Figs. 1–10 and 1–11).

Another significant concern is the use of a seat belt. It may be advantageous during activities that require good sitting posture (e.g., archery). However, considerations against its use should include the risk of falling and becoming trapped in the wheelchair (e.g., in sprint racing), thereby increasing likelihood of injury.

The Sports Wheelchair. The disabled individual who participates in wheelchair sports is always well advised to use a wheelchair other than his own chair. This reasoning is supported by 2 arguments: (1) a wheelchair designed for the sport engaged in and which may be adapted or modified to serve the individual's peculiarities provides a far greater avenue for the development and expression of a person's skills and talents, than a personal chair does; and (2) a sports wheelchair is economically feasible insofar as its use

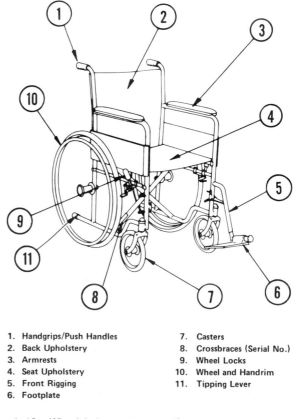

1. Handgrips/Push Handles
2. Back Upholstery
3. Armrests
4. Seat Upholstery
5. Front Rigging
6. Footplate
7. Casters
8. Crossbraces (Serial No.)
9. Wheel Locks
10. Wheel and Handrim
11. Tipping Lever

Fig. 1–10. Wheelchair terminology. (Courtesy of Everest & Jennings, 3233 E. Mission Oaks Blvd., Camarillo, CA 93010.)

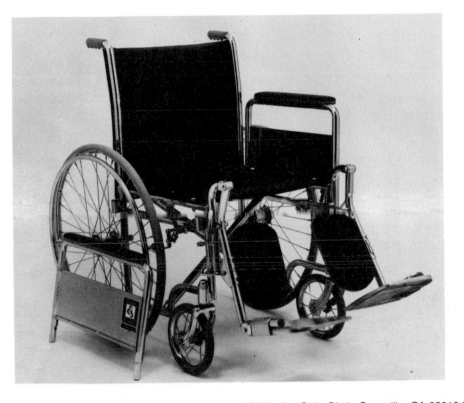

Fig. 1–11.   Standard wheelchair. (Courtesy of Everest & Jennings, 3233 E. Mission Oaks Blvd., Camarillo, CA 93010.)

saves wear and tear on the personal wheelchair upon which a person depends for everyday use (Fig. 1–12).

The sports chair is also becoming popular for everyday use because the light frame allows for easy maneuverability which in turn conserves energy. Pushing is more efficient due to the low back which allows for freedom of arm movement. As a rule, however, the more severely involved individual who needs specialized accessories such as inserts, etc. to maintain a solid seat and back is generally best served by using a standard chair. Motorized chairs (sometimes referred to as Power-Drive chairs) are used by the more severely disabled person who is unable to push a wheelchair. Means of control include: 1. arm and hand control, 2. breath control, and 3. chin control.

The following factors should be taken into consideration when designing a wheelchair for an athlete: wheel size, handrim size, seat position (vertical and horizontal), and trunk position. The type of sport will also dictate chair design. Track chairs, for example, are characterized by large wheels (70 cm), small handrims, and low seats with a forward leaning trunk position. This design allows maximum speed. Basketball chairs, on the other hand, are generally constructed with small wheels (61 cm), larger handrims (53 to 56 cm), and a higher, more upright seat position to enhance mobility and to put the player closer to the basket.[3]

Assess Considerations For Use Of Warm-Up Exercises In Wheelchair, i.e., Trunk Twisters, Arm Circles, etc.

Evaluate Limiting Factors, i.e., Contractures, Spasticity, And Weak Muscles. Assess The Possibility Of Incorporating Movement Exploration Activities.
Frequently, general warm-up exercises are performed prior to an activity period in physical education class or to increase flexibility prior to an athletic event. The goal is to center attention on 3 general areas of the body: the trunk, the arm-shoulder, and in some cases the legs. In some situations, each warm-up lesson used also has physical fitness implications, developing such fitness qualities as endurance and strength. It is conceivable that a wheelchair-user can perform exercises such as trunk twisters and arm circles with his normal peers. To achieve endurance, the individual can propel his wheelchair around the gymnasium for progressively greater distances as his overall conditioning improves. However, it may not be practical to consider using warm-up exercises for those limited by spasticity, severe contractures, and muscle weakness.

In elementary school, movement education is an important concept within the framework of physical education. Learning to manage the body leads to better control over gross motor movements. To achieve basic conditioning or movement experiences, the instructor can encourage self-exploration and spatial exploration by encouraging changes in position. In many instances, a scooter board, for example, could be used as a replacement for a wheelchair in an activity program if the child had good upper-extremity strength and trunk stability. This would enable the

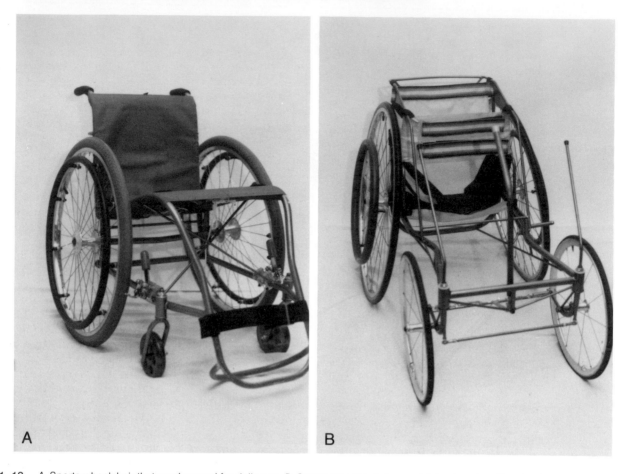

Fig. 1–12.   *A,* Sports wheelchair that can be used for daily use. *B,* Sports wheelchair for road & track racing. Note bucket-type frame. (Eagle Sportchairs courtesy of IDEA: Innovator of Disability Equipment and Adaptations, Inc., 1393 Meadowcreek Drive, #2, Pewaukee, WI 53072.)

child to participate in a greater range of motion and activity.

Assess Urologic Considerations. Chronic urinary dysfunction is common in patients with spinal cord injuries and tumors, myelomeningocele, and other developmental defects of the spinal cord. The problems associated with bladder incontinence are often overlooked, but concern should be demonstrated by any program leader who has direct contact with a patient or student who has bladder paralysis (inability to control emptying of the bladder). If urine is retained, some children will achieve continence with bladder pressure (Credé's method) applied every 2 to 3 hours. Some individuals use an indwelling catheter (a tubular instrument used to drain urine from the bladder). In some cases, boys can use an external condom (sheath or covering over the penis) attached to the leg for urine control. In addition, some individuals have a urinary diversion procedure (ileoconduit). Urinary diversions are indicated for tumor removal, congenital anomalies, and nerve defects or injuries that affect voluntary bladder control. A person who has a diversion must wear an ostomy appliance (collecting device) over an outside opening on the skin in the abdominal region of the body.

The program leader should demonstrate concern if a patient or student is using a catheter or ostomy bag. An adolescent who had dribbling of urine and soiling from a condom and leg bag during exercise would be embarrassed by his inability to remain dry and control his urinary functions. In general, the program leader should have a basic understanding of how to manage an individual with a neurogenic bladder problem. Immediate attention should be given to a patient or student who has a distinct odor and demonstrates an inability to remain dry and/or who shows poor hygiene by lack of concern for changing or emptying an appliance while away from home. Immediate attention and encouragement should focus on self-care and assurance that these problems are correctable. Effective management of an appliance should be maintained consistently before involvement in recreational exercise and physical education is allowed. Obviously, it is imperative that individuals refrain from physical activities involving impact or pressure to the site of the urinary collection appliance.

Evaluate The Effects of Wheelchair To Surface Of Playing Area. It is essential that a program leader make adequate adjustments according to whether a student or patient is maneuvering a wheelchair on a natural or unnatural surface. It is not uncommon to see footrests that are ineffective because they are too close to a playing surface. Low or defective footrests can scrape against the ground, terrain, or gymnasium floor, causing the wheelchair to tip forward. It is feasible to wrap and secure a towel around the footplates, thus protecting the floor from possible damage due to scraping.

Pneumatic tires are especially good in comparison to solid rubber tires for travel on soft or uneven surfaces. When pushing a wheelchair over grass or an uneven surface, an able-bodied person can provide assistance by tilting the chair backward and pushing forward so that weight is displaced to the back tires.

Assess Specific Performance Goals. Assess the functional motor capacity (range of motion, control of motion, strength, and active use) of the upper extremities by considering the following sequential steps:

Grasp and Release. If a student or patient can grasp and release objects, but cannot flex and extend his muscles (as seen frequently in cerebral palsy and muscular dystrophy), then certain adjustments must be made to compensate for the loss of motor patterns. For example, a dart game can be adjusted for distance: if the individual cannot grasp and throw, the target can be placed next to the wheelchair and the dart simply dropped onto the target. The instructor needs to observe carefully such limiting factors as muscle tightness or contractures, and hand prehension patterns (Fig. 1–13). Passive stretching may be recommended to produce the desired movements and promote relaxation. Additional support can be achieved by using a lapboard attached to the wheelchair to assist in maintaining the hands in a functional position. Quadriplegics can use numerous kinds of adapted aids in sports to compensate for loss of voluntary hand control.

It is not possible to discuss adequately all the extremity-bracing aids that are used to provide assistance to the affected extremity. However, when possible, the teacher/therapist should integrate his efforts closely with an occupational therapist to achieve common goals.

Flexion and Extension. Some persons (those with cerebral palsy, stroke hemiplegia, closed head injuries) exhibit a crude palmar grasp (opposition of the thumb and digits), but are able to flex and extend to some degree. For individuals with a crude palmar grasp (thumb flexed and adducted inside the palm with the fingers flexed over it), it is feasible to use grip prehension (digits curled about an object such as a pencil or a peg) to strike lightweight objects in table games or to push a ball down a bowling ramp.

For persons with no upper extremity involvement, the ability to flex and extend provides an important dimension in the selection of activities. Fundamental game skills such as striking, throwing, catching, and batting can be incorporated into the development of recreational and sports skills.

Trunk Flexibility. Every wheelchair-user should be evaluated in terms of trunk flexibility. Obviously, some individuals will have limited ability to bend at the waist while sitting in a wheelchair. This is often the case with patients who have recently had reconstructive surgery of the lower extremities and those who have incomplete knee flexion. In such cases, concern should focus on maintaining the normal range of motion of the upper extremities.

Individuals who have good trunk control and can bend at the waist in 2 directions (forward and lateral flexion) can be more independent. The patient or student should be assessed in terms of bending at the waist and touching the toes and bending to the side of wheelchair to retrieve an object from the floor. Additional flexibility provides opportunities for efficient movement patterns related to distance, time, space, force, speed, and direction in the use of implements and balls for activities.

Transfer. The instructor should observe the specific transfer techniques of a student or patient who has the physical capacity to perform such a movement.

A transfer consists of a person shifting or being shifted from one surface to another (wheelchair to mat) by means of a specified pattern of movements (Fig. 1–14). If a patient or student can transfer to and from a wheelchair, this should be encouraged whenever possible in order to improve or maintain functional independence. For example, in a weight training program, a paraplegic should be encouraged to perform a successful, safe transfer from the wheelchair to the mat or weight bench without assistance from another person.

Due to space limitations, the many various transfers will not be discussed. The transfer technique will depend upon the height, weight, agility, degree of involvement, and age of the individual. Transfers can be done with one or more able-bodied helpers for support, or performed independently depending upon the strength of the individual. The program leader should always consult with the attending phys-

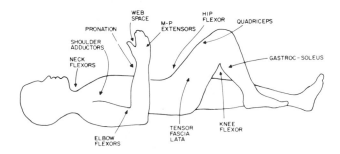

Fig. 1–13. Areas in which soft-tissue tightness most frequently occurs during prolonged immobilization or as a result of neuromuscular conditions. (From Krusen, M.: *Handbook of Physical Medicine and Rehabilitation,* Philadelphia, W.B. Saunders Co., 1966.)

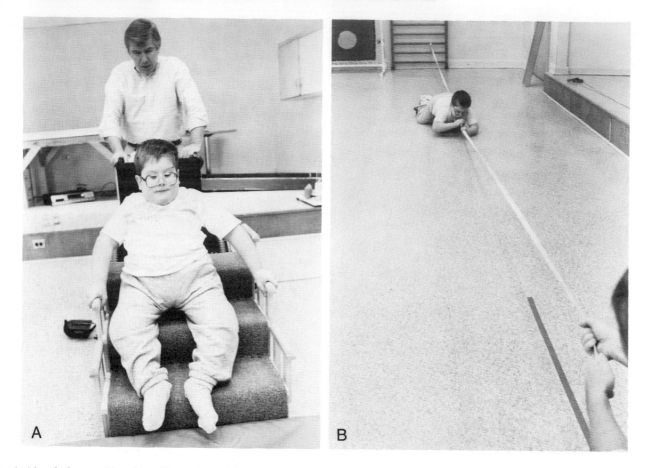

Fig. 1–14. *A,* 6-year-old patient with myelomeningocele transferring to a mat in preparation to engage in a physical conditioning/weight management program. When possible, it is important to focus attention to opportunities for physical development out of a wheelchair. *B,* In the horizontal rope climbing exercise, the patient is actively stretching and strengthening the arms while pulling himself on a gym scooter.

ical therapist to obtain further information on the type of transfer to be used. A few basic guidelines apply: (1) The chair must be locked for maximum stability during the transfer process and (2) the footplates are removed in most cases except for independent transfer to a bed or location of similar height.

Obviously, some persons can accomplish a transfer only with extensive assistance. Under certain circumstances, for example, transferring from a wheelchair into a swimming pool, assistance may be given by able-bodied persons, and, in such cases, it is suggested that every assistant have some knowledge and training in proper lifting techniques.

Some individuals with poor trunk control and sitting posture use seat inserts or special alignment accessories (Fig. 1–15). The program leader should consult with other professionals who are managing the patient to determine how useful the seat insert would be when the patient or student is sitting someplace other than in a wheelchair. (For example, a seat insert may be used for balance support while the student or patient performs from a sitting position on a mat.)

Concerns For Other Mobility Aids

The Quad cane which has 3 or 4 extensions at the bottom is a weight bearing device that provides the ambulator with a broad base of support. It provides more stability than a single floor contact point such as a standard cane. Some cerebral palsied ambulators with bilateral involvement use two Quad canes to assist in securing a more stable weight shift pattern. The hemiplegic with unilateral involvement (Fig. 1–16) uses the Quad cane to assist in ambulating with a more secure gait pattern. The non-affected upper limb which manages the cane is positioned in a normal walking position (to the side of the body).

A standard aluminum or wooden cane is more of a balance aid than a weight bearing device. Like the Quad cane, it can be used with patients or students who have unilateral or bilateral involvement. The standard cane is frequently used with ambulators who demonstrate a Trendelenburg/lurching-type gait (pelvis lowered on non-affected side when in weight bearing position) (Fig. 1–17). Frequently cane users exhibit enough weight bearing ability to stand for periods of time without support from the cane.

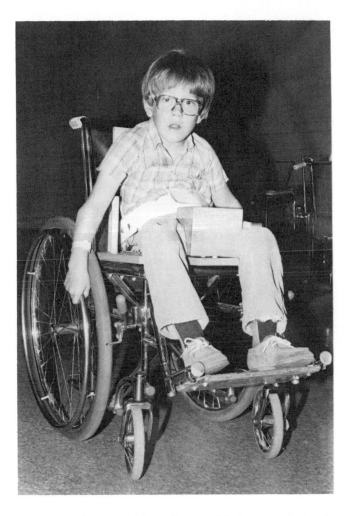

Fig. 1–15. Six-year-old boy, diagnosed to have cerebral palsy (spastic quadriplegia), with increased muscle tone in all extremities. Using the seat insert improved his pelvic mobility and back extension.

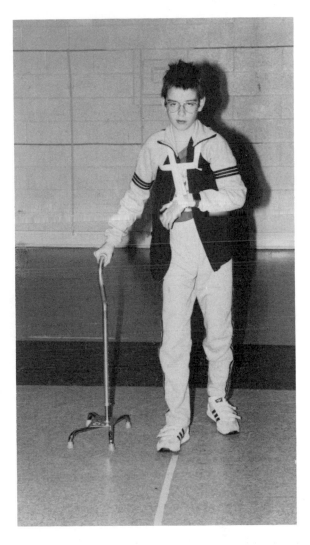

Fig. 1–16. This young boy had left hemiparesis secondary to closed head injury. Note four level rubber tip legs on quad cane that rest squarely on floor during walking motion.

Sample Assessment For a Cane User

Evaluate medical history, condition of the canes, and other concerns similar to a crutch-user. The instructor should take into account the user's functional ability. Remember, when a patient or student has unilateral involvement, the cane is always used on the strong side of the body. Similar to a crutch user, consult with other specialists to determine if the individual can use a standing device during physical activity periods. The cane tips should be inspected frequently to determine if their condition is suitable to maintain maximum security during physical activity programs.

Sample Assessment for a User of a Walker

The purpose of a walker (Fig. 1–18) is to provide balance support for independent mobility and standing. Ambulation using a pick-up walker is achieved by grasping the front horizontal bar or side bars, lifting the frame forward, placing it down, and then stepping forward. This type of walker is used fre-

quently with ambulators who demonstrate reciprocal leg action. Rolling walking aids with casters or front wheels are frequently used to aid gait training problems of cerebral palsy and multiple sclerosis. Generally referred to as a rollator, this type of aid conserves more energy than the pick-up walker, and speed control is more variable since the device is pushed.

Evaluate medical history, motor function of the user and gait pattern. Determine if the walker is adaptable to the working environment. For example, mobility problems can occur when using a walker on uneven terrain, loose carpets, etc. For some, it may be difficult to maneuver in close quarters. The instructor should also decide if the walker is to be used as a standing aid during physical activity periods. For example, the user may be able to hold onto the walker with one hand while freeing the dominant hand for throwing balls, etc.

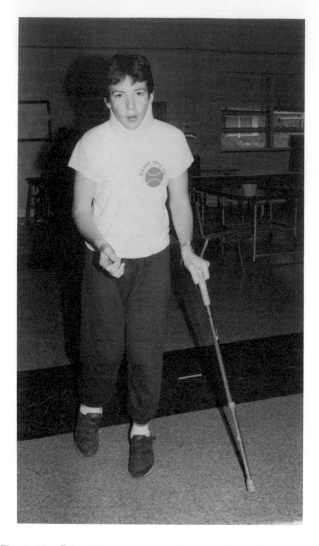

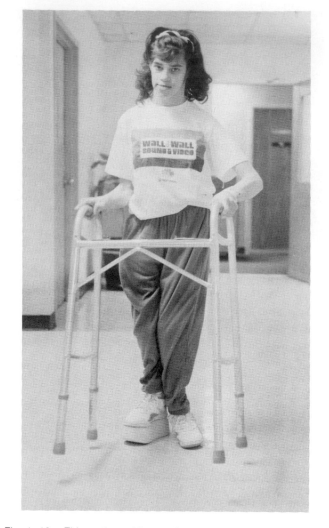

Fig. 1–17. This adolescent had a diagnosis of spastic quadriparesis secondary to cord compression at C1–C2 level. He had a fusion at that level. He was able to ambulate independently using a straight cane for support. Residual weakness of antigravity muscle strength was more pronounced on right side than the left and he had a tendency to walk in a mild crouched position.

Fig. 1–18. This patient with spastic cerebral palsy underwent a surgical procedure to correct right knee and hip contractures. Although weight shifting was difficult because of a built up shoe, she was able to ambulate for brief periods with a pick-up walker.

Early Intervention

Early intervention is the initiation of management and treatment for the child who demonstrates delayed or abnormal development.

The developmental processes that occur in the first year of life far exceed those of any other period except that of gestation. Research has demonstrated that the typical child has attained approximately 50% of his ultimate intellectual ability by the age of 4 years. Rapid changes in growth and development take place in the early years, and gross motor coordination develops more rapidly than mental function does before the age of two years. However, motor skills will not develop unless the child's neuromuscular system is sufficiently functional.

The therapist plays an important role in this program. Through the use of various treatment techniques and skills, he is able to work with the child and parent to plan sound strategies for the child's delayed or abnormal development. The therapist must be aware of the various procedures and techniques of early infant stimulation. Some of these techniques are discussed here. But, if a therapist is to provide optimum results, a short-term course covering the various techniques should be taken or reviewed.

There are many factors that should alert physicians to the need to refer children to an early intervention program.

Many children born to mothers with problems are strong candidates for the early intervention program. Some problems which mothers may have that could cause disabilities in their newborns are:

1. diabetes
2. extremes of maternal age
3. toxemia
4. drug addiction
5. use of certian medications
6. infections
   a. rubella
   b. syphilis
   c. intrauterine
7. tuberculosis
8. Rh or ABO sensitization

Problems that occur to either the newborn or the mother during the delivery can also cause disabilities in the newborn. Some of the problems related to labor or delivery are:

1. placental hemorrhage
2. prolapse of the umbilical cord
3. difficult delivery
4. intracranial injury
5. peripheral nerve injury
6. fractures

To complicate and add to the number of factors that can cause problems, the child also may be considered a high risk for the following reasons:

1. immaturity and low birth weight
2. high birth weight
3. postmaturity exceeding 43 weeks
4. multiple births
5. meningitis
6. blood disorders
7. respiratory distress
8. seizures
9. jaundice

It is important, therefore, in view of the many factors that can cause problems in the newborn, that as much information as possible be obtained prior to initiating any treatment program.

The information supplied by the physician is extremely important when dealing with the complex problems of a child who needs early intervention. This information should include the original assessment made by the delivery physician and subsequent assessments made by other physicians. If a copy of the child's hospital record can be obtained, it may supply some in-depth information unknown to the parents.

The Apgar Scoring Scale (Table 1–4) is useful in making a quick evaluation of a child immediately at birth. It is a scale that is used widely by many physicians and hospitals. Newborns normally score 8 or 9 within the first minute after birth. Lower scores that do not improve within the next few minutes indicate that the infant requires special attention immediately. Scores under 4 indicate that the infant's bodily functions are seriously depressed.

In addition to information from the Apgar scoring scale, any other early assessments and managements should be reviewed. The cardio-respiratory function of the child, including oxygenation of tissue without maternal and placental help, should be reviewed. Was there continuation of oxygen without more than a few minutes of interruption? The heart should beat between 110 to 160 times per minute. Was the child active at birth? This activity may be hindered in part by the maternal analgesia and anesthesia. Was the infant exposed to undue heat loss? Infants are vulnerable to heat loss. Newborns are affected by hypothermia, and additional heat loss may result in respiratory depression and hypoglycemia due to the body's utilization of energy to produce heat. The skin should be pink and not cyanotic, pallid or jaundiced. The circumference of the head should be noted as well as any blood pressure points. There should also be assessments of the abdomen, genitalia, extremities, eyes, ears, nose, and throat.

Most children are examined or evaluated by a pediatrician or pediatric neurologist the day after delivery or shortly thereafter. If a child has a problem that is easily detected, or of such magnitude that it is immediately observed or diagnosed by the delivering physician, then a specialist is usually called in immediately.

The assessment or evaluation performed by the specialist covers a wide range of tests and observations. The various procedures cited above are repeated, and first opinons are evaluated against present information. Special attention is given to the infant's nervous system. It is important to determine by testing various reflexes whether the nervous system is functioning properly. A few of the reflexes are noted below:

1. Oral reflexes:
   a. sucking—ability to suck such as on a nipple
   b. swallowing—ability to swallow liquid in the mouth
   c. rooting—movement of the head, mouth, and tongue toward a touch in the corner of the mouth or cheek. (Presence of the rooting reflex in an infant beyond 2 months of age indicates a possible developmental delay.)
2. Moro reflex:
   Test by holding the baby in the supine position and dropping the back of the head suddenly; or holding the hands and raising the baby's trunk off the table slightly, then releasing the child; or jarring the table or crib suddenly.
   The expected response is for the baby to cry and extend the arms, fingers, and legs, then return all extremities and fingers to a position of flexion against the body. This reflex is considered abnormal if elicited after the fifth month.
3. Asymmetric tonic neck reflex:
   With baby in a supine position, turn the head passively 90° to the right or left. The baby should respond by extending the extremities on the side

Table 1–4.
Apgar Scoring Scale

Sign	0	1	2
Heart rate	Absent	Below 100	Over 100
Respiratory rate	Absent	Slow, irregular	Good, crying motion
Muscle tone	Flaccid	Some flexion of extremities	Active
Reflex irritability*	No response	Grimace	Cry
Color	Blue, pale	Body pink, extremities blue	Completely pink

*Test by inserting the tip of a catheter into the nostril. (Courtesy of Virginia Apgar, M.D., and Smith, Kline, and French Laboratories, Philadelphia, Pennsylvania.)

the face is turned toward and flexing extremities on the opposite side. (Response to this reflex is considered abnormal after the fifth month.)

4. Grasp reflex:

A finger is placed in the palm of the baby's hand. The baby's hand grasps the finger. If the arms are lifted the baby tends to pull up and may support his weight. (Response to this reflex beyond the third month is considered abnormal.)

If any of the evaluated reflexes are uneven in strength of response on different sides of the body or if any response is asymmetric, some kind of neurologic dysfunction is usually suspected. Various other pathologic reflexes, if present, may also indicate the possibility of some kind of irregular neural function. A more complete description of reflexes can be found in a pediatric neurology or motor development text.

Normal motor development proceeds in an orderly fashion. As the nervous system develops, more areas are established that coordinate combined muscle activities.

Early motor responses of the infant are controlled primarily by reflexes. The highly coordinated movement patterns necessary for locomotion emerge from reflex patterns.

The normal development of children involves a series of successive stages. Within each of these stages are milestones of normal, or average, rates of change in social, intellectual, physical, and emotional development. The ranges of the various normal milestones can be predicted for the individual child, but there are still many questions to be answered regarding the development of a child from conception to maturity.

To discuss the normal growth and development of children here would not achieve the standards of previous research such as that by Gesell, Amatruda, Cratty, and Ayers. One of the excellent books on growth and development of children should be used as a reference guide when working in an early intervention program.

When a child is referred for treatment in an early intervention program, a complete evaluation should be made. The evaluation that is completed by the instructor or therapist should be reviewed in conjunction with the data that is sent by the physician or the hospital. If no data is obtained from the physician or hospital, then a case history should be obtained by a social worker, if one is available. Prenatal care, previous pregnancies, length of pregnancy, delivery, labor, and history that the parents/guardians can recall will provide information with which to establish a baseline.

The evaluation utilized by the instructor or therapist varies depending on the age or disability of the child. Some of the evaluations that could be used are:

1. Portage Guide to Early Education
2. Cerebral Palsy Assessment
3. Bellmawr Pre-School Program
4. Denver Developmental Screening Test
5. Gesell Developmental Schedules
6. Preschool Attainment Record (PAR)
7. Developmental Screening Inventory
8. Bayley Scales of Infant Development
9. Milani-Comparetti Motor Development Test

After a child is evaluated, a treatment program can be established, based on the case history, data from physician or hospital, and the evaluation.

The treatment program will be planned in a sequential manner, establishing what the child can and cannot perform. Then, with the knowledge of normal growth and development, goals can be developed and planned. The program must have the cooperation of the parents/guardians in order to be successful. The parents/guardians must continue the activities, exercises, and skills in a home program in addition to the therapy the child receives. A complete understanding of the order of goals and objectives must be explained to the parents/guardians. Their cooperation and assistance cannot be emphasized enough. Perhaps a hypothetic case will serve as an example:

A 3-month-old child is referred by a physician to the early intervention program. The data indicate that there were some earlier indicators of a problem. The score on the Apgar Scoring Scale was low, and some responses to the evaluation performed by the pediatrician were questionable. The child has had difficulty with head control, and does not appear to be using the right upper extremity as much as the left upper extremity. The right upper extremity is held close to the body most of the time. There were some problems with sucking and swallowing initially, but they seem to have improved. The child has not been very active and lies quietly most of the time.

After completing all the evaluation procedures discussed previously, you find basically the same responses, but your evaluation provides you with some additional facts. Your program is then based on both your findings and the findings obtained by the physician.

The child is begun on a series of activities and exercises to increase head control. One such exercise would be lifting the head and holding it up while the child is in a prone position. You could also move the head passively through a range of motion and have the child try to hold it. Objects could be placed above or near the head to obtain a lifting response. Exercises for the right upper extremity could include passive motion to all the joints in the various planes of motion. Try stimulating the right upper extremity with a brush or stroking it with your finger to elicit a response. Place various objects in the palm of the right hand to begin a grasp reflex if one is not present.

The above are suggestions for possible procedures. Naturally, the actual program depends on the disability of the child. The possible activities, exercises, and procedures will be limited only by the instructor or therapist who does not understand growth and development or have the imagination to vary the skills and activities and to assist the child and the parents/guardians.

A constant review of the growth and development patterns is an essential part of the program, as is the idea that every child responds differently, and adjustments must be made constantly to accomplish a satisfactory result.

Adapted Physical Education in the Public School Setting

Physical education is an important component of the curriculum in today's schools. The purpose of physical education is to promote the development of physical fitness, motor skills and abilities so children can learn to lead active and healthy lifestyles. The promotion of healthy lifestyles is equally important for physically disabled school-aged children. This population often needs physical education even more than able bodied students due to an increased incidence of sedentary lifestyles. This section will identify the important aspects of physical education including the legislative mandates that require physical education within the public school setting.

The federal legislation that primarily supports the inclusion of physical education for handicapped students within the public school setting are the Rehabilitation Act of 1973, P.L. 93-112 and P.L. 94-142, the Education of All Handicapped Children Act of 1975. The Rehabilitation Act is considered to be the civil rights act for disabled persons. Section 504 of the act states that "no qualified handicapped individual . . . shall be excluded from participation or denied the benefits . . . under any program receiving federal assistance". This includes nonacademic and extracur-

ricular activities and physical education. Another important law is P.L. 99–457, which provides federal assistance in the identification of pre-school-aged children and mandates appropriate educational services for handicapped children beginning at age 3.

The Education of All Handicapped Children Act stated that all children must receive a free and appropriate public education in the least restrictive environment. The law specifically indicates that specially designed physical education is a necessary component of special education. These physical education services are considered a direct service and must be provided to every handicapped child in the least restrictive environment. Direct services (i.e., required special education) are differentiated from related services. Related services must be provided, only if necessary to benefit from special education. Related services include physical therapy, speech therapy, occupational therapy and recreational therapy. These services must be provided for children aged 3 to 21 years of age. Page 4480 of the Federal Register states that special education means "specifically designed instruction at no cost to the parent, to meet the unique needs of a handicapped child, including classroom instruction, instruction in physical education, home instruction and instruction in hospitals and institutions".

Physical education is defined in the Federal Register as a term meaning the development of:

a. Physical and motor fitness
b. Fundamental motor skills and patterns; and
c. Skill in aquatics, dance, and individual and group games and sports including intramural and lifetime sports.

Another extremely important provision under P.L. 94-142 is the need for an individualized education program (IEP) for children needing special education. This is a written program specifically designed to meet the need of a child. The document is developed by the child's teacher, parents, administrators and professional staff responsible for the direction of the child's educational program. The content of IEP must include:

a. A statement of the child's present level of functioning;
b. A statement of annual goals, including short-term objectives;
c. A statement of the specific education and related services to be provided to the child, and the extent to which the child will be able to participate in the regular educational programs;
d. The projected dates for initiation of services and the anticipated duration of services; and
e. Appropriate objective criteria and evaluation procedures for determining, on at least an annual basis, whether the short-term instructional objectives are being achieved.

INDIVIDUALIZED EDUCATIONAL PROGRAM

DATE: _____

Name: __Brown, Alfred_____   Date of Birth:__January 2, 1970_____

Address:__411 Jefferson Avenue____   Present Condition/Placement:_CP Spastic (L)_
                                                                          Hemi
_____Hometown, N.J. 08000_____   Classification:_Neurologically Impaired___

                                      Instructor:_Ronald Adams - Alfred Daniel__

                                      Date of Parent/Guardian Contact:_11/10/79____

I.   INSTRUCTIONAL LEVELS:
     Individually prescribed instructional program for recreational therapy
     and/or Developmental Physical Education.

II. ANNUAL GOALS AND SHORT TERM OBJECTIVES:

     A. Annual Goals:
         1. Increase strength and range of motion of left upper extremity.
         2. Increase strength and range of motion of left lower extremity.
         3. Improve ambulation with quad cane.

     B. Short Term Objectives:
         1. Exercises to left upper extremity via exercise program, games or
            activities.
         2. Exercises to left lower extremity via exercise program, games or
            activities.
         3. Balance and stability when using cane for ambulation.

III. SPECIFIC SERVICES NEEDED AND EXTENT OF PARTICIPATION IN REGULAR PROGRAM:

         1. Recreational Therapy
         2. Developmental Physical Education
         3. All other classes in regular school program.

IV. RATIONAL FOR THE TYPE OF PROGRAM:
     Child Study Team recommendations via letter from Dr. Helen Smith,
        Pediatric Neurologist

V.   INDIVIDUALS RESPONSIBLE FOR IMPLEMENTATION OF IEP:
     Ronald Adams - Alfred Daniel

VI. EVALUATIVE CRITERIA:
     1. Report from Dr. Helen Smith, Pediatric Neurologist
     2. Manual muscle test
     3. Gait analysis

VII. ADDITIONAL COMMENTS:
     Child on medication, Dilantin for mild seizures. Seizures under
     control, none for the last year.

Fig. 1-19. Completed short IEP form.

INDIVIDUALIZED EDUCATIONAL PROGRAM

Name ___Brown, Alfred_____ Grade _5th_____ Date_____

Address _411 Jefferson Ave., Hometown, N. J. 08000_____ Phone _100-1234_____

School _Washington Elementary__ C.A. _10-4__ Name of Parent/Guardian _____

Date of Parent/Guardian Contact _11/10/79__ Specialists _____
                                            (R.T., O.T., P.T., Dev. P.E.) - Signature

Date

10/10/79 Psychologist _Louis Blue_____   10/7/79_ Physician _William White, M.D._

10/1/79_ Social Worker _Mary Green____   _____ Psychiatrist_____

10/4/79_ LDT-C   _John Johnson____   10/14/79 Neurologist _Helen Smith, M.D._

                                           _____ Specialists _____

I. INSTRUCTIONAL LEVELS

    Individually prescribed instructional program for Recreational
    Therapy and/or Developmental Physical Education.

II. ANNUAL GOALS AND SHORT TERM OBJECTIVES
     (Denote teacher(s) and schedule when applicable.)

     A. Annual Goals
         1. Increase strength & range of motion of left upper extremity.
         2. Increase strength & range of motion of left lower extremity.
         3. Improve ambulation with quad cane.

     B. Short Term Objectives
         1. Exercises to left upper extremity via exercise programs, games
            or activities.
         2. Exercises to left lower extremity via exercise programs, games
            or activities.
         3. Balance and stability when using cane for ambulation.

III. SPECIFIC SERVICES NEEDED AND EXTENT OF PARTICIPATION IN REGULAR PROGRAM

     1. Recreational Therapy
     2. Developmental Physical Education
     3. All other classes in regular school program

Fig. 1-20. Completed long IEP form.

-2-

IV. RATIONALE FOR THE TYPE OF PROGRAM

Child Study Team recommendation via letter from Dr. Helen Smith,
   Pediatric Neurologist

V. INDIVIDUALS RESPONSIBLE FOR IMPLEMENTATION OF I.E.P.

Ronald Adams
Alfred Daniel

VI. EVALUATIVE CRITERIA

1. Report from Dr. Helen Smith, Pediatric Neurologist
2. Manual Muscle Test
3. Gait analysis

VII. ADDITIONAL COMMENTS

Child on medication, Dilantin, for mild seizures.   Seizures under
   control, none for last year.

Fig. 1–20, continued.

This IEP helps insure school accountability for providing appropriate educational programs. This legislation further identifies the procedural safeguards that must be followed for placement and evaluation procedures. Parents have the right and obligation to take an active part in the development of the IEP. If the guidelines are not followed in accordance with P.L. 94-142, then the parents have the legal right and support to insure the programs are developed and followed. Though many states have similar state laws that parallel this legislation, it is imperative that parents are educated to their children's educational rights.

These legislative documents have greatly influenced the educational right and privileges of handicapped children. This has also had a positive effect on the opportunities for quality physical education programs in the public schools. It it important for all educators to realize that the legislative acts could potentially be modified or changed in years to come. As such, advocacy for the educational rights and privileges is a professional obligation that educators must realize.

Various IEP forms can be utilized (Figs. 1–19 and 1–20). The short form does not specify the various individuals involved and the dates of evaluations as the long form does. In addition, the long form allows one to go into depth regarding each category.

The following example of the use of an individualized educational program (IEP) for a specific disability may assist with the planning of future IEPs.

A 10-year-old child has spastic cerebral palsy with left hemiplegia. His intelligence is normal but he cannot function in a regular physical education program in a public

Table 1–5.
Project UNIQUE Physical Fitness Test Items
According to Major Participant Groups

Test Items	Normal, Auditory Impaired, Visually Impaired[a]	Cerebral Palsy[a]	Wheelchair Paraplegic Spinal Neuro-muscular[a]	Congenital Anomaly/ Amputee[a]
Body composition skinfolds	X	X	X	X
Muscular strength/endurance				
grip strength (strength)	X[b]	X[c,f]	X[g,h]	X[b,j]
50-yard dash (power-speed)	X	X[d]	X[d]	X
Sit-ups (power-strength)	X	—	—	X[i]
Softball throw for distance (power strength)		X[e]	—	—
Flexibility				
sit-and-reach	X	X	—	X
Cardiorespiratory endurance				
long-distance run	X	X	X	X

[a]Items may require modification or elimination for selected group subclassifications.
[b]The broad-jump may be substituted for grip strength tests as a measure of strength for these groups.
[c]Grip strengths measure power-strength for males with cerebral palsy.
[d]The dash measures power-endurance for individuals in this group.
[e]The softball throw is recommended for females only as a measure of power-strength.
[f]The arm hang may be substituted for grip strength tests for males.
[g]The arm hang or softball throw for distance may be substituted for grip strength measures (strength factor) for males.
[h]The softball throw may be substituted for grip strength measures (strength factor) for female participants.
[i]The softball throw for distance may be substituted for sit-ups (as a power-strength factor) when the sit-up would be considered inappropriate.
[j]Males may substitute the arm hang for grip tests (strength factor).

school. The child can ambulate with a wide-base quad cane. His left hemiplegia has caused some limitation of motion and strength in the left upper extremities, particularly the shoulder, elbow, and wrist. The left lower extremity also has some limitation of motion and strength in the knee, ankle, and foot.

The child must be evaluated to determine his strengths and weaknesses. This evaluation should include gross motor abilities, posture, gait, hand-eye coordination, foot-eye coordination, strength, and range of motion of the various joints. Standardized evaluation procedures should be utilized in order to have valid data for comparison. After completion of the various evaluation tools and a review of the results, an IEP can be produced with the cooperation of the parents/guardians and the various individuals responsible for the evaluations and follow-up program.

A completed short (Fig. 1–19) and/or long (Fig. 1–20) IEP form should become part of the child's permanent record. The IEP must be updated yearly, or more often if specific changes are to be made regarding the various programs offered to the child.

Project UNIQUE

Project UNIQUE was a field-initiated research project funded through the U.S. Department of Education to test the physical fitness of orthopedically and sensory impaired youth. The project was under the direction of Dr. Joseph Winnick and Dr. Frank Short, SUNY-Brockport, and completed in 1982. This project modified and extended the AAHPERD Youth Related Test of Physical Fitness for a variety of handi-

capping conditions. Testors were trained across the United States. These testors then tested adolescents aged 10 to 17 who were orthopedically or sensory impaired. Data generated from this study now provide basic performances on these tests of physical fitness that can then be compared with normal populations or intra-individual comparisons. These results were generated with valid and reliable measures of physical fitness (refer to Table 1–5).

The representative groups tested included: Visually Impaired, Auditory Impaired, Orthopedically Impaired. The orthopedically impaired population included congenital anomalies (poliomyelitis, bone tuberculosis, clubfoot deformities) or from other causes e.g., cerebral palsy, fractures or burns that cause contractures. Also included were spinal neuromuscular conditions subclassified as in the NWAA system. This group included spina bifida and spinal cord lesions. The cerebral palsy group was classified by the NASCP guidelines. The following other conditions were also considered: Arthritis, Multiple Sclerosis, Muscular Dystrophy, Osgood-Schlatters Disease, Scoliosis, Cystic Fibrosis, Diabetes, Cardiovascular Disorders, Respiratory Disorders and Arthrogryposis.

This study made a major contribution to the available assessment items utilized in recreation and physical education in regard to the physical fitness status of these populations. For additional information, see *Physical fitness testing and the disabled: Project UNIQUE*, Champaign, IL: Human Kinetics Publishers.

Table 1–6.
Disqualifying Conditions for Sports Participation

Conditions	Collision*	Contact†	Noncontact‡	Other§
GENERAL				
Acute infections: Respiratory, genitourinary, infectious mononucleosis, hepatitis, active rheumatic fever, active tuberculosis	X	X	X	X
Obvious physical immaturity in comparison with other competitors	X	X		
Hemorrhagic disease: Hemophilia, purpura, and other serious bleeding tendencies	X	X	X	
Diabetes, inadequately controlled	X	X	X	X
Diabetes, controlled				
Jaundice	X	X	X	X
EYES				
Absence or loss of function of one eye	X	X		
RESPIRATORY				
Tuberculosis (active or symptomatic)	X	X	X	X
Severe pulmonary insufficiency	X	X	X	X
CARDIOVASCULAR				
Mitral stenosis, aortic stenosis, aortic insufficiency, coarctation of aorta, cyanotic heart disease, recent carditis of any etiology	X	X	X	X
Hypertension on organic basis	X	X	X	X
Previous heart surgery for congenital or acquired heart disease¶				
LIVER				
Enlarged liver	X	X		
SKIN				
Boils, impetigo, and herpes simplex gladiatorum	X	X		
SPLEEN				
Enlarged spleen	X	X		
HERNIA				
Inguinal or femoral hernia	X	X	X	
MUSCULOSKELETAL				
Symptomatic abnormalities or inflammations	X	X	X	X
Functional inadequacy of the musculoskeletal system, congenital or acquired, incompatible with the contact or skill demands of the sport	X	X	X	
NEUROLOGIC				
History or symptoms of previous serious head trauma, or repeated concussions	X			
Controlled convulsive disorders#				
Convulsive disorder not moderately well controlled by medication	X			
Previous surgery on head	X	X		
RENAL				
Absence of one kidney	X	X		
Renal disease	X	X	X	X
GENITALIA**				
Absence of one testicle				
Undescended testicle				

*Football, rugby, hockey, lacrosse, etc.
†Baseball, soccer, basketball, wrestling, etc.
‡Cross country, track, tennis, crew, swimming, etc.
§Bowling, golf, archery, field events, etc.
¶Each patient should be judged on an individual basis in conjunction with his cardiologist and operating surgeon.
#Each patient should be judged on an individual basis. All things being equal, it is probably better to encourage a young boy or girl to participate in a noncontact sport rather than a contact sport. However, if a particular patient has a great desire to play a contact sport, and this is deemed a major ameliorating factor in his adjustment to school, associates and the seizure disorder, serious consideration should be given to letting him participate if the seizures are moderately well controlled or the athlete is under good medical management.
**The Committee approves the concept of contact sports participation for youths with only one testicle or with an undescended testicle(s), except in specific cases such as an inguinal canal undescended testicle(s), following appropriate medical evaluation to rule out unusual injury risk. However, the athlete, parents and school authorities should be fully informed that participation in contact sports for such youths with only one testicle does carry a slight injury risk to the remaining healthy testicle. Following such an injury, fertility may be adversely affected. But the chances of an injury to a descended testicle are rare, and the injury risk can be further substantially minimized with an athletic supporter and protective device.
(Courtesy of the American Medical Association.)

Medical Evaluation and Physical Basis for Exclusion from Athletics

PL 94-142 and Section 504 of the Rehabilitation Act indicates that individuals with handicapping conditions cannot be denied opportunities to participate in sports activities. To do this, playing rules need to be non-discriminatory. The questions then arise regarding the risk factors associated with granting such privileges. For example, is it sound judgment to permit an individual with a unilateral kidney malformation to play contact sports? After all, there is always the possibility of future injury to the remaining functioning organ.

Involvement in sports is a privilege and should be an individual choice, provided the individual can perform in all aspects of practice and competition without endangering himself or other participants.

The American Medical Association identifies the basic principles that assure protection against needless injury. The 5 safeguards are: (1) proper conditioning, (2) good coaching, (3) capable officiating, (4) proper equipment, and (5) adequate health supervision.

The primary consideration, however, must be the medical evaluation. A responsible evaluation should detect any physical limitations that would expose an individual to undue risk through participation in certain forms of athletics.

The disqualifying conditions listed in Table 1–6 are subject to evaluation by the responsible physician with respect to anticipated risks, the otherwise athletic fitness of the candidate, special protective, preventive measures that will be utilized, and the nature of the supervisory control. Disqualification does not necessarily imply restriction from all sports at that time or from the sport in question in the future. If the decision is disqualification, however, the physician vested by the school with the authority to disqualify should not be overruled by any other person. This is a direct and unavoidable responsibility, and the physician needs the full support of the institution and all personnel involved. Further considerations regarding a candidate's participation in athletics and recreational exercise are discussed in Chapter 4.

REFERENCES

1. Wright, B.: *Physical Disability—a Psychosocial Approach.* 2nd ed. New York, Harper & Row, 1983.
2. Annarino, A.: The five traditional objectives of physical education. JOHPER, *41*: June, 1970.
3. Walsh, K.: Wheelchair Kinesiology. Sports and Recreational Programs for the Child and Young Adult with Physical Disability. The American Academy of Orthopedic Surgeons, 1983.

BIBLIOGRAPHY

Annarino, A.: The five traditional objectives of physical education. JOHPER, *41*: June, 1970.

Ayres, J.: *Sensory Integration and Learning Disorders.* Los Angeles, Western Psychological Services, 1975.

Bobath, B.: The very early treatment of cerebral palsy. Dev Med Child Neurol, *9*:373, 1967.

Bromley, I.: *Tetraplegia and Paraplegia,* 2nd Ed. New York, Churchill-Livingstone, Inc., 1981.

Burden, R.L.: An approach to the evaluation of early intervention projects with mothers of severely handicapped children: the attitude dimension. Child, Care, Health and Development, *4*:171, 1978.

Caputo, A.J. et al.: Primitive reflex profile. Phys Ther, *58*:1061, 1978.

Chee, F.K. et al.: Semicircular canal stimulation in cerebral palsied children. Phys Ther, *58*:1071, 1978.

Cratty, B.J.: *Perceptual and Motor Development in Infants and Children.* New York, Macmillan Co., 1970.

Esposito, R.R.: Physicians' attitudes toward early intervention. Phys Ther, *58*:160, 1978.

Fiorentino, M.R.: *Normal and Abnormal Development, The Influence of Primitive Reflexes on Motor Development.* Springfield, Charles C Thomas, 1978.

Fiorentino, M.R.: *Reflex Testing Methods for Evaluating CNS Development.* Springfield, Charles C Thomas, 1963.

Fulkner, R.: *Therapeutic Recreation in Health Care Settings, A Practitioner's Viewpoint.* Greenville, N.C., Leisure Enrichment Service, 1984.

Goldberg, K.: The high-risk infant. Phys Ther, *55*:1092, 1975.

Hoskin, T.A., and Squires, J.E.: Developmental assessment: a test for gross motor and reflex development. Phys Ther, *53*:117, 1973.

Kantner, R.M. et al.: "Effects of Vestibular Stimulation and The Developmental Behavior of the Premature Infant." Dissertation, New York University, 1976.

Mason, E.W., and Dando, H.B.: Corrective Therapy and Adapted Physical Education. Introductory Handbook to Corrective Therapy and Adapted Physical Education. Association for Physical Mental Rehabilitation, Inc., 1965.

McAndrew, I.: Children with a handicap and their families. Child, Care, Health and Development, *2*:213, 1976.

Pringle, M.E. et al.: Survey of physical therapy provided to infants under three months of age. Phys Ther, *58*:1055, 1978.

Report on the University of Illinois Wheelchairs for Athletic Use: Rehabilitation-Education Center, University of Illinois, 1967.

Shivers, J., and Fait, H.: *Special Recreational Services Therapeutic and Adapted.* Philadelphia, Lea & Febiger, 1985.

Waechter, E., and Blake, F.: *Nursing Care of Children.* 9th Ed. Philadelphia, J.B. Lippincott Co., 1976.

A clarification of terms. JOHPER, *42*:1971.

Winnick, J. and Short, F.: *Physical Fitness Testing of the Disabled, Project Unique.* Champaign, IL, Human Kinetics Publishers, Inc., 1985.

Zimmerman, J.: *Goals and Objectives for Developing Normal Movement Patterns.* Rockville, MD, Aspen Publishers, Inc., 1988.

2 *Brief History of Therapeutic Exercise*

Innumerable theories and accounts have been proposed about prehistoric man's beginnings, ways of life, and evolution. Historians have explored Africa, the Near East, and the Far East. Archeologists have dug, uncovered, interpreted, and made assumptions. Cave drawings, fossils, and various other materials have prompted numerous theories concerning our ancestors. With these findings comes evidence of various forms of treatment for physical defects and the relief of pain.

ANCIENT CULTURES

Just where therapeutic exercise began is difficult to establish; however, most historians and archeologists agree that the Chinese, in approximately 2500 B.C., were one of the first groups to have attained a civilized state.

The Chinese practiced a series of light exercises called Cong Fu. These exercises bear a certain resemblance to the Swedish Ling system. The Chinese believed that disease derived from bodily inactivity. To prolong human life, mild forms of medical gymnastics were derived. These exercises were a combination of stretching and breathing to maintain organic function. The medical gymnastics were usually performed in a sitting or kneeling position.[1]

The Cong Fu reached its greatest popularity during the Chou Dynasty (1115 B.C.), when it was practiced in national schools throughout the country.

The ancient Hindus of India propounded many rules for medical and health protection, many of which were used until the time of the Crusades. Today, the best-known influence of the Hindus is Yoga, a system of physical and mental exercises designed to bring the body, the senses, and the mind under control.

THE GREEK INFLUENCE

The first Greek to write on the subject of remedial gymnastics was Herodicus, sometime after 480 B.C. A teacher, he developed a system of exercises based on geometry to correct various bodily weaknesses in his students. It was felt by many of Herodicus' students, however, that his exercises were too severe and strenuous.

One of Herodicus' students was "the father of medicine," Hippocrates, who has been credited with the writing of many books on exercise. In one, *On Articulations*, which Licht discusses very ably, Hippocrates

revealed a thorough understanding of muscles and their motions:

The wasting of the fleshy (muscle) parts is greatest in those cases in which the patient keeps the limb up and does not exercise it. Those who practice walking have the least atrophy.[2]

Hippocrates also advocated rapid walking to reduce obesity, exercising cautiously after long rest, and using exercises in a manner to which an individual was accustomed in order to remain healthy and strong.

Aristotle and Plato continued to carry forth the thesis of the relationship between exercise and health.

THE ROMAN ERA

Slowly, the Greek civilization crumbled and was succeeded by the powers of the Macedonians and then the Romans, who adapted Greek culture and knowledge for their own use.

Galen, born a Greek about A.D. 130, spent most of his life in the Roman Empire. A great philosopher and student of medicine, he served as a physician to the Roman athletes and to Emperor Marcus Aurelius. Galen wrote hundreds of books on various subjects. "In his book *On Hygiene* he classified exercises according to their vigor, duration, frequency, use of apparatus and the part of the body involved."[2] Galen divided his exercises into 3 specific groups: "group one were exercises to give muscle tone; group two were exercises for quickness, and group three, violent exercises."[1]

Of the Romans following Galen, one of the most famous is Caelius Aurelianus, an advocate of the use of suspensions and therapy with pulleys and weights. In his book *On Chronic Diseases*, he discussed various exercises performed with these devices to gain muscle strength and tone. He also suggested squeezing and gripping wax to gain strength of the fingers and hands for arthritic patients.

Other Romans did use exercise, along with a calculated diet, for health and medical reasons, but slowly most Romans became more sedentary. They decreased their physical activity and came to depend upon baths and massages to keep fit.

THE DARK AND MIDDLE AGES

As the Greek Empire fell, so crumbled the Roman Empire. The barbarian hordes from the North conquered and destroyed Roman civilization. Throughout Europe the strong offered the weak protection behind the walls of their fortresses in return for work and obedience.

The Christian Church remained intact and offered some leadership, but it taught renunciation of material things and concern with the soul and not the body. So the desire for preservation of the body was lost, and the "mortification of the flesh" was thought to improve one's sanctity. Practices such as flagellation and fasting were the exact opposite of the earlier attempt to promote good health. From the sixth to the eleventh centuries, games and sports were considered frivolous and undesirable. Since it was believed that man was placed on earth to suffer, medicine was practiced very little during this period.

Beginning in the fourteenth century, the Renaissance brought a renewed interest in the culture of the Greeks and Romans, including their sports and medicine. Around 1423, Vittorino da Feltre started a school for young noblemen in Mantua. He divided the teaching between mental and physical education. Although the school did not last long, it did influence the return of physical activity.

Hieronymus Mercurialis wrote a book, *De Arte Gymnastica,* in 1569. This was the first modern book on therapeutic exercise.

Mercurialis set the following principles for medical gymnastics:

1. Each exercise should preserve the existing healthy state.
2. Exercise should not disturb the harmony among the principal humors.
3. Exercises should be suited to each part of the body.
4. All healthy people should take exercise regularly.
5. Sick people should not be given exercises which might exacerbate existing conditions.
6. Special exercises should be prescribed for convalescent patients on an individual basis.
7. Persons who lead a sedentary life urgently need exercise.[2]

THE MODERN AGE

During the next 2 centuries, the use of various forms of exercises and treatments increased steadily. In the seventeenth century, Friedrich Hoffmann had the greatest influence on kinetic occupational therapy. He felt that occupational movements, such as cutting and sewing, and general everyday activities provided the exercise for gaining strength and good health.

Following Hoffmann, Nicolas André proposed exercises for correcting postural deformities in his book *L'Orthopedic.* However, it was Joseph-Clement Tissot in 1780 who stressed that a knowledge of anatomy was essential in prescribing exercises. Tissot advanced the work of Friedrich Hoffmann on occupational exercises, and he is credited with establishing the principles of occupational therapy. Tissot also began the use of adapted sports and recreational therapy. He vigorously opposed prolonged bed rest claiming that

it caused decubitus ulcers and the formation of kidney stones; but his recommendations for early treatment and movement for patients suffering from strokes were ignored. He also strongly advocated massage and passive movement for the arthritic patient as soon as it was tolerable.

Per Henrik Ling of Sweden had a great influence on the gymnastic movement in the nineteenth century. His exercise programs were used widely throughout Europe and the United States. Ling classified exercises into 4 categories: (1) pedagogic, (2) aesthetic, (3) military, and (4) medical. Medical gymnastics for the physically disabled came under 3 subheads: (1) active, exercises the patient did himself; (2) passive, exercises that someone did to the patient, without having the patient resist or assist; (3) duplicated, exercises in which the patient resisted efforts being made by someone else.

THE UNITED STATES INFLUENCE

Certainly the historical influence of the United States on physical education for therapeutic purposes is quite noteworthy. In the late 1700s notable people such as Benjamin Franklin, Thomas Jefferson and Noah Webster all proclaimed the need for physical activity for the improvement of health. In the 1800s the European influence on the need for physical activities for health impacted greatly on the schools of the country. Public schools began to require exercise for health of all students. Such Americans as Catherine Beecher, Dudley Sargent, and Edward Hitchcock were on the forefront of establishing exercise guidelines and prescribing exercise to ameliorate injuries and to restore health. In fact, in 1861, Dr. Edward Hitchcock, a physician and Director of Department of Hygiene and Physical Education at Amherst College, required all students to participate in exercise that was led by squad leaders and to the accompaniment of music. This practice is certainly in existence today with dance aerobics. Hitchcock noted through his work and research that student illness declined, as did class absenteeism, following mandatory exercise sessions. Dr. Dudley Sargent of Harvard developed individualized exercise programs for college students in the 1870s using anthropometric measurements and strength evaluations. This is another practice that has continued today. Sargent developed many of the exercise apparatus still being utilized today in gymnasiums across the country. Certainly early U.S. physical educators (trained physicians) influenced the utilization of physical activity and exercise as a means of promoting physical and psychological health.

World War I brought a major breakthrough in the use of therapeutic exercises and recreational activities to aid in the restoration of function.

Dr. Rudolf Klapp, in the 1920s, devised a series of creeping and crawling exercises for children with scoliosis. Phases of this technique were used until spinal bracing gained favor in the treatment of scoliosis.

World War II further advanced the use of therapeutic exercises in hospitals for restoration of muscle strength and function. Convalescent centers and long-term rehabilitation centers were established. Adapted sports and modified games for amputees, paraplegics, and those with other major disabilities became popular. One of the greatest contributions to therapeutic exercises to come out of World War II was progressive resistive exercise (PRE), a technique started by Thomas DeLorme in 1944. While stationed at a military hospital, Dr. DeLorme found that by giving increasing resistance to a muscle, it regained its strength faster.

In the 1950s isometric exercise entered into the area of therapeutic exercise as a result of the work of Hettinger and Muller[3] (1953). In isometric contraction, the muscle creates force against an immovable object. Essentially, the muscle does not change in length as in most contractions. Isometric contractions in strength training programs have been shown to be effective, however, less effective than more current types of resistance exercise programs. The utility of isometric resistance exercise is for improving strength for persons who are physically unable to move through an entire range of motion or when controlling weight is impractical or dangerous. It is convenient because no equipment is necessary.

Newer types of resistance exercise programs are being utilized today in therapeutic programs. These programs followed the work by DeLorme in the 1940s utilizing progressive resistance exercise to improve muscle size, muscle strength, and endurance. The newer techniques have been found to be beneficial particularly in rehabilitation. Isotonic exercise is defined as a strengthening exercise in which the muscle length shortens during exercise against a constant resistance. Equipment such as NK tables and Universal Gym are sophisticated versions of isotonic resistance. Variable resistance exercise is a method where the muscle moves through the entire range of motion similar to isotonic exercise, however, unlike isotonic the resistance varies through mechanical advantages so the muscle is exercised at near maximum force throughout the range of motion. Nautilus, Universal-DVR and CAM-2 are examples of equipment designed with variable resistance. Isokinetic is dynamic exercise in which the muscle is forced to move through the entire range of motion at near maximal resistance. This type of resistance is provided mechanically and the speed of movement is controlled during each repetition. Thus the person would move at maximal speed and the resistance applied is related to the speed of movement. This type of resistance has been used in the rehabilitation of stroke patients[4] and persons with selected neuromuscular disorders.[5,6] Machines such as Orthotron, Cybex and Kinetron are examples of isokinetic rehabilitation instruments.

Another concept utilized in therapeutic exercise is one of proprioceptive neuromuscular facilitation (PNF). PNF is a method used to improve range of motion, flexibility, and neuromuscular function. The theory is based upon stimulating the Golgi tendon organs and associated nerve endings. Typically the person maximally stretches the muscle prior to initiating or contracting a muscle against resistance.

Certainly the use of systematic and progressive exercise has been shown to be effective in therapeutic areas such as the prevention of cardiovascular disease and stress reduction. The physiologic and psychologic benefits of exercise are in our everyday world. Fortunately, the utilization of the same therapeutic benefits are being expressed for disabled persons. Consequently, much research is presently available in the literature as to the therapeutic benefits of exercise for disabled persons.

The utilization of sport as a rehabilitative form of therapeutic exercise has become a much accepted trend in many parts of the world. Successful participation in the sport area has resulted in numerous improvements in the health and well-being of disabled persons. This realization by the medical community has led to furthering the cause of sport for the disabled. Without question, the furthering use of exercise as a form of therapy will continue.

REFERENCES

1. Van Dalen, D.B., Mitchell, E.D., and Bennett, B.L.: *A World History of Physical Education.* New York, Prentice-Hall, Inc., 1953, pp. 25, 93.
2. Licht, S.: *Therapeutic Exercise.* Baltimore, Waverly Press, Inc., 1965, pp. 428, 431, 437–438, 454.
3. Hettinger, T. and Muller, E.: Muskelleistung and muskel training. Int Angewandte Physiol Arbeitsphysiol, *15*:111–126, 1953.
4. Glasser, L.: Effects of Isokinetic training on the rate of movement during ambulation in hemiparetic patients. Physical Therapy, *66*:673–676, 1986.
5. McCubbin, J. and Shasby, G.: The effects of isokinetic exercise on adolescents with cerebral palsy. Adapted Phys Activity Quart, *2*:56–64, 1985.
6. McCartney, N., Moroz, D., Garner, S. et al.: The effects of strength training in patients with selected neuromuscular disorders. Med Sci Sports Exercise, *20*:362–368, 1988.

BIBLIOGRAPHY

Clein, M.: The early historical roots of therapeutic exercise. JOHPER, *41*:1970.
DeLorme, T.L.: Restoration of muscle power by heavy resistance exercise. J Bone Joint Surg, *27*:645, 1945.
Fait, H.: *Special Physical Education: Adapted, Corrective, Developmental.* Philadelphia, W.B. Saunders Co., 1969.
Guthrie, D.: *A History of Medicine.* Philadelphia, J.B. Lippincott Co., 1946.
Joseph, L.: Gymnastics from the middle ages to the 18th century. Cibia Symposia, *10*:1053, 1949.
Krusen, F.H.: *Physical Medicine.* Philadelphia, W.B. Saunders Co., 1941.
Weston, A.: *The Making of American Physical Education.* New York, Appleton-Century-Crofts, 1962.

3 *History of Wheelchair Sports*

Not long ago, organized sports for the disabled, primarily wheelchair sports, were virtually nonexistent everywhere in the world. Perhaps a few better adjusted and more imaginative disabled individuals with a love for sports found themselves tossing a basketball around from their wheelchairs on some seldom used basketball court. Perhaps they might have found some pleasure in racing their wheelchairs against each other for the sheer sport of it. Many swam in private pools or pools operated occasionally for the use of the paraplegics strictly for therapeutic purposes. But before the advent of World War II, there were no known organized wheelchair sports.

Tragically, World War II brought home to most of the countries in the world disabled veterans: paraplegics, amputees, and other service-related casualties. These men, heroes to their respective countries, were looked upon in a new light. Before the war, the disabled were unfortunately regarded burdens to society if not to their own families. The war, with all of its horror, ironically enough brought to the disabled person something better than he had previously received. The disabled were now looked upon with a measure of respect (a major accomplishment) even if they were sometimes pitied members of society.

The aftermath of the war created an emergency situation for rehabilitation and vocational training centers, private and government supported, throughout the world. As part of the vast rehabilitation program, sports were suddenly seen by some as an important aid to rehabilitating the disabled veterans. Programs of wheelchair sports began at various Veterans Administration Hospitals throughout the United States. From the V.A. Hospitals in Birmingham, California; Richmond, Virginia; Staten Island, New York; Framingham, Massachusetts; Memphis, Tennessee; Chicago, Illinois; and the Bronx, New York, came a smattering of wheelchair basketball players. These veterans gradually adapted the rules and regulations of regular basketball to their own specific needs. More and more disabled men joined in the new wheelchair sport until finally several complete teams were officially organized. Thus, basketball became the first organized wheelchair sport in history.

Because of the great distances that wheelchair teams had to travel to play in competition with other wheelchair teams and because of the problems and expense involved in wheelchair travel, the wheelchair teams often competed with and beat teams composed of able-bodied players who strapped themselves into the wheelchairs for an exhilarating new kind of basketball experience. The game was as exciting as regular basketball, if not more so, and without doubt it took more stamina and skill to play.

As the interest in the sport grew, the range of disabilities of the participants also increased. Added to the list of war-injured were those disabled because of polio, amputations, and other orthopedic disabilities.

In 1946, with wheelchair basketball still in its infancy, an effort was made to boost public awareness of wheelchair athletics. The Flying Wheels team of Van Nuys, California, toured the United States, leaving unbelieving and amazed citizens in their wake. The result of this important tour of the country by the Flying Wheels was twofold. First of all, it furthered interest in and support for wheelchair sports in general. Secondly, and most importantly, it stimulated those who actually saw the wheelchair team in action to realize that if a disabled person could summon the strength, courage, and skill to play basketball from a wheelchair, there would be virtually no limits to the capabilities of this same individual, if properly trained, as an employee. This same beneficial thinking has been the backbone of wheelchair sports enthusiasm to the present day.

During 1947 and 1948, new wheelchair basketball teams appeared: the Pioneers of Kansas City, Missouri; the Whirlaways of Brooklyn, New York; The Gophers of Minneapolis, Minnesota; the Bulova Watchmakers of Woodside, New York; the Chairoteers of Queens, New York; and the New York Spokesmen of Manhattan, New York. All added to the growing popularity of the wheelchair games.

In 1949, a giant step in the growth of wheelchair basketball took place. Tim Nugent, Director of Student Rehabilitation at the University of Illinois and coach of the Illinois Gizz Kids team, organized the first wheelchair basketball tournament. Invitations to participate in the tournament were extended to all wheelchair basketball teams throughout the United States. The success of this organized tournament gave new direction to the growth of wheelchair basketball. During the planning stages of the tournament, administrative details were such that, because of the delegation of responsibility and the many people involved in the planning, an organization was formed, under the direction of Tim Nugent, which emerged as the National Wheelchair Basketball Association.

Table 3–1.   Wheelchair Sports Chronology

1945—Earliest known wheelchair basketball game in the U.S., played by war veterans at California's Corona Naval Station.

1948—First Stoke Mandeville Games for the Paralyzed, held in Aylesburg, England, with 16 British ex-servicemen competing.

1949—First Annual Wheelchair Basketball Tournament, in Galesburg, Illinois, at the University of Illinois campus. Won by the Kansas City Rolling Pioneers.

¶National Wheelchair Basketball Association formed.

1952—First international wheelchair athletic tournament, held at England's Stoke Mandeville. No U.S. athletes among 130 competitors.

1957—First National Wheelchair Games in U.S., at Adelphi College, New York, with 63 competitors.

¶National Wheelchair Athletic Association formed, organized by Ben Lipton, of the Bulova School of Watchmaking.

1960—First International Games for Disabled (Paralympics) held in Rome, with 21 countries represented.

1967—First Pan American Games for spinal injured athletes.

¶National Handicapped Sports and Recreation Association formed.

1974—First women's National Wheelchair Basketball Tournament held in U.S.

¶First National Wheelchair Marathon, in Ohio, won by Bob Hall, 2:54.5.

1975—Bob Hall, a post-polio paraplegic of Belmont, Massachusetts, first athlete to enter the Boston Marathon in a wheelchair, finished in 2:58, 790th in a field of 2392.

1978—George Murray is the first person in a wheelchair to beat the nondisabled winner in the Boston Marathon.

1979—U.S. Olympic committee sets up Handicapped in Sports Committee.

1980—Olympics for Disabled held in Holland with 2000 athletes participating.

1981—First National Veterans Wheelchair Games, McGuire VA Medical Center, Richmond, Virginia.

1983—Seven wheelchair racers finish the Boston Marathon in under two hours. (Curt Brinkman of Utah was first sub-two hour marathoner in 1980.)

1984—Two wheelchair races added to Los Angeles Olympic Games, the women's 800 meters (won by Sharon Hedrick of the U.S.) and the men's 1500 (won by Paul Van Winkle of Belgium, with Randy Snow of the U.S. second).

¶George Murray is first wheelchair athlete on the Wheaties box (Doug Heir gets on the box in 1986).

1985—George Murray breaks the four-minute mile in a wheelchair (3:59.4), at the 29th National Wheelchair Games, Edinboro, Pennsylvania. Jim Knaub is less than two seconds behind; Marty Ball, 48, competing in his 25th National Games, clocks a 4:09.3.

1987—Candace Cable-Brookes wins the Boston Marathon for a record fifth time; Andre Viger was Boston's first three time men's winner; John Brewer wins quad division for seventh time. Candace and Andre among six wheelchairs involved in crash at start of race.

¶Rick Hansen finishes 24,901-mile round the globe Man In Motion tour, raising $10 million for spinal research and treatment programs.

1988—The U.S. overwhelmed its closest rival, West Germany, by 268 to 189 medals in 8th Paralympics in Korea. Great Britain came in third with 179.

Courtesy of Spinal Network, PO Box 4162, Boulder, CO, 80306

In 1948, on the front lawn of the National Spinal Injuries Centre of the Stoke Mandeville Hospital in Aylsburg, England, Ludwig Guttmann introduced Europe's first organized wheelchair sports program. In what Dr. Guttmann termed the Stoke Mandeville Games, 26 paralyzed British patients, injured in World War II, participated in archery in an unhurried way. The Stoke Mandeville Games were originally founded for both complete and incomplete paraplegics.

Dr. Guttmann expanded the range of wheelchair sports. He was instrumental in adding such wheelchair events as lawn bowling, table tennis, shot put, javelin throwing, and the club throw. Basketball replaced net ball, and, by 1960, he had added fencing, snooker, and swimming. After 1960, weight lifting was introduced.

The Stoke Mandeville Games were successful. As in the past, the psychologic benefit of developing self-confidence in the disabled participant became increasingly apparent.

In 1952, the first international games were held at Stoke Mandeville. The Netherlands accepted an invitation to meet in direct competition with the British team. From 1952 on, wheelchair sports could do nothing but mushroom.

In the early 1950s, Dr. Guttmann traveled to the United States. While in the States, he met with Benjamin H. Lipton, Director of the Joseph Bulova School of Watchmaking, a tuition-free school for the disabled. Ben Lipton, in addition to coaching the Bulova Watchmakers' team, was then responsible for spearheading the growth of sports for the disabled in the United States. Dr. Guttmann and Mr. Lipton discussed the future growth of wheelchair sports and the possibility of a United States team traveling to England to participate in the Stoke Mandeville Games.

South America entered the sports arena in the late 1950s. After the crippling polio epidemic which hit South America in 1957, Miss Monica Jones, a physiotherapist, aroused the interest of polio victims to enter the Stoke Mandeville Games in the basketball competition.

In 1956, recognition was given to Dr. Guttmann's work by the International Olympic Committee. The Olympic Committee awarded those persons directly associated with the International Wheelchair Games the Fearnley Cup, lauding the social and human value derived from the wheelchair sports.

Each year saw the addition of teams from more countries to the Stoke Mandeville Games.

In the United States, preparatory plans for entering the International Games were under way. In 1957, Ben Lipton pioneered and launched, in cooperation with the Paralyzed Veterans Association of America and Adelphi College (now Adelphi University) of New York, the first National Wheelchair Games in the United States. The United States National Wheelchair Games, patterned after the Stoke Mandeville Games in England, introduced for the first time the 60-, 100-, and 220-yard dashes on the macadam race track, the 220- and 400-yard shuttle relays, and in subsequent years, initiated discus throwing and slalom racing.

In 1958, the National Wheelchair Games Committee organized the National Wheelchair Athletic Association (NWAA) for the prime function of establishing rules and regulations governing all wheelchair sports in the United States except basketball, which had its own national association.

As the United States National Games increased in scope in the number of disabled persons participating (Fig. 3–1), the time seemed ripe for the United States to enter international competition. A comprehensive wheelchair team was selected from the winners of the National Wheelchair Games competition, and the first United States team, under the direction of Mr. Lipton, was financed with the cooperation of interested individuals, organizations, and teams, including the participants themselves. As a direct result of these financial effects, Mr. Lipton incorporated an organization known as the United States Wheelchair Sports Fund. Along with the fund incorporators and directors, General Omar N. Bradley, Dwight D. Guilfoil, Jr., Robert L. Raclin, and Robert C. Hawkes, Mr. Lip-

ton laid out the purposes of the Wheelchair Sports Fund. The purposes, as incorporated, were:

1. To encourage disabled persons using wheelchairs to take part in sports activities, and to foster growth of organized competitive sports and recreation for handicapped in the United States.
2. To foster and advance understanding and better relations between the United States and other nations through the medium of international wheelchair sports and recreation activities and programs.
3. To solicit and collect funds for these purposes

Not only did 1960 mark the United States' entry into international competition, but it also marked the first time the wheelchair games were held close in time to the Olympic Games. Immediately after the Olympics in Rome, the city hosted another set of international athletes—wheelchair athletes from all over the globe who were greeted by the Pope and who held their international contest, which they referred to as the Paralympics (Olympics for paraplegics).

The Paralympics are held every fourth year, frequently in the same city as, and immediately following,

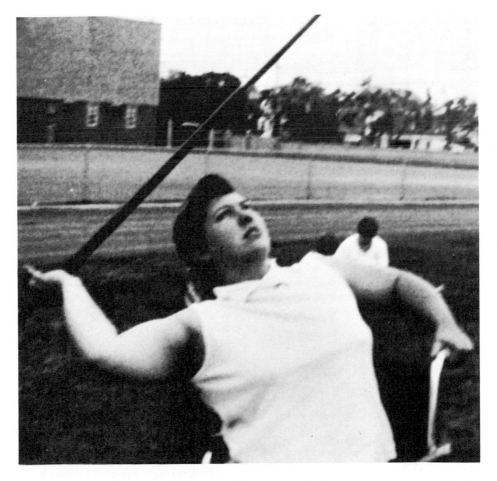

Fig. 3–1.   Rosalie Hixson, a premier field event star in the early 1960's throwing the javelin (courtesy of Louis Neishloss).

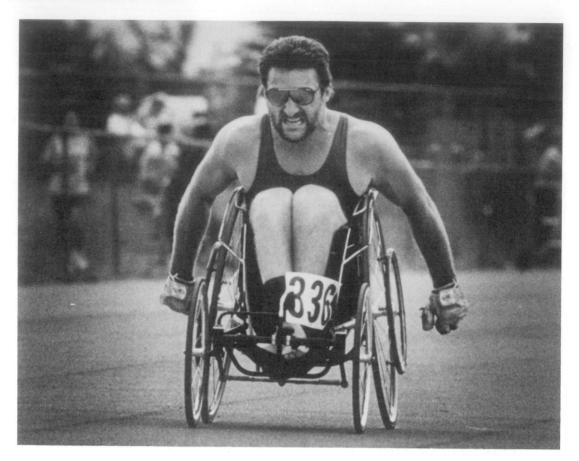

Fig. 3–2. Track event at the 7th National Veterans Wheelchair Games in Ann Arbor, Michigan—1987. Equipment excellence as seen in this road racing wheelchair has opened up new performance standards (courtesy of PVA Publications).

the Olympic games. In 1976, at the Torontolympiad, blind and amputee athletes were allowed to compete for the first time. In the 1980 Olympiad, athletes with cerebral palsy were allowed to compete for the first time.

One historic feature in the mid 1970s was the inclusion of wheelchair athlete, Bob Hall, who competed in the Boston Marathon (1975). It was at this time that the wheelchair sports movement took on a new dimension. Tied to the development of wheelchair road racing, efforts were concentrated by the athletes themselves in improving the design and construction of the racing-model wheelchair. With the necessary change in the rules approved by the NWAA, wheelchair design advanced dramatically (Fig. 3–2), producing performance results that were unthought of a decade earlier.[1] Present day growth has led to the development of "high technology" in the lightweight sports wheelchair (refer to Chapter 1).

A number of sports and recreational organizations were formed in the 1970s and 80s. Sports organizations included the United States Association for Blind Athletes (1976), National Association of Sports for Cerebral Palsy (1978), and United States Amputee Athletic Association (1981). Additional organizations

included Handicapped Scuba Association (1974), Wheelchair Motorcycle Association (1975), National Foundation of Wheelchair Tennis (1976), and National Wheelchair Softball Association (1976), to name a few. Other organizations were formed earlier and still continue to coordinate and regulate guidelines for assisting disabled persons to achieve excellence in their chosen activities. Two instrumental groups are the North American Riding for the Handicapped Association (NARHA) established in 1969, and the National Handicapped Sports (NHS), which was organized in 1967 as the National Handicapped Sports and Recreation Association. NARHA coordinates various training programs at different levels of training for instructors of disabled riders. NHS has made contributions in developing Aerobics/Physical Fitness programs, and has been instrumental in organizing regional and national ski championships.

Junior wheelchair sports are rapidly gaining attention and developing at a phenomenal pace. One new focus of attention has been the NFWT Wheelchair Sports Camp Program. Started in 1981 with a single camp in Mission Viejo, California, it has spread to numerous cities throughout the country. In each camp, children and youth receive special instruction from world-class athletes in their chosen sports interests. In addition, the youth movement is expanding rapidly through the efforts of the NWAA. The NWAA Junior Program organizes competition for youths through age 18 on the local, regional, and national level.

Media coverage is of paramount importance for the future growth of sports for the disabled. It has only been in the past few years that newspapers, radio, and television in the United States, the Orient, and Europe have accepted wheelchair sporting news on a regular basis. Public relations work and exposure at major sporting events is at a new high. It is only through publicity that the impact of the amazing and varied abilities of the disabled can be brought to the attention of the public.

The future of wheelchair sports is unlimited as more sponsors come to the forefront of the action. For example, the annual National Veterans Wheelchair Games (in its tenth year in 1990) is gaining in popularity. Sponsored by the Paralyzed Veterans of America and hosted at various locations, the games attracted approximately 500 athletes in 1989 and the number of competitors will continue to grow. International growth has been unbelievable. Even cultural exchanges are taking place to spread the meaningful exposure of the sports movement. This type of support was magnified by the Organized Sports Development (ASO) USA who organized a goodwill trip in 1987 for a northern California All-Star Wheelchair basketball team to travel to the Far East to play teams from China. Even today more than 30 years after their inception, new sports are being developed for the disabled. To illustrate, tennis was introduced to Stoke Mandeville Competition in 1987 with 10 countries fielding teams. It is important to introduce new sports into the competitive arena as it stimulates a more comprehensive outlook for the athletes and their interests. New goals are being reached as the pursuit of excellence reaches profitable results. To illustrate, at the 1988 Paralympic Games in Seoul, Korea, the United States sent 376 athletes and they amassed an incredible 268 medals (Table 3–1). At the 1989 Stoke Mandeville Games, the United States contingent of 58 athletes won 71 medals to its closest competitor, Great Britain, which won 64 medals.

Considering the gains of the wheelchair sports movement in recent years, there are still inroads to be made. Classification standards for competitive athletes need universal approval and acceptance. A greater and more complete financial structure must be realized. More people must be encouraged to give their time, if not their money. Wheelchair sports must be accepted on an equal basis with sports for the able bodied. Great strides have been accomplished in these areas over the past few years. The wheels are rolling, there is a great deal of ground to be covered, but in the final analysis, the trip can only be worthwhile.

Recently, the NWAA has undergone substantial organizational changes and is now a federation or umbrella organization which coordinates the efforts of the National Wheelchair Shooting Federation, Physically Challenged Swimmers of America, U.S. Wheelchair Table Tennis Association, U.S. Wheelchair Weightlifting Association, Wheelchair Archery Sport Section, and U.S. Wheelchair Athletics of the USA. The NWAA coordinates multi-sport competitions involving these sports on the regional, national and international level.

REFERENCES

1. Labanowich, S.: The Physically Disabled in Sports. Sports 'N Spokes, vol. 12, no. 6, 1987.
2. PVA Publications, Wheelchair Sports, Competitive and Recreation. 1989.

BIBLIOGRAPHY

1. Labanowich, S.: The Paralympic Games: A Retrospective View. Palaestra, vol. 5, no. 4, 1989.

4 *Survey of Prevalent Disorders*

Before reviewing the various types of sports, games, and exercises suitable for the physically disabled, it is necessary to define and discuss some of the common physical defects in children and adults. Knowledge of each defect and the procedures of treatment for it will contribute to an understanding of the therapeutic value of the physical activity recommended for those with the specific disability. For each physical defect there are brief discussions of the following:

- Description of disability
- Incidence
- Treatment
- Program implications
- Exercises

Various handicapping conditions will be discussed in this chapter. To clarify further the following classifications have been broken down into three distinct groups.

Individuals with physical disabilities include those with orthopedic conditions that limit functional efficiency and motor output. Included in this group are conditions such as paralysis, amputations, progressive muscle disorders, limited joint disorders, and other body-mechanic deviations. Some persons are ambulatory, and others nonambulatory. Some orthopedic impairments are temporary while others are permanent.

Persons with health impairments have chronic or acute problems that tend to lower energy levels and physical activity output. Many lack muscular strength and cardiorespiratory efficiency. Included in this group are such conditions as sickle cell anemia, chronic lung disease, and obesity.

Those with sensory impairments have unique problems associated with communication skills which frequently affect educational endeavors. This group would include the deaf, hard of hearing, and visually handicapped.

ABNORMAL POSTURE AND SPINAL DISORDERS

Rapid physical and emotional growth during adolescence makes children particularly vulnerable to certain illnesses that affect the developmental process. Some of these relate to the development of the spine and result in such deformities as idiopathic scoliosis (a lateral curvature of the spine), kyphosis (an abnormal convexity or backward curvature of the spine), and Scheuermann's disease (a degeneration of one or more of the growth or ossification centers in the vertebrae, followed by regeneration or recalcification), otherwise known as juvenile kyphosis or vertebral osteochondrosis. Unfortunately, these deformities are rarely identified in their initial stages, for despite the fact that good posture is basic to healthy growth, little attention is given to it in most physical examinations and education programs. However, in the firm belief that early detection may prevent serious medical problems later in life, more and more doctors and physical education teachers are urging local school systems to provide thorough postural evaluation for all children—particularly during the eleventh and twelfth years of age because of the accelerated growth beginning at this level.

Scoliosis

Scoliosis is a lateral curvature of the spine (Fig. 4–1). Depending on the cause, there may be just one curve or both major and minor curves. Scoliosis may be *fixed* because of muscle and/or bone deformity, or *mobile* because of unequal muscle contraction.

Terminology

It is appropriate to begin this discussion by defining some of the common terms associated with the disorder.

Major Curve. The major curve is the primary structural curve in the deformity; usually, there is a minor curve above and below the major curve.

Minor Curve. The minor curve (sometimes called a *secondary*, or *compensatory*, curve) occurs as the result of the primary curve.

Functional Scoliosis. This type of curvature of the spine is caused chiefly by faulty growth or poor posture habits. On forward flexion, the lateral curve will disappear.

Structural Scoliosis. In this type, changes in the anatomy of the vertebral body and its facets (small flat surfaces on the bone) have taken place. On forward flexion, the curve shows fixed lateral deviation and rotation.

Major Types

There are 3 major types of scoliosis (congenital, paralytic, and idiopathic); however, emphasis will be placed on adolescent idiopathic scoliosis, since it is the

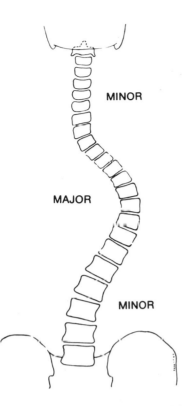

Fig. 4–1. Diagram of spine showing the major and the usual minor curves in scoliosis. (Adapted from Hoppenfeld, S.: Scoliosis. Philadelphia, J.B. Lippincott, 1967.)

most common type. Approximately 80% of all scoliosis cases seen in the average orthopedic practice are in the idiopathic group.

Idiopathic scoliosis is the most common and least understood type. The cause is unknown and may develop at any time during growth. This type of scoliosis is broken down into 3 chronologic groups:

1. Infantile: birth to the age of 3.
2. Juvenile: ages 4 to 9.
3. Adolescent: age 10 to the end of skeletal growth.

Incidence

Structural scoliosis is a relatively common deformity of the musculoskeletal system, affecting from 0.5 to 2.0% of the general population.

Screening surveys indicate that curvatures of the spine such as scoliosis and kyphosis occur in 10% of the adolescent population.[1] Adolescent idiopathic scoliosis accounts for 90% of all idiopathic scoliosis and occurs about 8 times more frequently in the female than in the male.

According to the recent Utah Study, the prevalence of college-aged women with a visible scoliosis is somewhat higher than the national norm for the younger 10- to 15-year-old group. A lateral deviation of the spine was visible in 12% of the subjects (3,210 female college students who were screened over a 3-year period). The study suggests the possibility of late development of scoliosis among teen-age girls.[2]

Treatment

An initial examination should reveal pertinent facts about causative factors. The factor of heredity should be ascertained, since it is certain that some forms of scoliosis are hereditary. In addition, it is important to note when the child first started menses if the patient is a girl, as most patients are, and also to determine if any siblings or relatives have had scoliosis in the past. It is extremely important to determine the progression of the deformity. Roentgenograms are taken for the purpose of documenting the extent, the degree, and mobility of the curves.

Some lateral curvatures resulting from functional scoliosis may be cured by exercises and appropriate correction of nutrition and rest habits. Functional scoliosis is discussed further in Chapter 5.

Treatment for structural scoliosis is directed at straightening the spine and stabilizing it in the corrected position, preventing progression of the curve. In addition to relieving pressure from the concave portion of the curve, this treatment improves cardiopulmonary function.

Side-bending roentgenograms distinguish structural from nonstructural curves by establishing the flexibility and passive correction of the vertebral deformity. A flexible curve of 5 to 10 degrees does not justify treatment other than a roentgenogram taken while the patient is standing and a careful follow-up. A curve of 15 to 20 degrees should be investigated by making supine, voluntary, side-bending roentgenograms. If the curve does not reverse itself when bent to the side of the convexity, there are structural components. Without efficient treatment, the curve will become rapidly worse during a growth spurt. In most instances, scoliosis progression slows when the patient reaches skeletal maturity.

Management of scoliosis consists of close observation with periodic assessment of progression of the curve by visual inspection and radiographic examination combined, in most cases, with an exercise program. The Milwaukee brace was widely accepted as the standard brace for spinal deformities for a number of years. More recently, however, a variety of underarm braces have been used (Fig. 4–2). The thoracolumbar Boston module is now a popular orthosis and is described further in this section. A Milwaukee brace or an orthoplast jacket is used for skeletally immature curves of 20 to 40 degrees. External bracing must be used in conjunction with a daily exercise program.

Milwaukee Brace

The Milwaukee brace consists of a molded pelvic portion of plastic, front and metal uprights, and a ring encircling the neck. A pressure pad is attached to the metal uprights which applies corrective force to the apex of the curve. The brace is frequently used when there is a curve with an apex above T7 or T8. Initially, the brace is worn 23 hours a day, 7 days a

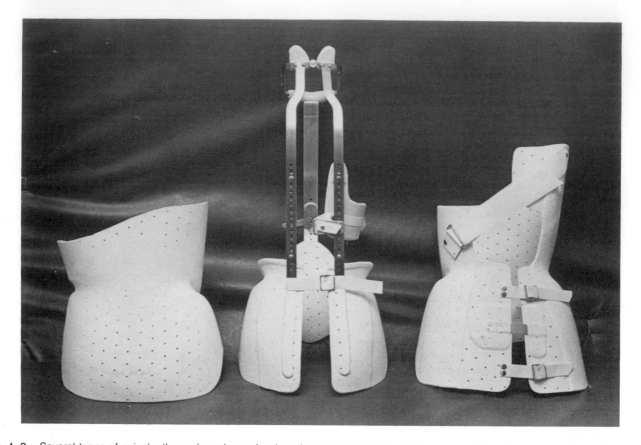

Fig. 4–2.   Several types of spinal orthoses have been developed to treat curvatures of the spine. Left to right posterior views of underarm brace for thoracolumbar curve, Milwaukee brace, TLSO (thoracolumbosacral orthosis), sometimes referred to as the "Boston Brace" for thoracic curve.

week, with time out for a daily bath and swimming. It is worn until the patient reaches skeletal maturity.

One of the most controversial questions is when and how rapidly to wean the patient from the brace. Idiopathic curves behave differently. Some stabilize early during brace treatment, long before skeletal maturity. Others do not. The most reliable evidence of skeletal maturity is the closure of the ring apophyses of the vertebrae. Stable curves of 25 degrees or less usually do not progress when weaning is started a little early. If curves increase when the brace is removed, the brace must be worn longer. The stability of correction must be demonstrated in a radiograph of the vertebrae taken at the end of a proposed period of time while the patient is standing without the brace. The patient must accept the fact that weaning from the brace depends upon the radiograph(s). If the roentgenogram shows no worsening of the major curve, the patient may remove the brace for 3 hours once or twice a week. The free time is gradually increased at the discretion of the orthopedic surgeon. However, if the patient takes more free time than is permitted, the patient and parents must be told that there will be some loss of correction. This will be evident in the roentgenogram. If the loss is significant, immediate fusion is the best solution.[4]

Orthoplast (Underarm) Jacket (TLSO Brace)

A jacket made of orthoplast has been successfully as an alternative to the Milwaukee brace in the treatment of mild scoliosis. This type of orthosis is gaining in popularity, but associated problems such as muscle atrophy and reduced vital capacity while wearing the jacket need further study.

The Boston or TLSO brace is a common orthoplast orthosis for idiopathic scoliosis (Fig. 4–3). The brace prevents relapse into deformity. Hall feels that a safe guideline for treatment with an orthoplast jacket would be a curve with an apex at T-10; for a curve with an apex at T-8 patients should be warned that if control is not good, it will be necessary to add the metal uprights. In the short-term follow-up of patients who have been out of the Boston brace for 2 years, the results are similar to those that are expected after use of the Milwaukee brace.[5] That is, 2 years after the end of brace-wearing, the curve has returned close to its original figure. This, of course, means that bracing should be restricted to curves under 40 degrees. The only exception to this seems to be the juvenile curves, which respond rather quickly to the brace and have maintained their correction. Wearing time will vary from 12 to 23 hours a day depending upon degree of spinal curvature.

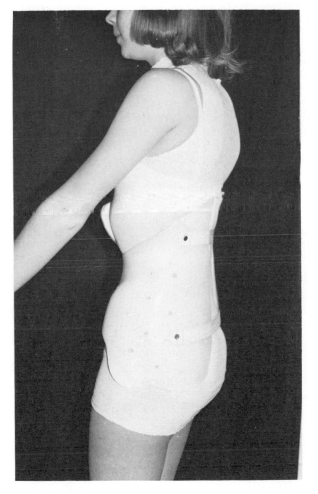

Fig. 4–3. Boston brace—a low-profile brace to correct idiopathic scoliosis. (Courtesy of John Hall, M.D.)

Low-Profile Orthoses

With the development of modern thermoplastics, low-profile braces have been widely used to improve a moderate, flexible, lumbar or low thoracolumbar curve. Basically, a low-profile brace is a passive, snugly-fitting girdle with posterior and lateral extensions. A low-profile brace with an axillary extension is used for thoracic curves whose apexes are no higher than T-8. In the low-profile brace, most of the correction results from the significant pressure of the pads.

Program Implications

Technological advances in the state of spinal orthoses have changed considerably in the last few years. This includes brace design, fabrication, and indications for wearing time. Some patients (depending upon skeletal maturity and degree of deformity) are initially treated while wearing the brace/jacket for 16 hours a day, while others are required to follow a 23-hour wearing schedule. Because of this, the program leader should consult with treatment personnel (orthopedist or physical therapist) to determine whether the patient needs to wear the brace/jacket during physical exercise. The following section focuses on the full-time (23-hour) wearer.

Graded activities on the low balance beam are especially valuable for children who have just been fitted with a brace, because such activities aid in the development of kinesthetic awareness skills and help the wearer to compensate for anatomic distortions by requiring her to perform rotating or revolving motions with her body in positions in which forces are equally distributed on either side of a base of support. This form of remedial exercise can be initiated in a hospital, rehabilitation center, or outpatient clinic during the brace fitting period and carried on for an indefinite period of time in the regular school physical education program if the child needs further training in balance and coordination skills.

Participation in physical education class is encouraged after the child returns to the regular school. However, the instructor should excuse the brace-wearing student from certain exercise and activities that require a flexible back. These activities would include tumbling and flyaway and somersaulting apparatus dismounts that involve heights. Milwaukee brace- or orthoplast jacket-wearers should *never* be allowed to act as human stabilizers in such activities as pyramid-building and dual stunts. Sports with maximal contact on impact (football, lacrosse, and wrestling) and track and field events such as pole vaulting, the running broad jump, and the high jump, should also be excluded from the brace-wearer's program.

A wide range of sports and games is permitted. Sports like volleyball, tennis (Fig. 4–4), and basketball include frequent movements and mobilize the trunk in extension. Skiing (on moderately steep slopes), ice skating, and roller skating are excellent activities for maintaining dynamic balance and correct posture. Small craft activities, horseback riding, dancing, bicycling, archery, bowling, badminton, table tennis, and a few track events such as short dashes and relays are perfectly acceptable. Gymnastic activities, including those performed on uneven parallel bars, still rings, and horizontal bars, are also recommended if the fundamental skills are developed through logical, graded sequences.

Many orthopedic surgeons will allow their patients to remove the brace/jacket for interscholastic sports competition. Others allow the brace to be removed for one-half to 1 hour to allow participation in regular physical education class. It is important to note, however, that children are always encouraged to remove the brace/jacket for 1 hour in the evening for bathing and out-of-brace exercising. Some orthopedic surgeons feel that allowing a patient too much freedom will only lead to bad habits, and as a result, patients will become negligent in maintaining a good brace-wearing program by taking the brace off for functions other than athletics and physical education.

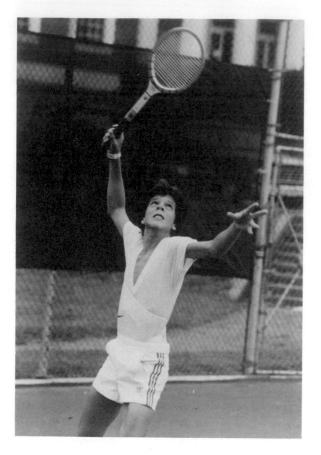

Fig. 4–4. This 15-year-old athlete wore his underarm jacket during interscholastic varsity tennis meets.

In a study by Drs. Benson, Wolf, and Shoji, it was indicated that the adolescent wearing a Milwaukee brace might actually benefit from time spent in constructive physical activity of up to 5-hours' duration while out of the brace.[6] It is possible to allow a competing athlete more time out of the brace while participating in sporting events. However, each child is different in both progress and severity of curvature, and there possibly would be reasons to preclude athletics for some individuals. It is unreasonable to believe that all brace-wearers with well-muscled bodies and supple spines can remove their braces for competitive physical activities and not adversely affect their scoliotic or kyphotic spines.

Individuals wearing orthoplast jackets will obviously have more opportunities for developing motor control, because neck mobility is not constricted as it is by Milwaukee braces. This is greatly significant because increased neck mobility enhances ocular management of objects in space which is helpful when pursuing balls in racquet sports, baseball, and volleyball. Upper trunk mobility is enhanced, which is especially important for adolescent girls who perform various tumbling stunts as in cheerleading (Fig. 4–5). Another important factor is that the jacket provides

improved cosmesis and is less objectionable in appearance than the Milwaukee brace.

Weight lifting is a controversial and potentially dangerous activity. There is evidence that weight lifting can damage vertebral end plates and growth cartilage in developing vertebra in the adolescent spine. Military presses or erect type standing presses should be discouraged. However, stress forces to the spine can be eliminated when doing bench press routines. Still, it is recommended when lifting from the supine position to use multiple repetitions with less than maximum weight (8 to 12 reps per set). Weight training under proper supervision with mechanical devices, pulleys, etc. where no free weights are used is reasonably safe with low potential for injury or stress to the immature spine.

The Milwaukee brace, or the orthoplast jacket, may be removed for swimming, an activity that is an excellent medium for strengthening key postural muscles and for improving general body mechanics.

Most physicians agree that the transient compression of the spine associated with diving is not harmful. However, diving is not an acceptable substitute for swimming. Too often adolescents dive continuously without concern for spending their out-of-brace time actually swimming. Furthermore, it is not unusual to observe adolescents performing uncoordinated acts from a diving board such as "belly flops" and "cannonballs." It is believed that the amount of force applied to the immature spine when entering the water while performing uncoordinated dives is potentially dangerous and may cause back pain syndromes.

Active participation in regular school programs is strongly recommended, for in addition to the desired achievements in her physical characteristics and abilities, the brace-wearer needs contact with her peers, diversion, and respect as an individual. The physical education teacher can do much to promote a healthy personality in his pupil by treating her as a normal student, encouraging social contacts with her peers, and providing an opportunity for emotional release through physical activity.

Particular reference should be made to the female athlete. The teenage years are a period of rapid and marked physiologic and emotional changes. It is obvious that involvement in athletics provides opportunities for psychologic and social development. In the opinion of most orthopedic surgeons, the brace or jacket should not be a barrier to sports activities and competition, and every effort should be made to assure a female athlete's participation in the sport of her choice. This opinion is based on the assumption, however, that the female athlete has sufficient strength and skills to perform her desired activity competently, and that she is well enough conditioned to withstand stresses, torques, and shocks without applying stress to the spinal column. As a rule, most parents of female athletes insist that their daughters remain activity conscious and continue to participate

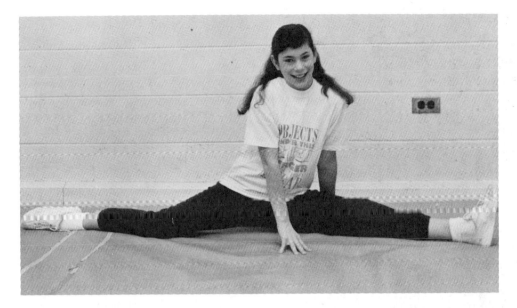

Fig. 4–5.   Most brace wearers can generally identify with normal adolescent tasks. This girl with idiopathic scoliosis is an active cheerleader and can master the required stunts while wearing and complying with the required brace wearing treatment program.

in athletics provided that safety is assured and the activity is within medical guidelines.

In terms of regulations concerning the wearing of a brace or jacket in popular female interscholastic sports, the National Federation of State High School Association rulings indicate the following: In gymnastics, there are no restrictions on the wearing of the brace or jacket provided that it does not aid the gymnast in her performance. In field hockey, there are no restrictions concerning the wearing of a brace or jacket except that the officials have discretionary powers to disqualify a player if, in their opinion, the device might harm other players.

Internal Instrumentation

One common surgical procedure is done with Harrington rods. Internal fixation is done with rods that obtain spinal correction by means of distraction and compression. The rod acts as a spacer, and the spine is fused over the segment spaced by the rod (Fig. 4–6). A postoperative immobilization cast or brace is worn until solid fusion is achieved (generally 6 to 12 months).

Another surgical procedure includes Luque rods which incorporate use of multiple wires around long rods laid along each posterior laminar surface. This type of instrumentation is used primarily for patients with neuromuscular scoliosis and for patients with complete neurologic deficits.

Program Implications

Postsurgically, the patient is usually encouraged to engage in early movement, stretching and ambulation, and in most cases an active exercise program will assist in decreasing postsurgical complications.

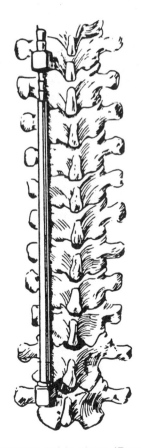

Fig. 4–6.   The Harrington rod in place. (From Physically Handicapped Children, A Medical Atlas for Teachers. Courtesy of Eugene Beck, M.D.)

During the first couple of days after surgery, the patient will demonstrate some stiffness due to the encasement of the trunk within a cast or brace. This, coupled with the added weight of the cast or brace, causes the patient to have a tendency to use the extremities as short levers (shorter stride in walking, etc.). Balance is often lost easily, however, progress is generally rapid after the patient develops sufficient antigravity strength.

During the cast or brace wearing period (which generally ranges from 4 to 12 months), patients are encouraged to participate in safe, low impact recreational games such as table tennis and badminton. Walking should be encouraged and increased in time and distance as tolerated. Stress forces to the spine should be minimized. Some patients complain of pulmonary decompensation associated with brace or cast confinement which results in shortness of breath during physical activity.

After the cast or brace is removed then a precautionary period of reduced activity is recommended. At this time, swimming, walking, and gentle stretching exercises are useful. High impact stress should be eliminated until at least 6 months postsurgery. Collision sports are obviously not recommended.

Therapeutic Exercises

Postoperative lower-extremity range of motion exercises are recommended for spinal fusion patients. Deep breathing exercises are recommended for patients in a postoperative cast or brace. They are also important for the Milwaukee-brace or orthoplast jacket patient, because they aid in correcting the thoracic lordosis and the rib hump. As the child inhales deeply and forces her back against the major pad, the torso derotates.

Appendix A
Exercises for deep breathing
Exercises 142 through 145
The properly constructed brace corrects the posture, but exercises are desirable to maintain muscle tone. A physical therapist is a great help during the first week of wearing the brace and at regular intervals thereafter.

Appendix A
Exercises for scoliosis
Exercises 147 through 155
Exercises on the balance beam are encouraged for patients who are adjusting to wearing Milwaukee braces, or orthoplast jackets. The balance beam is an excellent tool for testing precision of movement. It can teach the students the value of good posture as an expression of personality.

Appendix E
1. Stationary balance exercises
   Exercises 1 through 8
2. Movement balance exercises
   Exercises 1 through 12

Scheuermann's Disease

Scheuermann's disease (juvenile kyphosis) is an accurate and fixed kyphosis developing during puberty, its active course lasting for 2 or 3 years. It is caused by a wedge-shaped deformity of one or more vertebrae that show certain changes. Early symptoms are fatigue, vague pain in the thoracic spine radiating laterally toward both loins and subsiding with recumbency, and kyphosis of gradual development.

The cause is unknown. Ferguson reported the theory that excessive pressure on the vertebral body causes compression and gradual reduction in the caliber of the bony channels through which the vessels course.[7] Reduction in circulatory flow results in aseptic necrosis, particularly at the ends of the body that succumb to pressure.

Another theory suggests that Scheuermann's disease is a disturbance of epiphyseal growth by protrusion of the intervertebral disks through deficient cartilage plates. Defects in the cartilage end plate, due to various causes, including endrocrine, permit the bulging disks to penetrate into the soft yielding spongiosa.

Incidence

The absolute incidence of Scheuermann's disease in the general population is not known. The disease is equally common in both sexes. The age of clinical manifestation is generally between 13 and 17 years, occurring somewhat earlier in girls than in boys.

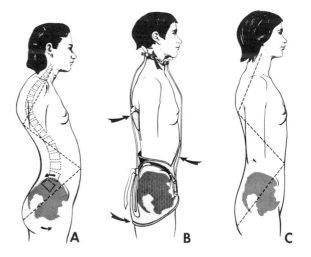

Fig. 4–7. Correction of excessive kyphosis of the thoracic spine and lordosis in the lumbar region. *A,* The pelvis is tilted in the direction of the arrows to improve the lordosis. The dorsal rounding is corrected by hyperextension exercises. *B,* The improved position is held by the Milwaukee brace, which produces holding forces at the arrows. The pelvic tilt and flat lumbar spine are maintained by the kyphos pad above, the lower edge of the girdle below, and the apron above the abdomen. The improved dorsal rounding is maintained by the abdominal apron, the kyphos pad, and the neck ring. *C,* The improvement achieved after Milwaukee brace treatment is indicated by the more obtuse angles formed by the broken line, as compared with *A.* (Courtesy of Walter Blount, M.D.)

Treatment

The most effective method of treatment is the Milwaukee brace (Fig. 4–7). With the close fit of the upright bars, the kyphosis can be effectively corrected by distraction forces and by increasing the pelvic tilt and decreasing the exaggerated lumbar lordosis. Usually the brace is worn continuously for approximately 12 months until there is radiologic evidence of healing; then the brace is used only at night for another 12 months.

Various forms of anterior jackets without upright bars are being used as corrective appliances, but these will not be discussed here.

Program Implications

The implications for scoliosis also apply to Scheuermann's disease.

Case History: A 13-year-old girl, who enjoyed athletics in school and had received the President's Physical Fitness Award, illustrates how the wearer of a Milwaukee brace can continue to participate in the physical education program. When first seen in the out patient department at the Children's Rehabilitation Center, University of Virginia Hospital, she had pain in her back and poor posture and was stooping. An examination revealed that she had some tenderness over the dorsal spine but full range of motion and only a slight amount of fixed kyphosis. Radiographs showed rather advanced Scheuermann's disease, with a narrowing of one disk space. The girl was fitted with a Milwaukee brace and started hyperextension exercises during her hospital treatment. She tolerated the brace well and continued with regular physical education activities at school, including exercises on the high balance beam (Fig. 4–8). She became a capable performer on the high balance beam and perfected a five-minute routine to music for a gymnastic exhibition.

Therapeutic Exercises

The exercises that are outlined in the section on scoliosis would be beneficial for Scheuermann's disease, also (Fig. 4–9).

Spondylolisthesis

This entity should not be confused with Scheuermann's disease. Spondylolisthesis is anterior or posterior slipping or displacement of one vertebra on another. Most frequently the fifth vertebra is displaced on the sacrum (Fig. 4–10).

Spondylolisthesis is classified according to degree of displacement of the vertebra on the vertebra below. In grade I, the displacement is 25% or less of the anteroposterior diameter of the vertebra below; grade II between 25 and 50%; grade III between 50 and 75%; in grade IV, greater than 75%.

Children and adolescents may have dysplastic or isthmic types of spondylolisthesis. The former is secondary to congenital defects in the lumbosacral joint, and the latter usually results from a fatigue factor combined with hereditary elements.[8]

Treatment

Early detection is important as seen in lateral roentgenograms. Healing may occur with proper immo-

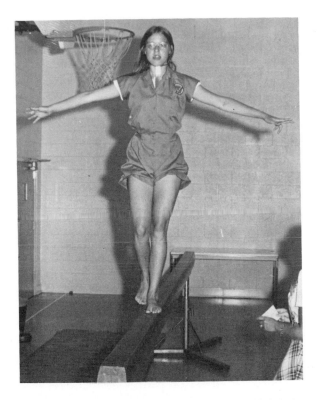

Fig. 4–8. Milwaukee brace wearer performing on high balance beam.

bilization of the low back with a Boston type brace system. Symptomatic relief is possible with abdominal strengthening and hamstring stretching exercises.[8]

Individuals with significant slips or evidence of progressive slipping, when symptomatic, usually require surgery. Most surgeons prefer fixation of the unstable spine by posterolateral and posterior fusion.

Program Implications

Most athletes with grade I spondylolisthesis are competing without pain and are unaware of their defects. As the young athletes approach grade II spondylolisthesis, or greater, they start to obtain structural

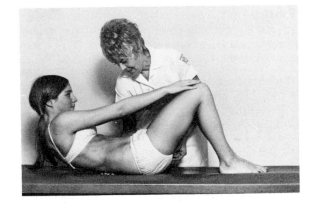

Fig. 4–9.   Sit-ups with pelvic tilt. As long as the girl wears the brace, the movements of her torso will be limited.

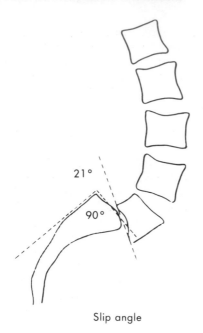

Slip angle

Fig. 4–10. Angle of slipping, formed by intersection of line drawn parallel to inferior aspect of fifth lumbar vertebral body and line drawn perpendicular to posterior aspect of body of first sacral vertebra. Fusion is recommended when slippage exceeds 25% and the child is symptomatic, or with slippage of 50% or more in the growing child regardless of symptoms. (From Boxall, R., et al. Courtesy of J Bone Joint Surg *61A*:479, 1979.)

changes with vertical sacrum, loss of extension of the hips, tight hamstrings, and are usually eliminated from the more competitive sports. There are examples of football players in the NFL, and in other vigorous sports, with grade II vertebral slippage, or greater, but these are unusual and these individuals may have chronic low back difficulties.[9]

Weight lifting is somewhat controversial, but if the patient is asymptomatic then participation is usually safe if the necessary precautions are taken. It is generally best to wear a lumbosacral support and to refrain from hyperextending the lumbar spine. Bench presses are usually safe, but standing free lifts should be avoided.

If surgery is indicated, then patients may return to sports after satisfactory bone healing. Participation in gymnastics and heavy contact sports is not usually recommended.

Therapeutic Exercises

Spinal and abdominal muscular rehabilitation is often recommended for patients with minimal problems. Refer to section on Low Back Pain for guidelines.

Several stabilization techniques are used to fixate an unstable spine, and postsurgical exercises will depend upon the type of fusion or procedure and recovery course to be followed. The therapist will be guided by a physician in determining the proper exercise regimen to be used.

Low Back Pain

Affections of the low back are common and often are brought to the attention of medical practitioners and physical education teachers. Low back pain may be caused by a number of factors such as ligamentous and muscular strains, abnormalities of the bony structure of the low back, or lesions of the lumbar intervertebral disks. In some cases low back pain is imaginary, and referral to a psychiatrist may be the treatment of choice. The major cause of low back pain, mechanical stress, is termed lumbosacral strain. Further discussion will be limited to this dysfunction, since it is the most frequently encountered condition that is associated with back pain.

Reference is made to the reason for occurrence of pain. The structures of the lower back have nerve endings that can become a source of painful stimulus. In the common low back injury, the pain may arise from damaged muscles, ligaments, or discs (jelly-like cushions between the vertebrae). Disc injuries come in many varieties, from minor damage to the outer ring of the disc (anulus) to more severe damage to the disc called a rupture. In a ruptured disc, the anulus is torn and the softer center of the disc is pushed out. A ruptured disc is also called a prolapsed or a slipped disc. Pressure on a spinal nerve by a damaged disc or other structure can cause pain that moves down the leg into the buttock, thigh, calf, or foot. This pain is known as sciatica.[10]

Treatment

The initial treatment is typically a combination of bed rest, medication (pain relievers, muscle relaxants, anti-inflammatory agents—not steroids) and heat. Occasionally, a back support may be prescribed for up to 6 weeks. If pain persists, other diagnostic tests are performed such as x rays, a myelogram (x rays with injected dye) etc. to determine other causative effects. Surgery to remove excess bone or extruded disk material and/or to fuse together two vertebrae may be required in more severe cases.[11]

Program Implications

Preventative measures should be encouraged whenever possible. For example, proper training techniques, protective equipment, and conditioning are important preventative steps for athletes. For the school-age student, postural training should be encouraged in physical education class. The best preventative medicine is to teach a unit on the principles of body mechanics in class, particularly in junior high school.

Many low-back injuries are caused by failing to use the longest and strongest muscles of the arms and legs properly. Severe strain is often placed on the antigravity muscles (erector spinae group) of the vertebrae when the body is incorrectly positioned to lift objects. One cardinal rule is to work as closely as possible to an object that is to be lifted or moved, bringing the center of gravity close to the object being moved.

Another rule is to use a wide base of support when stability of the body is required while lifting an object.

Certain athletic activities such as handball, tennis, bowling, and golf should be curtailed if an individual has persistent low back pain.

Martial arts as a healing process demands attention. Most chronic low back pain is the result of muscle tension, particularly in the area extending from the lower back to the back of the knees. The kicking and stretching as done in martial arts activates this area. It has been recognized that the Korean form, Tae Kwon Do, emphasizes the use of legs, probably more so than the other Oriental types, in self defense. This includes leg raises (done in warm-ups) and kicks of all kinds such as the front snap, roundhouse, side and back kicks and leg sweeps. This form of exercise stretches the low back and the hamstring muscles of the upper thighs, an important concentrated area to mobilize to reduce chronic stiffness and pain.[12]

Therapeutic Exercises

Finneson suggests that an understanding of the role played by the principal muscle groupings upon the lumbar spine is mandatory in planning a low back exercise program.[13] Four factors need to be considered:

1. The specific postural impairment manifested by the patient.
2. Pre-exercise evaluation of the strength and flexibility of the principal muscle groupings.
3. The special action each of the various exercises exerts upon the muscle groupings.
4. The degree of muscle strength and flexibility demanded by each exercise in accordance with the limitations imposed by the patient's present clinical status.

A physician should prescribe, in writing, the type and duration of exercises. Lifting and bending are forbidden during the rehabilitation period.

Appendix A
Exercises for lower back
  Exercises 18 through 27
Exercises for the abdominal muscles
  Exercises 32 through 42

AMPUTATIONS

An amputation may be defined as the removal of a limb or part of a limb. Amputation may be the result of an accident or it may be necessary as a lifesaving measure to arrest a disease. A small but significant number of individuals are born without a limb or limbs or with defective limbs that require amputation.

Causes of Amputation

For the purpose of this discussion, amputations will be classified into 4 categories:

Congenital. Absence of all or part of a limb at birth is not an uncommon occurrence. These anomalies may be confined to the digits or may be so involved as to produce a child with complete absence of all 4 extremities. Amputation may be indicated for those born with defective limbs, but it is not always recommended, since some individuals rely on the malformed part to help control the prosthesis.

Tumor. In some cases an amputation may be required to arrest a malignant condition. A part of a limb may be removed, but in most instances the entire limb is amputated.

Trauma. A traumatic amputation is the result of a sudden physical occurrence which may either remove the limb or cause such extensive damage that the only surgical procedure possible is to remove the damaged area. Accidents involving automobiles, farm machinery, and firearms account for many amputations.

Disease. Diseases that cause circulatory problems, such as diabetes and arteriosclerosis, may become serious enough to require amputation of a limb (usually the leg). In these cases not enough blood circulates through the limb to permit body cells to replace themselves; therefore removal of the limb, or a part of it, is indicated.

Classification of Amputations

Amputations are generally classified according to the level at which they are performed (Fig. 4–11). Amputation performed through a joint is called disarticulation. If the surface wound is not covered with skin, it is referred to as an open amputation; one that creates a residual limb suitable for an artificial limb is termed a closed amputation.

Incidence

Although the exact number of amputees in the United States is difficult to estimate, it is generally agreed that numbers fall within the 350,000 range. Lower-extremity amputations are twice as common as upper-extremity amputations.

The ratio of congenital to acquired limb losses in children varies from area to area, but clinical data indicate a congenital to acquired ratio of 2:1.

Treatment

The first important phase in the treatment program is the period after surgery and before the fitting of the prosthesis. Three of the major responsibilities are (1) care of the residual limb, which includes massage to aid in the reduction of the residual limb size; (2) bandaging to aid shrinkage and hold the dressings in place; and (3) after the residual limb heals sufficiently, exercise of the residual limb to strengthen muscles and mobilize joints.

The prosthesis is usually selected by a consulting team consisting of the orthopedic surgeon, prosthetist, therapist, psychologist, and others. The personal and occupational needs of the patient must be taken into consideration.

The patient will usually follow an intensive course of training to learn to function as well as possible with the prosthesis. The time required for training de-

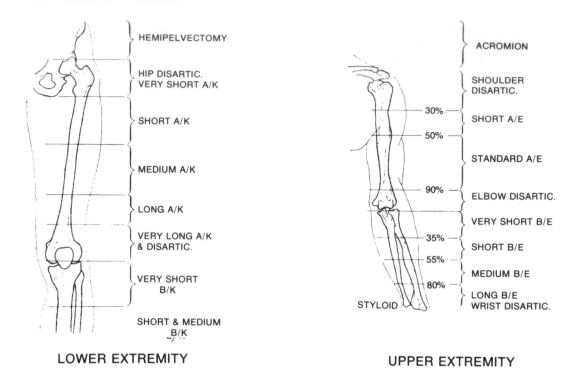

LOWER EXTREMITY   UPPER EXTREMITY

Fig. 4–11.   Classification of amputation. (From Artificial Limbs, 7:1963, National Academy of Sciences—National Research Council.)

pends upon the physical condition of the patient and the complexity of the prosthesis.

Care of the Residual Limb

Even under ideal circumstances, the residual limb, when fitted with a prosthesis, is subjected to certain conditions that may lead to physical disorders making the use of a prosthesis impossible. Lack of ventilation, as a result of encasing the residual limb in a socket with impervious walls, causes an accumulation of perspiration and other secretions. Bacteria can then lead to infection, and the solid matter, although the quantity may appear to be insignificant, can result in abrasions and the formation of cysts. For these reasons cleanliness of the residual limb is of the utmost importance, even when sockets of the newer porous plastic laminate are used.

It is equally important that any skin disorder of the residual limb receive prompt treatment because even apparently minor disorders can rapidly become disabling. Not only should the amputee see a physician for treatment, but he should also see his prosthetist; it may be that adjustment of the prosthesis will eliminate the cause of the disorder.

Upper-Extremity Devices

No artificial arm can duplicate the movements of the fingers and thumb of a normal hand. The main objective is to maintain function or substitute for lost function.

The residual limb is used as a source of energy for control of the prosthesis except in shoulder-disartic-ulation and forequarter amputations. Force and motion can be obtained by means of a cable that is connected between the prosthetic device and a harness across the chest or shoulders.

The occupational therapist will use training techniques that help the patient develop skill in activities of daily living, such as eating, grooming, and toilet care. Vocational training may also be introduced.

First, the patient is shown how the various mechanisms are controlled. He then practices these motions until they can be performed in a graceful manner and without undue exertion.

The art/science of prosthetics has been aided by modern technology (Fig. 4–12A). Such is the case with the myoelectric arm which is free of harness and cable systems. Electric arms and hands rely on biofeedback techniques which are taught by skilled prosthetists. Design operation includes activating nerve signals from the muscles in the amputee's residual limb to operate mechanical joints that move at the wrist and fingers.

Hand Substitutes—Terminal Devices

Split hooks are much more functional than any artificial hand devised to date. The arm amputee must rely heavily upon visual cues in handling objects, and the hook offers more visibility. The hook also offers more facility in grasping and can be more easily put into and withdrawn from pockets than a device in the form of a hand. Therefore, the hook is used most often for amputees who require manual dexterity.

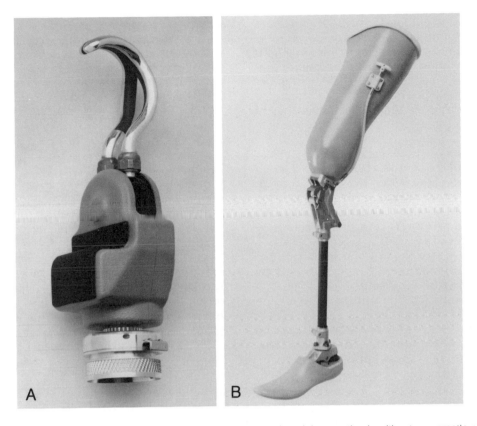

Fig. 4–12. Advanced prosthetic designs include (A) Ultra Roelite endoskeletal modular prosthesis without a cosmetic cover and (B) newest electronic terminal device, called the NU-VA Synergetic Prehensor. It is a myo-electrically controlled device which allows proportional movement (open-close) of the hook fingers. (Courtesy of Hosmer Dorrance Corp.)

Lower-Extremity Devices

One of the main objectives in training the lower-extremity amputee is to enable him to walk as gracefully as possible. A patient with Syme's operation (amputation at the ankle) needs a minimum of training, since his necessary ankle action is provided by making a heel of sponge rubber for his prosthetic foot. The average below-knee amputee will require somewhat more training, though, unless other medical problems are present, he usually will not require an extensive amount. The patellar-tendon-bearing below-knee prosthesis is suspended by a cuff or strap around the thigh, and weight is taken through the residual limb by the socket that covers the tendon below the patella. Extensive training is usually required for patients who have lost the knee joint. Patients with amputations of both legs will require more extensive prosthetic training, and most will need at least one cane to aid in walking.

A number of methods for suspending the above-knee artificial leg are available. For younger, healthier patients, the suction socket is generally chosen. In this design the socket is simply fitted tightly enough to achieve sufficient suction between the residual limb and the socket to lift the leg from the ground.

An array of advanced components can be combined which result in an advanced prosthetic system uniquely designed for each patient. In each system it is imperative to have a proper socket design. It is important for a socket to be muscle contoured as well as bone contoured with full consideration to vascular flow, so it is not impeded. Other considerations include alignment and quality of materials used in fabrication (Fig. 4–12B).

Program Implications

The task of a therapeutic recreation specialist in a clinical/hospital setting is to provide the amputee with a well-balanced program of body-awareness activities. It is important to instill confidence in the individual so that he can adjust to his limitation. A carefully planned program of sports and games that offers some early success can increase the confidence of the amputee and enhance his acceptance of the prosthesis. One important aspect to observe during the training period is how much enthusiasm the child has for learning motor skills with the aid of the prosthesis. Obviously, some children will be highly motivated; others will have serious body-image problems.

One method for developing prosthetic awareness skills is through formal training during which the patient responds to specific exercise commands of the occupational or physical therapist. The other method is through therapeutic recreation where unconscious movements are used to enhance prosthetic awareness skills. For example, a unilateral below-knee amputee can develop a feeling of security with his prosthesis by participating in games and sports that require constant change in pace, or unanticipated changes in position, as in dodge ball, badminton, and tennis.

Initial prosthetic training in a clinical environment aims to increase the length of wearing time and to promote functional habits. Another strategy especially with elementary school age children is to use travel or obstacle course routines (Fig. 4–13). For example, by challenging the lower-extremity amputee with various movement related problems requiring skilled maneuverability, the recreationist can assess functional usage or prosthesis control and coordination. Travel design can be structured to focus attention to balance, symmetry of posture and making position and postural changes. Similar prosthetic awareness concepts can be introduced to older children and adolescents incorporating ball handling games.

The amputee will need to make an adjustment to himself and others when he returns to public school. It must be assumed that some amputees may need provisions for enrollment in an adapted physical ed-

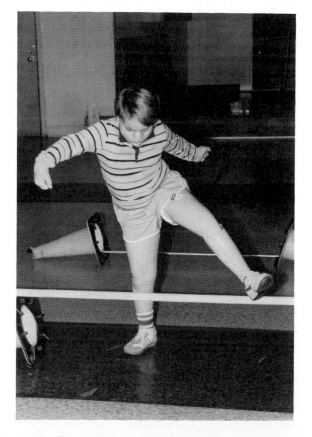

Fig. 4–13. This young amputee is employing strategies to learn efficient movement habits in a travel/obstacle course game. Movement competencies were assessed by the therapist during the recreational session.

ucation program. For example, an amputee especially with an above knee amputation may not have devoted sufficient time in a clinical setting to adjust to a new prosthesis or discover new levels of physical well-being. For this reason the student needs to go through an adjustment period that includes slow, but challenging movement experiences. The physical education teacher can help guard against needless anxieties and help the amputee to withstand the psychologic trauma of amputation by making him conscious of belonging to the group.

The physical education teacher should observe the amputee for any changes that might occur in the quality of movement as the result of some underlying problem. The teacher may need to suggest modification of an activity for the following reasons:

1. If normal walking patterns change for a lower-extremity amputee, or if there are signs of an obvious gait deviation (abducted or rolling gait, significant limp), then there is a possibility that the person has outgrown the prosthesis or that excessive wear has taken place.

2. Any unusual appearance of the residual limb (upper or lower extremity) may need immediate attention. The residual limb is subject to irritations, blisters, and cysts caused by bacteria and perspiration that accumulate when the prosthesis is worn.

3. The prosthesis (upper or lower extremity) should be in good working order. If for some reason there is a malfunction or breakdown, the student should be excused from further participation in physical activities. The prosthesis should be repaired as soon as possible to insure safety and quality of performance skills.

The unilateral amputee can participate in most areas of competitive organized athletics, and he should be encouraged to participate within the limits of his capability. Physicians should encourage the child to participate in sports, and his parents should permit such participation. Baseball is a popular sport, and many below-elbow amputees have had fitted special baseball glove attachments fitted to their prosthesis (Fig. 4–14). Some prefer to put the baseball glove over the terminal device.

In contact sports (football, soccer, ice hockey, wrestling) a hook-type prosthesis should never be worn, but in many competitive sports with little or no contact, such as baseball and golf, the active use of a prosthetic terminal device is almost essential. In other activities (tennis, badminton, and track and field events such as shotput, discus, and javelin throwing) wearing an upper-limb prosthesis may help maintain balance and timing. In sanctioned USAAA field events, a prosthesis is worn if the competitor wears one for everyday use. No crutches or other assistive devices are allowed.

The Super Sport hand (Fig. 4–15) provides a new dimension for upper-extremity amputees who are interested in participating in ball sports. The terminal

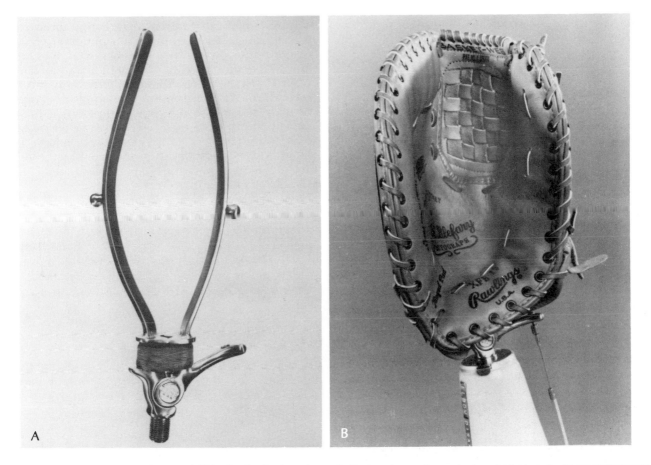

Fig. 4–14. Baseball glove attachment. *A,* This simple attachment permits the wearing and use of a baseball glove for those amputees who enjoy playing the game. Made of stainless steel, it is designed to provide gripping action in the thumb and forefingers of a baseball glove. *B,* Knobs permit the glove to be secured to the fingers of the device. The glove attaches to any Hosmer-Dorrance wrist. Hosmer-Dorrance products are available from any Certified Prosthetic Facility.

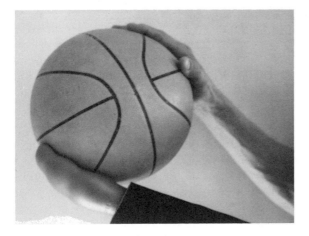

Fig. 4–15. The Super Sport hand. This sports prosthesis duplicates many biomechanical functions of the normal hand, allowing improved performance in ball handling and tumbling. (Courtesy of Therapeutic Recreation Systems, Inc., 1280 28th St., #3, Boulder CO 80303-1797.)

device is passive, not cable activated, and is helpful in ball control when used in opposition to an anatomic hand or another terminal device.

Activity designed terminal devices for prostheses and assistive devices specific to recreational and organized sports are varied and numerous for upper-extremity amputees. Still, considering the many options, some amputees prefer to use a regular prosthesis with standard terminal device, while others prefer to dispense of the prosthesis during involvement in physical activities. The decision to use specialized equipment often depends upon the level of the amputation. For example, a below-elbow amputee would be best served with a prosthetic device designed specifically for golf to enhance upper-limb mobility and control. The above-elbow amputee would find the device to be of less benefit.

The lower-extremity amputee can make similar choices of wearing a prosthesis or not, and some even prefer to use a wheelchair during organized sports. Some amputees prefer to compete with their able-bodied peers and act on their need for "normality" during recreational sports. Such is the case in (stand-

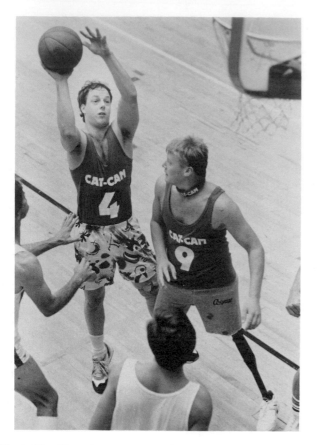

Fig. 4–16. Above-knee amputees (No.'s 4 and 9) playing "stand-up" basketball. (Courtesy of George DePontis, Creator of CAT-CAM team.)

up) basketball where the amputee wears a prosthesis with proper suspension and material covering for stump protection as opposed to hopping without a prosthesis or engaging in wheelchair basketball (Fig. 4–16).

The participation of juveniles with uncomplicated unilateral amputations in competitive interscholastic athletics is possible and desirable. The same is true for students with some types of bilateral amputation. In permitting participation, it is important to do so in ways that do not disadvantage able-bodied competitors. The following is a listing of the rules coverage regarding artificial limbs and the amputee athlete in interscholastic sports.

From 1966 through 1977, below-knee amputees were not permitted to play interscholastic football. Because of public controversy and efforts by sports-medicine specialists, and partially because of new materials used in prosthetic devices, the restriction was removed in 1978.

Artificial Limbs*

Baseball: Prosthesis may be worn. (Interpretation: the prosthesis must be properly padded and void of exposed metal or any hard material.)

*Interpretation made possible by National Federation of State High School Associations.

Basketball: Each state association may authorize the use of artificial limbs which in its opinion are no more dangerous to players than the corresponding human limb and do not place an opponent at a disadvantage.

Field Hockey: Artificial limbs which, in the judgment of the state association, are no more dangerous to players than the corresponding human limb are permitted provided they have a soft covering or are padded with at least ¼-inch closed cell, slow recovery foam rubber padding. Upper limb prostheses and above-knee leg prostheses are discouraged. Hinges shall be lateral and covered by leather.

Football: Each state association may authorize the use of artificial limbs which in its opinion are no more dangerous to players than the corresponding human limb and do not place an opponent at a disadvantage.

The following criteria are recommended as a guideline to follow in determining the legality and suitability of wearing an artificial prosthesis in a contact sport.

1. Restricted to below-the-knee prosthesis. No artificial hand, arm or above-the-knee prosthesis should be permitted.
2. Metal hinges restricted to the lateral and medial surfaces and covered with leather or padding (similar to that required on approved knee braces).
3. No metal in front of the knee unless properly padded.
4. Prosthesis should be wrapped with a minimum of ½-inch high-density polyurethane or foam rubber.
5. Approval of an orthopedic surgeon, or physician associated with a juvenile amputee clinic, is recommended.

Boys Gymnastics: Are allowed, but if it presents an advantage, there will be a 2.0 deduction in the score.

Girls Gymnastics: There is nothing in the rule book on this, as this has not been a big problem in girls' competition. However, they do follow the boys' rules when a question arises.

Ice Hockey: Artificial limbs which, in the judgment of the rules administering officials (state association office), are no more dangerous to contestants than the corresponding human limb and do not place an opponent at a disadvantage, may be permitted.

Soccer: Artificial limbs, which in the judgment of the State High School Association are no more dangerous to players than the corresponding human limb and do not place an opponent at a disadvantage, may be permitted. Upper limb prostheses and above-knee leg prostheses are discouraged. Hinges shall be lateral and covered by leather. All permissible artificial limbs shall be covered by at least ½-inch (0.0127 m) foam rubber padding.

Softball: Prosthesis may be worn. (Interpretation: the prosthesis must be properly padded and void of exposed metal or any hard material.)

Swimming and Diving: Not specifically addressed in rule book. It is assumed they would be removed and case book rulings indicate that adjustments should be made accordingly (i.e., swimmer with only one leg is given permission to start in the water).

Track and Field: No specific coverage.

Volleyball: Artificial limbs which, in the judgment of the state association are no more dangerous than corresponding human limbs, are permissible provided they are covered by at least ½-inch foam rubber padding (or ¼-inch closed cell, slow recovery foam rubber).

Wrestling: Artificial limbs, which, in the judgment of the state association office, are no more dangerous to a contestant than the corresponding human limb and do not place an opponent at a disadvantage, may be permitted. Also, if a contestant wishes to wrestle wearing an artificial limb, he must weigh in with the artificial limb.

Many amputees avoid swimming because of psychosocial prejudice. However, this is one of the better activities for increasing endurance and promoting better physical conditioning, and it should be encouraged, particularly for lower-extremity amputees. Also, swimming does not tend to traumatize the residual limb area. Plastic waterproof prostheses are available for recreational swimming. However, no prosthesis is allowed in sanctioned USAAA swimming events.

Downhill skiing remains one of the most popular sports for the leg amputee. Through skiing, the amputee can move with speed, grace and ease, and challenge the steepest slopes to be found. The use of an outrigger (short ski, a Lofstrand or similar crutch, and a hinge device which connects them) increases the base of support and provides balance for the lower-extremity amputee. It is especially useful to an above-knee amputee who uses his non-involved leg for this type of "three-tracking" method. Below-knee amputees can ski with or without a prosthesis. The bilateral below-knee amputee can "four-track" with two prostheses and two outriggers. Bilateral above-knee amputees often prefer the option of using a sit ski. Upper extremity amputees often use the Ski Hand (Hosmer-Dorrance) which fits over the ski pole and substitutes for the missing grip hand, or an AT-Ski-TD (refer to Chapter 8, section on skiing).

New advanced prosthetic systems have been developed for above-knee amputees. One example is the CAT-CAM (contoured adducted trochanteric controlled alignment method.) In the system, the ischial bone is not pounding on the flat, hard shelf. Amputees can enjoy sports and more strenuous activities due to the greater stability of the bones within the socket.

The O.K.C. or Oklahoma City running knee can be used with the CAT-CAM system. It utilizes aerospace-material cables to snap an artificial knee back in place after each running step. This provides above-knee amputees the opportunity to run step over step rather than using the hop and skip running gait. The O.K.C. system supplies a dynamic force to the shank, much as the quadriceps does in the normal human during running (Fig. 4–17A).[13a]

Commercially available prosthetic feet are now designed to conserve energy and enhance performance skills in recreational and sport activities. One example is the Flex-Foot which utilizes graphite fiber composite technology to store energy (Fig. 4–17B). The Flex-Foot uses the entire distance from the tip of the toes to the end of the residual limb for function. Another special prosthesis is the S.A.F.E. (stationary attachment flexible endoskeletal) foot which is designed to simulate the natural shape and action of the human foot. It is especially popular with golfers since the foot will stay flat on the ground during the tee off motion. Another alternative is the Seattle Foot. It is made of thermoplastic material and cosmetically mirrors a normal foot. Two components are featured—a spring assembly which stores energy and foam through which the natural push-off motion for running is simulated.[14]

It is possible for many bilateral amputees to participate in recreational sports and achieve the same success as their normal peers. Scuba diving, spin and bait casting, riflery, and archery are activities needing little modification.

Therapeutic Exercises

Therapeutic exercises are utilized to strengthen and stretch specific muscles or groups of muscles; to maintain or increase the range of motion of the joints above the amputation, and generally to prepare the individual to use the prosthesis.

Upper-Extremity Amputations

A. Above the elbow

The opposite shoulder girdle must be exercised and strengthened to prepare the individual to use his prosthesis.

Appendix A
1. Exercises for the upper back
   The stump will be used as an entire extremity.
   Exercises 1 through 8, 12, 14 through 17
2. Exercises for the shoulder
   The stump will be used as an entire extremity.
   Exercises 125, 126, 127, 129, 130, 132, 138
3. Exercises for the head and neck
   Exercises 139, 140, 141

B. Below the elbow

Appendix A
1. All exercises listed above in section A, *Above the Elbow*
2. Exercises for the elbow
   The stump will be used as an entire extremity.
   Exercises 118, 119, 120, 123

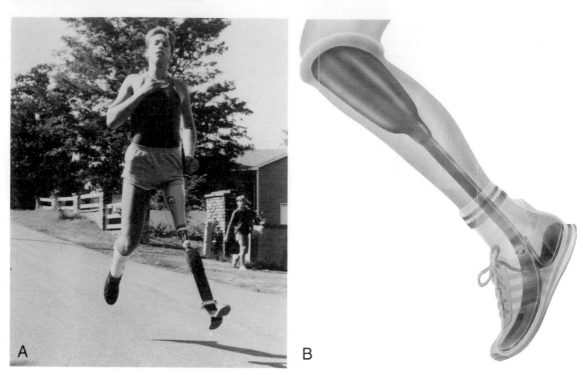

Fig. 4–17. *A,* Runner equipped with a sports belt, a flexible socket, an Oklahoma City running knee with an internal sports cable, and a carbon fiber Flex Foot. (Courtesy of Sabolich Prosthetic and Research Center, 1017 N.W. 10th St., Oklahoma City, OK 73106.) *B,* Showing full length carbon fiber strut for energy storage and release. (Courtesy of Flex Foot.)

Lower-Extremity Amputations

A. Above the knee

The entire uninvolved lower extremity must be exercised. See Exercises for the hip, knee, ankle and foot in Appendix A (Exercises 43 through 95). In addition, the following exercises, with the residual limb used as an entire extremity, are beneficial:

Appendix A
1. Exercises for the lower back
   Exercises 18 through 22, 25 through 31
2. Exercises for abdominal muscles
   Exercises 32 through 42
3. Exercises for the hip
   Exercises 43 through 57

B. Below the knee

The residual limb will be used as an entire extremity
1. All exercises listed above in section A, *Above the Knee*
2. Exercises for the knee
   Exercises 64 through 69, 71, 72

General Exercises

Weight-training activities are encouraged for lower-extremity amputees; however, adaptation in lifting techniques is usually required. Isometric, isotonic, and active resistance exercises can be used depending upon each individual case. Several terminal devices are available to assist the upper-extremity amputee in manipulating dumbbells and barbells. A certified prosthetist can assist in this area. Readers are encouraged to read the article by Radocy[15] for further information on the subject.

Competitive Sports

The United States Amputee Athletic Association (USAAA)

The USAAA is the governing body of amputee sports in the United States. In addition to sanctioning amputee competitions, the USAAA holds an annual Open National Amputee Championships featuring a wide variety of sports. Individual sports include weightlifting, swimming, table tennis, track and field, air pistol, air rifle, and archery. Team sports include volleyball, track and swimming relays, standing and wheelchair basketball. The USAAA amputees compete while wearing their prosthesis except for the A1 and A9 classifications.

Classification System

There are four upper extremity and four lower extremity classifications.

Double AK—A1	Single—A2
Double BK—A3	Single—A4
Double AE—A5	Single—A6

Double BE—A7   Single—A8
Combined lower and upper amputations—A9

Amputee-based classifications modified by the International Sports for the Disabled for winter sports is different, but due to space limitations will not be discussed. Readers are encouraged to read other sources for information on the subject. Sports include alpine and nordic skiing, biathlon, sledge downhill, sledge racing, and sledge hockey.

Many lower extremity amputees engage in wheelchair sports sponsored by the National Wheelchair Athletic Association (refer to section on spinal cord injuries for details). Even though an amputee may not be totally confined to a wheelchair, he can compete due to a permanent physical disability of the lower limb. Bilateral above the knee amputees find wheelchair events to be popular as they fulfill their needs to have a solid base of support for their trunk musculature.

AUDITORY IMPAIRMENTS

Hearing loss may be classified in terms of the site of the lesion as either conductive, sensorineural, or central. Conductive hearing loss is caused by lesions in or obstructions of the external ear or the middle ear where sound is reduced before it reaches the inner ear. An example of this type of hearing loss is otitis media. Sensorineural hearing loss is caused by lesions of the structures that receive and transmit the sound stimuli. This type of impairment is often irreversible. Central hearing loss means the individual can hear, but cannot understand what he hears. For example, a result of this type of impairment can often be traced to a CVA (stroke) patient. With a central auditory processing problem, a person has normal hearing sensitivity, but is unable to cope with filtered information such as in a noisy environment.

Causes of deafness are often associated with multiple handicaps. Implications of additional handicaps pose a more complicated picture especially in terms of social and emotional adjustment issues, and educational programming. Discussion will not focus on this population group.

Types of Impairment
Persons with hearing impairments fall into two distinct classes based upon the time at which hearing was lost.

Congenital Impairment. The most frequent condition is congenital impairment. The term implies that the individual was born with a hearing deficit. Contagious diseases, such as rubella, mumps, and influenza in the pregnant mother are causes of deafness in infants.

Acquired Loss or Sudden Deafness. A number of causes are accepted by most investigators as possible reasons for this type of hearing loss. Included are hereditary disorders and certain childhood diseases, such as meningitis, encephalitis, measles, mumps, and influenza. Other relatively rare causes may include head trauma, brain tumors, vascular disorders, etc.

Some etiologic factors go unrecognized and the cause is unknown. However, a certain percentage of these may be hereditary deafness as a result of an inability to historically trace hereditary patterns.

Early diagnosis is essential. An audiologic examination can provide evidence of a hearing loss and information regarding the severity of the problem (determined in terms of hearing threshold levels) and site of the lesion. Levels of hearing impairment can be identified as mild, moderate, severe, or profound. After identifying the problem it is important to determine the means of communication (sign language, speech reading, total communication, etc.) to be used.

Incidence
Today, in the United States, it is estimated that approximately 15 million adults and 3 million children have some degree of hearing loss. In the United States and other parts of the world for which statistics are available, between 5 to 7% of school-age children have some degree of hearing loss. About 50% of all cases of deafness are due to genetic causes.

Treatment
Some of the specialties involved in the diagnosis and treatment of auditory disorders in children are otolaryngology, pediatrics, neurology, speech pathology, child psychiatry, and audiology. Recommendations to the parents for treatment procedures and special training programs will usually be made by specialists in one or more of these fields.

Children with a mild hearing impairment usually do not wear a hearing aid and are engaged in integrated programs. Hearing aids are prescribed on an individual basis, but most frequently are used by those who have a moderate hearing loss. Those with moderate to severe hearing loss need to be served in the least restrictive environment; however, this is not always a public school classroom. Children with profound hearing losses are frequently best served in residential schools where they are taught manual communication based on the American Sign Language system. Various placement alternatives are often possible; however, there is a trend to use public school education (such as done in self contained classrooms) with special education teachers.

Program Implications
To clarify again, the terms deaf and hard of hearing are used conclusively to distinguish each group when discussing program implications. It is not unusual for the deaf population to experience widely different needs for adapting their environment in comparison to an individual with a mild hearing loss who can usually be integrated with regular peers in physical activity programs. To add further, the deaf person must be more acutely aware of using vision for communication.

Persons with auditory impairments can participate in all athletic games that are played by hearing individuals. Many special schools for the deaf offer competitive team sports, such as wrestling, swimming, basketball, and football. Various other sports like tennis, badminton, bowling, and volleyball require little or no modification for the deaf.

Many children with auditory impairments like to explore their immediate environment, and they often engage in compulsive movement to satisfy their curiosity. The motor characteristics of each child vary considerably, ranging from severe incoordination and balance problems to rigidity and random movements. Winnick suggests: It seems fair to conclude on the basis of completed research that the deaf, as a group, are inferior to the hearing on static and dynamic balance and motor speed. However, there appears to be little or no difference between hearing and deaf children in motor maturation as reflected by sitting and walking ages and other indicators of motor proficiency. Differences between the deaf and hearing are probably the result of malfunctioning of the semicircular canals.[16]

Many children with hearing impairments will be enrolled in regular school physical education classes. The teachers must be sure that directions and explanations are clearly understood by the hard-of-hearing student. Otherwise, he cannot realistically be expected to function as a participant in a concentrated program of sports and games. When speaking to a child with a hearing aid or to a child who depends partly on lipreading, the teacher should face the child at close range. It is important to speak slowly and distinctly without exaggeration of facial movements or tone. The student will often rely on normal hand gestures for cues. Use of written cues is also helpful in improving communication. The physical educator should remember that the hearing aid is an amplifier. If a teacher is having difficulty communicating with a student, then the problem might be solved by moving closer, thereby improving the channels of communication. Butterworth suggests, if there are several deaf children in class, the teacher may elect to use one of the formations[17] (Fig. 4–18).

It is important to remember that children with impaired hearing learn by seeing. In group relays or squad formations, it is best to have the hard-of-hearing individual near the front of the line so he can lipread well. Games in a circle formation are recommended, because this allows the child to see what his classmates are doing.

Basic movement skills are introduced to children in elementary physical education classes. These offer each child a way of expressing, exploring, and interpreting himself and of developing his capabilities. Every physical educator should be concerned about the relation of the hearing-impaired child and his movements to the physical environment (gymnasium, playground, or other area) in which he moves. Specialized skills that should be developed include rhythmic activities, stunts, tumbling, and fitness. Other skills can be identified as apparatus types and include climbing ropes, horizontal ladders, and activities on jumping boxes and bounding boards. One safety rule that should be stressed is the removal of a hearing aid during vigorous physical activity. This provides a safer environment for appropriate movement; however, the teacher must remember that he is removing the child's only warning system. In such cases, it is best to organize a buddy system for the child. The hearing-impaired child can depend upon a buddy to relay commands or demonstrate a skill. Working with partners in this way is often successful and offers the hearing-impaired child a better opportunity to move with competence and manage himself and his pieces of apparatus without interfering with other children.

Some team games such as lacrosse, soccer, basketball, and football are played over a wide area. Some problems may occur for the hearing-impaired players of such games because he will not hear warnings or a whistle. Also, these sports require a change of direction so that the player will not always be facing the referee to perceive cues to stop play. It is suggested that the closest teammate act as a middleman to inform the hearing-impaired player of the referee's decision. Generally, it is best to instruct the player and his teammates about a system of special signals that will be used during the athletic contest. This way all team members can focus their attention on a few visual cues instead of spending time on the court or field trying to explain decisions. Also, this method will

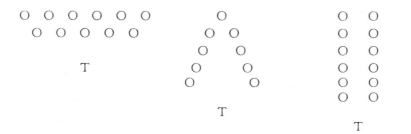

Fig. 4–18. Class formations which provide a direct view of the teacher's face. (Reproduced from Palaestra 4 (3), 30 with permission of Challenge Publications, Ltd.)

keep the contest moving at a desirable rate of speed without a needless delay in the action.

Good sportsmanship is a vital link to the development of social skills, and the instructor must eliminate the so-called barriers of confusion. Lengthy explanations and constant changes in rules and regulations must be avoided. Students with impaired hearing may show impulsive behavior, and lack of cooperation may be due to their inability to comprehend directions and rules.

In terms of adapting rules in competitive sports, it has been reported that deaf and hard-of-hearing runners and swimmers can gain equality in starts by increasing the caliber of starting pistols and putting the gun in down rather than the traditional up position. The National Federation of State High School Associations makes exceptions to this statement:

The *down* position for the gun in track events is acceptable in some cases, but it is not acceptable when the starter's position is some distance from the finish line (timers position). The timer must immediately detect the smoke from the starter's pistol and therefore, the gun is fired in a "raised position" to get an accurate timing.

Other adaptations are used for swimming than using a larger caliber pistol which would be disrupting in a pool area. These include:

1. Starter explains to the swimmer ahead of time that when he says, "Swimmers, take your mark," he will raise the arm without the starting device. He will lower the arm as the starting device is discharged. (The deaf swimmer is often moved closer to the starter.)
2. A timer on the lane with a deaf starter raises his arm, lowers it on the starting signal.
3. A timer on the lane taps the deaf swimmer's foot on the starting signal.

Guidelines for the Student with a Hearing Aid
There are different types of hearing aids; body hearing aids where the controls are kept in a shirt or blouse pocket, and behind the ear (BTE) which are more cosmetically appropriate are two examples. Wearing of stretch bands is useful in keeping BTE hearing aids in position during active physical exercise. Also, hearing aids molded to fit the inside of the ear are becoming popular.

A hearing aid is part of the real world of sound to a hearing-impaired child. It is not only the moral but also the legal responsibility of the physical education teacher to exercise all precautions necessary to avoid accidents and injury to the hearing-impaired player, and to provide for the welfare of all students involved. Certain guidelines should be followed for 2 specific reasons: to allow the hearing-impaired child to achieve maximum benefit from his hearing aid and to eliminate needless breakdowns of the instrument.

1. A harness should be worn, allowing the hearing aid to be positioned conveniently and securely.

2. The physical education teacher should always keep a spare battery in case a replacement is needed. It is always best to contact the parents and request their support for this type of service in case of an emergency.
3. The student should remove the hearing aid during vigorous play periods. It should be locked in a desk or locker after it is taken off. When outdoors, it is important not to place the hearing aid in the grass or expose it to temperature and humidity changes. Excessive moisture will cause the battery to corrode.

It is important to point out that the ultimate responsibility for the hearing aid belongs to the parents. The student will have general knowledge about the care and management of the hearing aid. However, in no circumstances should a physical education teacher try to repair a defective instrument.

Precautions
The most evident motor problem of children with peripheral deafness is disturbance of balance due to reduced functioning of the semicircular canals. The instructor should limit climbing and apparatus work for safety reasons if the child with peripheral deafness has balance difficulties, although there need be no limitations if the child has no such difficulty.

Some persons with a history of ear, nose, and throat problems should avoid exposure to low temperatures and excessive wind and water. If exposure is required, it is recommended that they wear proper clothing or ear plugs to protect their ears.

Note: It is never safe to assume that the use of a hearing aid will provide a person with hearing acuity within the normal range.

Therapeutic Exercises
No specific therapeutic exercises are needed unless otherwise indicated by a physician.

General Exercises
1. General exercises and weight training are beneficial to the individual with auditory impairment.
Appendices B and C
2. Balance beam exercises for general balance, coordination, and change of direction may also be indicated. They are useful for children with auditory handicaps, because the kinesthetic awareness skills that are developed aid in body control for those children who have difficulty maintaining balance due to a damaged semicircular canal.

Appendix E
1. Static balance exercises
Exercises 1 through 8
2. Dynamic balance exercises
Exercises 9 through 12

Competitive Sports

American Athletic Association of the Deaf (AAAD)
The AAAD is affiliated with the United States Olympic Committee and sanctions state, regional, and

national sports. It also promotes the participation of United States athletes in the World Games for the Deaf and other international competitions in various events.

Summer game events include track and field, basketball, cycling, football (soccer), gymnastics, team handball, wrestling, swimming, table tennis, tennis, shooting, and volleyball. Winter games include downhill and slalom skiing, combined alpine events, long distance races and relays.

The Social Elements of Competition

Deaf athletes must become as skillful at their special forms of communication and orientation as they are at performing a sport itself. In most cases, communication among deaf athletes is done by signing (Fig. 4–19). A small minority will use speech as their means of communication. Whether it is desirable for the deaf to compete in sports against hearing teams is a matter of debate. Always a concern is how the deaf athlete can receive communication from game officials, and in some cases, hearing opponents as well. Generally speaking, there is some deprivation of the social aspects of competition. On the other hand, competition with hearing teams is often desired to increase the level of competition and to test the quality of deaf athletes under such conditions.

Stewart reports, for the deaf athlete, competition amongst hearing people also implies competing against social stigmatization and dealing with a limited range of communication opportunities. Ultimately, a deaf person must decide if the rewards of competition with hearing people outweigh the costs of social iso-lation. For many, the rewards are insufficient and sport for the deaf provides a desirable alternative to their dilemma.[18]

OTITIS MEDIA

Otitis media means infection of the middle ear. By definition, otitis media implies fluid and exudate in the middle ear, a cavity that usually contains air. It is primarily a disease of childhood. One reason children are more susceptible is that the eustachian tube is shorter and wider in children than in adults.

The causative organisms in most instances gain access to the middle ear from the nasopharynx through the eustachian tube. Obstruction of the eustachian tube impedes drainage and traps secretions and bacteria in the middle ear. The offending agents that appear most commonly are the pneumococci, Hemophilus influenzae, or the hemolytic streptococci.

The usual history of otitis media in the younger child is that of a cold for several days complicated by a fever, commonly up to 104°F. Earache is the most frequent complaint, but it is not always present in children over 3 years of age. Other symptoms of respiratory tract infection such as sneezing, cough, and sore throat are frequently present with acute otitis media. Every child who has significant fever or ear pain during or after a cold should be seen by a physician, because visual examination of the eardrum is the only satisfactory way to diagnose otitis media or any other bacterial complication. It is of extreme importance to obtain visualization of the eardrum and to know what is and what is not normal.

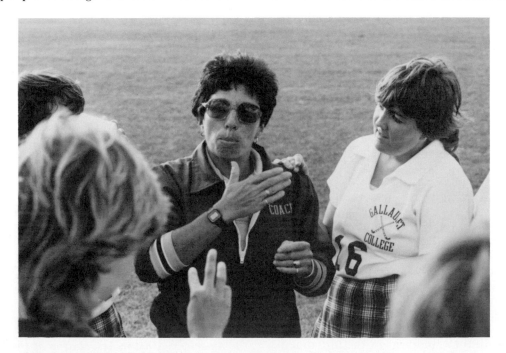

Fig. 4–19. Gallaudet field hockey coach talks strategy via sign language method of communication. (Courtesy of Gallaudet College, Washington, D.C.)

Serous otitis media is a condition that is noninfectious, but there is a collection of fluid behind the eardrum. It is referred to as a "silent" problem because the child is generally asymptomatic except for a hearing loss.

Incidence

Otitis media represents one of the most frequent illnesses of childhood. There are indications that 10% of all children under 15 years of age experience an attack of acute otitis media annually and that upwards of 15% of children under 10 years of age experience an attack each year.[19]

Treatment

The selection of antibiotics for the treatment of otitis media depends on the offending agents. Ampicillin appears to be the oral antibiotic agent that is most often used to eradicate the principal organism. Oral antibiotics are generally taken over a 10-day period. Penicillin is also used, particularly with older children, because pneumococci or group A streptococci may be presumed to be responsible. Follow-up examinations should be performed to determine whether the eardrum is normal. In serious cases, repeated reassessment by audiometry is highly desirable.

As a general rule, if a chronic problem continues after 6 months of antibiotic therapy, and if a moderate hearing loss persists, then pressure equalizing (PE) tubes are inserted into the tympanic membrane to allow for drainage of fluid behind the eardrum. Children may be required to wear the PE tubes for a period of 4 weeks to a couple of years, but generally not beyond the age of 8.

Myringotomy (clean elliptical incision of the tympanic membrane) may be performed to relieve pressure. These forms of treatment are used only in severe cases of otitis media and are not indicated as routine procedures.

Program Implications

In most cases the child will be treated in a physician's office and allowed to return to regular school activities in a short period of time. The large majority of children with otitis media will be in kindergarten through second grade. Parents sometimes tend to be overly cautious and fear that vigorous physical activity and outdoor play in cold weather will aggravate the middle ear infection. Some physical education teachers are reluctant to allow the student to participate in activities that require a variety of movements and rapid changes in position such as apparatus activities and tumbling for fear of aggravating the condition. However, these are misconceptions: most physicians agree that there is no need to restrict physical activities during the period of time a child is on antibiotic treatment once the child is free of symptoms and his temperature has returned to normal.

Some diminution of hearing occurs in all cases but may not be noticed or complained of by the student.

Olmstead reported that significant hearing loss persists for some weeks or months after otitis media.[20] The physical education teacher needs to be sensitive to this problem, and, if a significant hearing loss is evident, preferential positioning in squads or formations may be necessary so the student can hear auditory commands.

Swimming merits special discussion. Hoekelman states:

The advice so often given that children with recurrent or chronic middle ear infection refrain from swimming is based on the theory that pressure changes that occur in the nasopharynx secondary to immersion in deep water may cause displacement of air and bacteria from the nasopharynx through the eustachian tube into the middle ear. This is probably a valid assumption. However, children who refrain from diving (head first or feet first) and confine their swimming to the surface of the water or just below it should not be at risk from pressure changes.

If a perforation in the ear drum is present, swimming should not be allowed, since water and bacteria will easily enter the middle ear through the ear canal. Ear plugs with or without a bathing cap will not prevent this with sufficient regularity to warrant their use. If one can guarantee that the child will not immerse his or her head while 'swimming' in shallow water, this can be permitted. Ear plugs may be helpful for the child who complains of 'water in the ear' during or after swimming, but do not affect the pressure changes in the nasopharynx and middle ear mentioned above.[20a]

Swimmers using PE tubes should wear swim plugs or molds to prevent moisture from entering the ear canal, and should not submerge their head under the water.

OTITIS EXTERNA (SWIMMERS EAR)

This condition is the inflammation or infection of the external canal or the auricle of the external ear. It is often associated with swimming when water remains in the external ear canal. Symptoms vary from mild pain to a low grade fever with discharge, and partial hearing loss. A physician should be consulted, and frequently treatment consists of antibiotic eardrops in combination with cleansing of the ear.

Physical activity guidelines are similar to that already described under Otitis Media. Again, it should be reiterated, if permission to swim is allowed, total reliance on premolded earplugs is not always achieved because they are not watertight seals.

Therapeutic Exercises

No specific therapeutic exercises are needed unless otherwise indicated by a physician.

CARDIOVASCULAR DISORDERS

The heart (Fig. 4–20) and the network of blood vessels through which the heart services every cell in the human body, bringing oxygen and nutrients and

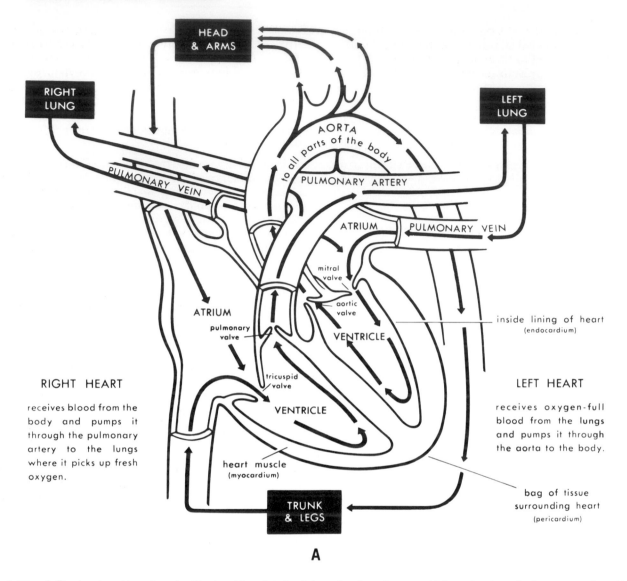

HEAD & ARMS

RIGHT LUNG

LEFT LUNG

AORTA
to all parts of the body

PULMONARY ARTERY

PULMONARY VEIN

ATRIUM

PULMONARY VEIN

mitral valve

aortic valve

inside lining of heart
(endocardium)

ATRIUM

pulmonary valve

VENTRICLE

RIGHT HEART

receives blood from the
body and pumps it
through the pulmonary
artery to the lungs
where it picks up fresh
oxygen.

tricuspid valve

VENTRICLE

LEFT HEART

receives oxygen-full
blood from the lungs
and pumps it through
the aorta to the body.

heart muscle
(myocardium)

bag of tissue
surrounding heart
(pericardium)

TRUNK & LEGS

A

Fig. 4–20. *A,* The heart and how it works. The heart is a fist-sized, four-chambered pump which contracts and relaxes more than 100,000 times a day, during which time it pumps about 4,300 gallons of blood through 60,000 miles of arteries and capillaries. (Courtesy of the American Heart Association.)

removing wastes, are both vulnerable to a broad complex of diseases and disorders called cardiovascular diseases. Cardiovascular diseases accounted for 991,300 deaths in 1985 (47.6% of all deaths). More than one in four Americans suffer some form of cardiovascular disease.[21]

There are more than 20 forms of heart disease and many forms of blood vessel disease. The most common heart and blood vessel diseases result from one or more of the following disorders:

Atherosclerosis

Arteriosclerosis (hardening of the arteries) is a condition in which the inner linings of the arteries become hardened, thickened, and roughened. Atherosclerosis, a form of arteriosclerosis, is probably the most important single cause of cerebral insufficiency and

strokes because of its effect on the arteries that supply the brain. Additional information is documented in the section on cerebrovascular accidents.

Hypertension

This condition, often called high blood pressure, is believed to result from constriction of the smallest arteries which increases resistance to blood flow.

Drugs can chemically control blood pressure levels. Relaxation, weight reduction (if the person is overweight), and lessening of salt intake are additional treatment measures. With proper medication, most persons can work and live normal lives, and even participate in some athletics.

Congenital Heart Defects

There are 35 recognized types of congenital heart malformations, most of which can be corrected or alleviated by surgery. Congenital heart defects are malformations in the structure of the heart or the large blood vessels near the heart. Although they are present at birth, some heart defects reveal no symptoms until later and may not be discovered until childhood or adulthood.

In addition to a yearly medical examination, the adolescent with congenital heart disease may need to be screened for his ability to participate in competitive sports. If there is doubt regarding the cardiac status, the advice of a pediatric cardiologist should be solicited. If the defect is mild, i.e., a small atrial or ventricular septal defect, team sports may be allowed, but if the defect is of greater severity, this type of activity should be avoided. Functional murmurs should be labeled as such and the erroneous diagnosis of a congenital cardiac defect removed. Since certain defects may worsen during adolescence, the patient with conditions such as aortic coarctation or aortic or pulmonary stenosis requires close observation. It may be advisable for the asymptomatic adolescent with one of these problems who has not undergone cardiac catheterization in a cardiac center to have this procedure performed for full delineation of the cardiac defect.

Further information regarding recreational recommendations for patients with heart disease is listed in Table 4–1.

Heart Murmurs

A heart murmur consists of auditory vibrations that are heard between normal heart sounds. Vibrations are started by one of 3 mechanisms: (1) Increased flow through normal or abnormal valves; (2) forward flow through a constricted or irregular valve into a chamber or vessel larger than the valve; (3) regurgitant, or backward, flow through an incompetent valve.

Not all murmurs mean heart trouble. Before any restrictions on activity are made, the diagnosis should be confirmed. Functional, or innocent, murmurs are vibratory or buzzing sounds heard as the result of a physiologic disturbance. The murmurs characteristically radiate poorly, and are not loud unless there is increased cardiac output because of fever or excitement. The second type of murmur is an organic or structural murmur, which is usually the result of heart disease (congenital or acquired).

Heart murmurs may be audible in any child sometime during youth. Schaeffer and Rose state that in their personal experience "roughly 85%" of young athletes have audible normal ejection-type murmurs.[22] These murmurs are poorly transmitted, and change in intensity with change of position and from one examination to the next. Therefore, it is essential to perform a comprehensive cardiovascular examination in order to determine if a murmur is due to a hemodynamic (movement of the blood) abnormality. Any situation that increases cardiac output will usually also increase the intensity of both murmur and

cardiac activity. Therefore, fever, anxiety, and recent exertion will commonly alter an otherwise normal cardiovascular examination. If this is the case, the youth should be reexamined when the exciting circumstances are no longer present. From this brief discussion of the evaluation of a murmur, it should be evident that auscultation alone is inadequate for proper diagnosis—the examination must also include inspection and palpation.

When there is a definite or suspected cardiovascular abnormality, the individual should have a chest roentgenogram and an electrocardiogram. If these 2 studies are normal, there is little likelihood that a significant cardiovascular defect exists. However, a normal roentgenogram and electrocardiogram may appear in the presence of mild acyanotic congenital heart defects, e.g., mild aortic stenosis. The physician who continues to have doubts should request further evaluation by a qualified cardiologist who has experience in treating youths with cardiac problems. Furthermore, any youth who has a recognized cardiac defect should have an evaluation by a cardiologist prior to participation in sports.[23]

Some overcautious parents and pediatricians needlessly force children with minor or questionable heart defects to become "cardiac cripples". In effect, unnecessary restrictions produce undue fragility, harmful overprotection, and undesirable health and personality traits. Premature excuses from physical activity should not be allowed. Unfortunately, many parents misinterpret the diagnosis of an innocent heart murmur and inform school officials that their child has a heart problem. The physical education teacher should check the school health record of the child to determine the nature of the murmur, and if it is described as an innocent or functional murmur, then the child should be treated normally.

With the availability of accurate noninvasive methods for making a precise diagnosis in virtually all subjects, it is no longer acceptable to restrict children from participation in athletics or physical education class. The Pediatric Cardiology Department at the University of Virginia Medical Center has found the form seen in Figure 4–21 useful in conveying thoughts on exercise participation to the schools.

Two conditions which generally preclude athletic participation include:*

Marfan Syndrome. This condition is a dominantly inherited connective tissue disorder with multisystem involvement. The typical clinical picture is that of a slender patient with long, thin extremities, arachnodactyly, hyperextensible joints, chest deformity, and dislocated lenses. Mitral valve prolapse and aortic dilatation, often with aortic insufficiency, are the major cardiovascular abnormalities. In the absence of aortic or mitral insufficiency, the cardiovascular examina-

*Permission to reprint from Pediatric Cardiology Update, Summer, 1987. Dept. of Pediatrics, Children's Medical Center of the University of Virginia.

Table 4–1.
Activity Guidelines for Common Heart Defects

Defect	Recreational Restrictions	Examples of Allowable Recreation
AORTIC INSUFFICIENCY		
Mild, with normal ECG and heart size	NONE	All recreational activity is allowed
Moderate, with cardiac enlargement	MILD	All but those requiring violent, prolonged exertion
Severe, without signs of QRS-T angle abnormality on ECG	MODERATE	Baseball, volleyball and non-competitive activities
Severe, with signs of QRS-T angle abnormality on ECG	SEVERE	Golf with cart, bowling, walking, swimming at own pace
AORTIC STENOSIS[1]		
Mild, with or without surgery	NONE	
Moderate, with or without surgery	MILD	All recreational activity is allowed
Severe, with or without surgery[2]	MODERATE	All but those requiring violent, prolonged exertion
		Baseball, volleyball and non-competitive activities
ATRIAL SEPTAL DEFECT		
Unoperated or successfully operated, with normal pulmonary artery pressure	NONE	All recreational activity is allowed
Unoperated or successfully operated, with pulmonary hypertension but pulmonary artery pressure <.50 systemic	NONE	All recreational activity is allowed
With severe pulmonary vascular disease[3]	MODERATE	Baseball, volleyball and non-competitive activities
CHRONIC CONGESTIVE HEART FAILURE	SEVERE	Golf with cart, bowling, walking, swimming at own pace
COARCTATION OF THE AORTA		
Unoperated, without severe systemic hypertension and no significant aortic valve disease	NONE	All recreational activity is allowed
Postoperative, with normal blood pressure and no significant aortic valve disease	NONE	All recreational activity is allowed
MITRAL INSUFFICIENCY		
With little or no cardiac enlargement	NONE	All recreational activity is allowed
With moderate to marked cardiac enlargement	MODERATE	Baseball, volleyball and non-competitive activities
MYOCARDITIS, ACTIVE	SEVERE	Golf with cart, bowling, walking, swimming at own pace
PATENT DUCTUS ARTERIOSUS		
Unoperated or operated, with normal pulmonary artery pressure	NONE	All recreational activity is allowed
Unoperated or operated, with pulmonary hypertension (pulmonary artery pressure <.50 systemic)[3]	NONE	All recreational activity is allowed
Unoperated or operated, with severe pulmonary vascular disease[3]	MODERATE	Baseball, volleyball and non-competitive activities
PROSTHETIC VALVE REPLACEMENT	MODERATE	Baseball, volleyball and non-competitive activities
PULMONARY STENOSIS		
Mild to moderate (peak systolic gradient <50 mm Hg) with or without surgery	NONE	All recreational activity is allowed
Severe (peak systolic gradient >80 mm Hg)	MODERATE	Baseball, volleyball and non-competitive activities
TETRALOGY OF FALLOT		
Postoperative, right ventricle-pulmonary artery gradient < 50 mm Hg without outflow patch	NONE	All recreational activity is allowed
Postoperative, right ventricle-pulmonary artery gradient <50 mm Hg with outflow patch and pulmonary insufficiency	MILD	All but those requiring violent, prolonged exertion
VENTRICULAR SEPTAL DEFECT		
Unoperated or operated, with normal pulmonary artery pressure	NONE	All recreational activity is allowed
Unoperated or operated, with pulmonary hypertension (pulmonary artery pressure <.50 systolic)[3]	NONE	All recreational activity is allowed
Unoperated or operated, with severe pulmonary vascular disease[3]	MODERATE	Baseball, volleyball and non-competitive activities
OTHER MILD FORMS OF HEART DISEASE not requiring surgery and without natural history of progressive disability	NONE	All recreational activity is allowed
OTHER SEVERE DEFECTS not operated or amenable to surgery	SEVERE	Golf with cart, bowling, walking, swimming at own pace

[1]Definition of severity by gradient not included because of individual patient variability.
[2]Patients with severe aortic stenosis may or may not have ECG abnormalities.
[3]Restricted to low altitude, except airplane travel.
(Courtesy of the American Heart Association)

DIVISION OF PEDIATRIC CARDIOLOGY
DEPARTMENT OF PEDIATRICS
UNIVERSITY OF VIRGINIA MEDICAL CENTER

HOWARD P. GUTGESELL, M.D., DIRECTOR
MARTHA A. CARPENTER, M.D.
FRANK DAMMANN, M.D.
KAREN S. RHEUBAN, M.D.
DOROTHY G. TOMPKINS, M.D.
EDWARD D. OVERHOLT, M.D.

MAILING ADDRESS
DEPARTMENT OF PEDIATRICS
BOX 386, UNIVERSITY OF
VIRGINIA MEDICAL CENTER
CHARLOTTESVILLE, VA 22908
TELEPHONE (804) 924-9119

TO WHOM IT MAY CONCERN.

_____ IS FOLLOWED IN THE PEDIATRIC
CARDIOLOGY CLINIC OF THE UNIVERSITY OF VIRGINIA HOSPITAL WITH A DIAGNOSIS
OF _____.

OUR RECOMMENDATION(S) REGARDING EXERCISE ARE AS FOLLOWS.

☐ NO RESTRICTIONS (INCLUDES INTERSCHOLASTIC ATHLETICS, CONTACT SPORTS)

☐ MODERATE EXERCISE (INCLUDES REGULAR PHYSICAL EDUCATION CLASSES, TENNIS, BASEBALL)

☐ LIGHT EXERCISE (NON-STRENUOUS TEAM GAMES, RECREATIONAL SWIMMING, JOGGING, CYCLING, GOLF)

☐ PHYSICAL EDUCATION CLASSES NOT RECOMMENDED

☐ REQUIRES HOME-BOUND TEACHER

ADDITIONAL COMMENTS _____

_____

_____

_____

_____

THIS CLINIC WILL BE GLAD TO SUPPLY FURTHER INFORMATION IF NECESSARY.

_____ M.D.

_____

Fig. 4–21. Exercise prescription form.

tion may be normal, although aortic dilatation can be detected by echocardiography.

The presence of the Marfan syndrome is generally considered a contraindication to athletic participation and the physician screening prospective athletes should be familiar with this condition. However, it is apparent that *most* tall people do *not* have Marfan syndrome and the diagnosis should not be made indiscriminantly. A detailed family history and appropriate laboratory testing can usually clarify the diagnosis.

Hypertrophic Cardiomyopathy. In a review of cardiovascular findings in young athletes dying suddenly and unexpectedly, hypertrophic cardiomyopathy was the most common underlying condition. This is likewise a familial disease and the family history often reveals cases of syncope or sudden death in adolescents or young adults. Many individuals are asymptomatic in childhood and a murmur or hyperdynamic cardiac impulse may be the only clues to the diagnosis. The electrocardiogram is usually abnormal. Echocardiography demonstrates the specific intracardiac abnormalities and is the diagnostic procedure of choice. The risk of sudden death is such that athletic participation is strongly contraindicated.

Many youths with congenital and rheumatic heart defects that do not cause hemodynamic impairment are capable of full, active interscholastic competition. Activity guidelines for the more common heart defects seen in children and adolescents are listed in Table 4–1.

Rheumatic Heart Disease

Rheumatic heart disease is usually acquired in childhood or adolescence as a result of one or more attacks of rheumatic fever. The heart structures that most often suffer permanent damage are the valves. The heart contains 4 valves (Fig. 4–22). When healthy,

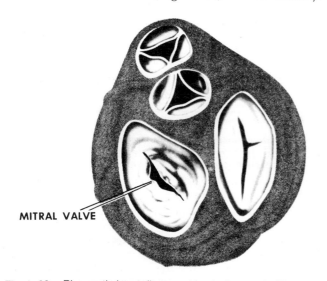

Fig. 4–22. Rheumatic heart disease with mitral stenosis. (Courtesy of the National Heart and Lung Institute.)

MITRAL VALVE

they allow blood to pass through them in one direction only. When the delicate valve leaflets become inflamed as a result of rheumatic fever, 2 things happen:

1. During the healing process, scar tissue may cause portions of the affected leaflets to become fused together. This restricts leaflet motion, reduces the effective opening of the valve, and thus impedes blood flow. The condition is called valvular stenosis (Fig. 4–22).
2. The leaflets may become shrunken or deformed by scar tissue. As a result, they fail to close properly, or they may be so weakened that they collapse under pressure and allow backflow of blood. This is known as an insufficient, or a regurgitant, valve.[24]

Incidence
Modern antibiotic therapy has sharply reduced mortality of rheumatic fever and rheumatic heart disease. For example in 1950, more than 22,000 Americans died of these diseases in comparison to about 6,200 in 1985. According to the American Heart Association, the prevalence rate includes approximately 2,150,000 persons (adults and children) still living with rheumatic heart disease.

Treatment
With the development of advanced life-support techniques, surgeons can now operate with direct vision, carefully cutting the leaflets free, removing excess scar tissue or calcium deposits, and, where necessary, replacing one or more damaged leaflets with artificial ones made of various synthetic materials.

With the recent improvements in artificial heart valves and procedures for their installation, the risk of valve replacement surgery has steadily decreased. Currently, more than 80% of patients with severe aortic or mitral valve damage can be saved, and their condition improved, by valve replacement operations.

Program Implications
Many physicians agree that most children who have had rheumatic fever do not need to have their activities limited when they return to school; however, some children may require a restricted activity program. The student should not participate in regular or adapted physical education classes until written permission is obtained from the physician.

We recommend that the postrheumatic fever patient who has specified activity restrictions follow the guidelines set forth by the Committee on Exercise, American Heart Association, for returning to physical education class:

Highly competitive game situations or activities that demand burst of energy, sudden rapid movement, or body contact are to be avoided initially.

Activities requiring effort against heavy resistance, such as weight lifting at near-maximum exertion and isometric exercises, do little to improve cardiovascular function and are not recommended, since they provoke an excessive, possibly dangerous pressor response. The subject should be told not to perform the Valsalva maneuver (prolonged effort with a closed glottis) while exercising.

In most cases the child is allowed to participate in competitive sports within 6 months after his return to school. In such cases, rather than occupying the position of middleman between student and physician, the physical education teacher should send the student directly to his cardiologist with a "letter of recommendation" based on the teacher's observation of the individual in class. Most physicians will make the necessary tests and then approve participation in the sport if there is no obvious reason against it.

Too often children who have recovered from rheumatic fever are labeled as heart patients when no apparent heart damage has occurred. The physical education teacher has a responsibility to include the student in some form of physical activity to minimize the danger of having the child begin to feel different from his peers. The teacher must use both good judgment and, if necessary, objective measurements, such as the subject's heart rate at specific work levels, to regulate the intensity of the exercise program. Adequate rest periods should be enforced; however, in most cases, the student will draw his own conclusions and rest when he becomes tired.

Exercise

In some cases, the student returns to physical education class with instructions to follow a calisthenic program outlined by the therapist who helped manage the child during his convalescence. If possible, the therapist or instructor should follow the instructions and review the student's progress with the physician or therapist at periodic intervals.

It is important to distinguish between aerobic and anaerobic exercise. During aerobic exercise, a steady supply of oxygen is delivered to the exercising muscles. According to Cooper, to be effective exercise must be carried out long enough to train both the skeletal muscles and the cardiopulmonary system, and this can be done only if the exercise is aerobic.[25] Aerobic activities include rope-jumping, jogging, and cycling. Anaerobic exercise is short-lived and characterized by short bursts of effort, such as in sprinting. Anaerobic exercise causes an accumulation of lactic acid, and the large oxygen debt causes the subject to reach a point of exhaustion early. This type of exercise is not beneficial in cardiovascular training programs.

Therapeutic Exercises

A controlled general conditioning program to re-educate the heart muscle may be recommended.
Appendix F

General Exercises

All exercises should be approached gradually with slow, but progressive increments. General balance, co-ordination, and fitness related exercises may be useful depending upon the rate of recovery status and/or physical condition of the individual. Weight training may be recommended in some cases.
Appendices B and C

CEREBROVASCULAR ACCIDENTS (CVA OR "STROKE")

The brain is an intricate mechanism, extremely dependent upon proper blood flow. Any major interruption of the blood circulation through the brain usually results in a cerebrovascular accident (CVA), commonly referred to as a "stroke". The overt physical sign of a stroke is usually hemiplegia (complete paralysis of one side of the body) or hemiparesis (partial paralysis of one side of the body). Keeping in mind that the right side of the brain controls the left side of the body, and vice versa, any damage on the right side of the brain results in left hemiplegia (paralysis of the left side of the body), and damage on the left side of the brain results in right hemiplegia (paralysis of the right side of the body).

An interruption of the brain's blood supply usually is due to a cerebral thrombosis, hemorrhage, or embolism. A thrombosis is a blood clot that forms within a major blood vessel of the brain and gradually slows or stops the supply of blood to a particular area. A cerebral hemorrhage is the bursting or rupturing of a blood vessel, usually an artery in the brain, which results in bleeding in and increased pressure on an area of the brain. A cerebral embolism is the result of a blood clot or fatty material that enters the arterial bloodstream somewhere in the circulatory system and eventually lodges in a vessel in the brain, thereby interrupting the blood supply to the area of the brain supplied by that vessel (Fig. 4–23).

Some of the problems that one might see in patients who have recently had a stroke are as follows: incontinence of bowel and bladder, partial memory loss, and psychologic problems, most commonly in the form of depression. Some victims of strokes will have hemianopsia (loss of vision from ½ of the visual field). Right hemiplegics tend to lose the right half of the visual field and left hemiplegics tend to lose the left half. Many stroke patients learn to compensate for this problem by turning their heads; however, in some cases, patients cannot make this adjustment. This is referred to as neglect, which means, basically, that the patients neglect objects on one side. For example, they may not recognize their own arms or legs as a part of their bodies. Stroke patients tend to have difficulty in new learning situations, and they usually will have problems in generalizing information from one situation to another, but they usually are able to remember familiar situations. Some stroke patients suffer from emotional lability, which is a loss of emotional control. They may laugh or cry inappropriately and may, in fact, switch from laughing to crying with no apparent reason: there is usually no obvious relation-

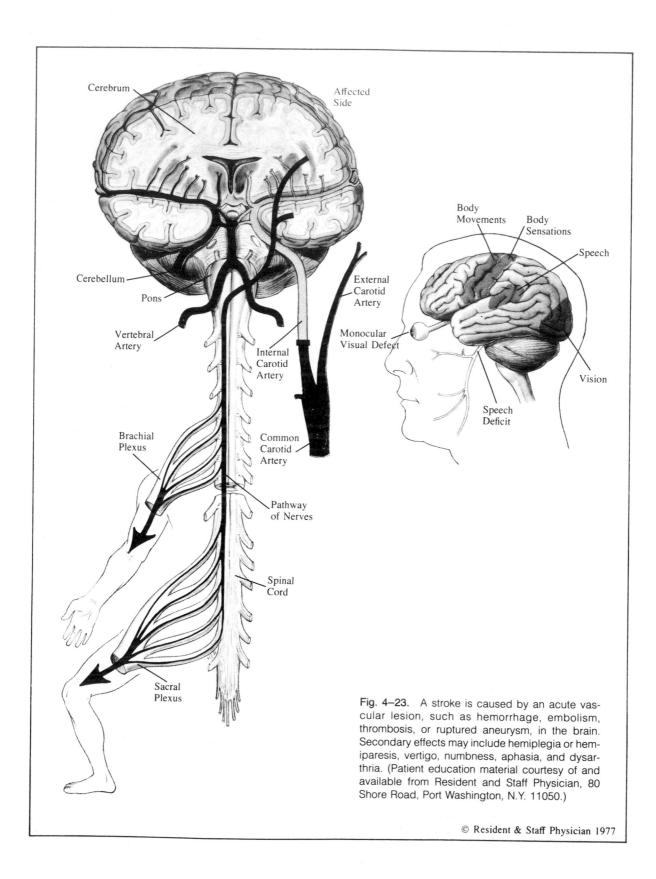

Fig. 4–23.   A stroke is caused by an acute vascular lesion, such as hemorrhage, embolism, thrombosis, or ruptured aneurysm, in the brain. Secondary effects may include hemiplegia or hemiparesis, vertigo, numbness, aphasia, and dysarthria. (Patient education material courtesy of and available from Resident and Staff Physician, 80 Shore Road, Port Washington, N.Y. 11050.)

ship between what is happening at the time and their emotional response.

Although many signs seen among stroke victims are similar, there are an equal number of dissimilar signs. There are no characteristics common to all right hemiplegics or to all left hemiplegics. However, there are basic signs that one usually sees. Left hemiplegics tend to have more problems with neglect than do right hemiplegics. They tend to have more difficulty with spatial, perceptual tasks and with understanding or using visual cues received from their environment. Many tend to be impulsive and careless in their actions, and often seem to be unaware of their deficits. They often show poor judgment and reliability, and speak with a confidence and normalcy that belies their physical disabilities.

Right hemiplegics suffer more often from aphasia (problems with speech and language). Many times patients have trouble speaking but are able to understand instructions given to them. Right hemiplegics have a tendency to be slow, cautious, and sometimes disorganized, especially when approaching an unfamiliar situation.

Incidence

The American Heart Association estimates that approximately 500,000 people suffer strokes each year. A rough guide suggests that of every hundred persons who survive a stroke, approximately 10 will be able to return to a normal lifestyle with no major impairment; 40 will have some mild residual disability; 40 will be severely disabled and require some type of special services; and 10 will need institutional care. Stroke victims can be seen in most age categories; however, the frequency of strokes increases with advancing age, and the major incidence is seen in those aged 60 to 65 and older.

Treatment

Immediately following a stroke, the first major concern is the survival of the patient. Upon hospitalization of the patient, medical management of the life threatening situation is the primary concern. Vital signs must be made as stable as possible, and numerous tests must be administered in order to diagnose the particular type of cerebrovascular accident that the patient has suffered, so that proper treatment can be started immediately. Treatment may take many forms, among which are the administration of drugs, anticoagulants, antihypertensives, and sometimes even surgery.

Rehabilitation of stroke patients should begin as soon as possible after control of the life threatening crisis is gained. Rehabilitation is accomplished best by a stroke rehabilitation team. The rehab team should include, in addition to physicians and nurses, an occupational therapist, a physical therapist, a therapeutic recreation specialist, a social worker, a speech pathologist, audiologist, psychologist, in some cases, and,

when appropriate, a vocational rehabilitation counselor.

Active and passive range-of-motion activities should be initiated very soon after the stroke. They may be done with the aid of the occupational, or the physical, therapist and may initially be performed at bedside. At the same time, careful attention should be given to skin care, and bowel and bladder management and retraining. As soon as possible, the patient should be moved to the sitting position and into a wheelchair, whereby he can reorient himself to his environment and attend the appropriate therapeutic sessions.

The basic goal of the rehabilitation team is to try to overcome as much of the lost body functions as is possible, and to retrain the patient in deficient areas. Retraining usually must be done in activities of daily living, ambulation, perceptual/cognitive motor function and, in some cases, language functions. Many patients do not recover from the losses they have suffered, and some continue to depend upon assistive devices such as wheelchairs, canes, or braces. The lower extremities tend to regain function before, and usually more completely than, the upper extremities. Some spontaneous recovery usually occurs, and it is the therapists' responsibility to help retrain and reintegrate the returning functional ability. If limbs remain flaccid for a long time after a stroke, the prognosis for return of function becomes quite poor. If no voluntary motor return takes place in a limb in 3 to 4 weeks, treatment is usually discontinued, and other training techniques are pursued in order to teach the patient to compensate for the lost function of that limb.

Program Implications

In programming treatment for the patient with CVA, the therapist must keep in mind the fact that no two patients are alike. Specific, individualized treatment programs, with appropriate goals and objectives, must be established and modified as needed. Stroke patients require a great deal of feedback from the therapist in the process of carrying out almost any task. Because the judgment and reliability of stroke patients is often poor, initially the therapist will need to remind them to do things such as lock their wheelchairs; and when they are moving in their wheelchairs, stroke patients may need to be warned not to bump into walls or objects in their path. Patients will need seatbelts to hold them securely in their chairs. Some patients naturally slump and slide out of their chairs, and others, forgetting that they cannot walk, attempt to stand up out of the chair and fall. Some patients have painful joints, and some have subluxations (usually in the shoulder) or contractures.

Because of these problems, the therapist should work a great deal on improving general strength and endurance. Activities need to be very limited initially, and gradually increased in intensity. As function begins to return to the leg, activities that require the use of the leg become important. Patients can work initially from a sitting position and be moved slowly to standing-type activities with an assistant standing by. Ball-kicking activities, especially those that require accuracy, are important in terms of reintegrating neuromuscular function in the leg. If a patient's balance is good, riding a 3-wheel-bicycle provides excellent treatment for strengthening the leg, increasing its range of motion, and improving the reciprocal leg movement activity.

The upper extremities, as indicated earlier, will probably improve much more slowly than the lower extremities. Initial activities usually emphasize gross motor movements and should improve strength and range of motion. If additional functions return, the patient should begin performing fine motor tasks. In working with both the upper and the lower extremities, especially of those patients who neglect one side, it is important to include activities that require the patients to cross their midlines and work on both sides of their bodies. As a general rule, when working one-to-one with a patient with unilateral involvement, it is a good practice to work from his affected side. This helps make him more aware of that side and aids in retraining him to use it again.

Many activities help the therapist in retraining the stroke patient's perceptual/cognitive motor skills and spatial awareness. Activities that require figure/ground discrimination, task analysis, learning generalization, and speech and language skills should be utilized. Initially the stroke patient may be easily distracted and must be worked with on a one-to-one basis in an isolated area. When possible, however, the patient should be involved in more social types of activity. This is important because the stroke patient has a tendency to become isolated and ignored.

When selecting specific activities for the stroke patient, the therapist should keep in mind the age of the patient and the type of activities most suitable for his age level. Many activities will have the treatment potential that the therapist needs and still be appropriate for the patient's age level. Therapists should not become discouraged when stroke patients seem to be depressed or to have volatile tempers, because this is a normal process of grief in reaction to the stroke. Patience is a must when working with stroke victims.

As patients begin to reach their maximum functional return and move toward discharge, hopefully back into the community, the functional therapist should make every effort to interest them in activities that they can pursue at home. Many patients return home and become isolated instead of returning to a normalized level of function in their community. The therapist should try to make contacts in the community to which the patient will return and find activities that are available for the patient to become involved in. Many communities have clubs for stroke victims which the therapist can contact before the pa-

tient is discharged. Many of these are run by local chapters of the American Heart Association or the local recreation department, and addresses can be secured from them.

Case History: This 16-year-old with sickle cell disease suffered left frontoparietal CVA with resultant right hemiparesis and dysarthria.

The patient made slow, but steady progress in his rehabilitation program. During the early phases of his treatment program perceptual-motor training drills were used to resolve problems associated with motor planning deficits and short-term memory concepts. Program selection was geared to improve reaction time and ability to make positional changes, stimulate trunk rotation, and improve right hand usage (Fig. 4–24).

Therapeutic Exercises

Therapeutic exercises are utilized to strengthen and stretch specific muscles or groups of muscles, and to maintain or increase range of motion.

Exercise for the upper extremities, lower extremities, and upper and lower trunk area can be passive, active assistive, active, or resistive. The type of exercise depends on the amount of paralysis and the areas of involvement.

The use of therapeutic exercises should be authorized in writing by a physician.

Appendix A
1. Exercises for the upper back
   Exercises 1, 2, 4, 6, 9, 10, 11, and 13
   If patient is unable to grasp the pulley in exercises 9, 10, 11, and 13 the hand can be held in place with an elastic bandage or similar wrap.
2. Exercises for the lower back
   Exercises 18 through 22
3. Exercises for abdominal muscles
   Exercises 32, 33, 34, 37, and 39
4. Exercises for the hip
   Exercises 43 through 53
5. Exercises for the knee
   Exercises 64 through 67, 69, 71, 72, 77 through 80
6. Exercises for the ankle and foot
   Exercises 81 through 86
7. Exercises for the fingers (These exercises can be done lying down.)
   Exercises 96 through 110
8. Exercises for the wrist (These exercises can be done lying down.)
   Exercises 111 through 115
9. Exercises for the elbow (These exercises can be done lying down.)
   Exercises 118, 119, and 122
   If patient is unable to grasp wand in exercise 122 the hand can be held in place with an elastic bandage or similar wrap.
10. Exercises for the shoulder (These exercises can be done lying down.)
    Exercises 126, 128 through 131

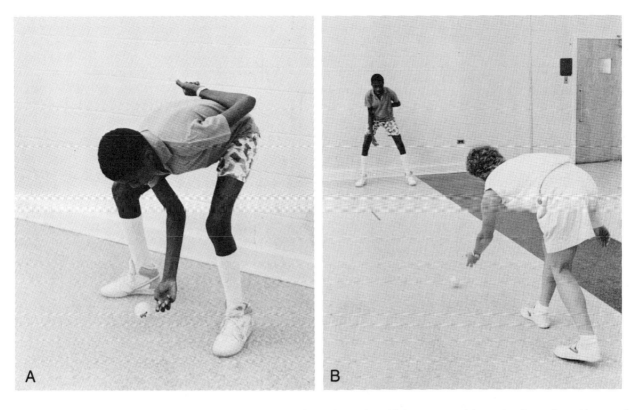

Fig. 4–24. It is not unusual for stroke patients to exhibit impaired proprioception which causes a delay or hesitancy in making a voluntary motor response. With this patient, it was useful to facilitate exploration of the involved right side while using ball handling activities. Lack of dexterity (note illustration B) and sensory stimulation were problems especially during activities that required functional hand usage.

Hand can be held in place by an elastic bandage for exercises 128 and 131.
11. Exercises for deep breathing
    Exercises 142 through 145

General Exercises

General exercises are beneficial to some patients who have suffered a stroke. Naturally the patients will need assistance and exercise should only be undertaken after permission is granted in writing by a physician.

Appendix B
Exercises 11, 12, 13, 16, 20, and 23

CANCER

Cancer is a large group of diseases characterized by uncontrolled growth and spread of abnormal cells. The American Cancer Society estimated in 1989 that about 1,000,000 people would be diagnosed as having cancer (excluding non-melanoma skin cancer and carcinoma in situ). The survival rate is improving, however, the incidence of cancer, and therefore, the number of deaths are increasing. A major reason for this is that lung cancer, one of the deadliest forms, is becoming increasingly common among women. Most lung cancers are caused by cigarette smoking with an estimated 155,000 new cases in 1989.

Various combinations of cancer drugs and new approaches combining drugs and chemotherapy, and chemotherapy with surgery have improved the survival rate. New technologies continue to improve and have made it possible to aid diagnostic and treatment procedures. For example, in computerized tomography (CT scanning) the use of sophisticated x rays can pinpoint the shape and location of a tumor. This isolates the specific location for radiation dosage while not affecting normal tissue.

Prevention to eliminate risk factors (smoking, occupational hazards, etc.) is important. In addition, cancer related medical checkups (pap test, breast detection, etc.) reduce cancer risks. Research involving good nutritional habits is an issue that is demanding more attention, although no direct cause-and-effect relationship has been established.

Further discussion is limited to 3 forms of cancer.

Cancer of the Breast

The breast is a glandular organ with many lobuli. Its secretions pass through collecting ducts to the nipple.

When the breast is diseased, a neoplasm is usually produced. This mass of tissue is always a source of alarm, because it may be malignant. Since the breast is considered, at least in Western cultures, a major ingredient in female beauty, a diseased breast causes great anxiety to the patient. These pressures or psychologic problems can play a major role in the treatment and rehabilitation of a patient who is suspected of having a breast tumor or who has undergone breast surgery; and the fear of disfigurement may prevent some individuals from seeking assistance when they detect a change in their breast.

The majority of disorders involving the breast are benign, even though it is also one of the primary sites of cancer. About 25% of all women have abnormal areas in their breasts at some time. Changes in the breasts often occur before the menstrual period begins. Other changes take place in breast tissue between periods.

Diagnosis
About 95% of all breast cancers are detected by women themselves. The American Cancer Society suggests that women establish a routine, monthly self-examination of the breast.

In addition to the monthly self-examination, a breast examination should be included in the annual physical examination. A breast examination should be done twice a year for women who have a family history of breast cancer.

There are many diagnostic procedures that can be performed before any major surgical procedure need be undertaken. Two common procedures are:

Mammography. In this procedure, a roentgenogram is taken of the breast without the injection of a contrast medium. Once a breast lump is found, mammography can help determine if there are other lesions in the same or opposite breast which are too small to be felt.

Biopsy. There are 2 types of biopsies: aspiration and incisional. In the aspiration procedure, a local anesthetic is given, then a needle is directed to the area to be tested. Tissue is drawn into the needle via suction, and the tissue is then tested.

The incisional method is usually accomplished under general anesthesia. Tissue is removed surgically and then tested.

Incidence
Cancer of the female breast affects 5 of every 100 women and rarely occurs in women under the age of 25. In 1989, 142,900 new cases of breast cancer were diagnosed, and 43,300 deaths were related to it, according to the American Cancer Society.

The prognosis for breast cancer depends primarily on the extent of the disease at the time treatment is begun, as well as the location and size of the lesion and the presence or absence of axillary node involvement, and the number and location of positive nodes.

Small lesions that have not metastasized have a 90% chance of being cured. If the cancer has spread, however, the survival rate is 60%.

Treatment
If the diagnostic procedures and the biopsy show a malignant tumor, a mastectomy usually follows. In a simple mastectomy, only the tumor, the overlying skin and the breast tissue are removed. In a radical mastectomy, the breast, including the overlying skin and the pectoralis major and minor muscle, are removed. Also, tissue that contains axillary lymph nodes is removed for examination.

In some cases, after surgery or instead of surgery, the patient may be treated with radiotherapy and/or chemotherapy. These types of treatment are considered by the physician and administered according to his evaluation of the patient's needs.

The diameter of a patient's arm may increase after a radical mastectomy. In addition, pain, edema, and the type of location of the incision and subsequent sutures may restrict motion.

Edema may persist due to the removal of lymph nodes, and the formation of scar tissue. These factors, along with pain, contribute to the loss of mobility of the shoulder and, sometimes, of the elbow and hand on the involved side.

Breast reconstruction is now becoming an important part of treatment and rehabilitation.

Program Implications
Active exercise should be done slowly and smoothly during the immediate postsurgery period and sports can begin at various stages after surgery. Restricted arm movement is common after breast surgery due to limitations of motion at the shoulder joint. Once the physician approves, low impact aerobics and swimming are often recommended to activate the involved shoulder joint. After a reasonable period of physical rehabilitation, the postmastectomy patient can engage in active games and sports. In most cases full strength and range of motion in the shoulder joint should return in approximately 2 to 3 months.

Therapeutic Exercises
Therapeutic exercises for the patient who is recovering from breast surgery should be done bilaterally, and emphasis should concentrate on active motion of both shoulder joints (Fig. 4–25).

Exercise programs should be initiated only when written permission is given by the physician. Care should be taken, at least in the early stages of recovery, if the patient has had a skin graft, or if the incision was closed with considerable tension.

Appendix A
1. Exercises for the upper back
   Exercises 1 through 17
2. Exercises for the fingers
   Exercises 96 through 110
3. Exercises for the wrist
   Exercises 111 through 117
4. Exercises for the elbow
   Exercises 118 through 124
5. Exercises for the shoulder
   Exercises 125 through 138
6. Exercises for the head and neck
   Exercises 139 through 141

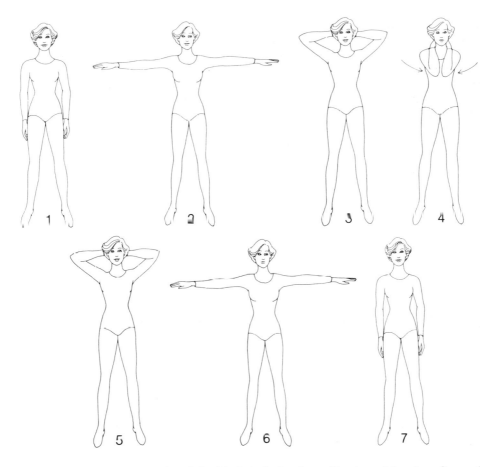

Fig. 4–25.   Elbow pull-in exercise to increase rotation of shoulder in both directions. (Courtesy of American Cancer Society.)

Leukemia

Leukemia is a disease of the blood-producing organs which is characterized by the uncontrolled production and growth of white blood cells or leukocytes. These immature leukocytes rob the body of its ability to fight infections and to form blood clots. In effect, the abnormal white cells affect the production of red blood cells and interfere with clotting; and they are also unable to fight infections.

The different types of leukemia are identified by the kind of white blood cell affected. The only form of leukemia that will be discussed here is acute lymphocytic leukemia (ALL), the form of cancer that is most common in children.

Acute Lymphocytic Leukemia

Lymphocytic leukemia is one of the 2 major types of leukemia. It involves the lymphocytes that are produced in the lymph nodes and bone marrow. Anemia, infection, and bleeding may occur as a result of bone marrow failure. When no leukemia cells are visible in the bone marrow or elsewhere, the disease is said to be in remission. When large numbers of leukemia cells are present in the bone marrow, the disease is said to be in relapse. The causes of the different types of leukemia are unknown. The symptoms of ALL are similar to many other diseases. The presenting signs include pallor, fatigue, fever, and pain in the bones and joints. Associated symptoms include increased susceptibility to infection due to the decreased number of white cells and hemorrhaging caused by the decreased number of platelets. Like other forms of cancer, a biopsy of the affected tissue is essential for diagnosis. Samples of marrow cells are obtained through aspiration or a bone marrow biopsy.

Incidence

An estimated 27,300 new cases of leukemia were reported in 1989, about half of them chronic leukemia. Although it is often thought of as primarily a childhood disease, leukemia strikes many more adults (25,000 cases per year compared with 1,800 in children). Acute lymphocytic leukemia accounts for about 1,800 of the cases of leukemia in children.[26]

Treatment

Prior to 1948, children with ALL had an average survival rate of only 3 to 4 months.[26a] Various new drugs have made it possible to extend the lives of children for many months, and in some cases, as long as 10 to 15 years. In some medical centers, optimum treatment has raised the survival rate to 75%. Most treatment protocols indicate 2 or 3 years of initial maintenance therapy. Then, if the patient is still in remission, treatment is discontinued. Various forms of chemotherapeutic agents have been used successfully, either one at a time or in intermittent combination therapy. The effect of therapy is to interfere with, or kill off, the leukemic cell population, thus allowing the normal blood-forming cells to repopulate the bone marrow and produce normal blood cells.

Nausea, vomiting, and anorexia occur frequently during chemotherapy. Another drastic side effect is alopecia. A patient may lose some or all of his hair, but it will regrow about 8 weeks after therapy ends. The decision to discontinue chemotherapy is made on the basis of several factors, including drug resistance, severe drug toxicity, or because all cancer cells have been destroyed.

In adults, acute leukemia is more resistant to treatment than in children, but improved modes of treatment are being developed, and the outlook for adults has improved.

Program Implications

Therapy is interdisciplinary, and, ideally, a therapeutic recreation specialist should be an important member of the team when the patient is receiving inpatient treatment in a hospital. Supportive therapy emphasizing psychosocial stimulation is important. The therapist should assess the patient's ability to cope with the disease and the emotional effects that often accompany the patient's treatment protocol. Two of the major difficulties in planning programs for the hospitalized cancer patient are the relentless routine of therapy and the drastic side effects of drug toxicity. Above all, the child with cancer should be made to feel as "normal" as possible. The child should be allowed to participate to his fullest ability, depending on his individual tolerance level.

Even though the patient with ALL must be given intravenous fluids and medications, he can often remain mobile for much of the time that he is hospitalized. Because he has routine periods of intravenous therapy, the patient is confined periodically to an IV pole. During these periods, the limb receiving IV infusion can be mobilized in physical activity provided that the form of recreational exercise is not too strenuous. Quiet and solitary play is often encouraged during these periods. It is important, however, to choose an IV site that hinders mobility least (such as the nondominant hand). Mild intensity activities are best for the patient undergoing active IV therapy, and in many situations this means playing sitting games which require little energy and endurance. It is important to emphasize that the IV solution should be filtering well and regularly before the patient engages in a recreational program.

The therapist often encounters patients who are using a heparin lock (Fig. 4–26A) (an intermittent catheter attached to the forearm). A solution of heparin, which is an anticoagulant, is flushed into the lock,

and travels to the tip of the needle, thus preventing it from clotting off. The lock remains in the vein and can be hooked up at anytime to start a new IV solution. For the following reasons the heparin lock is advantageous for children who require daily doses of chemotherapeutic agents: (1) it provides maximum mobility; (2) it minimizes the frequency of injections; (3) no special care, other than a sterile bandage, is needed.

A patient wearing a heparin lock can participate in a wide range of recreational activities. Two precautions are necessary: (1) a protective shield should cover the needle to protect it from external forces; and (2) activities that involve violent exertion and explosive body contact should be avoided to prevent the needle from being dislodged.

A lacrosse glove with protective interior padding to prevent friction (Fig. 4–26B) can provide adequate coverage during physical activity by a patient using a heparin lock. It has been used as successful protection in catching activities, floor hockey, and projectile-handling activities. Depending on the activity to be participated in, some materials should not be used for the protective interior padding. For example, the nonstructural surface of foam rubber provides insufficient protection when there is danger of external force to the site of the lock, as in such activities as catching a playground ball with both hands.

A number of moderately restricted activities are possible for patients using a heparin lock. Listed below are a few examples:

1. Archery (depending upon the location of the lock and the protective covering). Preventive care must take into consideration the whiplash of the bowstring against the forearm.
2. Volleyball (if a lightweight beachball is used in place of a regulation volleyball).
3. Basketball (if modified games are used in which there is no rapid or forceful passing and in which movement patterns are considerably slowed down. Examples are H-O-R-S-E, 21, long shots made from behind the foul line [2 points], short shots such as layups [one point], and free throw games).
4. Recreational games (such as darts, shuffleboard, billiards, table tennis, and badminton).
5. Swimming with protective equipment. No diving. (See Chap. 9 for information on protective devices.)
6. Marksmanship shooting (with a B.B. gun, pellet gun, pistol, or rifle).
7. Bowling (although each individual who throws with his affected arm should have his arm-swing motion assessed, because an explosive back-swing motion or forward release can dislodge a needle).
8. Low organization games, especially throwing and kicking activities, and catching games provided that a protective device is used over the

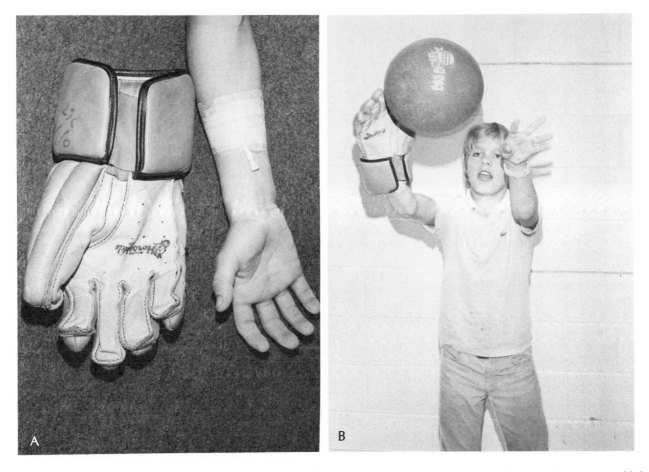

Fig. 4–26. *A,* Heparin lock and lacrosse glove. *B,* The glove provides protection from impact and allows freedom of movement with both hands.

lock when both hands are used for summation of forces.

9. Golf (putting games).

The therapist should know that the chemotherapeutic agents are carefully adjusted to the patient's tolerance. This generally means that the white blood cell count (WBC) is maintained between 2000 and 3000/cu mm, and that the absolute neutrophil count is maintained above 1000/cu mm. The normal WBC is 5,000 to 10,000/cu mm; in leukemia it may be more than 50,000/cu mm. It is helpful to review the medical chart frequently to maintain an awareness of blood cell counts.

When a child is discharged from a hospital, his schooling should certainly continue. Ordinarily the child can return to school if his white blood cell count (WBC) is about 2000/cu mm. If a child is in remission, then involvement in physical education class (either regular or adapted, depending upon the individual case) should be recommended.

The physical education teacher should be flexible in making adjustments whenever they are warranted. The child with cancer must explore, and come to terms with, being different in his appearance, experiences, and freedom to pursue physical activities.

Sometimes the child will feel perfectly normal, and at other times the drugs or the disease will force him to restrict his recreational exercise.

The child should regulate his own activity, but the teacher should be aware of symptoms that commonly preclude involvement in physical education classes. Dyspnea is a distressing symptom. Symptoms of anemia such as pallor, generalized weakness, and lack of strength and endurance are additional causes for concern.

Platelet counts may be low when the child is at home during chemotherapy; so, even if there is no visible evidence of bleeding, the parents should encourage their child to refrain from sports or activities such as football, soccer, bicycle riding, tree climbing, and skateboard riding, that may result in accidental injury. **Such information should also be forwarded to the physical education teacher.** This restriction may be more difficult for boys than for girls. One way of avoiding conflict is to explain to the child that when the platelet count is below 50,000 cu mm the cells needed for blood clotting are low. The child can then assume responsibility for tailoring his own activity. This also allows the child to resume normal sports when he learns that his platelet count has risen.[31]

Therapeutic Exercises

Specific therapeutic exercises are of little value unless there are particular weaknesses due to inactivity, or joint discomfort or tightness.

General Exercises

General exercises, weight training, balance beam, rehabilitation calisthenics, and stall bar exercises are beneficial in helping the child regain strength, muscle tone, and coordination. They must be initiated slowly under the approval of a physician.

Appendices B, C, and E

Hodgkin's Disease

Hodgkin's disease was first described in 1832 by Thomas Hodgkin, who characterized the disorder by enlarged lymph nodes, an enlarged spleen, and cachexia (a generally weak, emaciated condition). Hodgkin's disease can be defined as a malignant disease of the lymphatic system. Giant, multinucleated cells (Reed-Sternberg cells) are a diagnostic feature. If the disease follows an unrelenting course, lymphocytes (white blood cells) proliferate in a variety of abnormal forms and deplete the body of the normal cells it needs to fight infection.

The cause of Hodgkin's disease is unknown. The most common symptom of the disease is painless enlargement of lymph nodes, most commonly those in the neck. Fatigue, weight loss, and night sweats may be associated symptoms. Definite diagnosis can be reached only through clinical examination and laboratory tests. Unfortunately, it is common for several weeks or even months to elapse between the patient's first observation of symptoms and the diagnostic biopsy (a microscopic study performed on a specimen removed by surgery from an affected lymph node). As the disease progresses, it spreads through the lymphatic system, involving other lymph nodes, as well as the spleen, liver, and bone marrow. The patient often becomes anemic, and, because of blood changes, his body becomes less able to combat infections.

Stages

Clinical and pathologic stages of the disease are designated as follows, according to the Ann Arbor system of classification:

Stage I. Involvement of a single lymph node region (I) or a single extralymphatic organ or site (I_E).

Stage II. Involvement of two or more lymph node regions on the same side of the diaphragm (II) or localized involvement of an extralymphatic organ or site (II_E).

Stage III. Involvement of lymph node regions on both sides of the diaphragm (III) or localized involvement of either an extralymphatic organ or site (III_E) or the spleen (III).

Stage IV. Diffuse or disseminated involvement of one or more extralymphatic organs with or without associated lymph node involvement. The organs involved are identified by a symbol when cases are discussed.

The following two symbols are also used in discussion of cases:

A = Asymptomatic
B = Fever, sweats, loss of 10% of body weight

Incidence

Hodgkin's disease strikes about 9,000 Americans each year. The disease has an unusually age-specific incidence curve; one peak age group is 15 to 34, and the other is age 50 and over.

Treatment

Depending upon the stage of the patient's disease, the most effective treatment is to eradicate the malignant tissue. Therapy, however, must be individualized. Patients classified as Stage I, II, or IIIA are usually treated with radiotherapy. Chemotherapy is used for patients with widespread Hodgkin's disease. Combination radiotherapy and chemotherapy treatments often help patients with advanced disease. Careful evaluation and observation of a high proportion (90–95%) of patients who have survived disease free for 5 years shows that they are clinically cured of the disease.

Program Implications

Many of the program implications for leukemia also apply to programs for patients with Hodgkin's disease. It is important for therapists to plan therapeutic sessions around the treatment schedule of hospitalized patients. Unfortunately, the patient must cope with the limitations of the disease as well as the toxicities of the therapy. Frequently, patients receiving therapy in the morning experience a few hours of nausea and vomiting immediately following treatment, but recover by afternoon.

An appropriate recreational and physical education plan should be implemented through the joint efforts of the patient, his family, and his physician after the patient is discharged from the hospital (Fig. 4–27).

Therapeutic Exercises

Specific therapeutic exercises are of little value unless there are particular weaknesses due to inactivity, or joint discomfort or tightness.

General Exercises

General exercises, weight training, and balance beam, rehabilitation, and calisthenic exercises are beneficial in helping the child regain strength, muscle tone, and coordination. They must be initiated slowly under the approval of a physician.

Appendices B, C, and E

CEREBRAL PALSY

Cerebral palsy (CP) is a disturbance of muscular function that arises from destruction or congenital absence of upper motor neurons. The disability is

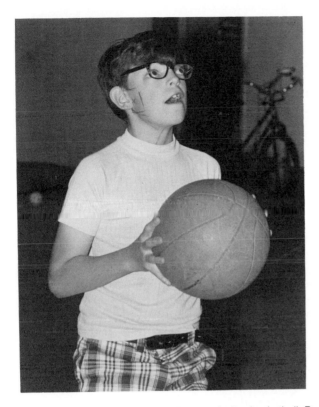

Fig. 4–27. Patient with Hodgkin's disease playing basketball. Radiation is one form of treatment for cancer. The effects of radiation that complicate a person's self-image include radiation markings (note illustration) and loss of hair (alopecia). Additional effects include fatigue, skin reactions, and gastrointestinal disturbances.

frequently complicated by the occurrence of a seizure disorder, behavioral disturbance, or mental retardation.

Causes

It is known that disease, injury, or malformation of brain cells can all produce effects identical to those of cerebral palsy. Since its exact cause is unknown, cerebral palsy is frequently classified by the time of life of its apparent onset. Different possible causes exist for each time period during which the disease may begin.

Prenatal (most frequent)
1. Functional disturbances of the mother, such as high blood pressure, kidney disease, or diabetes which may produce hemorrhages in the child's brain.
2. Incompatibility of maternal and fetal blood—Rh factor.
3. Infection in the early months of pregnancy.
4. Diseases of germ plasma that cause faulty development of the brain.

Natal (frequent)
1. Brain injury during birth from prolonged or difficult labor, or any condition that leads to lack of oxygen for the baby for more than a few minutes during delivery.
2. Premature birth.

Postnatal (less frequent)
1. Diseases such as whooping cough and encephalitis.
2. Insufficient oxygen in the blood, as in gas poisoning.
3. Trauma, such as cerebral stroke, gunshot wounds, or head injuries.

Types of Cerebral Palsy

There are 7 distinct types of cerebral palsy; however, only the 3 most prevalent—spastic, athetoid, and ataxic—will be discussed here. Characteristics of all the groups may occur together in any one person.

Spastic. Spasticity, occurring in approximately ½ of all cases of cerebral palsy, is characterized by hyperactive reflexes and contracted flexor muscles, which produce awkward and stiff movement. Mental impairment is often associated with this type of cerebral palsy.

Athetoid. Athetosis, seen in about ¼ of all cases, is marked by purposeless, involuntary, and incoordinated motions with varying degrees of tension. These movements cause the person to squirm or wriggle constantly. The extraneous movements are less severe when the individual is relaxed.

Ataxic. Ataxia, a less common type of cerebral palsy, is characterized by incoordination of activity or function, or both due to a disturbance of kinesthetic sense. The ataxic has to concentrate to keep from falling, and his swaggering gait resembles that of an intoxicated person. Muscle tone is poor in most cases.

The degree of involvement in cerebral palsy determines the movement capabilities and functional capacity. Ataxias are classified according to the extremities affected:

Monoplegia..................one limb
Paraplegia ....lower limbs
Hemiplegia ....both limbs on one side
Diplegia......................involvement primarily of both legs, with the arms affected to slight degree
Triplegia.....................three limbs, often both legs and one arm
Quadriplegia ....four limbs, legs usually spastic, arms dyskinetic (Fig. 4–28)
Double Hemiplegia ....all four extremities are affected, but lower limbs are less involved than the upper limbs
Tetraplegia ....all four limbs are equally involved
Total Body Involvement ...all four extremities involved as well as the trunk, head, and neck

Although the mentality of these children is likely

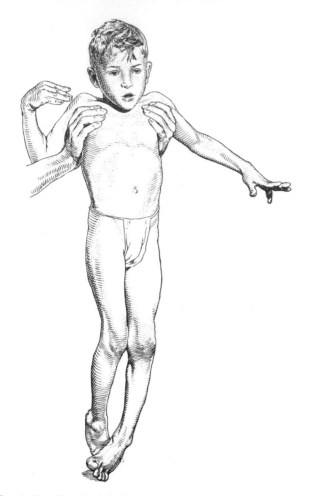

Fig. 4–28. Spastic quadriplegia in a child with cerebral palsy. (From Shands, A.R., Jr., et al.: Handbook of Orthopaedic Surgery. St. Louis, C.V. Mosby Co., 1963.)

to be affected, many have normal intelligence. With education and special training they may become useful citizens. There is an obvious discrepancy in the reports of the percentage of cerebral palsy with mental retardation; most medical records indicate that 35 to 50% of people with cerebral palsy are intellectually impaired. Even those with below-normal intelligence may be trained to earn a living or at least to care for themselves.

As a general rule, all hemiplegics will walk. Most diplegics will walk, but some may require assistance. A large number of quadriplegics and those with total body involvement will never walk and most will require a wheelchair or other form of sitting appliance.

Incidence
The generally accepted figure for the incidence is 7 per 100,000 births. About 75 to 80% will need medical and clinical intervention and special services.

Treatment
The course of treatment depends upon the extent of damage to the brain, its nature, and the age at

which it developed. The physical, mental, and emotional characteristics of each individual must be considered carefully because there is often a marked difference between the person's chronologic age, mental age, and physical development. Therapy should be started early, preferably as soon as the disability is recognized.

Treatment for cerebral palsy usually combines neurodevelopmental approaches, proprioceptive neuromuscular facilitation, and sensorimotor integration techniques. Mat activities consist of rolling, crawling, and knee walking. The treatment is also aimed at improving balance, righting reactions, and primitive reflexes (See Chap. 1, Early Intervention).

One important aim is training in self-help activities. Various therapeutic disciplines, such as physical therapy, occupational therapy, and therapeutic recreation, are directed toward improvement of motor function. Each discipline can complement the others by motivating the child and helping him to acquire skill in movement.

Vision and hearing are examined and, if necessary, treated. Speech training is often recommended to enable the child to make known his wants and to develop personal relationships with others.

Splints or braces are prescribed for some patients to prevent deformities and to aid in standing and walking. Many persons with CP have found it possible to participate in activities with the aid of braces.

Specific surgical procedures depend on the kind of deformity and the presence or absence of contractures. The goals of surgical intervention include:
1. Diminishment of muscle spasms through surgical procedures on motor nerves (e.g. neurectomy).
2. Correction of joint contractures and deformities.
3. Restoration of muscle balance by equalizing the power of opposing muscles (e.g., tendon transplants). Improvement in joint motion is the usual result.
4. Stabilization of poorly controlled joints through surgical procedures (e.g., fusion). An arthrodesis or an osteotomy is often used to treat uncontrollable structural changes in the foot. This is often done after soft-tissue surgery fails to maintain balance and stabilization.

Education plays an important part in the child's total habilitation and should be emphasized along with other aspects of this treatment.

Program Implications
The degree to which a child can participate successfully depends upon the extent of his physical and mental handicaps. Therapists, physical education teachers, and recreation leaders need to program activities that will overcome a child's specific deficits, including: (1) tone abnormalities (muscle tightness and imbalance), (2) sensory feedback problems (inability to know where limbs are in space), and (3)

incoordination of movement. Many children with severe involvement will need assistive devices to compensate for their lack of strength and poor neuromuscular development. Those with mild involvement may be able to engage in regular sports and games.

Motor deficiencies and perceptual inadequacies are common handicaps that need attention. Therefore, a sequence of motor activities should be introduced to provide for better movement skills. The therapist or instructor should stress slow, repetitive movements, because the child needs patient training in the performance of purposeful motor skills. Mass-movement activities accompanied by continuous excitement are contraindicated.

Since many children with cerebral palsy have a shorter span of attention than other children their age, a variety of activities should be encouraged and no one task continued to the point of fatigue. Often these children become visually preoccupied with stimuli other than with the motor task at hand. To prevent this, physical activities should be performed in a distraction-free environment.

Little information has been documented regarding program planning for cerebral palsied children who need remediation of visual-motor defects. The incidence of visual and ocular defects in children with cerebral palsy has been reported to be between 60 and 80%. Strabismus is the most common defect, occurring in 40 to 50% of cerebral palsied children. Strabismus (squinted or crossed eyes) is a condition in which the extraocular muscles are not balanced; therefore, the eyes cannot function in unison. Additional problems involved with strabismus include: (1) One eye that is used less than the other, resulting in poor vision in the seldom used eye; (2) a double image resulting from the absence of fusion; and (3) emotional problems due to taunting by others.

Different types of strabismus produce different effects on the eyes. The problem is often corrected before the child goes to school, but this is not always the case. A number of children go untreated or fail to follow the recommendations outlined for them by an ophthalmologist.

Children who have strabismus show a distinct inability to distinguish an object from its background or surroundings (figure-ground disturbance). Ocular tracking (eye movement following a moving target) is also difficult for them, particularly when small moving objects must be followed. If an ophthalmologist recommends it, a therapist or teacher can help strengthen the weaker eye by fixing a patch over the stronger eye. Training in visual-motor coordination is an important aspect of an adapted physical education program for the cerebral palsied. Training activities (games) can be introduced that stress accurate fixation on targets at near, mid, and far points in space. Children can develop effective visual guidance systems by using both sides of the body to throw, push,

and kick balls at wall targets and ground targets which are set at various distances.

Neuromuscular function in physical education class is dependent upon the child's level and quality of sensorimotor performance, the status of his postural reflexes, and his muscle tone. Regardless of the severity of his defect, every student integrates sensory information about the environment through visual, tactile, proprioceptive, and vestibular modalities. This integration provides the basis for the child's awareness of his body, its position, and its balance. It is also the basis for motor planning and the development of form and space perception.

The Bobath neurodevelopmental method of treatment for neurologic disorders is a popular form of motor therapy.[27] The method is directed toward the inhibition of abnormal reflex activity and the facilitation of normal automatic movement. Neurodevelopmental training (NDT) is a highly specialized field, and readers can refer to standardized texts for more detailed discussions on the subject of neurophysiology. Various opinions exist regarding whether a physical education teacher or therapeutic recreation specialist should follow a strict NDT program during physical activity sessions. Most authorities agree that physical education and recreational programming should focus on 2 general areas: (1) enhancing physical development through exploration of body parts and (2) emphasizing psychosocial growth instead of relying on strict neurodevelopmental methods which elicit desired movements through positional manipulation. It is critical, however, that the teacher or therapist understand some basic concepts of NDT. In general, the child should be positioned comfortably so that head, trunk, and pelvic control precede movements of the extremities. Proper postural positioning is important because it facilitates normal movement patterns and inhibits abnormal postural reflex patterns.

Zimmerman states that therapists facilitate and inhibit muscles every time they touch a patient. Choosing where and how your hands are placed maximizes the input to the appropriate alpha motor neurons and the chances for a successful motor response.

Examples of tactile cues are (1) facilitatory input to a muscle (tapping the quadriceps prior to active knee extension) and (2) a directional touch (tapping the arm forward as a reminder of proper alignment in weightbearing).

An example of a proprioceptive cue is joint compression (compression at the shoulder toward the palm in all fours) to facilitate upper extremity weightbearing.[28]

Through these efforts, basic performance skills and measurable goals can be achieved. Once definitive motor responses are identified, it would seem appropriate for a recreational or adapted physical education teacher to apply tactile and proprioceptive cues to reach desired objectives.

Many children with moderate to severe involvement will need structural changes in their environment to

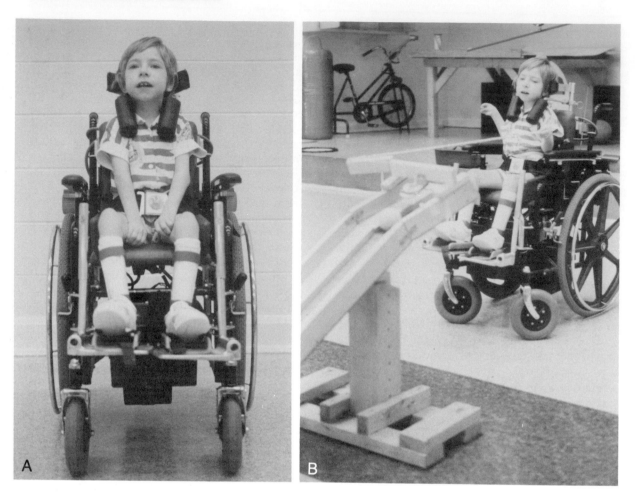

Fig. 4–29. A, This young girl with mixed cerebral palsy exhibits limited mobility of the trunk and shoulder girdles (usually protracted and in internal rotation). B, Adapted devices such as ramps and chutes are especially helpful in ball-related activities to compensate for lack of hand function. A quick release bar is opened creating space for the roll of the ball. It is activated by a volitional flexor pattern pull on a cord attached to the lever and hand. The device allows for independent operation during low organized games.

compensate for lack of strength and poor neuro-muscular development. Finnie[29] gives many practical suggestions for structuring the environment so that the child with cerebral palsy may comfortably explore his surroundings and engage in play. She suggests that a child who is severely restricted in movement be placed on a bolster or sloping board, because this allows the child to lie on his stomach with his head up and his arms forward in a position for functional use of the hands. The child will need continual help and encouragement from members of the family to touch, hold, and manipulate toys.

Movement experiences for the elementary school-aged child with CP are critical. Equipment adaptations to facilitate independence are often required (Fig. 4–29). Normally, at ages 6 and 7 a child appears to be in constant motion: wrestling, playing tag, tumbling, and running with other children. Unfortunately, cerebral palsied children are usually limited in their scope of movement due to varying degrees of motor involvement. Involvement in play must be stim-

ulated in part by members of the family (Fig. 4–30). Therapists provide assistance through a general guidance system, while offering suggestions for specific handling techniques and developmental growth. Many children with CP do not learn by spontaneous active curiosity. Consequently they need stimulation if their cognitive powers (attention span, ability to concentrate, audio visual discriminatory powers, etc.) are to be improved.

Programs in developmental play and sensory-motor training can be incorporated into therapeutic recreation and adapted physical education activities. Use can be made of various pieces of equipment (such as peg boards and sticks for copying patterns and teaching spatial relationships, and blocks of different sizes and textures for matching). Scooter boards are especially good for developing proficient muscular control while maintaining body symmetry. A tricycle is an excellent aide for stimulating hip flexor and extensor muscles and developing reciprocal patterns in the lower extremities.

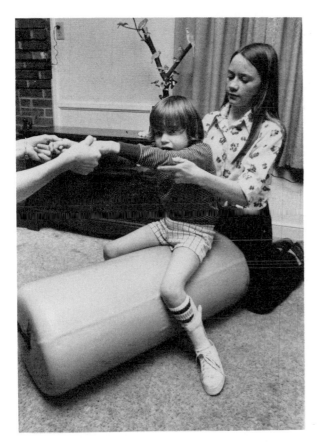

Fig. 4–30. Facilitation of equilibrium reactions through the use of a bolster. This 9-year-old child with cerebral palsy, spastic diplegic type, had the typical hyperactive reflexes with increased spasticity and involvement on the left side.

The person with hemiparesis needs particular consideration since physical education class and competitive youth sports often place him in situations that require normal peer relationships. Most students are integrated into regular school settings because their physical, emotional, and intellectual deficiencies are so mild that special treatment and educational techniques are unnecessary.

Unilateral involvement can include paralysis or weakness. Occasional pathologic reflexes are present on the affected side. A major physical problem of the lower extremity can be adduction of the leg at the hip joint, causing a flexion deformity at the hip. The calf muscles are usually very spastic, and the dorsiflexors on the foot are usually weak, leading to a plantar-flexion deformity of the foot. Occasionally, a short leg-brace is worn until there is control of dorsiflexion and eversion of the foot. In the upper extremity, the main handicaps are flexion of the forearm at the elbow, and hypertonia of the rotators of the forearm and the flexors of the wrist and fingers.

In evaluating the person, many observations can be made during the initial physical education or therapeutic recreation session. For example, is the affected hand used for holding, helping, transferring, playing, assisting the dominant hand, or is it completely ignored? This is an index, too, of the patient's intelligence, cooperation, independence, and motivation.

In selecting activities for elementary school children, the basic urges for adventure, social competence, and approval should be given the utmost consideration. Two-handed activities that can be encouraged are climbing, swinging, and hammering. Locomotor skills such as jumping, skipping, and hopping are good for teaching rhythm and improving balance. Kicking a ball is excellent training, because the child has to either kick the ball with his affected foot while his non-affected leg supports his weight, or kick the ball with his non-affected foot while his affected leg supports his weight.

The student with hemiparesis should participate in physical education class and in sports within the scope of his ability. Basketball, cycling, rowing, horseback riding, and billiards are activities that encourage the use of both hands. Throwing, kicking, and catching large balls stimulate bimanual activity and balance reactions from the affected leg.

Once the child reaches school age, program guidelines should be provided so he can participate successfully in group situations which foster learning, encourage self-expression, and help the child in social interaction with other children.

1. Excitement and tension must be avoided. Abnormal reflex patterns are frequently elicited by sudden noise, stress, or surprise. The classic Moro (startle) reflex is sudden extension or spreading of the upper extremities (hand signals should substitute for high shrill of a whistle).

2. Simplify the activity so that the cerebral palsied child can accomplish the task. For example, a ring-toss game can be adjusted for distance. If the individual cannot grasp or throw, place the target under foot and simply permit him to drop the ring on the target. Use lighter or heavier rings when necessary. Exaggerated stretch reflex patterns (when arm reaches forward or upward, it is jerked by the antagonists) are often present. A one-to-one relationship between child and instructor may be required in certain situations.

3. Free gross motor movements that aid in movement exploration are much better than those involving fine finger dexterity. Skill perfection should not be emphasized, but instead a program without complicated rules and regulations in which body-object-space relationships (grasp, release, joint flexion, and extension) are emphasized. Examples include bean bag games, ball rolling or throwing (with or without ramps) at targets, and kite flying. The spastic child typically holds the wrist and fingers in a fist due to hypertonic flexor muscles. It is important not to include activities that encourage or require a fisted hand.

Horseback riding is an increasingly popular therapeutic sport for cerebral palsied children. Self-control and mastery over a moving animal are important achievements for cerebral palsied children. In addition, the constant shifting and maintenance of sitting balance stimulates reflex and postural responses. Good body symmetry and head alignment are prerequisites for achievement, therefore the rider must be able to control his posture before he can develop the coordination patterns necessary for successful riding.

Swimming is an excellent activity for persons with cerebral palsy. Obviously, training in relaxation techniques while in the water is very important, and this is often done with the aid of flotation devices while the swimmer is in a supine position. Righting and supporting reactions are stimulated, and the resistance of the water stimulates static muscle control and activates resistive dynamic motions.

A cerebral palsied child may experience several hospitalizations for diagnostic evaluation, orthopedic management, and/or medical care. A therapeutic recreation specialist should be an important part of the integrated program of therapy. The therapist can engage the patient in play or recreational activities and still meet specific treatment goals.

Frequently, surgical treatment places a child with cerebral palsy in a hospital for a brief period of time. After the physician submits a postoperative plan, the therapist needs to concentrate on specific objectives, and in most cases, a general plan is coordinated with the specific objectives of physical and occupational therapy. Recreational programming can focus on the exercise objectives indicated by physical therapy, and at the same time it can complement occupational therapy by using games as techniques to improve coordination. One of the first goals of therapy is to overcome the persistence of infantile reflexes through positioning and relaxation. Next, the therapist needs to focus on specific physical and psychologic objectives. If standing is a major objective for the postoperative patient, games can be played while the patient is in the upright position. (Standing is often facilitated by the use of braces, casts, crutches and other standing appliances.) Manipulative activities (ball handling, bean bags, peg boards) that involve active upper extremity control and joint extension should be encouraged for the patient who uses a wheelchair.

Considerations for Controlling Spasticity

When working with patients with varying degrees of spasticity, it is important to maintain symmetry and work from the mid-line position. This is done to establish a base of support for better postural tone and controlled movements of the arms. Any attempts at rotational movements of the trunk will often increase abnormal tone and inefficient movement. Strapping of the legs or trunk might be useful to assist in controlling postural tone (Fig. 4–31) but should only be done after consulting with a physical therapist. The term fixation is often used to describe stiffening of whole body parts to execute a specific movement such as striking a suspended beachball. Spastic CP children use these compensatory patterns for stability and mobility. However, these types of movements are energy consuming and the instructor or therapist will need to monitor rate and degree of effort when performing a particular skill. Intermittent task oriented requirements should be brief and not extended for long periods of time without rest intervals.

Therapeutic Exercises

Cerebral palsy is a condition in which the child can have varying degrees of involvement. To further complicate the exercise program, there are different types of cerebral palsy such as spastic, athetoid, and ataxic.

The following exercises are listed to serve only as a guide. The instructor or therapist will not use all the therapeutic exercises but only those that will be beneficial in the total treatment of the child. Obviously, the type of cerebral palsy and general condition of the child must be considered before planning the exercise program. All of the exercises should be approved by a physician.

Appendix A
1. Exercises for the upper back
   Exercises 1 through 17
2. Exercises for the lower back and for the abdominal muscles
   Exercises 18 through 42
3. Exercises for the hip
   Exercises 43 through 63
4. Exercises for the knee
   Exercises 64 through 80
5. Exercises for the ankle
   Exercises 81 through 95
6. Exercises for the fingers
   Exercises 96 through 110
7. Exercises for the wrist
   Exercises 111 through 117
8. Exercises for the elbow
   Exercises 118 through 124
9. Exercises for the shoulder
   Exercises 125 through 138
10. Exercises for the head and neck
    Exercises 139, 140, 141
11. Exercises for deep breathing
    Exercises 142 through 146

General Exercises

There is no evidence to indicate that strength training leads to an increase in muscle tone or spasticity.

General exercises and weight training may be used for the child who is not severely disabled.

Appendices B and C

Crutches

Many children who have cerebral palsy will require braces and crutches for independent ambulation. The

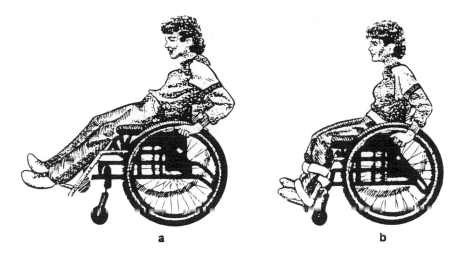

Fig. 4–31. *A,* Class III athlete demonstrating an extension pattern. *B,* Use of proper strapping can diminish extension problems. (Courtesy of Human Kinetics Publishers. From Boyd, R. and Grass, K., The Use of Strapping to Enhance the Athletic Competitors in Cerebral Palsy Sports. In Jones, J. (1988), Training Guide to CP Sports.)

type of crutch gait will vary with degree of involvement and the condition of the child.

Appendix D

Competitive Sports

The United States Cerebral Palsy Athletic Association (USCPAA)

The USCPAA governs sports opportunities for cerebral palsied athletes, and is an established subcommittee of the United States Olympic Committee. The USCPAA is dedicated to assisting local, state, and regional groups in conducting competitive meets from which outstanding athletes qualify for National Games. The outgrowth of achievement in the National Games leads to international competition.

Depending upon each individual case, some athletes participate in team sports, while others excel in individual sports. The three team sports are soccer, team handball, and boccia. Individual sports include archery, bowling, bicycling and tricycling, track and field (Fig. 4–32), horseback riding, swimming, rifle shooting, slalom, table tennis, and weight lifting.

It should be pointed out that the athlete with cerebral palsy may have an associated handicapping condition. It is possible that the motor deficit is not the most severe impairment. Other deficits may include learning disability, hearing impairment, visual impairment, and mental retardation to name a few. Grouped under multiply handicapped, athletes who are mentally retarded participate in Special Olympics as opposed to competing in USCPAA events.

Classification System

Class I. Quadriplegic with severe involvement. Limited functional ability necessitates use of a motorized wheelchair or assistance for mobility.

Class II. Quadriplegic with severe to moderate involvement. Wheelchair-user, often able to move chair with feet or very slowly with arms. Poor functional control of upper-body movements.

Class III. Quadriplegic with moderate involvement. Wheelchair-user, functional control and strength of upper-torso and extremities.

Class IV. Wheelchair-user, but good functional control and strength of upper-torso and extremities. Lower limbs have moderate to severe involvement.

Class V. May walk with assistive devices, and good functional control and strength of upper-torso and extremities.

Class VI. Quadriplegic with moderate to severe involvement, but able to ambulate independently. More involvement of upper-extremities.

Class VII. Hemiplegic with minimal to moderate involvement, but has good functional usage on non-affected side.

Class VIII. Hemiplegic with minimal involvement. Good balance and coordination skills.

Abnormal movement and posture are concerns to overcome for the cerebral palsied athlete. To achieve functional performance levels, proper alignment of the spine, pelvis, lower extremities, and in some cases the upper extremities needs special attention. For this reason, various strapping techniques are used to enhance competitive skills.

The typical pattern of movement elicited in cerebral palsy is the extension pattern characterized by hip, knee, and trunk extension, hip adduction and internal rotation, and ankle plantar flexion (toe pointing). This describes the position of an athlete who essentially ends up lying in his or her wheelchair when exerting maximal effort during competition (Fig. 4–31A). In turn, the angle between the athlete and his or her wheel axle is increased, and the ability of the athlete to provide a full stroke on the handrim is decreased. In conjunction with wheelchair design, strapping can be used to diminish these problems (Fig. 4–31B).[30]

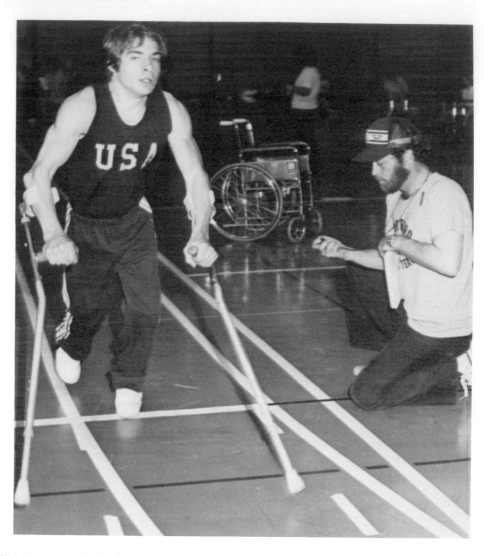

Fig. 4–32. Class V athlete with cerebral palsy completing a 400-meter race in the National Games. (Courtesy of the United States Cerebral Palsy Athletic Association.)

Various additional strapping techniques are used to control spastic patterns and athetoid movements, and to achieve safety requirements during competition but will not be discussed due to space limitations.

CHRONIC OBSTRUCTIVE LUNG DISEASE

The respiratory system (Fig. 4–33) is divided into the upper and lower tracts. The upper tract includes the nose, pharynx, larynx, and trachea; the lower tract is made up of the lung structure, including the bronchi. This discussion will be limited to the more common chronic obstructive pulmonary diseases: bronchial asthma, emphysema and chronic bronchitis, and cystic fibrosis.

The lungs are the organs of respiration for aeration of the blood. They are paired and occupy both halves of the chest cavity. The right lung is divided into 3 lobes: the upper, middle, and lower lobes; the left lung has 2 lobes: the upper lobe and the lower lobe.

Exchange of gases between the air and the blood takes place within these lobes. The air we breathe flows to and from each lobe of the lung through an airway that starts with the windpipe, or trachea, and then divides into two main branches called primary bronchi. From these, additional passages branch out so that the appearance of the structure is like that of a tree with its branches pointed in many directions; thus, the term *bronchial tree* is frequently used to describe this airway system.

In such a complex system, a number of problems can develop: ventilation can be impaired by mucus and other fluids which can block the passageways: the walls of the tiny air sacs (alveoli) can break down, forming internal spaces in which air becomes trapped; and infections and irritants can cause tissues to swell and close the air tubes.

Bronchial Asthma

Bronchial asthma is a disorder of the respiratory system characterized by dyspnea, wheezing, tightness

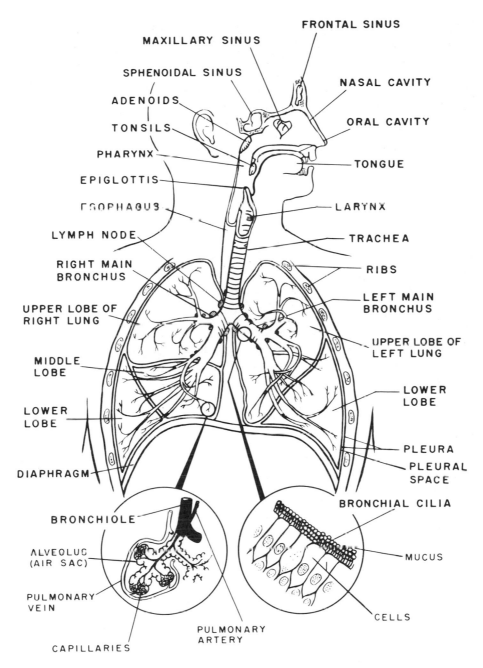

Fig. 4–33. The respiratory system. (Courtesy of the National Tuberculosis and Respiratory Disease Association.)

in the chest, and bronchospasm. Acute attacks may be short in duration, or they may be severe and last for days or weeks.

The primary disturbance in bronchial asthma occurs in the smaller bronchi and bronchioles, where there is spasm of the smooth muscle, or inflammatory edema of the mucosa, or both (Fig. 4–34).

Between attacks of asthma, the bronchi and the lungs resume their normal appearance in most cases, and permanent damage to the bronchi and lungs rarely occurs, even in patients who have had asthma for many years.

Causes

The nature of asthma is complex. With respect to cause, however, two types of asthma will be discussed here: allergic or extrinsic asthma and nonallergic or intrinsic asthma.

Nonallergic or Intrinsic Asthma

Nonallergic or intrinsic asthma usually occurs in adults with no previous history of allergy. No specific cause of the asthmatic attacks can be identified, but infection, fatigue, and emotional factors may precipitate an attack.

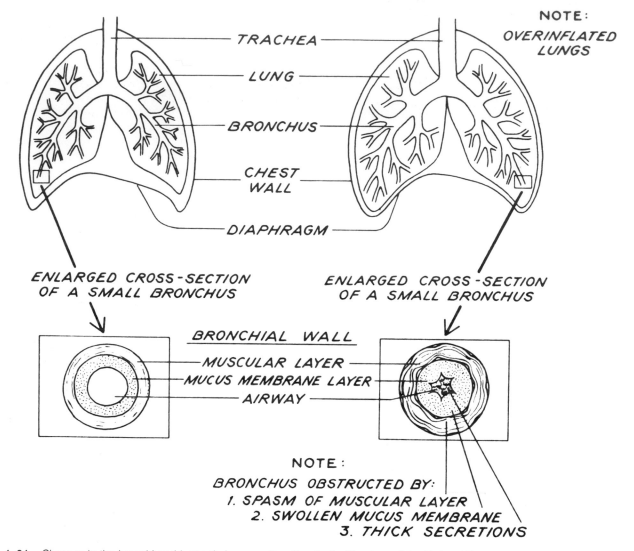
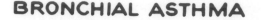

Fig. 4–34.   Changes in the bronchi and lungs during an asthmatic attack. (Courtesy of the National Tuberculosis and Respiratory Disease Association.)

Allergic or Extrinsic Asthma

Allergic or extrinsic asthma tends to occur in children and young adults with a previous history of allergy (sensitivity to a normally harmless substance) in the form of hay fever, hives, or eczema. The person becomes sensitized to some agent, such as pollens, dust, molds, drugs, animal hair, or a wide variety of other substances, and asthma develops.

Allergy-Provoking Substances. Program leaders should be aware of the causes of allergic bronchial asthma. Pollen, dust, molds, and animal emanations are the common allergens, but nonspecific factors such as cold air, high humidity, or respiratory tract infection can aggravate allergic bronchial asthma. Identification of the causative factors is important, as activities need to be carefully selected to eliminate exposure to an allergen and/or situation that will produce symptoms.

Pollen. The individual who is allergic to pollen is worse outdoors, better indoors. The asthma is generally worse on bright, sunny days, and the individual often complains of "itchy eyes". The pollen count is high from August until the first frost. Grass is a common offender in May and June.

Dust. The individual who is allergic to dust is worse indoors, better outdoors. The eyes do not itch; however, the individual tends to be worse after he goes to bed. The gymnasium mat or bed mattress are examples of prime generators of dust.

Molds. The individual who has an allergy to molds has more difficulty in damp weather and in the cool of the evening. The asthma is worse when the child plays in the grass. Seasonal peaks are summer and fall. The shower room is a prime generator.

Animal Emanations. Cats and dogs are the worst offenders. Horseback riding should be discouraged for those who are allergic to horse dander.

The Asthmatic Patient's Chest

A succinct description of the chest of the asthmatic (Fig. 4–35) is given by Gay:

As a consequence of the abnormal respiratory function, gross changes occur in the general structure of the asthmatic chest. The veins of the neck may be engorged. Repeated attacks produce deformity in early childhood before ossification of cartilaginous junctions occurs and the chest becomes fixed in an elevated distended position with marked increase in the costal angle. The sternum may become prominent, the ribs may assume a more horizontal position, and the anterior-posterior diameter may become equal to or greater than the lateral diameter. There is a tendency for the shoulders to become elevated and for kyphosis of the spine to become greatly exaggerated. As a consequence of the abnormally high value of the intrathoracic negative pressure, there may also develop a marked asymmetry of the bony structure of the right and left chests.[31]

Similar changes occur during the acute phase of almost any asthmatic episode, but they do not become fixed, except after a number of attacks, particularly in childhood. Essentially, the reason for the changes is the difficulty experienced during expiration.[32]

Incidence

It has been estimated that 23 of every 1,000 persons (2.3%) in the United States have bronchial asthma. The disease affects all age groups and both sexes.

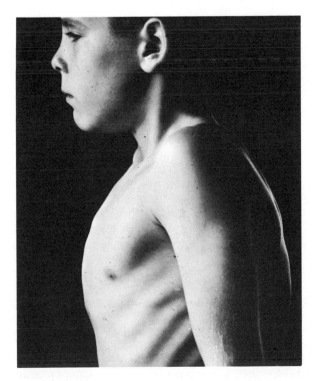

Fig. 4–35. Chest of an asthmatic patient.

Treatment

Hyposensitization injections to help develop antibodies against various substances may be of value for pollen-sensitive individuals, but elimination of environmental allergens is the primary objective. If this is impossible, then reduced exposure to the allergen by careful dust control or air conditioning is beneficial.

Bronchodilator drugs are often recommended to relieve bronchospasm. These include the xanthine derivatives, ephedrine, and corticosteroids.

The xanthine drugs, such as aminophylline, are the most effective medications for asthma. Side effects, which are usually brief, include nausea, vomiting, headaches, and restlessness.

Ephedrine is an effective bronchodilator and is often given separately, or in combination with xanthines. Epinephrine is another common drug that is often used if xanthine derivatives and/or ephedrine have failed. Epinephrine usually relieves obstruction by reducing edema and smooth muscle spasm.

Cromolyn sodium, a relatively new drug, represents an exciting advance in the treatment of asthma. Because the drug is prophylactic, it provides a radically new approach to patient management. It is the first drug that blocks the body from releasing the chemicals that lead to asthmatic attacks. Unlike the older drugs that counteract the chemicals once they have been released, cromolyn sodium prevents the mast cells from releasing their asthma-promoting chemicals. It should be noted, however, that cromolyn sodium has no effect on, and cannot be used to treat, an acute asthmatic attack. (See Table 4–2 for further information on cromolyn sodium.)

Corticosteroid drugs are frequently the only means of controlling persistent severe asthma when other therapeutic measures have failed. Some physicians find it necessary to place chronic persistent severe asthmatics on steroids to prevent permanent changes, similar to those that occur in emphysema, from taking place in the lung. Prolonged corticosteroid therapy can lead to serious complications: its interference with normal metabolism of protein and calcium steroids may lead to osteoporosis and spontaneous fractures.

There is general agreement among physicians that most children with bronchial asthma should attend regular school, since, when under proper control and with no residual pulmonary defect, the child needs no special facilities. However, in certain instances, special environmental facilities for rest periods, drug therapy, and other treatment may be needed.

Program Implications

Both physical and mental activities are useful to asthmatic children. Recent evidence indicates that most allergic asthmatics can participate in normal school physical education, community recreation, and sports programs. With proper medical management, the majority of asthmatics can participate in active

Table 4–2.
Suggested Drug Dosages for Exercise Induced Asthma

Drug	Dosage	Route of Administration	Time of Administration (Prior to Exercise)	Accepted at International Competition
Theophylline	5–8 mg/kg	Orally	1 hour	Yes
Dyphylline	15 mg/kg	Orally	1 hour	Yes
Theophylline-ephedrine combinations	½ tablet (5-10 years) 1 tablet (10+ years)	Orally	1 hour	No
Isoproterenol	14 micrograms/aerosol	Aerosol	5 minutes–30 minutes	No
Metaproterenol	20 mg/dose (12+ years)	Orally/Aerosol	1 hour	No
Terbutaline	5 mg/dose (12+ years)	Orally	1 hour	No
Cromolyn sodium	20 mg/dose	Inhalation	5–20 minutes	Yes

(Courtesy of the American Medical Association.)

sports. The risk of an asthmatic attack can be reduced by having the child take proper medication before exercise or by modifying the extent of work output through controlled exercise. Fatigue and emotional stress from athletic contests precipitate asthmatic attacks in some children, particularly those with non-allergic asthma, but, as a general rule, restrictions should be minimal, and activity should be limited only when the condition of the child makes it necessary.

With proper medical management, the majority of asthmatic children can participate in school physical education, although children with severe asthma should avoid sports involving body contact. Noncontact sports (e.g., tennis) and gymnastics (e.g., rope climbing, parallel bars) are recommended for the asthmatic child, depending upon his tolerance for duration of activity and intensity of effort. In a study by Verma and Hyde,[33] 316 physical education instructors described their experiences with asthmatic children and their methods of dealing with the problems exhibited by these children. The study showed that 98% of the instructors were permitting pupils to attend regular gym classes; 76% allowed students to limit activity by their own judgment; 47% provided exercises which they thought the children would tolerate. Many students use prophylactic bronchodilators prior to exercise.

Periodic reviews of the health of the asthmatic child should be made. Written records of periodic health evaluations performed by the pediatrician or family physician who is managing the patient should be on file in the office of the school nurse or physician. Physicians who care for asthmatic children can be more useful to their patients if they are familiar with the physical education and athletic programs in the school. Medical evaluation of the child with chronic or recurrent symptoms should include tests for allergens performed by a competent allergist who is also knowledgeable about the growth and development of children. Children who are predisposed to allergies may also be more prone to asthma during the seasons in which their allergens abound.

One of the most important results of asthma is the mental suffering and loss of initiative and confidence which arise from the physical handicap. Adaptation-conditioning or confidence-building activities, which are grouped under the term combatives, are encouraged for asthmatics with good kinesiologic skills. Judo is becoming a popular physical conditioning activity for asthmatics. In it, they are primarily taught graceful movement, proper body mechanics, and rapidity of action. All these factors lead to the conservation of energy, which is an obvious necessity for the asthmatic. It is felt that combatives, including karate and wrestling, aid the asthmatic in combating his disease as well as improving his adjustment to individual and group activities and to life in general.

Tumbling, vaulting, and martial arts are excellent activities for asthmatics. These activities are especially good for developing muscular flexibility, balance, agility, and coordination. The changes in body position that occur in these activities are therapeutically valuable, particularly at the end of expiration, because they loosen mucus in the bronchioles. However, it is important to remember that the intensity of these activities should be adjusted to the condition of the child. A sustained program with limited rest periods will often be exhausting for, if not hazardous to, asthmatics with low tolerance for exercise.

Swimming is an excellent activity because it combines use of all muscle groups with practical breathing exercises. It also improves physical development and thoracic expansion and helps prevent secondary deformities such as kyphosis and rounded shoulders with contracted pectoral muscles.

Precautions. Occasionally, a child with asthma may be fatigued by a previous severe asthmatic episode or other illness such as an upper-respiratory tract infection. Under such circumstances, the child is unable to maintain a normal level of exercise. In addition, secondary factors such as fatigue and general malaise frequently increase pulmonary hyperreactivity. Therefore, certain adjustments may be necessary in the daily routine. Participation in an adapted or individualized sports and recreation program should be encouraged until the child's condition is stabilized and under adequate control.

Parents and teachers should avoid making the child feel inferior or different from other children. Occasionally, asthmatic children display secondary emotional problems because of extended periods of pulmonary distress and for other reasons. Some children become timid or obsessed with their own problems, while others use their breathing problems as a means of coercion to gain attention and avoid competition at school. It is desirable, however, for asthmatics to participate in physical education activities with as little restriction as possible.

Some children use nebulizers to obtain prompt relief by self-administering epinephrine, or its equivalent, in aerosol form. The aerosols relieve symptoms quickly, but are dangerous if overused. The physical education teacher should be concerned if a student overuses or relies on a nebulizer during class activities. Under such circumstances the teacher should consult with the parents and physician to find out if a nebulizer has been prescribed and what the conditions are surrounding its use.

Exercise Induced Asthma

In some individuals, physical stress triggers asthmatic attacks. In these cases, the parasympathetic nervous system is thought to play a prominent role in bringing on the symptoms. Exercise induced asthma (EIA) is described as 5 to 8 minutes of sustained exercise (at maximum oxygen consumption and with a heart rate of up to 180 beats per minute) followed by significant bronchospasm during a 5- to 15-minute rest phase. This phenomenon has been reported in up to 95% of asthmatic children and in up to 40% of atopic, nonasthmatic children.[34]

If a person has a history of long-standing, exercise induced asthma, exercise involving intermittent exertion and inactivity, such as ball games, are more suitable than exercises that are uninterrupted, such as long distance track. Research clearly indicates that extended periods of full exertion, as in handball and tennis, are far more likely to produce EIA. In some cases, the occurrence of exercise induced asthma can be made less probable by: (1) general conditioning programs; and (2) intense warm-up periods prior to strenuous physical activity.

If a child with EIA who wishes to play contact sports can either limit his exertion to intervals of less than 5 minutes or work at a submaximal level, then asthma may not occur. One method of safeguarding against an EIA attack is known as the "limited participation

method." For example, a coach or physical education instructor could assign a player to a fullback position in soccer as opposed to a front line position in which sustained effort is required. This would place the player in a position requiring less work output, thereby lessening the risk of an EIA attack. However, this merely reduces the risk of an attack. There is no guarantee that a player participating at a submaximal level in a controlled situation will not have an EIA attack, because asthma can be aggravated by other nonallergic factors, such as infection or emotional stress, even during moderate exercise.

Because a high percentage of asthmatic children have EIA, the physical education instructor or activity leader should understand the aspects of drug therapy for EIA that relate to patient management. The following considerations are important: (1) prophylactic bronchodilators should be used prior to exercise; and (2) if administered promptly, adequate amounts of bronchodilators will abort an asthmatic attack or reverse a bronchospasm after it begins.

Table 4–2 provides basic information regarding the management of asthmatics who are limited by EIA.

Therapeutic Exercises

Breathing exercises can strengthen the respiratory muscles, provide better ventilation, and bring about a more efficient pattern of breathing. The asthmatic can be started on a diaphragmatic exercise plan after a physician has approved one. Concentration needs to focus on lifting the abdomen when inhaling. When exhaling, air needs to be expelled as slowly as possible.

Appendix A
    Exercises for deep breathing
    Exercises 142 through 146
The following exercises may be used as an adjunct therapy for asthmatics with general posture problems. These exercises are to be done between breathing exercises.

Appendix A
1. Exercises for the upper back
    Exercises 1 through 17
2. Exercises for the lower back
    Exercises 18 through 31
3. Exercises for abdominal muscles
    Exercises 32 through 42
A dry spirometer can be used to measure vital lung capacity at different pre- and post-exercise levels.

General Exercises

General exercises and weight training are recommended.

The exercises must be started gradually and increased according to the tolerance of the individual. The exercises will aid in building self-confidence and will encourage participation in future activities. General conditioning exercises are good because the focus of attention is away from the disease.

Appendices B and C

Emphysema and Chronic Bronchitis

Emphysema is by far the most common chronic disease of the lungs. Many victims are completely unaware that they have emphysema until after 50% or more of their lung function has been destroyed. In emphysema, the thin walls of the alveoli lose their elasticity and tear, causing large, inefficient air spaces. As a result, resistance to air flow increases, and breathing becomes progressively more difficult.

Exactly what causes the tissue destruction of emphysema is unknown; however, most reports indicate that cigarette smoking is the most significant factor in the development of the disease. Repeated exposure to lung irritants, polluted air, dusts, and molds are aggravating factors. Certain chronic illnesses, such as bronchitis, asthma, silicosis, and other chronic pulmonary problems, are also thought to favor the development of emphysema.

Some of the early symptoms of emphysema are wheezing and chronic coughing. Another symptom, dyspnea (labored breathing), may vary from mild distress after exertion to severe gasping episodes and cyanosis (blueness of the lips and skin caused by an insufficient amount of oxygen in the blood) even when the patient is resting.

Some forms of emphysema are usually not disabling. The disease ranges from mild to severe and is relentlessly progressive and seriously disabling only when an obstructive element is present with generalized involvement of the bronchial tree and the alveolar system. If emphysema is treated with proper care in the earlier stages, it often can be arrested.

Chronic bronchitis is an inflammation of the bronchial tree and the presence and persistence of cough and sputum. This condition coexists with pulmonary emphysema in many patients, and this group has been the subject of extensive research.

Bronchitis involves a thickening of the inner lining of the bronchial tubes, especially the large ones, which narrows the airways. Repeated irritation of the lining of the bronchial airways can destroy the action of the cilia (minute hairlike projections which sweep foreign particles and excess secretions out of the lungs) and cause excessive secretion of mucus. Coughing, which forces up secretions and which can be violent, may be the major symptom of the disease. The lung tissue may be damaged as the coughing and spitting become more frequent. In patients with advanced chronic bronchitis, airway obstruction is mainly irreversible because of structural damage to the bronchi.

Incidence

Adequate statistics on the prevalence of emphysema and chronic bronchitis are not available. It is thought that emphysema disables one out of every 14 wage earners over 45 years old; and emphysema is second only to heart disease as a cause of industrial disability. Emphysema strikes men about 7 times more often than it strikes women.

Treatment

Present therapeutic measures are aimed at arresting or slowing down the progress of emphysema or chronic bronchitis, relieving its distressing symptoms, improving the patient's general physical condition, and helping him make the best possible use of whatever lung function remains. As in the treatment of asthma, bronchodilators are often useful. Usually administered with inhalers, these drugs help to open up constricted air passages.

A number of portable oxygen devices have been developed for the ambulatory patient with emphysema, and some of them are compact enough to be carried in a pocket, briefcase, or purse. The oxygen output of these devices can be adjusted to meet the oxygen needs of the patient. Other mechanical devices are designed to assist the patient in breathing by increasing his intra-abdominal pressure. They are compact and light enough to be worn by the patient without interfering with his activity.

Program Implications

Emphysema primarily afflicts persons over 40 years of age; consequently, selecting of sports and games depends upon a number of factors. Naturally, the age of the individual and extent of lung damage will determine the type and amount of activity that he can tolerate without excessive fatigue. Quiet nonstrenuous activities, such as fishing, shuffleboard, lawn croquet, and billiards, are recommended, since many victims of emphysema have limited lung function. Each patient should know his limitations and rest whenever breathing problems develop. Social contact is essential in any recreational program for those with chronic lung disease.

Precautions. The patient with emphysema should not become nervous or excited since forceful efforts at breathing are likely to squeeze the airways shut, thus trapping more air in the lungs.

Therapeutic Exercises

Patients with emphysema and chronic bronchitis should be started on a breathing exercise routine after approval is obtained from the physician.

Appendix A
   Exercises for deep breathing
   Exercises 142 through 146

The purpose of training in breathing is to teach the patient maneuvers that can help him overcome some of the expiratory obstruction and facilitate emptying the lungs of air. Patients are inclined to expect improvement in lung function as a result of performing the exercises, so it must be explained that the techniques do not change the lung itself and are useful only as long as they are practiced. The patient is taught to inhale through the nose and then to exhale slowly, evenly, and deeply against pursed lips while contracting the abdominal muscles. The patient first learns to do this in the supine position, then in the sitting position, and, ultimately, while walking.

The following exercises may be used as an adjunct therapy for patients with posture problems.

Appendix A

1. Exercises for the upper back
   Exercises 1 through 17
2. Exercises for the lower back
   Exercises 18 through 31
3. Exercises for abdominal muscles
   Exercises 32 through 42

General Exercises

General exercises and weight training are recommended.

Appendices B and C

The exercises must be started gradually and increased cautiously. Careful consideration must be given to the patient's respiratory disorder.

Physical training consisting of daily walks at submaximal speeds improves the physical work efficiency of patients with chronic obstructive lung disease and allows them to perform a greater amount of work.

Cystic Fibrosis (CF)

Cystic fibrosis is a disease genetically inherited as a mendelian recessive trait, which means that both parents carry a gene for the disease. According to Mendel's law, this means that the condition may appear in one quarter of the children of such unions.

Cystic fibrosis is a disturbance of the exocrine glands (glands that secrete mucus, saliva, and sweat) which causes chemically, or physically, abnormal secretions. The underlying cause of the abnormal sweat, mucus, and saliva is not known.

The most serious effects of cystic fibrosis result from the mucus, which is unusually thick and sticky and which interferes with the functioning of the lungs and the digestive system. In the lungs, viscous mucus obstructs the smaller breathing tubes and leads to infection which can damage the airway walls and lung tissue. If the mucus blocks the ducts of the pancreas, enzymes needed for digestion cannot reach the small intestine, and the child will have foul-smelling, bulky stools and may suffer from malnutrition.

The most useful and reliable diagnostic test for cystic fibrosis is the sweat test, an analysis of the sodium and chloride concentration of the sweat. Sweat glands in a small area of the skin are stimulated by application of a dilute solution of pilocarpine and a weak electric current. Sweat is collected on a weighed gauze pad or filter paper under a plastic barrier. The sweat test has made diagnosis of cystic fibrosis relatively easy. Diagnosis is frequently made prior to 6 months of age, but it can be made at any age.

For many years, chronic undernutrition, with weight retardation and linear growth failure, has been recognized as a problem in most large cystic fibrosis clinic populations and, despite acknowledgment of its seriousness, was felt to be a natural consequence of the disease. More recently, there is some debate over the correlation of the severity of malnutrition and accelerated decline in pulmonary function. As lung disease worsens, a point is reached where the patient cannot ingest enough calories to maintain energy balance. Once progressive weight loss occurs, then reduced survival is likely. Over time, lean-tissue wasting might affect respiratory muscle strength, and also affect lung elasticity and immune function.[35]

The prognosis has improved dramatically, since children with CF in the 1950s often failed to survive until elementary school age. Today, more than half of the individuals with CF are living into their mid-twenties and beyond.

Incidence

Cystic fibrosis is the most serious lung problem affecting children in this country today. It occurs in approximately one in every 1,000 to 2,000 births. As many as 2 to 5% of the general population may carry the gene. The incidence is greatest among Caucasians and rare in black infants.

Treatment

As the effects on the lungs are usually the primary problem in patients with cystic fibrosis, treatment is directed toward assisting the child to remove the thick secretions of mucus from his lungs. Some of the treatment aids are as follows:

Aerosols. Aerosol therapy may be given by mask or nebulizer to relieve heavy secretions of mucus from the bronchi. In this type of therapy, various medications are deposited directly in the tracheobronchial tree. Medications may include water or salt particles, bronchodilators, decongestants, mucolytic agents, or antibiotics.

Postural Drainage. This type of physical therapy helps move mucus from smaller airways into larger airways where it can be coughed up. Postural drainage may be performed one or more times a day, often in the morning after awakening and before bedtime.

Digestive problems are controlled by supplements of pancreatic enzymes.

Clinical appointments are scheduled on a regular basis. Pulmonary function tests (Fig. 4–36), chest x rays, and arterial blood gas studies are often used to monitor the patient's pulmonary status.

Program Implications

Physical activity helps to prevent the accumulation of secretions in the lungs and is desirable if tailored to the extent of each individual's tolerance. Sports such as tennis, skiing, and golf, which strengthen the abdominal and shoulder muscles, are encouraged. Horseback riding, archery, and riflery are also encouraged primarily for their value in the development of good postural and breathing habits. Swimming is recommended by most physicians, although some urge the use of nose clips, and not all approve of diving.

Children in fair condition may be able to attend regular school on a full- or part-time basis. It is im-

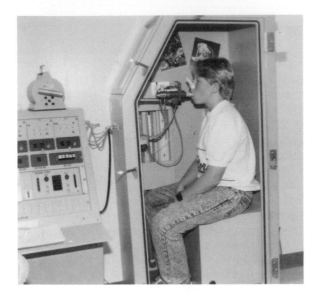

Fig. 4–36.   CF patient undergoing pulmonary function testing (PFT). PFT are two series of measurements that evaluate ventilatory function through spirometric measurements. (Courtesy of Cystic Fibrosis Foundation.)

portant to minimize restrictions and encourage participation in regular physical education activities. A program of sports and games can help the child win social approval from and acceptance by his peers. Obviously not all individuals will have the stamina to compete on equal terms with their peers.

Frequently, the child will manifest his anger, fear, and other emotions by resisting chest-physical therapy. Allowing children with cystic fibrosis to engage in normal activities (e.g., swimming) within their level of tolerance can help redirect these feelings, as well as improve respiratory function.

Participation in athletics can also promote body-image concepts through which the individual can adjust to his handicap and recognize his own limitations and strengths. Body contact sports should be evaluated on an individual basis.

Adams and Adamson report that trampoline tumbling is an excellent activity for children with chronic lung disease.[36] For children with cystic fibrosis, physical activity is an aid in preventing the accumulation of secretions in the bronchial tree. The bouncing associated with trampolining helps promote the cough reflex and improves drainage of respiratory tract fluid. Children with respiratory afflictions will breathe heavily and probably should not continue trampolining for more than 3 or 4 minutes at a time. An evaluation for a prophylactic program should include physical activity, and the trampoline is an excellent tool for assessing exercise tolerance.

CF patients are often admitted to a hospital or rehabilitation facility so that active infections can be systematically treated with high dosages of antibiotics for periods up to 2 weeks. Confinement to bed should be avoided if possible. The importance of this cannot be overemphasized. An expanded program of selected physical activities directed by a therapeutic recreation specialist is extremely important for psychologic and social reasons. In addition, the therapist should select games or activities that require short bursts of energy (e.g., running), because these games stimulate the cough reflex by changing the rate and volume of air flow through the bronchial tubes. (Further suggestions for IV patients are the same as those listed in the section on Program Implications for the Leukemic Patient.)

Precautions. Children may have slight, infrequent coughs or periodic coughing spells. At such times, the children should be allowed to excuse themselves from class so that they can cough up the mucus without focusing attention on their condition.

Sodium chloride supplements (salt tablets) should be available during vigorous physical activities, especially during outdoor play in hot weather.

Exercise

Exercise and its impact on CF continues to be a topic of interest and debate. Some patients and physicians believe that vigorous exercise and some sports (especially those involving multiple postural changes such as gymnastics and combatives) can produce positive effects by loosening mucous secretions. Exercise with an aerobic component such as aerobic dancing may produce similar results. Some dedicated persons with CF use exercise as prophylactic therapy and schedule their exercise sessions just prior to their chest physiotherapy sessions.

Exercise can improve physical fitness, but probably not lung function in CF. Orenstein et al. have studied patients who participated in a physical fitness training program. After 3 months of jogging 3 hours per week they showed that maximum work and fitness was increased but tests of pulmonary function were unchanged.[37] Orenstein adds further that limiting factors in exercise tolerance for CF subjects is different in comparison with persons who have normal lung function. Exercise tolerance is normally limited by the cardiovascular system before either the lungs or the musculoskeletal system reach their limits. In CF, respiratory function may be the limiting factor.

Therapeutic Exercises

Postural drainage with or without clapping and vibrating techniques has been used in the treatment of children with cystic fibrosis. The objective of this form of treatment is to aid in the removal of thick, sticky mucus that interferes with the function of the respiratory and digestive systems.

The treatment consists of placing the child in various positions so that the mucus can drain effectively from the lobes and bronchial segments and then be expectorated. Clapping and vibration of the chest wall are utilized during expiration only while the patient is in the drainage position. Coughing can be assisted by compressing the lower chest and abdomen with the hands while the patient is either in the drainage position or in a kneeling position on the bed or table, whichever is more comfortable for the patient.

The following exercises may be of some value to the child with cystic fibrosis.

Appendix A
  Deep breathing exercises
  Exercises 142 through 146

General Exercises

General exercises and weight training are excellent for the child with cystic fibrosis.

Appendices B and C

DIABETES MELLITUS

Diabetes mellitus is a hereditary or developmental disease characterized by impairment of the body's normal ability to metabolize or utilize food. The disease is manifested by abnormally large amounts of sugar in the blood and the urine. Insulin dependent diabetic mellitus (IDDM or Type I diabetes) is also known as juvenile diabetes and is the usual type found in children and young adults. It is caused when the pancreas does not make enough insulin. Adult onset diabetes or non-insulin dependent diabetes (NIDDM or type II diabetes) is most common in adults over 40 years of age. In this type, insulin is still made but it does not work very well in helping the body use sugar. Treatment may be limited to diet, weight loss, or medication to help the pancreas make more insulin. Exercise is important as it aids in the ability of the cells to utilize insulin. It also assists in maintaining weight control or reducing excessive weight by increasing energy expenditure.

Common symptoms of diabetes are excessive thirst, frequent urination, constant hunger, loss of weight, easy fatigability, changes in vision, and slow healing of cuts and bruises. Obesity is not so prominent a precedent to the development of diabetes in children as it is in adults, but it exists in occasional cases, and therefore it should not be ignored as an indicator of diabetes. Often in a mild case, only one or two of these symptoms may be present.

The patient's urine contains sugar and usually has a high specific gravity. Diacetic acid may also be present, indicating that acidosis exists. Analysis of the blood discloses a sugar content above normal, especially after meals.

Incidence

According to recent estimates, 3 million people in the United States are under treatment for diabetes. Children and adolescents comprise approximately 20% of the insulin-dependent diabetic population. It is estimated that about one child in 2,500 will have diabetes and that approximately 6,500 Americans become diabetic each year.

An apparent increase in the incidence of diabetes is partly due to improved methods of diagnosis and treatment. Diabetes is most frequently found in women past middle life, although no age group is exempt from the disease.

Treatment

Since the immediate cause of diabetes is insulin deficiency, treatment consists essentially in compensating for this deficiency. Practically every diabetic manufactures some insulin of his own (endogenous insulin). Treatment, then, involves adapting the patient's diet to his limited supply of endogenous insulin. If his supply of endogenous insulin is so limited that he cannot metabolize an adequate diet, then insulin (exogenous) should be administered.

There are many types of insulin, which will not be discussed in detail in this section. Examples of short-acting insulin are regular insulin (begins to act within ½ hour, and lasts 4 to 6 hours) and Semilente (begins to work in 1 hour and lasts about 12 to 16 hours). An example of long-acting insulin is NPH in combination with a protein, which lasts 18 to 24 hours. Ultralente is the longest acting and lasts 24 to 36 hours. The goal is to keep blood glucose levels as near normal as possible. In most cases, two shots per day are best for most diabetics.

Some individuals prefer to use an insulin pump (a small mechanical device that holds a syringe filled with insulin and small pump that infuses insulin at a slow rate over 24 hours). It is primarily used with diabetics who dislike or cannot be controlled on multiple injections.

Neglect of diabetes may lead to an increased risk of coronary disease, hardening of the arteries, cerebral hemorrhage, kidney disease, failing eyesight, gangrene, and diabetic coma. Whenever possible, it is desirable to hospitalize the patient for the period of adjustment.

Ketoacidosis

Ketoacidosis, or diabetic coma, is the almost inevitable culmination of uncontrolled diabetes. It is rare, but does occur when a severely diabetic person neglects his diet or fails to take his insulin. Most cases are needless, since coma can be prevented by proper management. Education of the patient and continual re-emphasis of the importance of early recognition and prompt treatment are essential.

Program Implications

Diabetics should be encouraged to participate in normal physical activities. Actually, exercise should be considered a duty, but it should not be forced on a patient just because he is a diabetic. Engerbretson states that a teacher or coach can expect to be confronted with three types of diabetics: the controlled and well-adjusted diabetic, the recently diagnosed diabetic, and the long-term diabetic who has become careless in the control of his disease.[38] It is imperative

Table 4–3.
Differential Diagnosis of Ketoacidosis and Hypoglycemia

Clinical Features		
	Ketoacidosis (diabetic coma)	*Hypoglycemia (insulin shock)*
Onset:	Gradual, over a period of days	Sudden
Symptoms:	Nausea	Fatigue
	Vomiting	Weakness
	Abdominal pain	Sweating
	Dyspnea	Tremor
	Dim vision	Sudden hunger
	High sugar in urine	Diplopia (double vision)
		Absence of sugar from urine
Treatment:	Both comas and serious insulin reactions require prompt treatment by a doctor. In case of shock the patient should be given fruit juice or sugar. Diabetic coma is a first-rank medical emergency; the response to initial treatment will serve as a guide to further treatment. If the diabetic becomes unconscious, he should be kept warm and sent to a hospital. A preliminary dose of 20 to 40 units of insulin, or more, should be given by the family physician or school nurse when a diagnosis of diabetic coma is made.	

that a child understand the disease and the theory of management before he attempts to become extremely physically active.

Adjustment to and management of diabetes in childhood often results in hospitalization. Those with overt diabetes should be treated not only for acute complications, such as ketoacidosis or a severe insulin reaction, but also to determine nutritional status, insulin requirements, educational needs, and psychosocial needs. Although not always possible in the hospital during the treatment period, it is distinctly advantageous to keep the child active for at least the first 2 or 3 weeks of the initial adjustment period. Participating in sports and games under the guidance of a therapist allows the diabetic to learn his tolerance for exercise and understand the need for activity restrictions related to his insulin and dietetic requirements.

The physical education teacher and the school nurse should keep records on all diabetics participating in physical education. The teacher should be familiar with the manifestations of ketoacidosis and hypoglycemia in case such emergencies arise (Table 4–3). Many times, diabetics recognize and treat their own reactions to insulin (this subject is discussed further in a later section). Good skin care is also important, and any break or opening in the skin should not be overlooked, but instead treated promptly.

Particular reference should be made to the sport of wrestling. Wrestling is one of the finest developmental sports, but it would have detrimental effects for a diabetic athlete, who, for example, might be encouraged to "make weight" for a competitive interscholastic meet. Under other circumstances a wrestler might be encouraged to lose weight rapidly in order to reach a lower weight class. This would be extremely dangerous for a diabetic, because purposeful weight loss or dehydration can trigger hypoglycemic reactions. The diabetic needs his calories, and a nutri-

tionally well-balanced diet should be encouraged at all times.

Studies by Drash and others indicate that many juvenile diabetics are below the norms in height and weight as well as bone age, and that they exhibit a slight delay in onset and progression of adolescent maturation.[39] An additional study by Etkind and Cunningham reports that, except in the 600 yard run/walk, the diabetic population performed significantly less well in the American Alliance for Health, Physical Education, Recreation, and Dance (AAHPERD) Youth Fitness test than the nondiabetic population did. In all tests that measure strength, agility, power, and endurance, e.g., sit-ups, pull-ups, and shuttle run, the diabetic performed well below the test norms.[40] This raises the possibility that lowered motor performance results from a decreased rate of physical growth and delayed maturation. Further studies are needed to prove this finding as well as to investigate the correlation between normal physical growth and the results of appropriate dietary control and insulin therapy. In any case, any deviation from appropriate norms during the adolescent growth spurt should alert the physician to examine his patient's diet and insulin requirements.

Because of the unusual stresses imposed by diabetes mellitus, children must learn to cope confidently within their limitations. Since the disorder involves altered energy metabolism, the diabetic requires close nutritional monitoring and appropriate adjustments in insulin dosage. Involvement in sports, games, and activities can help the young diabetic develop a positive perspective on his health. With this kind of positive feeling, the child should be secure enough to live a normal life—physically, psychologically, and socially.

Precautions

Hypoglycemia is undesirable and frightening. Teachers, coaches, and recreation leaders should understand why the balance between insulin, exercise, and food may become upset, producing an insulin reaction. A reaction may occur when a diabetic skips or partially eats his meals, exercises strenuously or continuously, or receives too much insulin because of an error in measurement (a rare occurrence). The diabetic usually recognizes early signs of hypoglycemia. If the diabetic is exercising when the signs appear—STOP! In addition, it is necessary to take quick acting sugar (sugar cubes or a regular soft drink) at the first sign of hypoglycemia.

The insulin-dependent diabetic either should not exercise at the time of peak insulin effect or should consume a carbohydrate snack about half an hour before exercising. If the child participates regularly in active sports, the physician may suggest extra food he can eat to give him more energy and prevent his blood-sugar level from getting too low. To minimize problems, the student's physical education period can be scheduled after the lunch period or after an established snack break.

A poorly-controlled diabetic who has consistent elevated blood glucose levels may not receive glucose lowering effects from exercise. If fasting blood glucose is less than 300 mg per deciliter, exercise will lower blood glucose levels. If fasting blood glucose is 300 to 350 mg per deciliter or more, exercise may cause blood glucose levels to rise. Diabetics in the 300+ range, or those with ketones in their urine, should not participate in vigorous physical activity until better control is achieved.[41]

Exercise

Although of general efficacy in the treatment of many chronic diseases, exercise is of specific value in diabetes because it promotes the utilization of carbohydrates, diminishes the requirement for insulin, and improves the circulation, thereby lessening the tendency toward arteriosclerotic complications.

There has been some controversy over the significance of exercise and metabolic control in insulin dependent diabetes mellitus. Many studies are insignificant because measurements related to frequency, duration, and intensity of exercise are inconsistent. Campaigne and others studied the effects of a regular physical activity program on metabolic control and cardiovascular fitness in young diabetic children. The experimental group of 19 children, ages 5 to 11 years participated in a 30-minute vigorous exercise program 3 times a week for 12 weeks. Studies indicated a decrease in Hemoglobin A and fasting blood glucose. Peak aerobic capacity also improved.[42] The investigation proved the fact that exercise can help accrue the same lifelong benefits as nondiabetics, with minimal risk taking concerns. This statement is also related to the fact that the diabetic children in the study were not in optimal control.

Cantu reports that diabetic marathoners who were interviewed indicated that vigorous exercise through daily running markedly enhanced diabetic control.

Exercise reduced their daily insulin requirements from 10 to 50%. In addition, during peak training periods of running approximately 50 miles a week, a marathoner commented on needing only one daily morning injection as opposed to needing two daily injections during offseason months in winter. This proves that sustained exercise is not a major risk taking event. Carbohydrate intake and/or insulin administration can be adjusted accordingly to meet individual requirements.[43]

It is also important to point out that exercise can increase the rate of insulin absorption, depending upon the site of administration. For this reason, runners should refrain from injecting insulin into their working thigh muscles. By injecting into the abdominal wall or arm the diabetic would eliminate the risk of a hypoglycemic reaction.

Therapeutic Exercises
No specific therapeutic exercises are indicated for diabetics unless the physician has outlined a particular medical problem.

General Exercises
General exercises and weight training would be beneficial, as previously mentioned.
Appendices B and C

SEIZURE DISORDERS (EPILEPSY)

Epilepsy, also referred to as seizure disorder, is the outward manifestation of a disturbance in the brain. It is not a specific disease characterized by a set of symptoms, but is rather a pattern of recurrent seizures. The causes are often unknown, but heredity, birth trauma, and other injuries of the brain are implicated in many cases.

As a result of public prejudice, ignorance, and superstition, many persons with seizure disorders are denied the opportunity to receive an education and to work, and many do not receive proper medical care. This group of people is often perceived as having gross brain damage, uncontrolled convulsions, psychologic peculiarities, and mental retardation. While only a small percentage are so severely disabled, this erroneous public image perpetuates fear and misunderstanding of the disorder.

The most accurate diagnosis and effective treatment of epilepsy is likely to be made by a neurologist (a physician who specializes in treatment of disorders of the nervous system). Various factors need to be analyzed such as the patient's history, use of drugs, drinking and smoking habits, and social or emotional problems.

After obtaining the above information, a neurologist can use a number of tests to determine the source of the problem. Included in the exam are tests of the senses (hearing, smelling, feeling, and tasting), reflexes, motor strength, and muscle power. Other tests may include roentgenograms of the skull, a spinal tap, and blood and urine samples. The electroencephalogram (EEG) is one of the most valuable tests used to diagnose and evaluate epilepsy. The EEG is a diagnostic tool which measures electrical activity in the brain. It is especially helpful because it can be used to confirm the physician's other findings. It is important to point out, however, that the EEG may be inconclusive in some cases, for 10% to 20% of epileptics have normal EEGs. Table 4–4 classifies the different types of seizures.

Types of Seizures

Absence (Petit mal). These attacks typically occur in childhood and adolescence. The seizures are brief but frequent periods of impaired consciousness. They are usually accompanied by rhythmic blinking of the eyes; sometimes the arms jerk. Usually the person with absence epilepsy does not fall down during seizures.

Tonic-Clonic (Grand mal). These seizures are the most common and are experienced by both children and adults. They are characterized by loss of consciousness, falling, and violent jerking of the head, arms, and legs. The abnormal muscle action may cause excessive saliva flow and vomiting, and the tongue may be bitten.

Complex Partial (Psychomotor). These seizures are periods of unusual behavior. The patient is usually in a trancelike or amnesic state, and in his mental confusion he appears to be acting out a bad dream. Such seizures occur in approximately one third of adult epileptics but are uncommon in children; children with this type of seizure frequently have severe behavior disorders also.

Incidence

Accurate statistics on the incidence of epilepsy are not available, principally because many people tend to conceal the disease and also because effective medical treatment has been developed comparatively recently. Some authorities estimate that 1 in 100 persons has a seizure disorder in some form; this figure indicates that between 350,000 and 650,000 school-age children in the United States have epilepsy.

Treatment

In recent years, excellent anticonvulsant drugs have been developed. In addition to being more effective in controlling or reducing seizures, the newer anticonvulsants have fewer undesirable side effects than the drugs used previously. Complete control of seizures with drug therapy is possible for about 50% of epileptics; partial control is possible for an additional 30%.

The various antiepileptic drugs will not be discussed in detail here. Phenytoin sodium (Dilantin) and phenobarbital are usually the drugs of choice for treating both generalized and partial seizures. Ethosuximide (Zarontin) is often used for generalized nonconvulsive seizures, especially petit mal. Temporal lobe seizures are difficult to control, and a combination of therapeutic drugs may be required. Medication should be taken regularly. Frequently attacks are triggered when medications are discontinued abruptly or taken irregularly.

In the past 15 years surgery has been recommended for some cases of epilepsy such as temporal lobe seizures or seizures caused by a tumor.

People with epilepsy should lead their lives as normally as possible. Anxiety tends to increase the frequency of seizures. Consequently, diversion appropriate to the age and ability of the patient should be provided to direct attention away from the illness. If his condition permits home care, the person with epilepsy should live at home rather than in an institution. If the person has adequate treatment and is mentally normal at the beginning of his illness, he can be expected to remain essentially normal throughout his life.

First-aid Procedures*

To help a person having a tonic-clonic (grand mal) seizure:

1. The important thing is to remain calm. The person having a seizure is not in peril although it may look like he is. A seizure is not a medical emergency, and there is no need to call a physician unless there is an injurious fall or seizures follow one after another without interruption.
2. Almost always the seizure will end by itself after a few minutes. In the rare case where it con-

*Courtesy of National Epilepsy League

Table 4–4.
Classification of Seizures

GENERALIZED SEIZURES WITHOUT FOCAL ONSET
  grand mal
  petit mal
  myoclonic seizures
  akinetic seizures

PARTIAL OR FOCAL SEIZURES, WITH OR WITHOUT GENERALIZATION
  partial or focal seizures
    motor seizures
    sensory seizures
  partial seizures with complex symptomatology—psychomotor or temporal lobe epilepsy
    automatisms
    visceral and autonomic, including olfactory and gustatory
    psychic (illusory, hallucinatory)
    affective symptoms

MISCELLANEOUS
  erratic seizures with inconsistent or changing patterns
  unclassified because of inadequate or incomplete information
  epileptic syndromes (classified separately because of the complex inter-relationship between the seizures and the neurological disease of which they may be the major symptom, such as hereditary myoclonus epilepsy and infantile myoclonic encephalopathy)
  other seizures of childhood, including febrile seizures

tinues longer than 15 minutes, a physician must be called; by administering appropriate treatments, he can terminate the attack. Nonmedical people should not attempt to ward off or stop the seizure. Do not try to restrain the convulsive movements and do not pour liquids into the mouth of an unconscious person. Do not slap or try to waken him.

3. If noticed in time, the person may be lowered to the floor. If his mouth is not yet tightly closed, place a piece of cork, rubber, or cloth between his teeth to prevent him from biting his tongue and cheek. Never place a spoon (or any other hard object) or a finger between his teeth. Do not attempt to pry open his mouth. Restrictive clothing at his neck, wrist, and waist may be loosened to make the person more comfortable. Place a pad under his head to help prevent injury from a hard floor.

4. When the seizure subsides, the person should not be left alone, as he may be confused for a while or require rest. Allow the person to lie down on his side to recover from the exertion of the convulsive movements.

Program Implications

Most people whose seizures are well controlled medically rarely have seizures during participation in athletic activities; however, certain safety precautions should be taken for those whose seizures have not been under full control for 2 years or longer. These people should not participate in activities that would result in injury if consciousness were lost, such as horseback riding, bicycling, rifle and pistol shooting, gymnastic apparatus work, and climbing activities. Swimming and boating are permissible with adequate supervision.

Opinion about the advisability of rough contact sports for children with epilepsy has varied. When the American Medical Association (AMA) supported physical exercise for convulsive disorders in 1968, they cautioned against participation in such sports as football, ice hockey, and lacrosse, noting that the possibility of sustaining head injuries might be hazardous to the person with epilepsy. However, the AMA revised this policy and now suggests that "serious consideration should be given to allowing participation if the seizures are medically controlled." Samuel Livingston, director of the Johns Hopkins Hospital Epilepsy Clinic, states that

to our knowledge, there are no studies reported in the medical literature which prove that chronic head trauma causes a recurrence of preexisting epileptic seizures, and over the past 34 years, we have observed at least 15,000 young children with epilepsy. Hundreds of these patients have played tackle football, some have participated in boxing, lacrosse, wrestling, and other physical activities which render the participant prone to head injuries. We are not cognizant of a single instance of recurrence of epileptic seizures related to head injury in any of these athletes.[44]

Individuals with bizarre forms of temporal lobe or psychomotor seizures, regardless of the frequency with which they have seizures, probably should be excused from body contact sports. Following a short seizure, people with these types of disorders generally return to normal activity almost immediately and have no knowledge of their attack. Fortunately, this type of seizure is encountered infrequently in children. Exclusion from participation in contact sports should also be considered for persons whose postconvulsive state is prolonged or typically includes markedly abnormal behavior.

Persons with akinetic seizures (sudden loss of voluntary muscle and postural control) may fall quickly to the floor during involvement in physical activities. Due to lack of postural reflexes, these people are unable to extend their hands to break a fall. Consequently, they may be instructed to wear helmets for cranial protection.

Livingston and Berman[45] state that many parents prohibit their children from engaging in physical activities because they fear that hyperventilation will precipitate a seizure. Hyperventilation is known to precipitate seizures in patients with absence (petit mal) epilepsy; however, we have observed that usual physical activities do not cause hyperventilation to a degree that can cause a seizure. Thoughtful judgment must be exercised in individual cases. However, the attitude that hyperventilation is medically unsound for seizure disorder patients should be dispelled. Also, to our knowledge, there is no unequivocal proof that fatigue resulting from sports or normal childhood physical activities has an adverse affect on the course of a seizure disorder.

The primary handicap of a person with a seizure disorder is social; emotional problems develop from fear of having a seizure, fear of being unconscious, fear of death, and fear of social stigma. Participation in regular group physical activities should be encouraged, as it promotes competitiveness, recognition, and social approval. People with epilepsy should engage in safe, nonstrenuous games and sports until they develop confidence in their ability to perform physical activities without injury. Permission to participate in competitive sports, in which injuries to themselves or others are possible, can be granted if the seizures are well controlled.

When planning a recreation program for a hospitalized patient with epilepsy, the therapist must consider the type and frequency of seizures involved. The patient should be ambulatory and permitted as much freedom as possible unless he has frequent uncontrolled seizures or other physical deficits. A therapist can often dispel fears and misconceptions about exercise by selecting appropriate games and sports. Extreme emotional or physical stress may precipitate a seizure, but some physicians emphatically state that no evidence clearly suggests that fatigue precipitates a seizure.

All therapists who work directly with hospitalized patients who have seizure disorders should be aware of the importance of their observations and know how to describe and record seizure activity specifically. This information is especially helpful to the managing physician who must control the drug dosage carefully and systematically.

Anticonvulsants are prescribed according to seizure type; therefore, it is necessary to know the type and frequency to determine treatment and control.

Very few people are trained in how to observe behavior, and it is essential for all those who come in contact with the patient—family, friends, teachers, employers, and allied health professionals—to be aware of the importance of their observations and to know specifically what to look for and record. Following are guidelines for describing and recording seizure activity:*

1. Environment or situation prior to seizure
   a. Fatiguing (too much exercise; not enough sleep night before)
   b. Stressful (argument with spouse, parent, sibling)
2. Seizure activity
   a. Warning (part of the seizure—begin recording time)
      (1) Fear
      (2) Headache
      (3) Unusual smell
      (4) Unusual noise
      (5) Unusual vision
      (6) Unusual feeling
   b. Record in proper sequence
      (1) How did activity begin (can begin as blank stare and be missed)
      (2) Did the individual fall; thrash; go limp; jerk
      (3) Did the individual lose consciousness
      (4) Did the individual make strange sounds or cry out
   c. What parts of the body were involved
      (1) Arms: right, left, both
      (2) Legs: right, left, both
      (3) Head: drop, turn to left or right; ache
      (4) Eyes: turn to right, left, up, down, blinking; were pupils dilated; did they react to light
      (5) Autonomic system: gastric disturbances; flushing of the face
   d. Did any of these activities take place during the seizure
      (1) Talk
      (2) Walk
      (3) Pick at clothes
      (4) Purposeless movement
   e. Miscellaneous activities
      (1) Teeth clamped

---

*Courtesy of Comprehensive Epilepsy Program, Department of Neurology, University of Virginia Medical Center.

      (2) Incontinence of bladder or bowel
      (3) Characteristics of respirations
      (4) Skin changes
   Record Time Activity Ends
3. Postictal phase (after seizure)
   a. Degree of alertness—to people, places, and things
   b. Degree of confusion—how long
   c. Was sleep necessary—for how long
   d. Any weakness in the extremities
      (1) Where
      (2) Degree
      (3) Length of time until full strength returned
      (4) Does the person remember anything unusual occurring prior to seizure
4. Did this seizure vary from past seizures?
   Recording information:
   a. Record date and time of day each seizure occurs.
   b. All who come in contact with an individual having seizures should be taught how to accurately record and keep records. The physician, family, school, and employer should be given this information on seizure activity and frequency.
   c. If you are not sure an individual is having seizures, observe that person for 5 minutes out of every hour for a day or two. (This is very helpful when identifying absence [petit mal] seizures.)

Precautions. The therapist or instructor working in sports, games, and activities should be aware of the first-aid measures to be taken in case of a seizure. Often, a warning sensation called an *aura* comes an instant before consciousness is lost in a tonic-clonic (grand mal) seizure. The aura can be almost any kind of unexplained sensation: a queer feeling, dizziness, numbness, or vague fear. When the person with a seizure disorder perceives an aura, the program leader can assist him to a quiet, inconspicuous place where he can lie down to prevent a fall. Unfortunately, not all persons with seizure disorders are forewarned of oncoming seizures by an identifiable aura.

Therapeutic Exercises
A well-balanced exercise program aids in reducing the likelihood of seizures; however, fatiguing exercises should be avoided. No specific therapeutic exercises are valuable unless the epileptic has a particular muscle weakness or physical problem. In such cases, the physician should recommend a series of exercises.

General Exercises
A general exercise program and weight training to increase organic function and neuromuscular coordination are usually helpful because many epileptics have been restricted in their physical development. Appendices B and C

HEMOPHILIA

Hemophilia is a hereditary disorder of the clotting mechanism that results from deficiency of a factor necessary for blood clots to form at a normal rate. The clinical problems result from the failure of clotting to occur in a normal way following trauma.

Although the deficiency is present from birth, the protected existence of the infant may delay suspicion of the disease until the child begins to crawl. Surgical procedures, such as circumcision, may lead to earlier detection. As the crawling infant explores his environment, a tendency towards bruising is noted. Baby teeth are usually cut without difficulty, but the early incisors may lacerate the tongue. Even mild blows to the body, particularly the head or the abdomen, may lead to fatal hemorrhage.

The major complication that becomes chronic and leads to disability is recurrent bleeding in the joints, or hemarthrosis. Relatively mild trauma to the joint can lead to hemorrhage into the joint space resulting in pain, warmth, and swelling. The knee is the most frequently affected joint, but the ankle and the elbow are also common sites. Once weakened by hemorrhage, a joint is more susceptible to subsequent hemarthroses.

Incidence

Hemophilia is inherited as a sex-linked recessive gene; therefore, except for rare instances, only males are affected. Deficiency of either of 2 blood proteins causes clinically similar diseases. Classic hemophilia, or hemophilia A, results from deficiency of coagulation factor VIII. Classic hemophilia is 5 times more common than Christmas disease, or hemophilia B, the result of factor IX deficiency. There are at least 20,000 males in the United States who have hemophilia. It occurs in 1 out of every 4,000 live male births.

Treatment

The hemophiliac is treated by infusing a clotting factor derived from human blood. Repeated treatments may be necessary for a single bleeding episode. Due to recent advances in treatment it is possible to have home therapy for suspected bleeding problems due to readily available plasma clotting factors in concentrated form.

Unfortunately permanent damage such as a contracture of a limb can occur unless clotting factors are administered soon after internal bleeding occurs. Management of musculoskeletal problems may include range of motion exercises or use of temporary splints. Surgical intervention may be the only reliable course of treatment for patients with severe joint involvement.

Program Implications

A carefully planned program of sports and physical education can play an important role in the total care of a child with hemophilia. Four specific problems can be effectively dealt with by such a program.

The first is the development of coordination. If, at an early age, the child is helped to attain as much motor coordination as possible, bleeding episodes due to clumsiness may be completely avoided. Although such a goal may be unobtainable by some, those who attain such coordination will be helped considerably.

The young child who has not yet suffered severe joint damage can be served in a second way. Sports and games designed to develop good general musculature can aid in protecting joints against bleeding due to trauma. Strengthening of specific muscle groups may also help in the rehabilitation of older patients. For example, repeated bleeding into a knee can lead to weakening of the joint capsule; disuse of that leg will result in weakening of the quadriceps muscles of the thigh. Strengthening of the muscles will result in a more stable knee and less loss of function with an acute hemarthrosis.

Perhaps the most important contribution of sports and physical education to a child with hemophilia is in the development of a healthy mental attitude toward his body. As the results of injury are feared by the parents from the day of diagnosis, the child is forbidden almost all of the activities associated with normal childhood. Although many families adjust admirably to the disease, others fail to find psychologically sound means of coping with the problem. There is a great possibility of psychologic damage that may lead to uncontrollable adolescent rebellion and even suicide. If, however, from early childhood, athletic skills are developed for sports in which the child can participate and if emphasis is placed on positive aspects, the child's adolescence will be much happier. Remarkably well-adjusted, active children have fewer bleeding episodes than their depressed, inactive counterparts.

The final area in which the therapist or instructor can play a role is in the rehabilitation of the severely disabled. For the child confined to a wheelchair or braces, morale can be considerably boosted by learning sports in which he can participate. If there is any hope for the return of function, games calculated to strengthen specific muscles are useful.

There are several general principles to follow in designing an athletic program for a child with hemophilia. It is appropriate to emphasize that the idea of athletics for children with hemophilia is a novelty and conflicts with many traditions. Such athletic programs should be carried out only in cooperation with a hematologist and orthopedic surgeon specially interested in hemophilia. Cooperation with an orthopedic surgeon is especially desirable in planning activities that avoid putting excessive strains on joints and muscles. Although specific sports will be discussed, programs should be individualized and planned with full knowledge of any risks.

It is desirable that the sport be competitive but not provide body contact. The element of competition is especially important to a child who is unable to compete in so many other areas of life. However, competition as such should not be emphasized, for, above all, sport should be fun for the child. Excessive demands in skill should not be made. The high probability of causing bleeding makes it essential that body-to-body contact (football) or body-to-object contact (tobogganing and skateboarding) be avoided.

Two sports that can be encouraged are tennis and swimming (without diving). Although hemarthroses of the shoulder may result from vigorous serving in tennis, they are unusual and treatable. Mild trauma may result from being hit by a ball, but this risk is small compared to the benefits from participation. Both tennis and swimming teach coordination and strengthen the musculature. Sports that strengthen shoulder and arm muscles are useful to a child who may later require crutches for ambulation.

Hemophilia is a variable disease, that is, the frequency of bleeding episodes varies greatly even in the same child. Restrictions should be made according to the severity of the disease. It is often difficult for the physician to decide to restrict activity because he realizes that this will induce a sense of total disability in the child. However, every child needs to understand his own capabilities and stay within the limits of desirable types and lengths of activity.

In summary, Boone[46] reports each hemophilic child differs in his physical abilities, the severity of his joint problems, and the frequency and kinds of bleeding episodes he incurs. His unique situation should be considered when a physical activity program is planned for him. For example, a child with severe ankle or knee problems is unable to run well; hence, track and field activities may keep his joints chronically irritated. However, he will be able to swim, bicycle, play golf, and perhaps tennis. In establishing his program, consultation with the child and his parents is encouraged, because they can describe the activities the child performs away from school.

Risk Related and Recommended Sports

Participation in sports carries certain risks for the hemophiliac. To add further to this discussion, The National Hemophilia Foundation has prepared an activity table that categorizes the risk factors associated with common sports.

For purposes of evaluation, sports activities have been divided into three categories:

Category 1. Recommended sports in which most individuals with hemophilia can participate safely.

Category 2. Sports in which the physical, social, and psychologic benefits often outweigh the risks. The vast majority of sports fall into this category. For each individual, the risk/benefit ratio must be evaluated, but today, for most youngsters with hemophilia, these are reasonable activities.

Category 3. Sports for which the risks outweigh the benefits for all hemophiliacs. The nature of these ac-

tivities makes them dangerous even for those without hemophilia.

Precautions

Bleeding episodes that resolve with a single infusion and do not interfere with normal daily activities should cause no increased concern. On the other hand bleeding episodes that require multiple infusions or forced bedrest, or leave the joint and/or muscles feeling stiff should signal the parents that the hemophilia clinic staff should be contacted before sports are resumed.[47]

Case History: This 16-year-old patient (Fig. 4–37) was fully capable of administering his own Factor VIII concentrates at home during bleeding episodes. However, he was hospitalized with hemarthrosis of the right knee after an injury of playing basketball. After a brief conservative treatment program he underwent arthroscopy surgery with partial synovial synovectomy. During the hospitalization period, he wore an immobilization splint during his recreational exercise sessions (Fig. 4–37). The postsurgical program was uneventful and he returned home on an aggressive strengthening and range of motion exercise program.

Therapeutic Exercises

Specific therapeutic exercises for the hemophiliac are difficult to outline because of the number of possible sites of irritation. Because one of the most common sites for irritation is the knee joint, exercises for it are beneficial (Fig. 4–38).

Table 4–5.

Activity	Category
Baseball	2
Basketball	2
Bicycling	2
Bowling	2
Boxing	3
Football	3
Frisbee	2
Golf	1
Gymnastics	2
Hockey	3
Horseback Riding	2
Ice-skating	2
Motorcycling	3
Raquetball	3
Roller-skating	2
Running and Jogging	2
Skateboarding	3
Skiing:	
Downhill	2
Crosscountry	2
Soccer	2
Swimming	1
Tennis	2
Volleyball	2
Waterskiing	2
Weightlifting	2
Wrestling	3

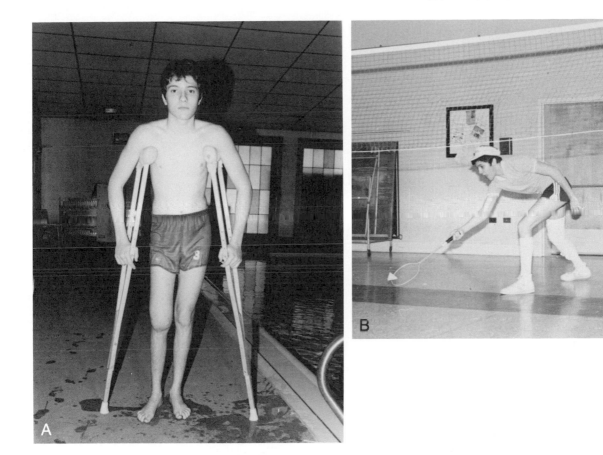

Fig. 4–37. *A*, Patient with hemarthrosis of right knee. Pre- and post-circumference measurements of the right knee were taken during daily hydrotherapy sessions. *B*, A leg splint was worn during recreational sports, and may be worn for 1 or 2 months following recurrences of knee hemorrhage.

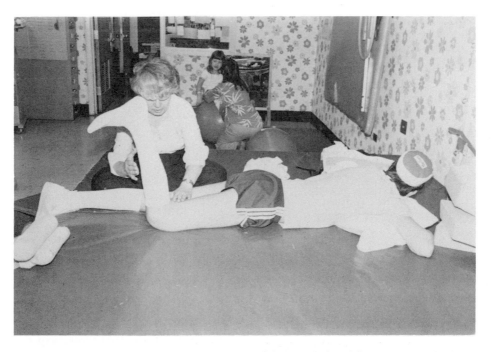

Fig. 4–38. Active and active assistive range of motion exercises to the right knee during daily sessions in physical therapy.

A similar exercise program can be started when other joints become involved. Start gently and progress to resistive exercises.

Appendix A

Exercises for the knee

Exercises 67 through 72, 74, 75, 76, 78, 80 through 83

General Exercises

After an acute stage is over, and as the patient's exercise tolerance improves, a program of general conditioning exercises are useful. This program will include a combination of proprioceptive neuromuscular facilitation techniques, manual resistance, and apparatus such as pullups, dumbbells, weight tables, treadmills, and bicycles.[48]

General exercises and weight training programs help to increase muscle tone, strength, and self-confidence. Caution must be observed to prevent overexertion and trauma to the joints.

Appendices B and C

Swimming is excellent for the hemophiliac.

HERNIA

A hernia is a protrusion of a loop or knuckle of tissue or an organ through an abnormal opening; usually it is a loop of intestine protruding through a weak area of the abdominal wall. The term *rupture* is occasionally used by nonmedical persons to describe a hernia.

If a hernia is present a lump or swelling may appear on the abdomen underneath the skin; however, swelling is not always present and may only appear when the individual is coughing, straining, crying, or lifting heavy objects. In some instances the only symptom is a swelling of the abdomen on one side of the body.

A strangulated hernia is one that is tightly constricted and requires immediate medical attention. If a hernia suddenly grows larger and will not go back into place, and there is pain and nausea, the hernia is strangulated.

Types of Hernias

The three most common types of hernias are discussed below:

Incisional Hernia

This type of hernia occurs when abdominal viscera (internal organs) protrude through the scar of a surgical incision. Persons who are obese or aged or who suffer from malnutrition are most susceptible to incisional hernias.

Inguinal Hernia

This type results from a defect in the structure of the inguinal canal; abdominal viscera escape through the deep inguinal ring, the inguinal canal, and the superficial inguinal ring into the scrotum (in males) or the labium majus (in females).

An indirect inguinal hernia is a congenital defect that is the result of the failure of a sac of the peritoneum to atrophy in utero as it should. This sac then remains as a mass in the inguinal region at birth (Fig. 4–39).

A direct inguinal hernia is acquired, often by men who are engaged in strenuous occupations involving heavy lifting. It may also result from a loss of abdominal muscle tone from old age or debility.

Umbilical Hernia

Umbilical hernias result from abnormal muscular structure around the umbilical cord. Some will close spontaneously; surgery is warranted if the hernia persists for more than 4 or 5 years. This type of hernia is most common in infants and children.

Incidence

Inguinal hernias occur more frequently in males than in females; they may be present at birth or may appear at any age thereafter. Unilateral hernias are found more often on the right side than on the left, but inguinal hernias may be bilateral.

Treatment

Herniorrhaphy is the operation performed for the repair of a hernia. The protrusion is replaced into the abdominal cavity, and the defect in the abdominal wall is repaired.

The temporary use of a truss (a device worn over the hernia) may be recommended by a physician. The truss applies gentle, continuous pressure and keeps the hernia reduced; however, it does not correct the hernia. The truss tends to move during activity, is difficult to keep clean, and may cause pressure and testicle atrophy in males.

Precautions. Most patients recover rapidly after a herniorrhaphy; however, the convalescent should avoid strenuous exertion, exercises, and heavy lifting until the physician allows such activity.

Program Implications

The delay of a herniorrhaphy for a young child, particularly if the child has been warned against participation in active sports and games, may hinder the development of a healthy body-image. The parents should be aware of this danger and of the desirability of early treatment.

Sports and games for children with hernias should be safe and nonstrenuous to prevent any unnecessary injury of the abdomen. Combative sports are naturally prohibited. Physical activities which limit intra-abdominal stress and utilize good posture techniques are recommended.

The pre-operative patient should avoid physical activities which place stress on the abdominal wall. This includes weight lifting, vaulting and jumping activities, and collision-type sports. Physical activities which limit intra-abdominal stress and utilize good posture techniques are recommended.

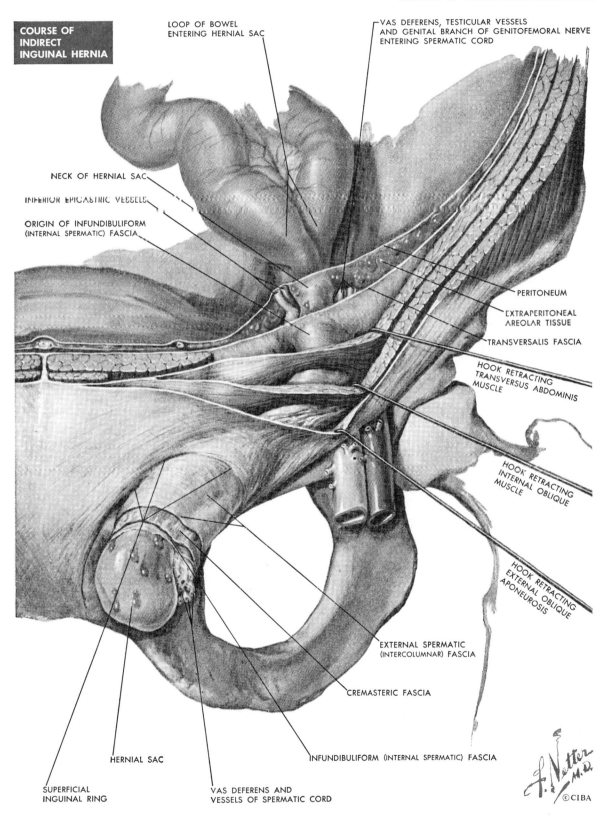

COURSE OF INDIRECT INGUINAL HERNIA

LOOP OF BOWEL ENTERING HERNIAL SAC

VAS DEFERENS, TESTICULAR VESSELS AND GENITAL BRANCH OF GENITOFEMORAL NERVE ENTERING SPERMATIC CORD

NECK OF HERNIAL SAC

INFERIOR EPIGASTRIC VESSELS

ORIGIN OF INFUNDIBULIFORM (INTERNAL SPERMATIC) FASCIA

PERITONEUM

EXTRAPERITONEAL AREOLAR TISSUE

TRANSVERSALIS FASCIA

HOOK RETRACTING TRANSVERSUS ABDOMINIS MUSCLE

HOOK RETRACTING INTERNAL OBLIQUE MUSCLE

HOOK RETRACTING EXTERNAL OBLIQUE APONEUROSIS

EXTERNAL SPERMATIC (INTERCOLUMNAR) FASCIA

CREMASTERIC FASCIA

INFUNDIBULIFORM (INTERNAL SPERMATIC) FASCIA

HERNIAL SAC

SUPERFICIAL INGUINAL RING

VAS DEFERENS AND VESSELS OF SPERMATIC CORD

Fig. 4–39. Coverings of complete indirect inguinal hernia. (From Netter, F.: Clinical Symposia. CIBA Pharmaceutical Company, 1968.)

General Guidelines in Postsurgical Activity Level and Return to Sports*

Initial consideration must be given to the incision area, and then further long-term study needs to be given to the type of sport, and its demands both in weight training and actual competitive stresses.

During the immediate postoperative period it is important to keep the incision area clean and covered until the sutures are removed. It is important to allow for an adequate recovery period to insure solid wound healing. In addition, it is important to refrain from undue stress to the area of repair in the abdominal wall. There are many kinds of abdominal hernias; a few are discussed below:

Ventral (Incisional) Hernia. This type is generally not common in athletes, but if it occurs then it could be debilitating for a long period of time, lasting from 3 to 6 months. In some cases, complete exclusion forever from collision sports may be recommended.

Inguinal Hernia (Indirect). This will be the most common type to be encountered. Children—Return to normal activities in 2 to 3 weeks. Adults—Graded exercises of mild intensity including walking during the first week. Advancement to moderately intense activities including bicycling by the 6th week, and return to noncontact sports by the 7th week. Depending upon the degree of surgery and rate of healing it is possible to return to contact sports in 8 to 10 weeks.

Inguinal Hernia (Direct). This type is not common in athletes. If it occurs, then the surgical procedure is more complicated than the indirect type. No strenuous activity before the 3rd week. Noncontact sports are generally allowed by the 8th week and contact sports by the 12th week.

Umbilical Hernia. Children—3 week excuse from physical education class. Adults—Graded convalescence including walking by the 1st week and bicycling by the 4th week. Noncontact sports are generally approved by the 7th week and contact sports by the 8th week.

The timing of the repair of a hernia in an athlete should be discussed. Obviously the physician should screen athletes for hernias during the pre-season when physical examinations are required. If detected, the hernia should be repaired before participation in sports.

Hancock suggests that the professional athlete must make his or her own decision in the matter unless incarceration or strangulation has already occurred. If the hernia is small (not tight) ring, the repair could be delayed for the rest of the season as long as the athlete, trainer, coach, and team physician all concur and keep the situation under close observation.[49]

Therapeutic Exercises

Some physicians recommend special exercises to strengthen the abdominal wall in preparation for a hernial operation.

---

*Adapted from Hancock, C. How I Manage Hernias in the Athlete, The Physician and Sportsmedicine, *11*, No. 8, Aug. 1983.

Appendix A
Exercises for abdominal muscles
Abdominal ptosis (sagging of abdominal contents) often accompanies a hernia. Postural, relaxation, and breathing exercises are therefore encouraged.

General Exercises

General exercises to regain muscle tone and strength are encouraged.

Exercises for the upper and lower extremities are helpful, provided that no excessive strain is placed on the abdominal muscles.

HIP JOINT DISORDERS

The ball-and-socket structure of the hip joint allows a wide range of motion that is exceeded in no other joint of the body except the shoulder. Of all the joints, the hip is most deeply situated and the bones fit so closely that much force is required to pull them apart. Two common conditions that affect the hip during childhood are Legg-Perthes disease and slipped femoral epiphysis. Within the last few years, some new methods of treatment have placed the child back in school even during the treatment phase and permitted him to perform some physical activity. Thus, it is important to keep abreast of the latest developments in treatment so that informed decisions can be made regarding limitations on movement and exercise. It is the responsibility of the physical education teacher to plan suitable programs while staying within the framework of medical guidelines and safety.

Legg-Perthes Disease

Legg-Perthes disease (osteochondrosis of the capitular epiphysis of the femur), a disease in the hip of the growing child, is characterized by degeneration of the top of the thigh bone due to a circulatory disturbance. The causes of the disease are not definitely known, and even though it occasionally is present in more than one child in a family, no definite familial or hereditary relationship has been substantiated. Injury apparently is usually an incidental factor, aggravating the disease rather than causing it. The disease generally runs a definite course lasting from 1 to 3 years, always healing, but with some residual deformity.

Stages

Incipient. During the onset, or incipient, stage the first and most common complaint is a limp. There is some pain but usually not enough to prevent walking. There are also muscle spasms and limitation of movement, especially in adduction, abduction, and rotation of the hip. The spasms and limited motion usually disappear with bed rest, but they return if weight bearing is resumed. If the child continues to bear weight with the affected leg, atrophy of the thigh and shortening of the femur will result.

Aseptic Necrosis. This is the active stage and it usually lasts from one to 3 years. During this period the head of the femur degenerates and will continue to degenerate if the leg is allowed to bear weight. During this period treatment must be continued, although there is no known method that will reduce the time for which the disease runs its course.

Regeneration. During the healing, or regeneration, stage, the head of the femur regenerates, and the bone slowly returns to a relatively normal state. The head seldom returns to a completely normal shape, but the hip socket usually adapts to any changes. The head may be flattened, irregular, and enlarged, and the femoral neck widened and shortened (Fig. 4–40). There may be some permanent shortening of the diseased leg; however, this can be corrected by a small lift placed on or in the shoe.

Catteral's Classification System—Prognosis for Legg-Perthes Disease

There are specific classifications of disease involvement for the child with Legg Perthes disease, and these are known as Catteral's classifications. This classification system is dependent upon the amount of femoral head involvement in the particular child's disease process. In Class I, only one-fourth of the femoral head is involved and there is no evident fragmentation. In Class II one-half of the epiphysis is diseased, with still no fragmentation of the femoral head. In Class III three-fourths of the epiphysis is involved and there is noticeable fragmentation and degeneration, and finally the entire femoral head is involved in Class IV. The Catteral's Classification system is the most important factor in the prognosis of Legg-Perthes disease, and is an essential factor when deciding upon treatment mode for the child. A child with Class III or IV involvement is considered "at risk", and will definitely have a worse prognosis than the child with Class I or II involvement.

Incidence

Legg-Perthes disease may occur in children between the ages of 3 to 12 years; however, about 80% of the cases are in those between the ages of 4 and 8. Approximately 80% of the patients are boys. Only one hip is affected in 90% of the cases, but in 10% the disease is bilateral.[50]

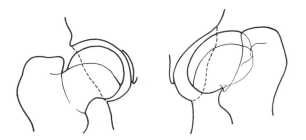

Fig. 4–40. Normal hip and Legg-Perthes hip. (From J Bone Joint Surg, 32-A:774, 1950.)

Treatment

Treatment methods vary among physicians. However, the Pediatric Orthopedic Society has studied this problem in depth, and their consensus is that containment of the femoral head in the acetabulum (cup-shaped cavity in the hip bone into which the head of the femur fits) during the healing stage with or without weight bearing, leads to the best roentgenographic and clinical results.

Methods

Methods of treatment for Legg-Perthes disease have included various modalities including combinations of observation, recumbency, non-weight bearing (abduction braces and slings) and containment surgery. The choice of treatment programs has been a matter of debate over a number of years and will not be reviewed here.

Abduction bars and braces are used to contain the femoral head in the acetabulum. This form of treatment is often used with patients in group III and IV by Catteral's classifications who do not have severe involvement. Prior to receiving the brace, many patients are required to be in traction to increase range of motion and relieve signs of synovitis. Based on the range of movement they permit, braces may be divided into 3 classes: (1) abduction braces and casts permitting no knee flexion and necessitating crutches, (2) abduction braces permitting knee flexion and (3) trilateral hip abduction brace. Although locomotion is somewhat awkward the containment principle is followed. However, many physicians have reservations about using abduction braces without knee flexion because without movement the knee joints become quite stiff. Thus, residual problems caused by stresses and strain in the knee are common. Prior to receiving the brace, many patients are required to be in traction to increase range of motion and relieve signs of synovitis (Fig. 4–41).

One common ambulatory orthosis used throughout the country is the Scottish Rite Brace (Fig. 4–42). Used widely since 1974, the orthosis maintains adequate 40 to 45 degrees of abduction of each hip. A slightly flexed posture is assumed during ambulation and contributes to coverage. Advantages of this orthosis include its durability and almost unlimited activity permitted to the wearers.

In more serious cases in which total involvement is diagnosed, surgical intervention is needed to completely cover the affected femoral head by lengthening the acetabulum. Many physicians feel that osteotomies (surgical cutting of the bone) have not been defined well enough to be used routinely in the treatment of Legg-Perthes disease. However, children with "head at risk" over six years of age seem to have better results following surgery than when treated by weight bearing containment orthoses or not treated at all.

Surgical correction is often preceded by traction and, possibly, muscle releases. The surgical procedure

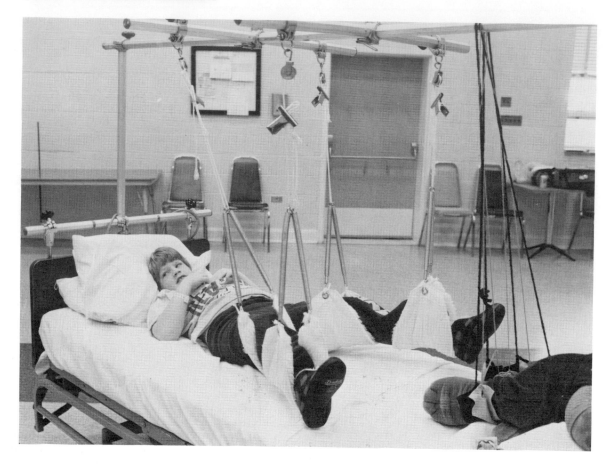

Fig. 4–41. Traction may be used to resolve the acute synovitis stage prior to receiving an abduction orthosis. The illustration depicts springs and slings traction, which eliminates gravity and promotes active motion to increase hip joint range of motion.

is usually followed by an innominate osteotomy or a varus osteotomy. The patient is in a cast for approximately 9 weeks, a period which is followed by physical therapy to regain range of motion in and muscle strength around the knee and hip joints. In most cases, the patient is fully active within 16 to 24 weeks after the operation.

Program Implications

Children will be confined to a hospital for a brief period if traction or surgical correction is the chosen treatment. A therapeutic recreation specialist should introduce a number of activities that challenge the patient's visual and tactile senses. Many children with Legg-Perthes disease were once active and excelled in gross movements. Postoperatively, the patient will have limited movement because his affected limb or limbs will be fixed in a cast to immobilize one or both lower extremities to the trunk. Activities that stress spatial relationships and pressure changes through movements of the upper limbs are recommended. Suggested activities include ball throwing and catching games, dart throwing, table games (to challenge cognitive skills), and miniature t-tether ball. Two important goals are the promotion of a good mental

attitude and the provision of an outlet for surplus energies.

A suggestion for planning a program for the child with Legg-Perthes disease was made by Puthoff:

The adapted or recreational phase of the program is to aid the child in participating in activities within his range of motion during treatment and providing him with opportunities to learn activities which will permit him to be a part of his peer group in physical activities. The child will no doubt have more success in closed skill activities in which he will not have to react to changing external environments and can attend to developing as good a pattern of movement as possible. One such adaptation is permitting the child to strike a stationary ball instead of a moving one in any of the games and team sports. Other times, open skills can be modified somewhat by changing the speed in which the child must respond. Permitting the child to catch or hit the ball on the second or third bounce instead of the first may be the only handicapping needed in a low level game or activity. With the heavy braces and crutches, open skills which would call for the child to adjust his movement patterns to fit an unpredictable series of environments would certainly limit his success in most activities. Some traditionally open skills may be adapted, however, to be more closed thereby giving the child greater chance for success. Bowling, archery and basketball foul shooting are examples of closed skills.[51]

One task of physical education is to teach students how to make changes within themselves. The only limitations to the student's activities should be those that are imposed upon him because of his anatomic defect. Most physicians support the principle that children in abduction braces and casts can participate in any activity that will not aggravate the condition. Most accidents occur when the child challenges his ability to react quickly. Students wearing abduction appliances cannot change direction or adjust position speedily. Thus, the physical educator should *not* introduce activities that require speed and agility.

One common abduction orthosis that deserves attention is the Scottish Rite Brace. The child wearing the brace can engage in a number of challenging activities including roller skating and bicycle riding. The brace is worn continuously, but can be removed for swimming which is an important outlet for stimulating hip joint range of motion. However, some physicians prefer the swimmer to use an inner tube to prevent weight bearing. Contact sports, distance running, and jumping are contraindicated. Ball kicking is often difficult because the kicking foot is positioned away from the midline of the body. To compensate, many brace wearers will run to gain speed so body momentum aids in kicking power to substitute for loss of complete leg action. The most important consideration is that patients are allowed almost unlimited activity and minimizes the psychologic effects of long-term brace wear.

Bowen reports that once reossification of the femoral head begins, the brace is removed and activities are progressed. However, it is recommended that no contact sports, prolonged running or jumping be allowed until the subchondral bone of the epiphysis is formed. At that time the patient may resume full activities. After healing, an occasional patient may complain of locking or giving out of the hip and an osteocartilaginous loose body should then be considered.[52]

The child who returns to school after vigorous surgical correction will have restricted activity. A modified program is usually allowed for the first 6 months. During this period, gymnastics, tumbling, contact, and combative sports are not recommended. A program of corrective exercises and activities to strengthen the quadriceps and hamstrings is indicated. Six months after surgery, the child is usually free to engage in full vigorous activity, including running and bicycling.

Activities to promote body-image should be included in the physical education program for children with Legg-Perthes disease. Generally about the time a child is 7 years old he should have a fairly accurate perception of the relationship of his body parts, the relationship of his body to external objects, and the

position of his body in relation to gravitational forces.[53] The inclusion of a significant amount of time spent on movement exploration is warranted for these children. This helps them explore themselves in their environments and learn their movement capacities both during treatment and post-treatment phases. Another benefit of movement exploration is that it involves no competitive pressures.

Precautions. Physical education instructors, particularly those in elementary schools, should be aware of the early signs of Legg-Perthes disease. Any child between the ages of 5 and 12 years who complains of a limp and pain in the groin or the knee, particularly during vigorous activities, should be suspected of having the disease. The hip should be carefully examined for limitation of motion and for pain and spasm during motion.

Case History: A 10-year-old boy with Legg-Perthes disease in the left hip was initially treated with an abduction brace. After 2 years, the brace was removed and he subsequently developed a left-leg limp which progressed to a flexion contracture. Four months later he underwent an innominate osteotomy and his left leg was placed in a hip spica cast for 2 months. He was then admitted to the Kluge Children's Rehabilitation Center at the University of Virginia for pin and cast removal and range of motion exercises.

Assorted recreational activities were incorporated into the patient's therapy plan to satisfy his continuous interests in physical activities (Fig. 4–42). Another goal was to convince the patient that he needed to adhere to a crutch management program. Therapy sessions concentrated on exploring the use of axillary crutches as aids to support and balance during physical activities.

Therapeutic Exercises

Most physicians advocate the use of exercise during the active and healing stages of the disease in order to maintain range of motion, prevent severe atrophy, and aid in the physiologic development of both the involved and the uninvolved hips. Exercise programs should be initiated only if a written order is given by the physician.

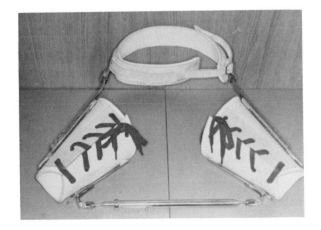

Fig. 4–42. Scottish-Rite abduction orthosis. (Photograph courtesy of Wood W. Lovell, M.D.)

Appendix A
1. Exercises for the upper back
   Exercises 1 through 17
2. Exercises for the lower back
   Exercises 21, 22, 25 through 31
3. Exercises for abdominal muscles
   Exercises 37 through 42
4. Exercises for the hip
   Exercises 43 through 57
5. Exercises for the knee
   Exercises 64 through 69, 71, 72, 77, 78, 79
6. Exercises for the ankle and foot
   Exercises 81 through 86
7. Swimming exercises listed above can be done in pool. The buoyancy of the water reduces the body weight on the avascular femoral head.

General Exercises
Weight training in the supine position can be helpful, provided that the hip is protected against undue stress.
Appendix C

Crutches
Crutches are used when a child is placed in a sling device to prevent the involved extremity from bearing weight. The crutch gait used should be a 3-point gait.

This gait pattern is also used for post-surgery patients (see Fig. 4–43).
Appendix D

Slipped Femoral Epiphysis

In the disorder of slipped femoral epiphysis (adolescent coxa vara) the epiphysis, either gradually or suddenly, slips downward and backward in relation to the neck of the femur. The cause is unknown; however, it is likely that trauma, angle of the epiphyseal plate, and hormonal abnormalities are important factors. Slipping of the upper femoral epiphysis occurs often in 2 types of children: (1) the Fröhlich type of adolescent with a female distribution of fat and sexual underdevelopment, and (2) the very tall, thin, rapidly growing adolescent. Most authorities think that the slips occur during the abnormal growth spurt of adolescence and are caused by growth hormone rather than a female sex hormone.

Early symptoms of the disorder include slight discomfort about the groin, usually after activity. Stiffness and a slight limp may also be present. As the slip progresses, a Trendelenburg type of gait develops (the patient's trunk leans toward the affected side as weight is borne on the affected limb), and the lower limb becomes externally rotated. During the chronic stage of slipping the pain increases in intensity, and the limp becomes more pronounced. Any child between 10 and 18 years of age who presents with pain in the hip, even if radiologic signs appear to be negative, should be examined, and further radiographs should be taken 4 to 6 weeks later.

Incidence
Slipping of the upper femoral epiphysis is most likely to develop in older children and adolescents from the age of 9 years to the end of growth. It is more common in boys than in girls. There is approximately a 30% chance of the second hip becoming involved subsequently.[54]

In a study in Connecticut, the annual incidence per 100,000 persons under 25 years of age was 3.41, while in New Mexico it was 0.71. Blacks were found to be more likely to develop slipped femoral epiphysis than Caucasians. Estimated incidence rates in Connecticut were 7.79 per 100,000 black males, 6.68 per 100,000 black females, 4.74 per 100,000 Caucasian males, and 1.64 per 100,000 Caucasian females.[55]

Treatment
Conservative treatment such as bed rest and traction to prevent further displacement is not effective. When the slip is slight and the position acceptable, internal fixation devices (pins) are inserted across the epiphyseal plate to help correct displacement and maintain correction until bony union between neck and epiphysis has taken place (Fig. 4–44). To provide freedom from weight-bearing, the child ambulates with crutches using a 3-point gait with toe-touch with the affected limb. Full weight-bearing is generally allowed in 3 to 4 months. General follow-up, with repeated clinical and radiographic examination of the opposite hip, is essential until the epiphyseal plate on the affected side is closed.

Program Implications
Physical education teachers and therapeutic recreation specialists are concerned with the extent of physical activity during the presence of internal fixation devices such as Knowles pins. It has been postulated that there is some weakening of the bone due to pins; however, little research has been done in this specific area. Fractures of the femur below metal fixation devices have been reported. On the other hand, many pins become enclosed in the bone, and this could actually strengthen the bone. Southwick states that if roentgenograms show no evidence of reaction or dissolution of bone around the metal and show essentially normal bone mineralization and normal appearing thickness to the cortex of the bone and if more than 3 months have elapsed since the placement of the pins, it would seem to be reasonable to allow children to carry on normal physical education activities, including contact sports.[56] Children should be trained and conditioned gradually to carry out sports activities and they should be checked to see if they have reasonably good coordination. Improving coordination and skills should not necessarily be considered an end but rather a means to another end—namely, the ability to participate in physical activity. If evidence of mineralization or resolution around the pins were present, then participation in sports activities would be unsafe.

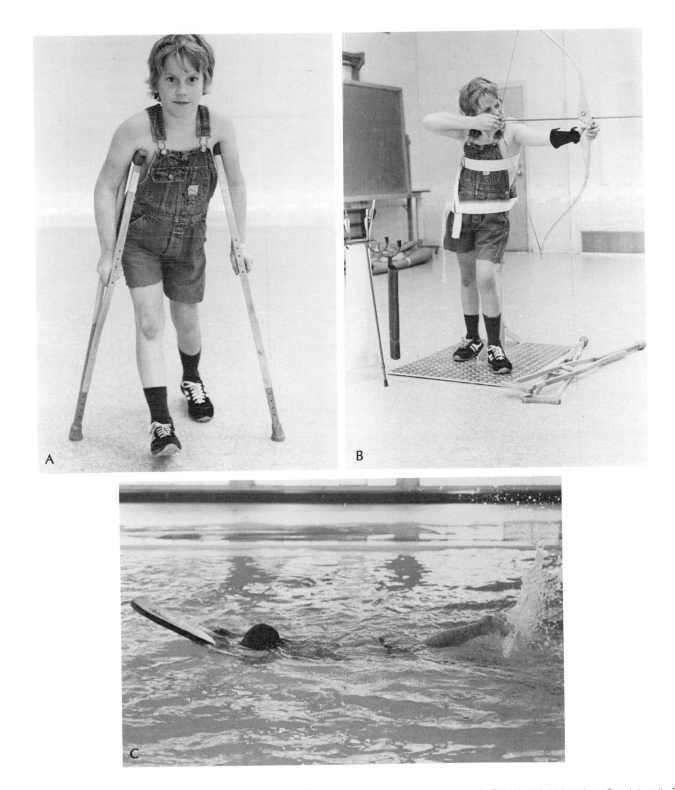

Fig. 4–43. Patient with Legg-Perthes disease during rehabilitation program following surgery. *A*, Partial weight bearing, 3-point gait. *B*, Involvement in archery while increasing standing balance and tolerance with support of standing platform. *C*, Exercises for hip joint range of motion.

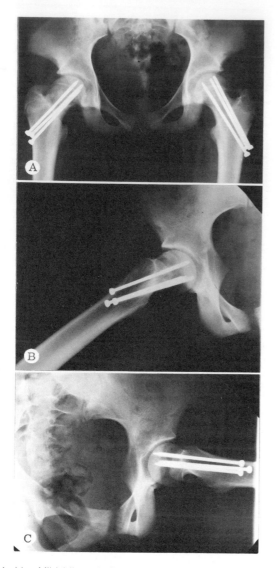

Fig. 4–44. Mild bilateral slipped capital epiphysis. Fixation with threaded Knowles pins. *A,* Anteroposterior view. *B,* Lateral view, right hip. *C,* Lateral view, left hip. (From Tronzo, R.G.: Surgery of the Hip Joint. Philadelphia, Lea & Febiger, 1973.)

The most important part of an adapted physical education program for children who have had internal fixation devices inserted takes place during the 3-month postoperative period, at which time the student is required to walk with the aid of crutches. Therapeutic exercises to strengthen the quadriceps and hamstring muscle groups are important (later, isometrics can be used to accomplish the same purpose). Before starting a program, the physical education instructor should consult with the student's attending physician and physical therapist. The child should be encouraged to participate in safe, nonstrenuous activities. Popular examples of sports requiring mild exertion are weight lifting (without weight-bearing), shuffleboard, archery, and horseshoes.

Vigorous play and group competition provide satisfying experiences for adolescent children. Unfortunately, during the period of nonweight-bearing, children limited by slipped femoral epiphysis must curtail many spontaneous activities such as running and jumping. Popular group games that require excessive use of the lower limbs, such as touch football, volleyball, dodge ball, and kickball, must be omitted. Sports like tennis, soccer, and basketball that require speed of movement should obviously be avoided. Under no circumstances should contact or combative sports be allowed. Although a slipped femoral epiphysis is not a serious condition, it is easy for an adolescent to regress in his interpersonal relations during the time his activity is restricted. Peer prestige is often affected when an adolescent is required to walk with the aid of crutches. Fortunately, a slipped femoral epiphysis does not require prolonged immobility, and resumption of most physical education activities can begin after the 3-month postoperative period. The physical education teacher can reiterate this fact during the postoperative period when the student is performing therapeutic exercises. The student must be aware of the need to reach maximum physical potential under established safety controls to prevent further trauma to the hip joint area.

Some physicians have reservations about the shearing effect on the epiphyseal plate after placement of internal fixation devices. This effect is intensified by activities that require violent exertion or in which the impact of landing is on the hip joint. Falling can also be dangerous because of the impact it places on the hip, and obese children (obesity is a common physical characteristic of those with slipped femoral epiphysis), because of their greater mass without equivalent agility or strength, are injured more seriously by falls. Thus, every physical educator should carefully evaluate the instructions of the physician before allowing the student to participate in activities where the hip has to absorb shock, and where protective equipment is limited. The hip joint is exposed to a heavy gravitational load in activities such as trampolining, wrestling, judo, and pole vaulting. High jumping, for example, often involves twisting one leg and rotating the body in space; thus the shock force to the hip joint is considerable after contact is made with the surface.

Every physical education teacher and therapeutic recreation specialist should be aware of the association between males with Fröhlich-type builds and slipped femoral epiphysis. An obese boy with underdeveloped sexual characteristics is often not athletically inclined. He generally has trouble competing with his peer group and tends to withdraw from athletic activity. He is often maladjusted as a result of his poor self-image. Any student after puberty who is fat, has underdeveloped genitals, and has persistent pain in the hip or a limp should be assumed to have a slipped upper femoral epiphysis until it is disproven. In such cases, the physical educator can be of enormous help to the student by focusing on the need for good weight control habits. If the shear strength of the epiphysis is reduced and more weight is placed on the hip joint, there will be more of a tendency for slippage. The teacher can assist the physician by encouraging good exercise habits and monitoring a weight control program for a student with slipped femoral epiphysis.

Southwick feels that 3 months following removal of the Knowles pins is enough time for restoration of the strength of the neck of the femur if roentgenograms show evidence of large defects where the pins were placed.[56] Again, it is important for children with slipped femoral epiphysis to have adequate training prior to carrying out vigorous sports activities. The question about activities would have to be decided somewhat on the assumption that these children are in a growing age group and that their remodeling is taking place rapidly.

Therapeutic Exercises

Therapeutic exercises useful for the patient with slipped femoral capital epiphysis will vary; therefore, written permission must be obtained from the child's physician before any exercises are undertaken. The following exercises will be of value.

Appendix A
1. Exercises for abdominal muscles
   Exercises 32 through 42
2. Exercises for the hip
   Exercises 43 through 57
3. Exercises for the knee
   Exercises 64 through 69, 71, 72, 77, 78, 79
4. Exercises for the ankle and foot
   Exercises 81 through 85, 92 through 95

General Exercises

General exercises and weight training without weight-bearing are recommended to increase the strength of the upper limbs for crutch walking. Caution must be observed to prevent trauma to the affected hip joint.

Appendix B
   Exercises 3 through 8, 11 through 13
Appendix C

Crutches

Crutches may be recommended by the physician. The 3-point gait, with toe touch on the affected side, is the gait of choice when there is unilateral involvement.

Appendix D

INFECTIOUS MONONUCLEOSIS

Infectious mononucleosis (mono, glandular fever, "kissing disease") has been recognized for more than a century, but remains a medical mystery. It is an acute disease and the causative virus appears to be the Epstein-Barr virus (EB virus). The EB virus is usually transmitted by direct oral contact, but it can be transmitted by indirect transfer of saliva (for instance on a bottle passed quickly from mouth to mouth) and, on rare occasions, by blood transfusions. There is also evidence that transmission occurs as the result of droplet infections from the nose and throat from someone with the disease.

The incubation period is 20 to 30 days. The illness develops slowly and the symptoms include enlarged lymph nodes, sore throat, loss of appetite, and a fever ranging from 101° to 105°F (lasting from 5 to 14 days). Some people have a fleeting red rash that does not itch, and occasionally, flu-like symptoms such as arthralgia and diarrhea. Moderate splenomegaly is present in about half of the cases, and rupture of the spleen may occur spontaneously or from minor trauma. Blood smears taken during infection show lymphocytosis, atypical lymphocytes, and rising EB virus antibodies. Liver function tests sometimes show abnormal function.

Incidence

Infectious mononucleosis typically occurs during the late adolescent years: 70 to 80% of all documented cases have occurred in persons between the ages of 15 and 30. However, it is not unusual to find the disease in children between the ages of 11 and 14, although the infection apparently is not as severe in this age range. Various sources have reported that epidemics of the disease develop most frequently in college dormitories or military barracks.

Treatment

Once the illness has been diagnosed, the only effective therapy is symptomatic: rest and aspirin to relieve the effects and discomfort of fever, arthralgia, and sore throat.

Bed rest is usually required for a week or more, or until the clinical symptoms of the illness have subsided. Residual effects often leave the individual with generalized weakness for 2 months or longer.

Rest, accompanied by continual observation for unusual manifestations of the disease, is mandatory. Recovery of full strength is often slow. Plenty of fluid and a normal, well-balanced diet are additional considerations.

Program Implications

Because recovery of full strength is often slow, the child may require supervised activity for several months. It is important, then, that the child avoid overexertion and strenuous exercise (exertion or trauma may cause the spleen to rupture). Competitive sports should be avoided until recovery is complete. After the acute stage of the illness, the immediate goal is acquisition of a higher standard of health, and this can only be achieved through a slow, regulated activity program. Obviously, this should be undertaken in accordance with the physician's recommendations.

A word of caution is needed about the young athlete. The combination of inactivity and the residual effects of an acute illness creates a condition of generalized weakness and low vitality in the child. An active child who appears healthy and who has no acute symptoms will often want to become involved in organized competitive sports too soon. This is understandable, because the child, more specifically, the adolescent, values exercise in itself and as a vehicle for obtaining the approval of his peers. Under such circumstances, concerns should be expressed to the patient regarding the necessity of guarding against relapse and complications. Even during convalescence, the child may require periods of bed rest or relaxation until endurance and strength begin to return.

It follows, then, that the child should be informed that he will have considerable loss of muscle strength, endurance, and power after the acute illness subsides. Unfortunately, in both physical education and organized youth sports, the child's return to activity is not always gradual (this is especially true in sports that do not require aerobic power and demand maximal oxygen uptake such as baseball). Because of decreased work capacity, there is usually lowered level of performance if the child returns to activity too soon. Despite the child's wishes, or parents who adhere to an "immediate return to activity" ethic, the child should follow a gradual and systematic return to physical activity (Fig. 4–45).

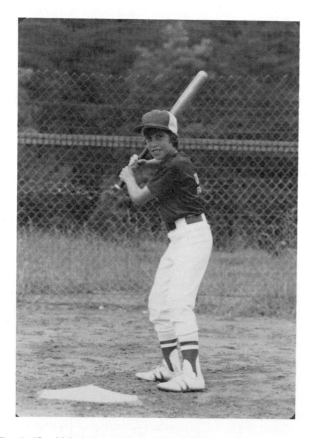

Fig. 4–45. Little League player with history of infectious mononucleosis.

It has been stressed that a child recovering from infectious mononucleosis will have limitations in physical, psychologic, and social development. Special considerations will be necessary when the student returns to school. The physical education teacher can provide encouragement and guide the student in appropriate activities. Activities should be underdone rather than overdone, and this may require involvement in an adapted physical education program. Activities that can be regulated easily in terms of energy expenditure are recommended (e.g., archery, shuffleboard, horseshoes). General conditioning through a program of exercises concentrating on rehabilitation calisthenics (see Appendix G) is helpful until improvement is noted in strength and endurance. Full recovery can be hastened by a carefully planned program of exercises and activities. Unfortunately, the length of the course of recovery is unpredictable. It is not uncommon for some weakness and tiredness to persist for 2 to 3 months after the acute symptoms have disappeared.

Case History: Just prior to his team's opening game, an 11-year-old Little League player had a period of fatigue, high fever, and swollen neck glands which lasted approximately one week. Originally, a nonspecific virus was diagnosed as the cause of his symptoms, but after a skin rash and an enlarged spleen developed, the physician was quick to make a definite diagnosis of infectious mononucleosis.

The player was on a program of restricted activity for 2 weeks, followed by a 2-week precautionary period which included a gradual return to normal activity. As a 10-year-old the child was chosen for the League All-Star team, but the following year the youngster never reached his potential because of the slow process of recovering from infectious mononucleosis. His batting average dropped dramatically, due in part to limited work output. His full work capacity did not return until 3 months after the diagnosis when he began to exhibit the strength, endurance, and coordination he needed to play as intensely as he had during the previous season. The following year, the child returned to his natural form, batting .550 and making the league All-Star Team.

OSGOOD-SCHLATTER DISEASE

This disease was first described by Osgood in 1903, and a few months later by Schlatter. The word "disease" is a misnomer, since the condition is not actually a disease. Essentially, the syndrome can be described as osteochondrosis (a disturbance of the growth, or ossification, center, which begins with degeneration or necrosis followed by regeneration or recalcification) of the tuberosity (structural protuberance) of the tibia. In other words, there is partial or complete separation of the tubercle from the tibia (Fig. 4–46). The condition is characterized by pain in the anterior aspect of the knee, tenderness and swelling of the patellar tendon, excessive enlargement of the tibial tubercle.

A comprehensive analysis of the data leaves little doubt that the cause of Osgood-Schlatter disease is

1 Patellar ligament
2 Partial avulsion of the
    anterior tibial epiphysis

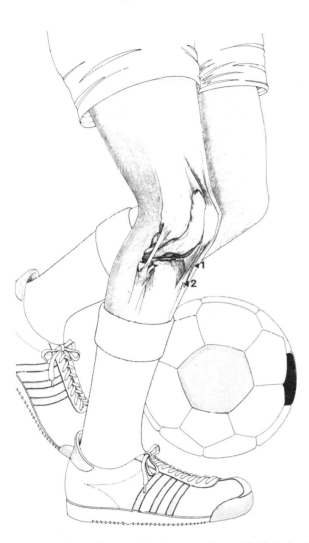

Fig. 4–46. Anatomic considerations in Osgood-Schlatter's disease. (Reproduced by permission of *The Physician and Sportsmedicine,* a McGraw-Hill publication.)

indirect trauma: sudden contraction of the quadriceps femoris concentrates force on a small portion of the incompletely developed tibial tubercle, and this produces an avulsion fracture (tearing away of part of a structure) which initiates the syndrome.[57]

Incidence

Active children, particularly boys, are predisposed to the condition during the rapid growth period of puberty. The age range in which the condition most commonly occurs is between 10 and 15 years.

Treatment

The outlook for recovery is good because the condition is self-limiting (Fig. 4–47). Treatment varies with the extent of the disease. Mild cases usually can be treated by restricting activities such as running and bicycling that require forceful use of the quadriceps femoris. This restrictive treatment is often sufficient to relieve symptoms. Some physicians recommend complete immobilization in a plaster cast for 6 to 8 weeks. Others inject corticoids into the tibial tubercle at the insertion of the tendon.

Surgery is used when conservative treatment fails or when symptoms recur, but details will not be discussed here. Generally, postoperative recovery includes 4 weeks of immobilization followed by a few weeks of rehabilitation.

Program Implications

Clinical manifestations include pain and swelling over the tibial tubercle; therefore, physical activities that impose a strong quadriceps contraction should be avoided. Kneeling, running, climbing, and shock absorbing activities such as jumping and gymnastics should be avoided. Active extension of the knee against resistance (soccer and kicking games) is painful and, obviously, contraindicated.

The major problem faced by the child with Osgood-Schlatter disease is basically that of accepting forced inactivity. Although the condition is only temporary, many active children, particularly during the early stages of restricted activity and treatment, have problems coping with the fact that they are physically inferior to their peers. It is important to encourage the child to substitute other activities as compensation for the physical restrictions imposed by the condition.

In moderate or severe cases of the condition, strenuous exercise and sports participation in regular physical education class may be curtailed for 3 to 6 months. Under such circumstances, an adapted physical education program should be instituted with adaptations made to suit the child's activities. It is important to keep the unaffected musculature highly toned. Sports such as archery, and riflery, and weight lifting are examples of activities that could be incorporated into an adapted program. It is important to emphasize that exercise is an important factor in the full recovery of the individual, both from a psychologic and physical standpoint.

The criteria that should be met before the individual returns to regular physical education classes are:
1. Normal range of movement of the knee.
2. Equal quadriceps strength in both affected and unaffected legs.
3. Asymptomatic evidence of the Osgood-Schlatter condition.
4. Ability to move freely without favoring the unaffected part.[58]

Therapeutic Exercises

A physician must prescribe the type and duration of exercise. Therapeutic exercises performed in the proper manner will help in achieving a normal range of movement of the knee as well as strength of the quadriceps muscle.

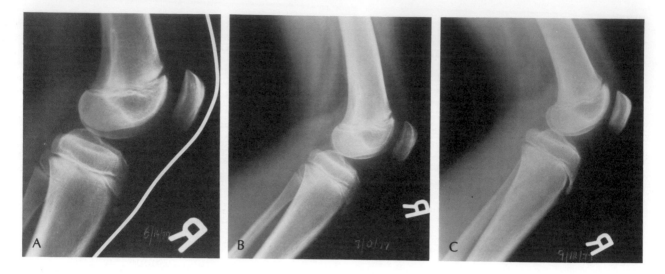

Fig. 4–47. Sequential films spanning 12 weeks which illustrate the normal healing process of Osgood-Schlatter's disease in a 9-year-old girl. *A*, Acute phase. Fragmentation of tibial tubercle is evident. Soft-tissue swelling in front of the tubercle has been outlined. *B*, Healing phase (one month later). Laying down of callus and bone bridging the fragment is evident. *C*, Healed tibial tuberosity (3 months after acute phase). Patient was fully active and asymptomatic at this stage. She was treated with a cylinder cast for 8 weeks and was on a partial weight-bearing crutch gait for another 2 weeks. (Courtesy of Mohinder A. Mital, M.D.)

The following exercises are to be used as a guide and should be approved by the patient's physician.

Appendix A
1. Exercises for the knee
   Exercises 64 through 69, 71 through 80
2. Exercises for the ankle and foot
   Exercises 81 through 91

General Exercises

General exercises, weight training, and general body building will help maintain muscle tone, strength, and range of motion of the unaffected musculature during the acute stage of the condition, and during the final stage of recovery they will help him gain strength to participate in the activities his tolerance allows.

Appendix B
Exercises 1 through 13, 16, 20
Appendix C
Exercises 1 through 4, 6, 8 through 20
When the condition is in the acute stage, perform exercise number 8 with the unaffected leg only.

KIDNEY DISORDERS

Acute Glomerulonephritis

Acute glomerulonephritis (inflammatory Bright's disease) most frequently affects children, boys slightly more often than girls. Symptoms include the presence of blood in the urine, headache, convulsions, generalized swelling or puffiness (especially in the face), high blood pressure, and malaise. Only the first of these symptoms is reasonably specific.

Complications during the acute phase of the disease may include renal failure, convulsions, or congestive heart failure, but all of these complications are rare. Even less commonly a patient may progress to chronic nephritis and slow, progressive renal failure.

The exact cause of acute glomerulonephritis is uncertain, but it is widely accepted that it is usually preceded by an infection with a Group A β-hemolytic streptococcus in the throat or on the skin or both.

Incidence

Glomerulonephritis is the most common form of nephritis in children. Its true incidence is not known, since many of the milder cases go unrecognized; it accounts for about 0.5% of hospital admissions of children. About ⅔ of the cases occur in children under 7 years of age. Although uncommon in children under 3, the disease has been observed in the neonatal period.

Treatment

Treatment is symptomatic. Drugs to lower the blood pressure and improve heart function may be used; in addition, methods to minimize renal failure may be beneficial. At best, most therapy is palliative, but the natural tendency of the patient is to improve.

Bed rest is usually prescribed during the acute phase as a general measure because of the severity of the illness, but it apparently has no specific value. Contrary to widely held earlier views, there is no evidence at the present time in favor of prolonged bed rest during convalescence, which frequently lasts up to one year. In general, the outlook is good for eventual complete recovery, and recurrences are rare.

Nephrosis

Nephrosis, lipoid nephrosis, and *nephrotic syndrome* are essentially synonymous terms for kidney disease characterized by albumin in the urine (frequently without other abnormalities of the urine), massive swelling due to fluid collection, particularly in the serous cavities, and low blood protein. Nutrition is usually poor, and malaise is common.

The cause of this disease in the vast majority of cases is completely unknown. It has followed bee stings, treatment with various drugs, and other specific events at times, but in general it begins insidiously and without any recognizable cause.

Incidence
The frequency with which nephrosis occurs is not known, an incidence of about 7 cases per 100,000 children under the age of 5 has been estimated, and nephrosis is more common in boys than in girls.

Treatment
Many months of treatment with adrenocortical steroids appears to be effective in most cases. Other forms of therapy are purely symptomatic, and particularly stubborn cases may be treated with certain anticancer drugs.

Bed rest or restriction of activity has been shown to be of no value in the management of this disease. Complete recovery occurs with adequate therapy in 70 to 80% of all cases. Some cases progress to chronic renal diseases with eventual renal failure. The disease is unpredictable in its course, and it cannot be assumed cured until at least 10 years have passed without significant abnormal findings.

Chronic Nephritis

Chronic nephritis is an all-inclusive term used to describe various degenerative renal diseases, most of which are poorly understood.

Chronic nephritis can be subdivided into several recognizable groups: Alport's syndrome, a hereditary form of nephritis associated with deafness; another less common form of hereditary nephritis; radiation nephritis; chronic renal deterioration following acute glomerulonephritis; chronic renal deterioration following nephrosis; nephritis associated with periarteritis nodosa and various other collagen diseases; and nephritis associated with Henoch-Schönlein purpura. The prognosis of these diseases ranges from very poor to very good. For those types of nephritis that cannot be clearly delineated the prognosis remains uncertain.

Program Implications
Usually contact sports are avoided during the convalescent phase to avoid trauma-induced hematuria. There is no apparent need for restricting other exercises, sports, or games if adequate rest periods are imposed.

When there is unilateral kidney malformation or related pathologic condition, many physicians recommend exclusion from contact sports to avoid injury to the remaining functional organ. The risk of a permanent disability is not a fair price to pay for the sake of athletics. In such cases the individual should be encouraged to compete in noncontact individual sports.

Therapeutic Exercises
Specific therapeutic exercises are of little value, unless there are particular weaknesses due to inactivity.

General Exercise
General exercise and weight training are beneficial in assisting the child to regain strength, muscle tone, and coordination.
Appendices B and C

Exercise Guidelines for Patients with Renal Disease
Chronic renal failure may result from other diseases. When medical management is exhausted, long-term hemodialysis is often begun. Treatment involves using a dialysis machine to filter the blood.

Dialysis patients are individuals with a persistent disorder that requires regular treatment. Regular exercise can help delay the onset of some of the metabolic and cardiovascular complications of the disease, and that alone should make it a major priority. Concentrate on exercises that maintain and increase flexibility and general muscle tone. Any aerobic program should be developed gradually and with supervision.[59] Control of hypertension is of utmost importance before engaging in sustained effort.

Medical permission should be granted before initiating an exercise program, and it is important to avoid exhausting exercise and competitive sports. On the other hand, for patients who do not have severe impairment in function it is important to avoid unnecessary restrictions and modifications of usual daily routines.

OVERWEIGHT AND OBESITY

Obesity (excessive fatness) in children is a great problem because it often leads to obesity in adulthood. Obesity may be defined as an excess of 20% or more above the ideal weight. An excess weight for height of 100 lbs. (45.4 kg) has generally been referred to as morbid obesity. Overweight may be defined as excess of 10% or more above the ideal weight. It is important to understand that overweight cannot be simply equated with obesity.

The American Medical Association has repeatedly warned that one of the prime predisposing factors of coronary heart disease and early death from myocardial infarctions is obesity. Overweight also increases susceptibility to other diseases, such as atherosclerosis, diabetes mellitus, joint disease, and gallbladder disease. Hypertension is twice as common in overweight people as in those of normal weight.

Obesity and heart disease are so widespread and so difficult to control in adulthood that many physicians favor preventive measures, particularly early childhood diet control, as the best way to focus in on the problem. Many experts on obesity think that eating and weight patterns are set in infancy. Another association with adipocyte size is the set-point theory of obesity. This theory is based on the assumption that the body has its own control system that regulates the amount of fat to be carried. The theory is based on the fact that each individual has an ideal biologic weight (the set point). Some people have high settings, others a low setting and a few have no setting at all. The significance of exercise is that it can be a safe way to lower the set point.

Many studies have shown that obesity runs in families and that apparently both genetic and environmental factors are involved. The role of heredity in influencing obesity has received attention in a number of research projects. Obese parents generally have obese babies. It is also known that body structure influences obesity and that skeletal proportions and muscle mass are hereditary characteristics.

The peaks of obesity are in early childhood and late maturity. This discussion concentrates on the obese adolescent.

In addition to the health risks, obesity may adversely affect the child's or adolescent's social relationships, school performance, and emotional adjustment. Obesity during childhood may also have greatly important effects on the development of emotional maturity, success in sports, and the attainment of physical fitness and maturity.

A number of nonhereditary factors contribute to obesity. Overeating by the adolescent or the young adult may result from either psychologic or physiologic needs, but usually overeating becomes more a habit than an expression of need, and the excess of caloric intake over caloric expenditure leads to accumulation of fat. It has been proved that physical inactivity is the most significant contributor to obesity. The life histories of obese children reveal that the tendency towards isolation and withdrawal often preceded the development of obesity, but obesity in an adolescent may lead to complete withdrawal and prevent him from making the necessary adjustment toward adulthood.

Incidence
Obesity is relatively common during pubescence and adolescence. It has been estimated that approximately 10 to 15% of the adolescent population of the United States is obese. One in every 4 women and one in every 5 men are at least 10% overweight by the time they are 20 years old.

Treatment
It is beyond the scope of this discussion to review all the alternatives for treating obesity. Short-term treatment is generally unsuccessful and a high degree of structure and constant supervision is required for a year or more to measure individual acceptance to treatment techniques. A monthly visit to a Weight Management Clinic is not the answer.

Family involvement is critical because there is a biologic correlation between parent and child obesity. For successful intervention to take place, issues regarding lifestyle, exercise, and dietary habits need to be addressed within the family constellation.

Studies show behavioral strategies (altering exercise and eating habits), and using a reward system for approval of maintaining self-control over intimidating factors show promising short-term results. Unfortunately, not enough research has been done to prove long-term effects with children and adolescents.

Nutritional instruction is very important. The diet should be based on nutritional needs, but the caloric intake may be safely reduced to 1,000 or 1,200 calories. The mother must help alter the child's eating pattern as well as provide emotional support whenever necessary.

The key to effective weight control is to keep energy intake (food) and energy output (physical activity) in balance. Obese persons will lose fat if they exercise properly and follow dietary restrictions. The so-called "crash diet" is not recommended, because it promotes poor eating habits and does not balance exercise and energy intake. Dieters often concentrate on counting calories and neglect the role of exercise. A weight-control program is a long-term process, and the overweight person must be properly motivated to break the habits that caused him to grow fat.

School based treatment is an encouraging form of intervention as documented by Seltzer and Mayer,[60] and Brownell and Kaye.[61] Since schools mandate attendance it seems logical that large numbers of obese students can be targeted for intervention. Cost can be minimized in comparison with clinical settings (where third party reimbursement is difficult to approve). In addition, children can be served before their obesity reaches a morbid state where medical intervention is required. Utilization of school personnel (teachers, physical education instructors, school nurses, food service staff, etc.) can encompass and facilitate the makeup of a comprehensive weight management team. Unfortunately most school systems resist such treatment because it is not a priority issue and it diverts away from traditional teaching habits.

Surgical intervention (gastroplasty, gastric bypass, dental splinting, and intragastric balloons to name a few) is warranted in some cases. However, it is difficult to compare advantages and disadvantages of the various procedures due to space limitations. In addition, long-term success rates of the different methods are lacking. This, coupled with the behavioral effects that potentially influence outcome, makes the subject matter difficult to interpret in a book of this type.

Tests and Measurements
The use of tests and measurements during programs for the control of obesity is essential. The data

serve as a guide for prescribing exercises for selected parts of the body.

Skinfold Measurements

Utilizing skinfold calipers to measure subcutaneous fat allows the physician, physical education specialist, or a therapist to get a reasonably valid estimate of overall percent body fat. This is achieved by using the sum total of the skinfold measures and inserting this information into an appropriate regression equation for the determination of body density. From the body density measure, the percent body fat can be estimated. This information is valuable in developing physical fitness program goals and objectives. It is important to recognize that body composition is an important component of health related physical fitness. Skinfold sites may vary according to the particular equation. However, typical skinfold sites for women include: (1) triceps skinfold at the midpoint between tip of the shoulder and tip of the elbow; (2) iliac crest skinfold at the apex of the iliac crest; and (3) thigh skinfold at the midpoint between the hip and the knee. Typical measurement sites for men include: (1) chest skinfold at a spot above and to the right of the nipple in a natural fold; (2) abdominal skinfold taken one inch to the right of the umbilicus in a vertical fold; and (3) thigh skinfold at the midpoint between the hip and the knee. Normative data for skinfold thicknesses are readily available in the literature.

The procedures at each skinfold site should include:

1. Hold the caliper between thumb and forefinger.
2. Mark a skinfold site with a felt-tip pen to insure reliable site location.
3. Grasp the skinfold and underlying fat between the thumb and forefinger, 6–8 cm apart, and lightly pull the tissue away from the body to allow measurement. Do not pinch the skin tightly. Be sure the skinfold site is taken in the natural fold of the skin.
4. Open the jaws of the calipers and place them over the skinfold site while maintaining the grasp on the skinfold. Have caliper dial face toward the tester for easy reading.
5. Close the calipers on the site slowly and allow the caliper tension to settle for 2–3 seconds prior to reading the measurement dial in millimeters. Record the measure.
6. Check the measurement by repeating the process three times to insure reliability of data. If the measurements are drastically different from one another, re-evaluate your technique and repeat as needed.

Girth Measurements

1. Test procedures
   a. Use steel tape to take all measurements.
   b. Take all measurements twice.
   c. Average measurements to the nearest ¼ inch.
   d. Record data on form.
2. Girth measurement sites
   a. Upper arm (dominant arm)—4 to 6 inches above (superior) elbow flexed 30 degrees.
   b. Bust—nipple level.
   c. Waist—umbilicus level.
   d. Hip—level of anterior-superior spine of the pelvis.
   e. Buttocks—just above (superior) gluteal fold.
   f. Upper thigh (dominant leg)—4 to 6 inches above (superior) top of knee cap.
   g. Calf (dominant leg)—4 to 6 inches below (inferior) knee cap (patella).
   h. Ankle (dominant leg)—just above (superior) ankle joint.

Weight Reducing Motivation Chart

Various line or block charts can be designed by the patient/student in collaboration with the instructor.

1. Procedure for hospitalized persons
   a. Weigh patient first day.
   b. Weigh patient every other day thereafter.
   c. Set goal at a loss of approximately 3 pounds each week.
   d. Record weight on chart.
   e. Record dates on chart.
   f. Document weights in chart after every weigh-in.
2. Procedure for regular school students
   Same as above except for the following:
   b. Weigh individual once a week.
   c. Set goal at a loss of approximately 1 pound each week.

Program Implications

There are many benefits from a properly conducted program of sports and games. Social, recreational, and physical values that aid total education and physiologic growth have been demonstrated and documented. Vigorous physical activity over a long period of time expends the most calories; therefore, whenever possible, endurance sports and games should be selected for the obese person. Physical activities that can be enjoyed regularly away from school facilities, such as swimming, bicycling, bowling, roller skating, or hiking, should also be encouraged.

Children not only like to achieve but also desire recognition of their achievement. Unfortunately, for many obese children, physical education class is a place where criticism and disapproval lead to frustration and lack of interest. Some children think that physical education is an activity for the athlete or "super-fit" person. Those who are moderately overweight can usually be accommodated in the regular physical education class, but morbidly obese children should be enrolled in an adapted class.

Every physical education teacher should understand how eager boys and girls are to be physically sound and possess bodies that are agile and attractive. Optimum development through movement is the key to a learning situation. Certain learning experiences need to be modified, or occasionally eliminated, in order to develop a program that has *value*. The rigid approach specifying conformance of all children to the same physical task is the most inappropriate approach. No child should be forced to perform movements beyond his own capacity.

Vodola recommends the aerobic circuit program for obese students.[63] The subjects are required to perform the following exercises for a 10-minute period without any rest interval: 100 side-straddle hops, 100 hops on the right foot; 100 hops on the left foot, 100 jumps on both feet, and running in place for 100 counts (left or right foot striking the floor). Students record the whole number 1 for a complete circuit plus 0.2 for each exercise beyond the circuit. Thus, if a subject completes 2 circuits and 2 exercises, his score is recorded as 2.4. The exercises and their duration can be varied, but the "overload concept" must be adhered to, i.e., the number of circuits completed within a certain time should be increased.

Attention should also focus on body- and self-image concepts. Many obese adolescents are unhappy and feel a sense of worthlessness. Some express strong feelings of resentment toward people who are slim. Additional behavorial characteristics include lack of maturity and self-confidence, and poor leadership qualities. Body- and self-image programs can include sessions on grooming, fashion, and physical fitness. Participation in sports and games that offer early success can also improve body-self-image concepts.

The efforts to reduce weight must be based on an understanding of the approximate caloric cost of recreational exercise and athletics. A long range, low caloric intake needs to be coupled with a sensible exercise program.

The preferred forms of exercise for obese subjects are those that use large muscle groups. In general, the target heart rate will be in the 130 to 140 BPM range for most adolescents. To add further, resting and exercise pulse rates should be monitored at each session. Intensity of effort needs to be carefully controlled especially at the beginning of the program. It is often necessary for the instructor to jointly monitor pulse rate recordings with the adolescent to assure accurate measurements. (For example, taking the radial pulse as the exercise subject takes the carotid pulse.) A wristwatch-style pulse monitor can also be used.

A sample exercise regimen in clinical settings or school physical education programs could include such activities as stretching/calisthenics, walking, bicycling, rope skipping, and swimming (Fig. 4–48). A few of the more common exercise modalities are listed below which reflect on the specific needs of the obese.

Calisthenics/Stretching (Flexibility Exercise). This form of exercise is good and highly recommended because it slowly prepares the individual for an aerobic workout. Body temperature is slowly increased as is blood flow to the working muscles. It also pre-vents injuries to muscles and other tissues. In addition, it can be used for strengthening specific areas where muscles are weak. For example, using bent knee sit-ups for weak abdominal muscles. Another advantage is that the pulse rate is slowly increased, allowing for a safe entry into a more vigorous aerobic activity. Caloric expenditure may vary from 2 to 7 K Cal per minute depending upon intensity of output (Fig. 4–48A).

Bicycling. This exercise modality can be used successfully in weight management programs. The cardiovascular system can be taxed, if done on an uneven surface. There is a lower incident rate than running in terms of leg trauma. Excessively obese subjects frequently demonstrate problems with shifting body weight on the bicycle seat to obtain a comfortable position for reciprocal pedaling action. If stress loads include cycling on uneven terrain, 300 to 400 K Cal can be expended in an hour.

Stationary (nonmotorized) bicycling is an excellent indoor activity. Some obese subjects can perform for 30-minute intervals without difficulty. By assuming a comfortable pedaling motion the subject can increase the heart rate and maintain it in a safe target zone. It is frequently necessary, however, to adjust the tension on the front wheel to increase stress loads which is helpful in providing a conditioning response. Stationary bicycling is a useful supplement for excessively obese patients who must limit their routine to walking and stretching exercise (Fig. 4–48B).

Aerobic Dance. Aerobic dance is especially popular with high school and college women and could be a useful supplement in school physical fitness programs. Adolescent girls tend to work harder and longer when exercising is done to the tempo of music. Also, motivation is often enhanced when done in groups. However, a basic routine (sometimes not the same as other group members) needs to be adjusted for obese subjects so the target heart rate is not exceeded. Unfortunately, some instructors do not have the flexibility to arrange for this in a group class. Aerobic dance is a good conditioning activity and a continuous 30-minute session can expend 200 to 250 K Cal.

Walking. This is a highly recommended activity for both moderate and extremely obese individuals. It is a safe activity and the performer can regulate a safe heart rate pattern through the duration of the walking course. A consistent stride should be maintained followed by a rhythmical arm swing motion. Another advantage is that the activity can be done virtually anywhere without the need for special equipment, *without concern for skill and coordination*. Walking should be a routine activity that is consistently used in weight management (school and home) programs. Initial programs should concentrate on 20 to 30 minutes of walking a day. One hundred K Cal can be expended by walking one mile, providing intensity of effort is sustained (Fig. 4–48C).

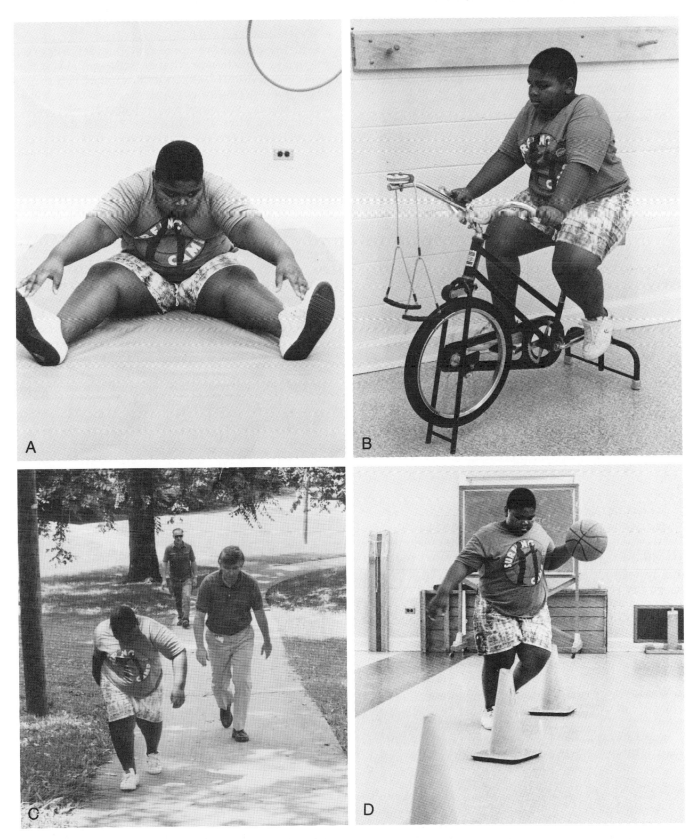

Fig. 4–48. Eleven-year-old obese patient following a 30 minute aerobic circuit program. *A*, stretching exercises; *B*, stationary cycling; *C*, sustained walking. Note the obese youngster setting pace in the front, and *D*, conditioning skill drill.

In summer weight control camps and adapted physical education programs, pedometers have been helpful in gauging progress for adolescents. It also promotes an appreciation for a systematic self-monitoring system through which workouts can be documented on a daily basis.

Running/Jogging. This popular activity should be used with caution. Initially, it should not be used for moderately and excessive obese subjects. Many of these individuals have pronated feet and internal rotation of thighs and legs causing an inability to absorb shock. In general, the activity is too traumatic to the ankles and knees. Mildly obese subjects could possibly use running in combination with walking during the initial stages. From a positive standpoint, a significant amount of calories can be burned up in a short period of time, 500 to 600 K Cal an hour, depending upon speed.

Rope Skipping. This is a good aerobic exercise, but requires a certain amount of skill and coordination. The legs, arms, shoulders, and back muscles are all activated during the course of the activity. Another positive feature is that it can be done almost anywhere without concern for space. The excessively obese performer may have difficulty due to lack of jumping ability, and it could be stressful to ankle, knee, and hip joints. Rope skipping needs to be started slowly while working for 30 seconds, then rest. Jump and rest workouts (4 to 8 minutes) should continue as conditioning improves. With sustained effort, the activity can expend 75 to 100 K Cal during a 10-minute period.

Swimming. This activity is especially good for the obese population because all major muscle groups are used in a non-gravity environment. One major obstacle is the accessibility of pools, which for many subjects is a problem. Another concern is cosmetic issues because obese individuals need to be comfortable with the swimming attire that is worn. If swimming is sustained with continuous movement then it is possible to burn 350 to 400 K Cal per hour.

Some obese subjects lack the coordination to become effective swimmers using a variety of strokes. Other alternatives include Hydro-Aerobics using aquatic-type calisthenics and water jogging. The main consideration, of course, is to reach a desirable target heart rate.

Weight Training. This modality is popular with adolescent boys. Obese adolescents often reflect on their added weight to strength issues so it can be an important adjunct to aerobic programs. Dumbbell and barbell weights can be used to improve muscle strength and endurance and protect the body from loss of lean body mass. It is possible to use weight training in a circuit training program where it is one of many stations interspersed with aerobic type activities during a 30 to 45 minute workout session.

Exercise

The five primary reasons why exercise is important for weight reduction are that exercise may (1) increase energy expenditure, (2) counteract ill effects of obesity, (3) suppress appetite, (4) increase basal metabolism, and (5) minimize loss of lean tissue.[64]

The long slow distance concept of exercise is stressed for obese persons because body fat stores become the energy substrate of choice after 30 minutes (providing intensity level is high). The question then becomes how much exercise is needed to produce a significant change in body fat stores. One factor is the age and build of the individual. A normal weight adult male may carry between 15 and 20% body fat and a female 20 to 25%. In comparison, a highly trained athlete such as a marathon runner may have only 5% body fat. Obese individuals may have upwards of 40% body fat. Clearly, the longer the duration and the heavier the intensity of the program, the greater will be the amount of fat lost. One crude estimate suggests that an exercise program of 3 sessions per week (45 minutes per session) consisting of an activity equal to jogging will produce a weight loss of about 0.5 kg per month without any forced restriction of intake. Exercise intensity should be sufficient to expend 300 or more Kcal per session.[65]

Contraindications

1. Activities in which body weight must be lifted, for example, rope climbing, high jumping, exercises on chinning bar, pushups and head stands, are contraindicated. A heavier body mass is a mechanical handicap, and the majority of obese children will not have the agility or strength to perform these activities.
2. Activities that require sustained exercise in hot, humid weather are contraindicated. Most obese persons will have difficulty participating under these conditions because of thick, ill-conducting layers of adipose tissue that interfere with their work capacity. Activities that precipitate a sweat will also cause chafing of the skin, particularly in the upper thigh and arm regions.
3. Team games that require agility and ability to carry on muscular effort over a large playing area, such as basketball and soccer, should not be played by people with morbid obesity. The person has a difficult time transporting his heavy body mass and easily becomes fatigued. If he is placed in a position in which he is unable to keep up with his teammates, then he loses a feeling of self-worth and confidence. This can have a profound effect on later participation in physical activities.

Precautions. Blood pressure monitoring before and after exercise may prove helpful, particularly for persons not accustomed to regular exercise. High blood pressure is known to be a complication of obesity and a major risk factor for cardiovascular disease.

Therapeutic Exercises

There are no specific therapeutic exercises indicated, unless suggested by a physician.

General Exercises

General exercises and weight training are beneficial to overweight individuals, provided that both are used along with a well-balanced diet. Gradually increase the amount of exercise as the patient's tolerance increases.

Appendices B and C

Precautions. An examination by a physician and written approval for admittance to a weight training program are required. Certain medical problems may exclude some individuals or limit their degree of participation.

OSTEOGENESIS IMPERFECTA

Osteogenesis imperfecta (OI) is a rare genetic disorder of the generalized connective tissue which mainly affects the skeletal system. The Sillence Provisional Classification is used for identifying types of OI. The four genetic types are distinguished for use in genetic counseling and to identify those who may become affected by persistent hearing loss later in life. The classification system will not be discussed in detail, but it identifies the four types to the degree of bone fragility, and other areas of involvement such as affected teeth, sclerae of the eyes, and potential for hearing loss. This classification scale replaces the old system which described types into two categories: Congenital (at birth) and tarda (late onset). Readers are encouraged to read other sources for a more detailed description on the classification system.

Bone fragility is a common characteristic and fractures occur frequently in the long bones of the body. Although the fractures heal, there are often secondary problems that occur such as loss of stature and bowing of the legs. Fractures are variable; some individuals have only three or four during their growth years while others have numerous ones which heal in poor alignment. The incidence of fractures decreases after puberty.

Other medical considerations include a high incidence rate of respiratory infections, cardiopulmonary complications, diaphoresis (an excessive amount of perspiration), scoliosis, and umbilical and inguinal hernias.

OI children possess normal intelligence and have the ability to attain a high level of independence depending upon their mobility limitations. Prognosis for a normal life expectancy depends upon the severity of the disability. Cardiopulmonary problems are the usual causes of death.[66]

Incidence

While the exact number of persons affected with osteogenesis imperfecta is unknown, the estimate suggests between 10,000 to 30,000 persons. Males and females are equally affected and no racial predominance is evident.

Treatment

When necessary, bracing of the lower extremities is required to improve mobility. Stabilizing the knees by use of long leg braces for standing is helpful for children who have reasonable alignment, but inefficient muscle tone. It is suggested that weight bearing should be attempted only in lightweight containment type braces after surgical alignment of the lower extremity bones. Long-term immobilization after surgery or fractures should be avoided as much as possible.

Treatment for scoliosis is often done with the use of body jackets. Some physicians have reservations about this because the bracing can produce additional defects in an already deformed thorax. When the spinal deformity is severe, then spinal fusion with Harrington rod instrumentation is often necessary.

Program Implications

With the constant fear of fractures, it is quite natural for parents and younger children to be somewhat overprotective and fearful of exploring physical activities. Millar describes an important distinction between activity levels. He contends that physical activities started at an early age, are essential for OI children. So much so to the degree that one should run the risk of fractures in order to encourage physical activity. The reason for this is that the bones respond to stress by increasing their density so that one finds oneself between the limits of too little activity, and too much activity.[67]

The ability of the ambulatory child (not wearing long leg braces) to participate in sports and games will depend upon the severity of the condition. In each case, the child should use preventative measures and not engage in collision or high impact (wrestling, touch football) or speed related activities (skateboarding) where there is a high risk of exercise related fractures. Some children with OI wear helmets, knee pads or other protective gear when engaging in active recreational activities and this should be encouraged whenever possible. However, some children feel self-conscious about using protective equipment because of feeling "different."

Those who are wheelchair-users will often need special considerations including use of adapted equipment to compensate for limited strength and mobility. It is with this group that enrollment in an adapted physical education is often necessary in the public school setting. One main concern for the physical education instructor will be how to adapt programs and equipment for the individual who is limited by short, deformed upper-limbs. Weakness of the skeletal muscles and hypermobility of the joints will frequently require the participant to use specialized equipment (Fig. 4–49). For example, a Uni-Cue spring loaded

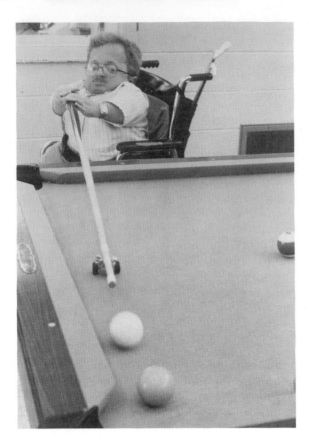

Fig. 4–49. OI patient using wheeled cue rest in billiards.

cue stick may be needed in billiards, or a ramp for pushing a ball instead of throwing a ball in bowling. Whatever the low impact activity, the instructor should be accustomed to the many self-help devices associated with recreational exercise. Equipment aids are also useful to students with OI who use motorized wheelchairs because many in their group have minimal trunk control.

The psychosocial aspects of OI need to be considered. With the constant fear of fractures, children are often overprotected by their parents and others. This sense of overprotection often leads to a fear of trying new physical activities. For this reason, a certain amount of security needs to be developed in the physical education teacher or recreation leader. For this to occur, education on safe handling techniques becomes an important issue. Methods to insure safe lifting practices in transferring to and from a wheelchair is especially important to learn. This is often done in collaboration with the parents. Once the bonding process between parent and child is lessened, then there is a good chance that independent habits can be developed through safe physical challenges.

Swimming is a non-weight bearing activity, and most OI children can become independent swimmers. From a practical viewpoint, involvement in this exercise medium overcomes the fear of gravitational force affecting an unstable bone structure. In addi-

tion, swimming is a popular competitive event for OI athletes competing in Les Autres sports.*

Therapeutic Exercises

After surgery for long bone deformities or fractures it is advisable to follow a postoperative range of motion exercise program at a time specified by the physician.

A systematic strengthening program is often recommended. Certainly caution would be necessary with resistance exercise. However, the safety factor may be increased by utilizing isokinetic and omnikinetic resistance devices.

General Exercises

A flexibility program of progressive static stretching is particularly useful for wheelchair-users.

Swimming to promote cardiovascular endurance and upper-body strength is recommended.

PROGRESSIVE MUSCULAR DISORDERS

The most common muscular disorder is muscular dystrophy. There are also a number of rather uncommon conditions in which the conspicuous feature is muscular weakness and lack of muscle tone. The hereditary pattern of transmission varies with the different types of progressive muscular disorders. The characteristics of all the diseases discussed here are similar and physical education and therapy programs are identical to those appropriate for persons with muscular dystrophy.

Muscular Dystrophy

Progressive muscular dystrophy is an inherited disease of unknown cause characterized by degeneration of the striated muscles. Little is known about the defective gene; most investigators believe it to be biochemically defective but as yet the nature of the defect is unknown. There are at least 3 well-defined clinical types of muscular dystrophy; classification depends

---

*The United States Les Autres Sports Association (USLASA) is the national governing body of athletes who are limited by various locomotor syndromes (static and progressive). International sports competition is governed by the International Sports Organization for the Disabled (ISOD).

Example of eligible Les Autres competitors include ankylosis, arthrogryposis, Guillain-Barre syndrome with permanent motor paresis/paralysis, muscular dystrophies, polyarthritis (i.e. juvenile), osteogenesis imperfecta, and various other locomotor disabilities. This is by no means an exhaustive source of disability groupings who fit the Les Autres category. Readers may write to the USLASA for a listing of other disability groups who are eligible for competition.

Sporting events include track and field, swimming, wheelchair team handball, table tennis, air weapons, weight lifting, sitting and stand-up volleyball, wheelchair and standing basketball. Athlete classification is rather complicated and defined differently in various categories depending upon the event. The ISOD and USLASA have a "minimum permanent disability" standard that must be met in order to qualify for competition. Write to the USLASA for details.

chiefly on the age of the patient at onset, the presence of pseudohypertrophy (increase in muscle size without morbid enlargement of cells), and the particular muscles first affected.

Common Types

Facioscapulohumeral. This form progresses slowly and often remains static for years after mild to moderate involvement of the hip muscles. The onset is usually about the time of puberty, and occurrences are equally distributed among both sexes. Weakness of the facial musculature may be the first involvement, and the patient has difficulty closing his lips, progressive weakness of the shoulder girdle and muscles of the upper arm follows. The course is slow with moderate disability, and some patients live virtually without symptoms for a normal life-span.

Limb-girdle. This form is indistinguishable from the facioscapulohumeral type except that there is no facial involvement. The onset is usually in childhood, but can be as late as the early third decade of life. The initial weakness occurs at the pelvic girdle, and less frequently at the shoulder girdle muscles. The rate of muscular wasting varies, but usually the patient is severely disabled and dies in the fourth or fifth decade of his life.

Childhood. This type of muscular dystrophy, also known as pseudohypertrophic muscular dystrophy or *Duchenne's muscular dystrophy (DMD),* was first described by Duchenne in 1868. It is the most progressive, most serious, and most common of all the dystrophies. DMD is transmitted as an X-linked recessive trait. It is transmitted through the female and predominately affects male offspring. Up to 50% of male children may develop the disease, while 50% of female children may carry the defective gene.

DMD tends to manifest itself in the following clinical course: (1) onset of symptoms between 3 and 5 years of age; (2) progressive muscle weakness, wasting and contractures involving first the pelvis and then the pectoral girdle, sparing the cranial nerve muscles; (3) hypertrophy of the calf muscle in most cases; (4) loss of independent ambulation by the ages of 9 to 11 years; (5) slowly progressive generalized weakness and scoliosis during the teen years; and (6) respiratory failure before the third decade.

Laboratory studies are used to confirm a diagnosis of DMD. One specific study involves the enzyme creatine phosphokinase (CPK). All constituents of a normal muscle cell are retained within its membrane. In dystrophy, where muscle tissue breaks down, the membrane becomes unusually permeable, and substances originally contained within the cell leak out into the blood serum, and are found there at higher levels than normal. Since CPK is confined almost exclusively to muscle, a leakage from this tissue can be assumed to be responsible when abnormally high levels of CPK are observed in blood serum. Elevation of CPK to 25 to 50 times the normal level is a helpful diagnostic sign in confirming DMD. As the disease progresses, CPK activity eventually decreases, but it usually remains high while the patient is ambulatory.

The CPK test has been utilized in recent years to detect carriers of DMD. Testing for carriers is approximately 70% effective and is done with female siblings of patients or sisters of known carriers of DMD.

The first weakness is in the muscles of the pelvis, abdomen, and hip and results in lordosis (abdominal and gluteus maximus weakness) and waddling gait (gluteus medius weakness). As weakness of the hip muscles progresses, the patient, in order to rise to a standing posture, must first straighten the hip and knee, then extend the trunk by pushing upward with the hands sequentially on the knees, thighs and hips (Gowers' sign, Fig. 4–50). Weakness gradually spreads to the trunk muscles, shoulder girdle, and finally to the hands and feet. Asymmetrical weakness of the back musculature may result in varying degrees of scoliosis in the late stages. The progressive weakness of the muscles of the legs during the period of rapid skeletal growth may produce contractures and foot deformities if adequate preventive measures are not taken.

Other forms of muscular dystrophy—the distal limb variety, the type localized in the ocular muscles, and congenital types—are rare and specialized.

Incidence

Definite data on actual prevalence are not available, but most authorities estimate that 150,000 to 200,000 persons are afflicted with muscular dystrophy in the United States. It is one of the most serious disabling conditions of childhood, since more than half of those affected are between the ages of 4 and 15 years.

Treatment

The lack of an effective therapeutic agent multiplies the problems of management. There is no convincing evidence that medication or a combination of medications will retard the inevitable degeneration of muscle. It is necessary to maintain active exercise whenever possible. Range-of-motion exercises are helpful to prevent contractures and tight muscles. Muscle tightness occurs early in the triceps surae, hip flexors, hamstrings, toe flexors, forearm pronators, and wrist and finger flexors.

Most children with DMD will need to wear long leg-braces by the age 7 or 8 years. Bracing is generally employed when daily walking time has decreased to less than one hour. Under such circumstances, many patients can achieve a stable gait with braces for at least 3 years. However, braced ambulation may not be suitable for all children. Each case should be assessed separately to rule out any attitudinal, mental, or physical problems that would interfere with successful bracing. The use of a standing platform or a standing table can adequately facilitate independent functioning from a standing position during selected

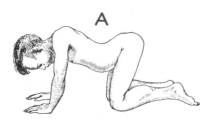

Fig. 4–50. Progressive muscular dystrophy. Characteristic method of rising to a standing position, the arms being used to push the body erect (Gowers' sign). Note the increased lumbar lordosis, relaxed shoulder girdle, and enlarged calves. (From Shands, A.R., Jr., et al.: Handbook of Orthopaedic Surgery. St. Louis, C.V. Mosby Co., 1963.)

periods of the day. Lower extremity bracing is usually not successful after long periods of restriction to wheelchair level.

When the child needs a wheelchair fulltime, an ankle-foot orthosis may be necessary in order to prevent ankle and foot deformity. Because of the degeneration of the postural muscles, mainly the extensor muscles of the back, careful observation should be made concerning scoliosis. A tight-fitting jacket made of plastic or fiberglass is usually of value. Surgical procedures to correct deformities of the spine are generally avoided because of the detrimental effects imposed by immobilization.

Various types of forearm orthoses and overhead slings have been utilized to maintain range of motion of the upper extremities for wheelchair-bound patients. The devices are often helpful in improving activities of daily living.

Pneumonia is the most common life-taking condition in muscular dystrophy. In advanced cases, the child has restricted pulmonary function with reduced vital capacity. Respiratory care in a hospital is often necessary to combat the effects of this life-threatening situation. The utilization of postural drainage, intermittent positive pressure breathing, and vigorous antibiotic therapy is necessary.

Treatment for muscular dystrophy is basically supportive in nature. Obesity hampers all forms of management and deters effective independence during both the ambulatory and the wheelchair stages. This hazard must be fully understood and appreciated by the family, because prevention of obesity is far easier than reduction of weight, especially with dystrophic children, who have reduced capacity to expend energy.

Stages of Functional Ability*

1. Ambulates with mild waddling gait and lordosis. Elevation activities adequate (climbs stairs and curbs without assistance).
2. Ambulates with moderate waddling gait and lordosis. Elevation activities deficient (needs support for curbs and stairs).
3. Ambulates with moderately severe waddling gait and lordosis. Cannot negotiate curbs or stairs, but can achieve erect posture from standard-height chair.
4. Ambulates with severe waddling gait and lordosis. Unable to rise from a standard-height chair.
5. Wheelchair independence: Good posture in the chair; can perform all activities of daily living from chair.
6. Wheelchair with dependence. Can roll chair but needs assistance in bed and wheelchair activities.
7. Wheelchair with dependence and back support. Can roll the chair only a short distance; needs back support for good chair position.
8. Bed patient. Can do no activities of daily living without maximum assistance.

An appropriate wheelchair should be introduced to the patient once stage 4 is reached. The patient can learn to transfer from wheelchair to bed and toilet and reverse and thus be independent for a significantly longer period of time.

The patient in the wheelchair (stages 5 to 7) becomes gradually less efficient in performing activities of daily living as the illness progresses. In stage 7 the weakness has involved the trunk to such a degree that the patient cannot maintain a satisfactory wheelchair position without the assistance of a back brace. Often the improved posture provided by the brace enables

*Courtesy of the Muscular Dystrophy Associations of America, Inc.

the patient to handle the chair with much greater efficiency. It is essential that the wheelchair patient (stages 5 to 7) and the bed patient (stage 8) be given the physiologic and psychologic benefits of achieving erect posture by the use of either an appropriate brace or a tilt table.

Peroneal Muscular Atrophy (Charcot-Marie-Tooth Disease)

Peroneal muscular atrophy causes a progressive muscular atrophy which first is noticeable when the patient is between 12 and 50 years old. It ordinarily begins with symmetrical atrophy and weakness of the muscles that extend and turn the foot. This results in clubfoot. In time, most of the leg and foot muscles become involved, as do the muscles of the hand and forearm. In some instances the arms may be involved before the legs.

Amyotonia Congenita (Oppenheim's Disease)

This rare disease is present at birth and characterized by extreme muscle weakness owing to the failure of development of the motor nuclei of the cranial nerves and the motor cells of the spinal cord. Sensation is not affected. The condition is generally believed to be either static or subject to gradual improvement.

Friedreich's Ataxia

This is a comparatively rare familial degeneration of the spinal cord and cerebellum of unknown cause. Onset usually occurs when the patient is between the ages of 6 and 15 years, and the disease is characterized by unsteady gait, foot deformity, involuntary rapid movements of the eyes, and curvature of the spine. There is weakness of the muscles of the trunk and legs.

Program Implications

Duchenne muscular dystrophy is characterized by progressive degeneration and weakness. Participation in physical activities will obviously depend upon the child's stage of involvement and functional capacity.

Ambulatory Child

A shift caused by lordosis and forward tilting of the pelvis occurs in the center of gravity of the child with DMD when he is between the ages of 5 and 8 years; and this is the period when walking balance is impaired. Because of lack of muscle power in the back, the body is arched beyond normal limits to maintain extension. In addition, the gait is slow; movement is a swinging forward rather than a stepping forward motion. Under such circumstances, balance is precarious and the nearest touch will upset the child. It is impractical to expect children with DMD of early childhood age to follow standard patterns of development. Basic locomotor skills, such as skipping, hopping, and jumping, which emphasize balance and

rhythm, will be difficult or impossible. Nonlocomotor patterns such as stooping and bending are also difficult to perform without losing balance. Many children will have to hold onto something when performing certain types of game skills, such as striking or kicking. It is essential that activities that require speed of movement (running relays, chase and tag games) and tests of strength (push ups, standing long jump) be avoided.

Children with DMD must find their own center of gravity and adjust their balance accordingly. Surprisingly, many children exhibit a good awareness of position in space. The reason for this is that they learn, and then replicate over and over again, positions and movements to maintain their balance. Losing and regaining his balance causes the child to stay within a vertical axis, and this causes maintenance of a vertical continuum, because positioning of the body segments is consistent. This is unlike normal children between the ages of 5 and 8 years who constantly change and alternate ways of performing motor tasks because their performance is not interpreted properly or because they become discouraged over the outcome. Therapeutic recreation specialists and physical education instructors should understand that many dystrophic children will display good kinesthetic motor awareness because of the consistency of their motor responses. Because of limited muscle power the dystrophic child has minimal strength to throw objects at ground targets. This limits his range of space for performing motor tasks. For this reason, throwing bean bags in boxes or balls in trash cans are simple, low organization games in which children with DMD often excel. It is also important to maintain a child's existing range of motion through bilateral movements so that both upper extremities can contribute equally to production of force and maintenance of balance. Throwing and catching lightweight balls (beachball, Nerf ball) to promote elbow extension and forearm supination should be encouraged.

A young child will want to participate, and should be included, in some physical education activities, especially those of a social and recreational nature. By modifying rules, area of play, method of locomotion, and type and size of equipment, participation is possible in many activities. As long as they experience success, children with DMD should participate in regular play activities. It is important to point out, however, that these children cannot be classified as "normal" just because they are ambulatory. Many will not have sufficient strength or balance to participate in regular physical education class. Some authorities in physical education have reported that children with DMD should participate in activities until they show signs of normal fatigue and stages of exhaustion. This conflicts with the opinions of many physicians who believe that children with DMD should know their fatigue level and stop before they reach it. It is believed that upon reaching fatigue, the affected muscle leaks CPK, which is presumed to be responsible for degeneration of muscle.

During periods when children are wearing long leg-braces, many will be using a standing table or platform for support. Balls of varying weight, bean bags, Frisbees, any object that can be thrown at a target, should be encouraged. Activities that include extensor power (throwing) and flexor power (catching) are recommended. Allowing the child to create rhythms by beating drums, clashing cymbals or using other rhythmic instruments can provide pleasurable opportunities for expressive movement. The rhythm can be varied with different tempos. In most instances, early instruction or experience is performed at a slower tempo; and the tempo is increased after the movement patterns have been learned.

Wheelchair-user Child

By the age of 12, most patients use a wheelchair. An appropriate program of adapted sports and games can prevent atrophy due to disuse of muscles and keep muscular power at as high a level as possible during the progressive phases of muscular dystrophy and atrophy. Slow and careful teaching of fundamental motor skills is important, as the patient finds it increasingly difficult to perform physical activities without learning new ways of doing the tasks. Since the muscular involvement becomes almost bilaterally symmetrical, it is important to include activities that maintain the existing range of motion in both the upper extremities. (Parachute play and throwing a beachball or playground ball from the overhead position are examples of such activities.) However, for some children with severe deformity contractures and little muscle power, active exercise is limited or impossible. Simple grasp-and-release games or table games may be the only activities that are possible under such circumstances. Arm suspension slings are of great help to these children, not only for allowing more movement, but for offering a means of exercise.

Since the finger flexor muscles are one of the last groups affected by the disease, it is imperative that program selection include use of the fingers for manipulation. Effective digital control is crucial in certain activities such as table shuffleboard and air-riflery. Dystrophy children often excel in these two activities, which are manifestly helpful in promoting emotional well-being during the later stages of the disease. Assistive devices are often necessary to compensate for loss of arm muscle strength. Ramps are especially useful for individuals with limited arm movement. Bowling and billiards can be adapted for most any disabled child, regardless of the level of his functional ability.

Upon arrival of adolescence, many individuals with muscular dystrophy will start to contemplate their uncertain future. For a wheelchair-user, it is at this stage that peer relationships need to be developed and/or maintained. Group participation skills need to be strengthened. This is often best accomplished in an environment that challenges others who have a like or similar disability such as seen in a residential camp setting. Unlike the wheelchair bound person who has good upper body strength, the equation of overcoming physical challenges is not as realistic for the individual with DMD. Simply stated, he is more dependent on others to assist in meeting recreational and personal needs (Fig. 4–51). Unfortunately, this will occur on a predictable course that involves coping with new compensatory skills.

Case History: An 11-year-old boy had Duchenne's muscular dystrophy which was diagnosed when he was 3½-years-old. He walked with a marked equinus deformity and lumbar lordosis (both characteristic patterns), but had fair quadriceps strength. Occasional complicating factors were substernal pressure (chest constriction) and tachycardia, which were not always associated with exercise. At the time of his admission to the Kluge Children's Rehabilitation Center at the University of Virginia, therapeutic recreation activities consisting of low organization games from the upright position were used to facilitate adjustment and tolerance to his new long leg-braces (Fig. 4–52).

Lifting

In assisting a muscular dystrophic child to his feet, it is best to stand directly in front of him. Put your arms around his lower back and lock your hands so that as he rises his upper trunk is free to sway back as you pull forward near the hips. This helps the patient to "lock" his hips. It is sometimes necessary to place a hand over the sacrum and forcibly push the pelvic girdle forward. *Never try to lift a muscular dystrophic child under the armpits.*

Precautions

Persons with progressive muscle disease tend to stay away from physical exertion. They would rather watch an athletic contest than try to expose their weak bodies to mild forms of physical exercise. Don't pamper—but don't push. It is unrealistic to urge the child beyond his physical capabilities. Forcing him into such situations only serves to heighten his feeling of inadequacy.

Care should be taken that no muscle group has to strain to perform a movement. No resistance other than gravity itself should be used, and as soon as the muscle shows sign of strain, gravity should be neutralized and assistance given to the muscle. Exercises should be done once or twice a day for 4 to 6 counts only. Avoid having the patient exercise at times when he may be tired, such as right after school or late at night.

Exercise

The effect of exercise on DMD needs consideration. Charash states,

Exercise has value in DMD for recreational purposes and for the favorable modification it may exert upon contractures. There is no evidence which would support the view that muscle strength in muscles which have not been clinically affected in dystrophy would be preserved as a result

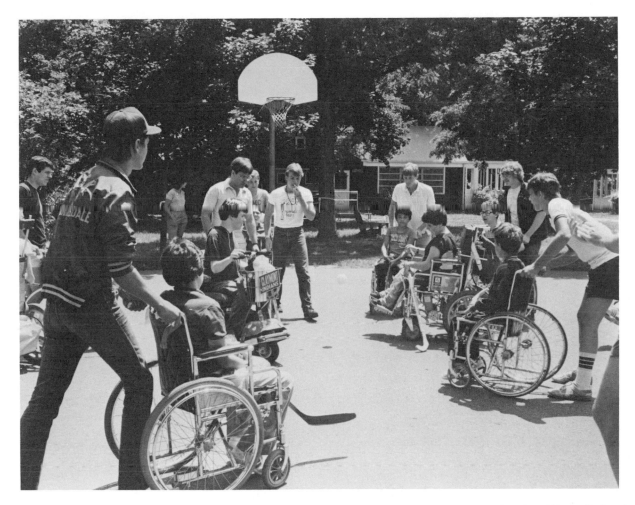

Fig. 4–51. To facilitate a feeling of sustained effort without fatigue these MD campers are enjoying a game of hockey. Able-bodied assistants push the wheelchair players (most are in stage 6 of functional ability) who are responsible for manipulating their own sticks, thereby overcoming total reliance on external controls. MDA chapters throughout the country support summer camping programs for children with dystrophy and related disorders. (Courtesy of Muscular Dystrophy Association.)

of exercise. Most clinicians recommend that patients remain active within the framework of their capability depending on the stage of the dystrophic process without producing undue fatigue.[68]

Any physical activity program that helps dystrophic children become more active and independent is a great boost to their morale. However, somewhere between complete activity and even the slightest fatigue is the range in which a child with DMD must pursue his way of life.

Therapeutic Exercises

The child with progressive muscular dystrophy (facioscapulohumeral, pseudohypertrophic, and distal types) has slowly progressive muscular weakness. Specific therapeutic exercises will not restore the use of affected muscles. However, a great deal can be accomplished in a supportive fashion to maintain ambulation and range of motion. Specific therapeutic exercises can be utilized, depending on the areas of involvement. For example, hip exercises would be of

use to a child with pseudohypertrophic muscular dystrophy.

Joint motion should be tested prior to initiating a stretching and exercise program. Quite often there is a better preservation of flexor strength.[69]

Other conditions associated with hypotonia and muscular weakness can also be treated with therapeutic exercises, depending on areas of involvement.

Appendix A

It is a good rule to consult the physician prior to planning any exercise program.

General Exercises

General exercises and weight training should be continued as long as possible. Watch carefully for signs of early fatigue.

Appendices B and C

RHEUMATOID ARTHRITIS

The term *arthritis* means inflammation of a joint, a condition marked by pain, heat, redness, and swelling.

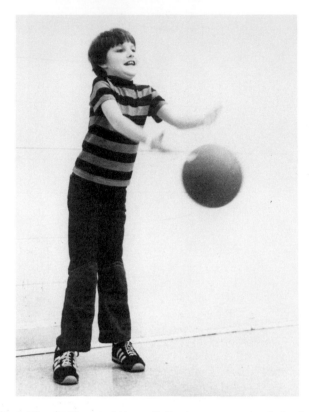

Fig. 4–52.   An 11-year-old boy with Duchenne muscular dystrophy participating in low organization games.

However, the word has become a popular label for a number of different joint abnormalities with many possible causes.

Rheumatism is a disease marked by painful inflammation of the connective tissue structures, especially of the muscles and joints. There are many different types of rheumatism; some forms are serious, others less serious.

Arthritis can be very disabling and permanent joint damage can occur over time (Fig. 4–53). However, with early diagnosis and treatment, major complications can be prevented. Most arthritics combine medication (primarily aspirin) with exercise to maintain joint integrity. Similar treatment is used in osteoarthritis (degenerative joint disease). Osteoarthritis is the result of lasting joint degeneration and unlike rheumatoid arthritis, individual joints are locally affected and inflammation is rarely a problem.

Children are also afflicted with rheumatoid arthritis and further attention will concentrate on this group. When reviewing physical activity considerations, certain implications may also apply to the adult group, knowing that daily exercise is essential in maintaining joint mobility.

Juvenile Rheumatoid Arthritis

There are several distinct subgroups of the disease and readers are encouraged to read other sources of information on the subject. However, a few variations are listed below to clarify further the many manifestations that are involved with the three known forms of Juvenile Rheumatoid Arthritis (JRA).

Systematic JRA

Ratio: Girls/Boys are almost equal. Variable temperature peaks are common frequently with shaking chills. A rash is frequently present, and occurs most often during febrile periods. Many joints are affected and can be a major long-term problem.

Pauciarticular JRA

There are two sub-types, one mainly seen in boys and the other mainly in girls. In most patients, the knees, ankles, and elbows are involved. With some boys, severe hip and spine disease are associated problems of late disability. Some children (usually girls) can have ocular damage. This form of eye inflammation is termed iridocyclitis which requires early diagnosis and treatment. Pauciarticular arthritis is a mild form of JRA which lasts only a few days and results in excellent recovery.

With early diagnosis and treatment, severe crippling can usually be prevented, and permanent damage can be kept to a minimum if the condition is kept under control.

Polyarticular JRA

Girls are more frequently involved on an 8:1 ratio. Many joints are involved, especially the small joints of the hand. About half of the children have arthritis in the neck, hips, or shoulders. Low fevers may be present in some children. It is estimated that 40 to 50% of all children with JRA will have this form.[70]

Incidence

Approximately 40,000,000 persons have arthritis. According to estimates, as many as 250,000 children in the United States may have some form of arthritis. Girls are affected more frequently than boys. It has been estimated that at least 75% of children with JRA, perhaps more, will eventually enter long-term remission without any significant joint damage.

Treatment

Anti-inflammatory drugs, such as large doses of aspirin, may be used to control pain and stiffness. Every patient with rheumatoid arthritis should be given a good trial of adequate dosages of salicylates first before any other drug therapy is attempted.

Steroid therapy for rheumatoid arthritis is usually administrered as a last resort when other agents fail to control the clinical manifestations. Although steroid therapy is used only under special considerations, swelling and stiffness of joints are reduced.

Gold compounds have been used in the treatment of rheumatoid arthritis. In many cases, treatment with gold dramatically improves the functional capacity of the patient. Gold compounds are administered by intramuscular injection. The course of treatment usu-

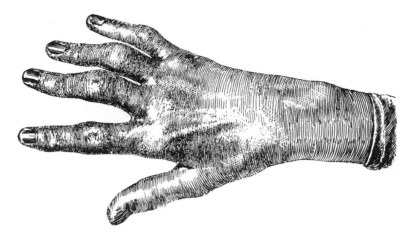

Fig. 4–53. Rheumatoid arthritis of the hand, early stage. Note enlargement of the proximal interphalangeal joints (after Duncan). (From Shands, A.R., Jr., et al.: Handbook of Orthopaedic Surgery. St. Louis, C.V. Mosby Co., 1963.)

ally starts with weekly injections, and after a specified time, the interval between injections is lengthened to 2 to 4 weeks for an indefinite period.

Splints or casts may be recommended to give joints added rest and to help prevent contractures. The longer a joint remains bent or in flexion, the greater the possibility that it will stay that way. Canes and crutches may also be used to assist weight-bearing joints.

Various orthopedic operations on joints can be effective in preventing some deformities, in relieving pain, and in improving overall function.

Physical therapy has no curative effect in arthritis, nor does it alter the course of the disease process. The objectives of therapy are to mobilize joints, improve their functioning and prevent or minimize disabilities.

Program Implications

Sports and games must be safe and nonstrenuous, since rheumatoid arthritis is systemic, fluctuating, usually progressive, and a cause both of physical disability and of pain. Obviously, the extent of joint damage is a major factor in determining what types of activities are to be performed.

It may be necessary to hospitalize the patient at times because of severe flare-ups of rheumatoid arthritis. The therapeutic recreation specialist will need to follow 3 important rules when outlining a program for the hospitalized patient:

1. There must be frequent consultation between the physician, the physical therapist, and the occupational therapist to review the functional status of the patient.
2. Physical activities must be restricted to prevent damage to the joints.
3. There should be frequent rest periods; however, the amount of rest needed will depend on the severity of the disease.

Usually the physician will prescribe and advise treatment for the individual to follow at home. Even

those, including children with juvenile rheumatoid arthritis, who need little medical care will need to follow certain general principles about recreational and physical education activities. Strenuous and combative sports and games are usually not recommended because vigorous activities may increase pain and damage to the joints. Individual or dual sports are generally recommended to allow the participant to develop confidence in his motor skills. Many assistive devices are available that can reduce stress on the joints and enable the individual to participate with his normal peers.

Most children with rheumatoid arthritis can attend regular school and engage in regular physical activity, but some considerations may be necessary in a classroom setting to eliminate joint stiffness. The students should be allowed to move about frequently instead of sitting in one position for a long period of time. These children should be enrolled in physical education class, provided that the activities do not aggravate their condition. The physical education teacher should be sensitive to the feelings of children with rheumatoid arthritis. The reaction of some children to active physical movements will be that of apprehension and doubt. This is especially true for those with a long history of arthritic symptoms. It is not uncommon to see children with rheumatoid arthritis who are self-conscious of their inadequacies. These children are usually fearful of body contact (football) and shock absorbing activities (tumbling) where impact to the joints may aggravate their condition. Children who have been inactive during the greater portion of their lives will need to be motivated to participate in physical education class, even during a period when their arthritis is in remission.

Sports and games should be modified to reduce stresses and strains on affected joints. Tennis, for example, can maintain and aggravate the active inflammation imposed on knee joints by rheumatoid arthritis. In order to reduce weight-bearing on persistently inflamed knees, the ambulatory arthritic can play the modified version of tennis called target tennis, which is played from a stationary position, or table tennis. Suitable activities include golf, angling, billiards, riflery, creative dance and shuffleboard.

Physicians maintain that each joint should be used at maximum range of motion and strength consistent with the disease process. Two frequently prescribed forms of recreational exercise are swimming and bicycling. Swimming promotes joint mobility in a non-weight bearing environment, and to achieve maximum results the water temperature should be between 83° to 89°F. Muscle strength can be maintained or increased as the water provides resistance to movement. Bicycling is often recommended to stimulate movement in the ankle, knee, and hip joints. The rotary action related to the pedaling motion keeps the joints mobile, providing the terrain is consistent with the effort and condition of the cyclist.

Precautions. Medical literature has depicted the arthritic as a person who often has difficulty in forming satisfactory relationships with people and who shows strong control of all emotional expression. Persons with rheumatoid arthritis, including children, suffer from a severe, well-masked anxiety state. A well-defined program of sports and games can help release pent-up anger. A good relationship with the program leader may have important psychotherapeutic benefits. Once the instructor or therapist has ascertained the individual's own motives and goals, any movement in the direction of the attainment of such goals serves as reinforcement. The program leader may need to set modest goals and reward the person on any small but significant gains.

Therapeutic Exercises

A physician must prescribe the type and duration of exercise, as well as the joint movement desired. Therapeutic exercises performed in the proper manner will aid in improving joint motion, stability, and function.

The following exercises are to be used as a guide and should be approved by the patient's physician.

Appendix A
1. Exercises for the upper back
   Exercises 1 through 17
2. Exercises for the lower back
   Exercises 18 through 31
3. Exercises for abdominal muscles
   Exercises 32 through 42
4. Exercises for the hip
   Exercises 43 through 63
5. Exercises for the knee
   Exercises 64 through 80
6. Exercises for the ankle
   Exercises 81 through 95
7. Exercises for the fingers
   Exercises 96 through 110
8. Exercises for the wrist
   Exercises 111 through 117
9. Exercises for the elbow
   Exercises 118 through 124
10. Exercises for the shoulder
    Exercises 125 through 138
11. Exercises for head and neck
    Exercises 139, 140, 141
12. Exercises for deep breathing
    Exercises 142 through 146

NOTE: Exercise should be done when there is the least amount of pain and stiffness. If taking a prescriptive pain medication, plan the workout when the drug is having the most effect. Range of motion exercises should be done even when the slightest amount of pain is present. If the joint is hot, inflamed, swollen, red or tender to touch, move it gently through its range of motion. If in doubt, contact the physician or therapist to find out how to adapt the exercises.

General Exercises

General exercise programs and mild weight training are beneficial when the rheumatoid arthritis is not acute.

Appendices B and C

SPINA BIFIDA

Spina bifida is a congenital anomaly characterized by a developmental defect in one or more vertebral arches through which the contents of the spinal canal may protrude. It usually occurs in the lumbar region, but it may be present at other levels of the spine.

Types

Three types are discussed here: spina bifida occulta, meningocele, and myelomeningocele, with hydrocephalus, which is an associated deformity.

Spina Bifida Occulta

Spina bifida occulta is a defect in the fusion of the posterior neural arch (Fig. 4–54). It is usually asymptomatic, is occasionally detected by x ray, and does not require treatment. The skin and spinal cord are normal.

Meningocele

This condition occurs when the meninges (coverings of the spinal cord), in a sac composed of the dura mater and arachnoid and filled with cerebrospinal fluid, protrude through a defect in the spinal cord (Fig. 4–55). The condition is rarely associated with neurologic disability, and its only danger is rupture of the sac with resultant ascending infection of the spinal fluid (meningitis). Surgical closure is required to prevent this complication.

Myelomeningocele

This condition occurs when the sac protruding from the defect includes both the meninges and por-

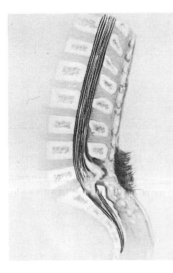

Fig. 4–54. Spina bifida occulta. (From West, J.S.: Congenital Malformations and Birth Defects. Baltimore, Williams & Wilkins, 1954.)

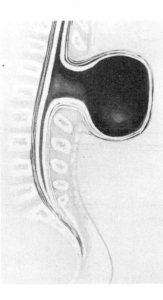

Fig. 4–55. Spina bifida with meningocele. (From West, J.S.: Congenital Malformations and Birth Defects. Baltimore, Williams & Wilkins, 1954.)

tions of the spinal cord (Fig. 4–56). It is the most common type of spina bifida, is always associated with some degree of neurologic deficit, and requires early surgical correction.

Further discussion will be limited to those patients with myelomeningocele, since it is the most common and most important, occurring 4 or 5 times as often as other types.

The nature and degree of involvement depends largely upon the location of the spinal cord lesion. Sacral myelomeningocele causes little involvement, with weakness confined to the feet; midlumbar lesions affect legs and feet; and lesions in the high lumbar area or above cause paresis (partial paralysis) of the muscles throughout the lower extremities.

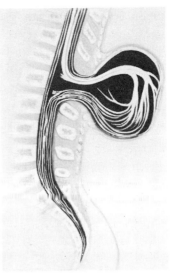

Fig. 4–56. Spina bifida with myelomeningocele. (From West, J.S.: Congenital Malformations and Birth Defects. Baltimore, Williams & Wilkins, 1954.)

The feet may be deformed because of intrauterine paralysis, and joints of the ankles, knees, or hips may be immobile.

As the nerves to the urinary and anal sphincters from the lumbosacral spine are involved in most cases, sphincter disturbances represent the most difficult part of management.

Hydrocephalus
Hydrocephalus, or water brain, is an associated deformity in 90 to 95% of children with myelomeningocele.[71] Hydrocephalus is caused by an inadequate absorption of cerebrospinal fluid and might either be present at birth or may develop later, usually within the first 6 weeks of life.

Treatment should be started as soon as the clinical manifestations are observed, before damage to the brain itself occurs. Surgery is required for the installation of a shunt to drain off the fluid; several shunting (diversionary) procedures are now in use (Fig. 4–57). The 2 most commonly used shunts are those leading directly into the bloodstream (ventriculoatrial) and into the abdominal cavity (ventriculoperitoneal).

Incidence
Myelomeningocele, or spina bifida cystica, is one of the most common birth defects and a rather frequent cause of disability in infancy and childhood. Statistics show an incidence of 1 to 3 cases in every 1,000 births.

Treatment
Although the disease is neither difficult to diagnose, nor, fortunately, to treat, the newborn infant with a myelomeningocele confronts the patients and physician with serious problems in management.

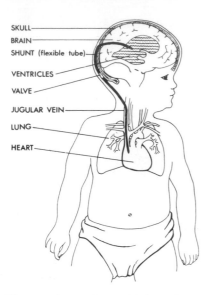

SKULL
BRAIN
SHUNT (flexible tube)
VENTRICLES
VALVE
JUGULAR VEIN
LUNG
HEART

Fig. 4–57. Diagram of a ventriculoatrial shunt. Cerebrospinal fluid, under abnormally high pressure in the brain, is redirected into the jugular vein above the heart by means of a small flexible tube. (Courtesy of Foundation for Child Development.)

Vigorous treatment of the myelomeningocele child within the first few months of life is important. Some physicians recommend immediate closure of the sac; others wait longer to see if the child will survive. Early closure results in marked decrease in both central nervous system infections and neonatal mortality. A neurosurgeon might perform the shunting first, with closure of the sac to follow. Prompt attention to the surgical covering of the myelomeningocele and the surgical prevention or arrest of hydrocephalus are the two most important steps in the early treatment plan.

The combination of paralysis, urinary and bowel incontinence, and absence of sensation in the affected parts constitutes a multiple disability; however, with the successful management of these problems and correction of orthopedic deformities, many individuals are able to successfully complete school and pursue careers.

Treatment is directed toward helping the child make maximum use of the unafflicted parts of his body and minimizing his disabilities. Most children can learn to walk with the aid of braces and crutches at about 4 years of age.

A urologist should be consulted for information and advice about bladder and bowel training, and most children with spina bifida should be able to master the procedures by the time they reach school age. Children with neurogenic bladder dysfunction are often taught intermittent self-catheterization. This allows for self-control of urinary functions. The patient catheterizes himself (or his parents perform the procedure) with a rubber catheter 5 to 6 times a day. Important features in bowel training are adequate diet, regular meals, a regular time for emptying the bowels, and exercise, including walking. In cases in which upper urinary tract damage is impending or has already occurred, the urologist may recommend a urinary diversion surgical procedure. This is used as a last resort when more conservative measures, including intermittent catheterization, fail to preserve good kidney function.

Care must be taken to prevent obesity, malnutrition, and secondary contractions. Any infection should be promptly treated with antibiotics. If the child is mentally normal, he can become a useful member of society.

Program Implications

Attendance at a regular school should be encouraged if the child has sufficient intellectual skills. Frequently, however, because of the need for continual neurosurgical, urologic, and orthopedic consultations and procedures, allowances for frequent absences from school must be made. The normal child who is 5 to 8 years of age uses an increasing variety and complexity of movement in his play. Unfortunately, due to lack of motor dexterity, many myelomeningocele children cannot participate in common childhood play activities such as climbing, jumping, tumbling, tag, and hopscotch. However, it is between the ages of 5 and 8 years that the greatest percentage of children with myelomeningocele learn to walk. These children especially need to be accepted by their peers and to belong to a group.

Eye-hand coordination is poor in many children with spina bifida. There is reason to believe that this is due in part to lack of normal experiences and not simply to neurologic damage.[72]

Elementary school physical education teachers should assist classroom teachers in analyzing the perceptual-motor capabilities of myelomeningocele children. Many have difficulty following 2-part directions and are unable to organize verbal directions and memorize concepts. Often, because of specific inborn or environmental characteristics, progress in various types of skills is uneven. For example, a child often develops normal cognitive abilities, but experiences problems in motor behavior; or he may have difficulties with perception, while progressing nicely in the verbal area. For children with body perception problems, a specific remedial program should be instituted. Adjustment of movement to distances, sizes, positions of objects and amounts of force applied to various projectiles should be encouraged. Low organization games that enhance eye-hand coordination and motor planning should be encouraged. Beanbags, yarn balls, and playground balls are important tools for experimentation. Object management (throwing and catching) and visual-motor activities that involve aiming and coordinating body parts are recommended. Also, since many children demonstrate inconsistency in their hand preference, it is important to use activities that contrast body sides.

More research needs to be done on the perceptual skills of both hydrocephalic and nonhydrocephalic myelomeningocele children. Gressang[73] studied 29 children, all of whom had myelomeningocele, to determine whether a significant difference existed between the performance of nonhydrocephalic and hydrocephalic children on a series of 4 perceptual-motor tests. Twenty subjects had hydrocephalus and had required surgical shunting procedures. The median age was 5 years 10 months. All participants had scored at the borderline (70 I.Q.) or above on psychometric testing or had a developmental quotient of 80 or above. The hydrocephalic children scored higher on all 4 tests.

A number of myelomeningocele children have difficulty processing information effectively, and visual cues help them organize and accumulate usable data. The teacher or therapist often must implement visual techniques to help the children understand basic concepts. For example, the program leader can color circles on a blackboard or set up bowling pins to identify the total number of points scored in a game. In this way the child can conceptualize and use visual stimuli to fixate at specific points, and thus reinforce learning. In this way, visual impressions can be used to compensate for deficits in auditory perception. Also, research has often associated distractibility with children who have hydrocephalus. Often, it is necessary to repeat directions. The child can repeat both directions and the intended response, if it is something he is expected to remember.

Physical activities that develop as much strength as possible in the shoulders and arms should be encouraged. Children with a lesion at the L4 or L5 level have enough motor power present for hip flexion and hip adduction; consequently, they should be encouraged to perform unilateral motor tasks such as throwing balls and striking objects from a standing position. Due to varying degrees of involvement, some children need to use one crutch for support while their dominant upper-extremity is free for propulsion. These activities help to develop nonlocomotor skills (body movements done while stationary) because they force the children to react to equilibrium and postural changes. Such skills are especially helpful for children who are effective household ambulators, but need additional work on developing standing balance and tolerance. In many instances, long leg-braces are used for ambulation, but it is often difficult for the child wearing such braces to perform motor skills from a standing position. For individuals with a thoracolumbar lesion or at L1 or L2, use of a wheelchair during participation in sports and games allows a certain amount of independence and prevents excessive fatigue. Children in wheelchairs can participate in "running" activities in their wheelchairs. Relays are good for both fitness and social objectives, and the wheelchair-bound student should be encouraged to participate. Distance can be modified to equalize competition. For example, the wheelchair racer can start first, and the distance between him and the second runner can be shortened. After this modification, normal play can resume and runners can complete action until a point is scored (Chapter 6).

Swimming is an excellent activity. The buoyancy of the water often permits a person with physical disabilities to acquire skills he could not acquire without the support of the water.

By secondary school age, most myelomeningocele children are independent in their activities of daily living. Unfortunately, many stop ambulating due to the amount of energy that must be expended to lift their body weight and the weight of their braces or crutches from one place to another. Walking with braces and crutches can be a laborious procedure, thus many individuals prefer to use a wheelchair. Using a wheelchair during participation in sports and games enables the person to achieve a certain amount of independence and prevents excessive fatigue. Sports such as archery, weight lifting, and physical exercise programs such as chair-obics, which promote active use of the upper extremities, should be encouraged (Fig. 4–58).

The United States Les Autres Sports Association's national competition is open to both wheelchair and ambulatory spina bifida athletes. Wheelchair athletes' results are kept separately from les autres while ambulatory athletes are considered as les autres. However, the USLASA does not offer the opportunity for international competition for the spina bifida group. Wheelchair spina bifida athletes must compete at NWAA sanctioned meets to qualify internationally.

Precautions. Because of poor circulation and absence of sensation, decubitus ulcers may develop very quickly. The instructor or therapist should instruct the child to inspect his skin for signs of pressure whenever he applies or removes his braces, particularly after participating in physical activities. If the child is enrolled in a public school physical education program, the school nurse can help in this phase of management.

Problems with incontinence can be a major social problem, especially if it occurs at school. Spina bifida children by the age of 7 with normal intelligence should be able to manage their own bladder appliances, protective pads and undergarments, and monitor regular bowel habits. However, some children require assistance with bowel and bladder management. A delegated person (school nurse, teacher) should assume the role of a responsible advocate in such situations.

Therapeutic Exercises

The exercises prescribed by the physician will depend upon the degree of involvement. The following exercises may serve as a guide for the spina bifida patient.

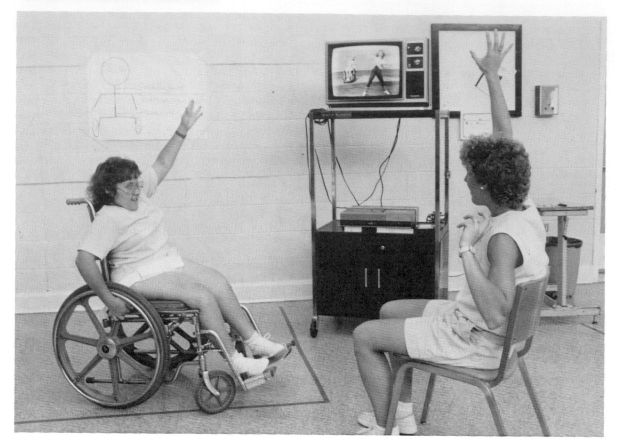

Fig. 4–58. Many adolescents with myelomeningocele, because of restricted mobility and lack of exercise, tend to have problems with weight management. With the increased popularity of wheelchair aerobics, aided in part by the many commercially available video tapes on the subject, it is possible to formulate desirable teaching objectives in a one-to-one or small group situation. Such programs can be utilized in a home exercise program or adapted physical education program at school.

Appendix A
1. Exercises for the upper back
   Exercises 1 through 17
2. Exercises for the lower back
   Exercises 18 through 31
3. Exercises for abdominal muscles
   Exercises 32 through 42
4. Exercises for the hip
   Exercises 43 through 63
5. Exercises for the knee
   Exercises 64 through 80
6. Exercises for the ankle and foot
   Exercises 81 through 95
7. Exercises for deep breathing
   Exercises 142 through 146

General Exercises
Resistive weight training exercises are useful for upper-extremity strengthening.
Appendix C

Crutches
Although his legs may be totally or partially paralyzed, the child with spina bifida is often encouraged to learn to walk with braces and crutches.

When crutches are recommended, the following sequences of gaits can be utilized.
Appendix D
No. 1
No. 4
No. 5
No. 6

TRAUMATIC INCIDENTS
Devastating injuries due to accidental causes (trauma) is the subject matter of this section. Although information on spinal cord injuries (SCI) is separated from head trauma, both are often related injuries in a separate incident (Fig. 4–59). In both, the resulting disability will vary according to the location of the damage. Due to space limitations information on

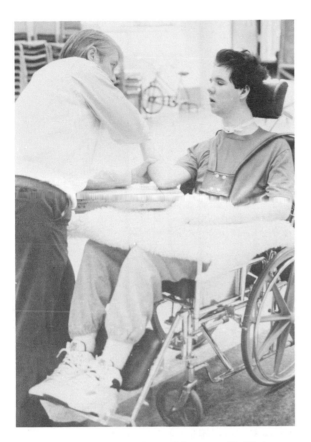

Fig. 4–59. Psychosensory effects of therapy with this trauma patient focused attention to alternating trials of moving right and left arms against resistance in arm wrestler's position. Head and eye control movement was also encouraged in relationship to location of therapist.

emergency and acute care management will be kept to a minimum. In the section on head trauma, many of the characteristics and treatment concerns are similar to those already described in the section on cerebrovascular accident (stroke) and will not be discussed in detail.

Case History: This 18-year-old patient sustained a closed head injury (from a fall) and spinal injury (C3–5 subluxation) resulting in quadriplegia (Fig. 4–59). He was admitted to the Kluge Children's Rehabilitation Center for intensive rehabilitation. Programming during recreational sessions focused on passive ranging of the upper extremities through various directional coordinates. It was important to challenge the patient in a game type situation. Consequently arm wrestling games were used to accomplish certain performance goals. The patient would facilitate volitional resistance to stretching at various points and then would actively move his arm away and return to midline when the elbow was supported by the therapist's hand.

SPINAL CORD INJURIES

The spinal cord is a fluted column about 18 inches long and about ½ inch in diameter (although its diameter diminishes considerably at its lower levels).

There are usually 31 pairs of spinal nerves branching out from the spinal cord and exiting from the vertebral canal through notches in the vertebrae. The 2 main functions of the spinal cord are to provide a center for reflex actions and to provide a channel for impulses to and from the brain. If the spinal cord is injured, it does not regenerate, and motor and sensory function are permanently disturbed below the level of injury (Fig. 4–60).

Nature of Injury

Depending upon the injury, an individual may suffer a complete or incomplete lesion. A complete lesion is one in which no sensation or motor function exists below the level of the lesion. Potential function is determined by remaining musculature, especially strength and function in the upper extremities. An incomplete lesion is one in which some evidence of sensation or motor function exists below the level of the lesion. Some individuals have progressive consistent return of muscle function (on a daily, weekly or monthly basis), however, return may cease at any time.

Following loss of sensation, the skin below the spinal lesion is particularly prone to pressure sores (decubitus ulcers), which are caused by interruption of nerve impulses to the skin and lack of blood supply to the tissues. Decubitus ulcers, which form primarily over bony prominences, become infected easily and heal very slowly.

Prevention of decubitus ulcers requires daily inspection of the skin in order to find and treat sensitive areas and frequent changing of position in the wheelchair or bed. The patient should keep a thick foam rubber cushion, or flotation pad, in the wheelchair for regular use.

Since paraplegics and quadriplegics cannot relax the urethral sphincter, the muscular valve at the mouth of the bladder, the retention of urine is frequent. If the bladder cannot develop enough pressure to overcome the resistance of the sphincter, infection of the urinary tract is likely, especially when the urine backs up into the ureters and kidneys. When the kidney pelvis is swollen with backflow, the condition is called *hydronephrosis.* Anyone who develops a bladder infection must interrupt his program of activities and receive intensive treatment to bring the infection under control.

A small rubber tube known as a catheter is placed in the bladder to control the flow of urine. The catheter may be open for constant drainage, or it may be clamped and opened only at regular intervals. Some men wear an external collecting device that drains into a leg bag. Enemas, suppositories, or mild laxatives may be used to evacuate the bowels and to lessen the possibility of complications from fecal impaction and incontinence.

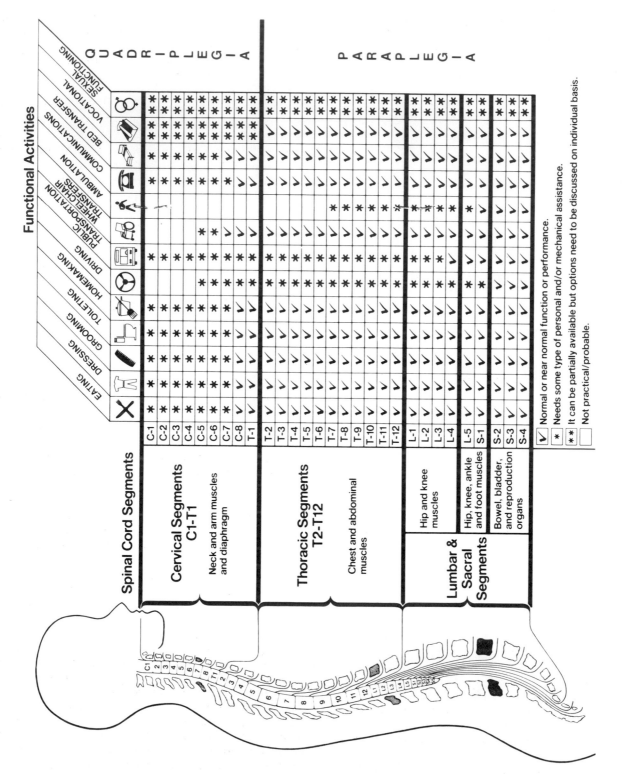

Fig. 4–60.   Functional activity for spinal cord injuries. (Courtesy of the Harmarville Rehabilitation Center, Pittsburgh, Pa. 15238.)

Paraplegia

Paraplegia is paralysis of both legs and the lower part of the trunk which may come as a result of damage to the spinal cord at the thoracic or lumbar level (see Fig. 4–60). Paraplegia can result from other disorders; however, this discussion is limited to traumatic paraplegia.

The use of crutches and braces enables some persons with paraplegia to walk. The use of a wheelchair is a distinct timesaver, since it allows the individual a greater sense of freedom. The main goal is to learn as much independence as possible (functional and vocational).

Quadriplegia

Quadriplegia is paralysis affecting all four limbs. Persons with high level cord lesions will frequently need some attendant care; usually they are unable to get from bed to the wheelchair and back again without assistance. A person with a lesion of the sixth or seventh cervical vertebra should be able to propel a wheelchair with minor modifications that will enable him to move around within his own home, and for traveling outside. Patients with lesions above the sixth cervical vertebra will need even more continuous care. The main goal is to learn wheelchair locomotion with as much additional movement as the individual problem and determination allow.

Mechanical breathing devices may be needed, especially for C-2 level quadriplegics.

Incidence

Estimates of the total population of people living with spinal cord injuries vary, but authorities generally agree that it is in the 250,000 range. It is seen more frequently in young males and frequently the result of motor vehicle accidents. More than half of all SCI accidents result in quadriplegia (53%) which shows no trend. The percentage of neurologically incomplete injuries has increased from 38% in 1973–74 to nearly 54% in 1983–84. This is explained, in part, by improved roadside emergency management.[74] On-site trauma care continues to improve, lending support for even further prevention of serious complete spinal cord injuries in the 1990s.

Treatment

After the initial therapeutic care period, the rehabilitation of a patient with a SCI is divided into 3 phases.

1. Psychiatric—To build up a sound mental attitude toward the disability. Therapeutic recreation is often introduced for the purpose of social stimulation.
2. Physical medicine—Physical therapy, occupational therapy, and corrective physical rehabilitation to assist in equipment needs, general strengthening and endurance exercises, ambulation, and activities of daily living.
3. Self-assistance—Actions taken by the patient and his family in cooperation with social workers and/or vocational counselors to solve the practical problems and enable the patient to live as normal a life as possible.

Skin care, nutrition, bladder and bowel training, and an exercise program are important aspects of a rehabilitation program. Rehabilitation may last 6 months for a quadriplegic and one to 3 months for a paraplegic. Constant medical follow-up is needed to avoid complications.

Functional electrical stimulation (FES) is an exciting research area. Various combinations of electrical stimulation with biofeedback and computers are used for walking and various other forms of exercise. However, considering the present state of experimental technology, it is still too early to evaluate results since only a small majority of the spinal-injury community have taken advantage of the treatment benefits.

Spinal regeneration experiments are also a focus of attention. The problem of regrowth and regeneration still eludes researchers. Efforts have promoted regeneration of the nerves but have been unable to solve problems associated with reconnecting functions of the spinal cord above and below the injury site.

Many paraplegics and quadriplegics have attended schools and colleges with great success. Vocational rehabilitation programs are available for those who need training in new occupations.

Program Implications

A number of individuals with spinal cord injuries are admitted to medical and rehabilitation centers. During the first awareness of the effects of spinal cord injury, the patient begins to deal psychologically with the injury. The patient's early reaction, especially during hospitalization, is often depression. During this period, a therapeutic recreation specialist can provide intervention therapy through supportive sessions that concentrate on psycho-social development. The 2 main objectives of such a recreation program would be: (1) to facilitate the individual's adjustment to his disability; and (2) to encourage self-expression through the process of resocialization.

When medical orders permit, the paraplegic can perform most physical activities from a wheelchair, and paralysis of both legs should not hinder participation to any great extent. It should be noted, however, that the process of achieving upright posture may require several weeks. Special attention should be given to strengthening upper-extremity muscle groups and to stretching muscles that have become shortened through disuse. It is important that weakened muscles not be strained by overwork during the active treatment stage. The quadriplegic will frequently need to use adapted devices when participating in sports and games, since involvement in all 4 limbs constitutes a major problem.

Body-image development is important, and the therapist must first introduce a carefully planned, graduated program of sports and games that offer early success. Possible muscular weakness and lack of endurance are important factors to consider when beginning an activity program for the paraplegic or quadriplegic. Popular clinical sports include swimming, archery and table tennis.

Every therapist and instructor should assess his patient's adjustment to peers and desire to overcome the acquired disability. Many victims of spinal cord injury find ways to use equipment and/or adapt to situations despite their limitations. Some will react with frustration or be overly cautious in approaching new activities.

If the paraplegic returns to a public school program, he should be treated as an independent individual, and he should be accepted naturally. The student should participate in physical education class unless his doctor has requested his exclusion. Social activity should not be forced upon the student, particularly if he is still adjusting to his disability; however, there is no need for a paraplegic or a quadriplegic to feel totally dependent. In some situations, the instructor may recommend exercises for upper extremity strengthening instead of regular physical education activities. As important, physical fitness development should be encouraged.

In general, the physical education program should be modified to focus attention on the arms. Weight training is an example of an activity that could be easily incorporated in a secondary school physical education program. Bench-press exercises develop muscles of the upper limbs and chest, particularly the pectoral and triceps muscles. When heavy resistance is used, spotters are required to assist in the placement and removal of the weight (Fig. 4–61). A personal progress record is helpful. The amount of weight

lifted and the number of repetitions should be recorded.

The quadriplegic will most likely need to be enrolled in an adapted physical education program. Those with a mid-level cervical lesion (C-5) can use various strapping techniques, gloves, or a wrist splint with a slot in the palmar surface to hold objects (Fig. 4–62A). Those with ultra-high lesions will need to use a mouth stick and/or head piece with control attachment (Fig. 4–62B) to manipulate objects. Skilled electronically operated devices with "puff and suck" tubes (refer to Chapter 8) are also used, but generally customized for each individual case.

Adapted physical education programs are expanding services to include instructional units on developing skill competencies in wheelchair sports. This more recent focus of attention is due, in part, to the growth of the junior wheelchair sports movement. However, the teacher must be knowledgeable and broaden his scope of understanding about rules, wheelchair technology, etc. to maximize skill sequence teaching techniques. In some cases, the ability to adapt instructional methods to the paraplegic is not totally different than teaching a sport unit to a nondisabled student (for example, archery).

Sport skill teaching will often focus on individual sports (bowling, swimming, track). Ceccotti suggests creating an informal contract with the junior wheelchair athlete that includes general goals—e.g., track events should be participated in to increase fitness levels and cardiovascular endurance—and specific objectives, e.g., a thorough understanding of the wheelchair, including its parts, functions, maneuverability, and pushing techniques for velocity to improve track performance.[75] This would be an optimum teaching situation. Then too, a physical education teacher can

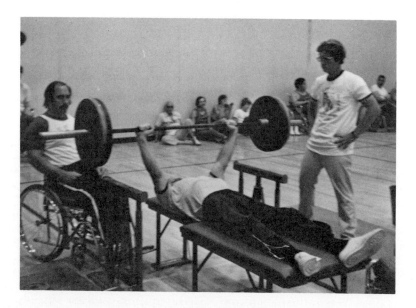

Fig. 4–61. Paraplegic performing bench-press exercise with barbells. (Courtesy of Jay Shearer.)

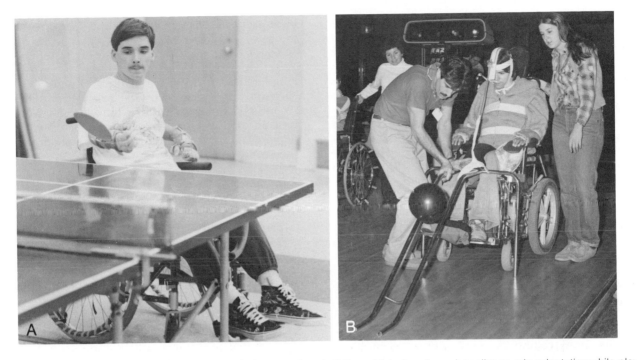

Fig. 4–62. Functional skill variations according to spinal cord lesion. *A*, C-5 quadriplegic using wrist splint as grip adaptation while playing table tennis. *B*, C-4 complete quadriplegic using head-push stick device to bowl independently. By using neck flexion the ball is pushed from the ramp stand. The individual was also respirator dependent with lack of arm function. (*B* Courtesy of F. Ceccotti, Alfred I. DuPont Institute of the Nemours Foundation, Wilmington, DE.)

gain additional pertinent information by consulting with related service personnel (P.T., O.T., etc.).

What appeared to be a trend in the 1970s is now a reality. This is, the spinal cord injured population wanted opportunities for choice, control, and mastery over recreational experiences. Many expanded beyond the view of athletics to experiment with new challenges. Many new opportunities, some still in the developmental stages, are available. These include chair-obics (wheelchair aerobics), racquetball, disk sports, self-defense programs, sit skiing, and water-skiing to name a few. Even skydiving is a viable alternative for someone seeking the ultimate challenge.

Particular attention should address the quadriplegic group. Even with the recent advances in recreational activities, quadriplegics are expanding their interests toward team oriented outlets, while looking beyond traditional wheelchair sports. In some circles, this trend is identified as alternative sports. For instance, quad rugby (refer to Chapter 8) has gained popularity as a substitute for wheelchair basketball. Persons with ultra-high lesions (C1–C3) in motorized wheelchairs are playing a modified version of soccer by attaching bumpers over their footrests. Players push a playground size ball over a court area in attempt to score goals.

Batavia[76] stresses the scarcity of active forms of recreation for high-level quadriplegics. He adds further the need for physical release, similar to that achieved by spinal cord athletes with less physical involvement.

As an alternative for nonpassive recreation, he discusses the therapeutic and recreational advantages of engaging in a new precision target game called Blow Darts (refer to Chap. 8). It should be pointed out that there are no NWAA sanctioned sports for the high level quadriplegic who uses a motorized wheelchair. Hopefully future research will focus attention to this group and examine methods of exploring alternatives for active engagement in physical exercise both from a recreational and competitive standpoint.

Functional Significance of Level of Spinal Cord Lesion

Management of the spinal cord injured patient is directed toward encouraging him to achieve the highest possible level of function within the limits of his disability. Eight critical levels of spinal cord severance and their effects on function are discussed here.

C-4. The quadriplegic has good use of sternocleidomastoids, the trapezius, and the upper paraspinal muscles. Shoulder girdle musculature is very weak, and no upper extremities function. The patient can learn to manipulate an electric wheelchair with a mouthstick. Externally powered devices are necessary to perform upper extremity functions.

C-5. The patient has function in the rhomboids, deltoids, and all major muscles of the rotator cuff, although they are only partially innervated. Elbow flexion is possible since the biceps and brachioradialis both remain partially innervated. Some shoulder functions, such as abduction, are possible. There is no muscular function in the wrist or hand. The patient is able to propel his wheelchair if projections are placed on the hand rim.

C-6. A significant amount of functional ability is present at this level. The rotator cuff mechanism is fully innervated. The critical function of elbow flexion is possible, and more power is available for shoulder flexion and abduction because the pectoral muscles are functional. Muscles of the wrist, nearly always the extensor carpi radialis, are functional. Slight wrist dorsiflexion is possible, allowing the patient to grasp large-handled, lightweight objects. This provides an important dimension of manipulation of such objects for recreational exercise as billiard sticks and golf clubs for putting. Transfers from wheelchair to bed and automobile are possible, and wheelchair propulsion is possible.

C-7/C-8. The quadriplegic with sparing of these segments has function in the triceps, finger extensors, and finger flexors (innervation varies in individual cases). A strong triceps enables the patient to stabilize the elbow in extension, an important factor in developing coordination and skills in the sports of archery and table tennis. The presence of finger flexors and extensors enables the patient to grasp and release. However, specific limitations are imposed by the weakness of the grasp. Therefore, activities requiring a tight grasp (J stroke in canoeing) are not recommended.

T-1. The T-1 paraplegic has full innervation of the upper extremity musculature. At this level, the patient has strength and dexterity in grasp and release, but trunk stability is lacking. Therefore, a seat belt encircling the chest wall is especially helpful for maintaining good sitting posture in forms of recreational exercise that require segmental alignment for skill development (as in archery).

With functional upper extremities, the patient should be able to transfer himself to the floor and return to his wheelchair without assistance.

T-6. The T-6 paraplegic has significant functional ability due to innervation of the antigravity muscles of the upper back, stabilized against the support of the pectoral girdle. Upper extremity strength including ability to sustain a tight grasp provides additional opportunities for recreational and therapeutic exercise (such as field events, bowling, and weight lifting).

With bracing, the patient can stand erect for specified periods of time, but, because of difficulty in maintaining an erect posture, ambulation is generally not considered a functional means of mobility.

T-12. The patient has good abdominal strength and function of all muscles of the thorax. However, there is still weakness of the lower back where lumbar musculature is not innervated. Good trunk control provides opportunities for various forms of recreational exercise including endurance activities that tax respiratory reserve (such as marathon racing, and swimming).

The T-12 paraplegic is completely independent in all activities of daily living. Ambulation with bilateral long leg braces is possible using a "2-point alternate", "4-point", or "swing through" gait, depending on the circumstances of each individual case. A wheelchair is often used as an alternate means of transportation depending upon specific environmental demands and the attitude of the individual.

Precautions

A person with a recent SCI is suddenly called upon to modify his concept of himself and his relationships to people and his work in accordance with the nature and extent of his disability. The program leader should expose his client to activities that have a high chance of success, thus building on the ability he has left and not on what has been lost. Different types of leisure-time pursuits should be introduced. Focus on the individual and positive reinforcement of his efforts may be necessary if success is not immediate. This type of program requires a one-to-one relationship between instructor and patient.

Spasticity is a quality of abnormal muscle tone below the level of lesion which is characterized by flexor patterns (hip and knee flexion and bending of the trunk) or extensor patterns (straightening out of limbs or trunk). Extreme physical effort, as in athletic competition, may precipitate spasticity, or it may result from other factors, such as temperature changes, bladder infection, or decubitus ulcers. Performance skills in athletics and physical education are obviously affected by episodes of spasticity. To counteract interference by spasticity, the program leader can stretch the involved limb. Some individuals are fully capable of using their upper-limbs to lift and reposition their own leg(s) to overcome spastic movements.

The high level quadriplegic (referred to as C4 and above) may have unique problems that should be addressed by a therapist, instructor, or coach. Hypotension resulting from vasodilation may be a problem that can preclude involvement in physical exercise. Low body temperature caused by the inability of the blood vessels to constrict efficiently is another concern that may require attention. Dehydration on hot days is a problem especially for athletes because the quadriplegic can sweat above the cord lesion, but not below the paralyzed part of the body. It is important to take salt tablets and drink extra fluids to avoid dehydration problems.

Exercise

Research has shown the quadriplegic to be somewhat limited by reduced physical work capacity (PWC). DiCarlo studied eight subjects in an 8-week aerobic conditioning program and investigated the effects of arm cycle ergometry training during progressive work loads. A sustained 12-minute wheelchair propulsion task was used to assess functional endurance capacity.

Results of the study demonstrated improvement in cardiovascular function (increased maximal oxygen consumption [Vo2 max.]), decreased resting heart rate, and increased PWC. The study also showed that arm cycling (with modifications to secure hands to pedals) is an acceptable mode of cardiovascular training, and is a viable substitute for other training methods (running, walking, or bicycling).[77]

The physical education teacher should encourage functional training programs in conjunction with exercises that promote upper-extremity strength. For example, the paraplegic should be encouraged to do at least one chair-to-floor transfer during his physical education period. It is important to consult with a physical therapist to determine the transfer of choice.

Therapeutic Exercises for Paraplegia

Therapeutic exercises for the paraplegic serve 2 purposes:

1. To maintain range of motion and prevent contractures of the involved areas.
2. To increase strength and range of motion of all uninvolved areas.

Exercises for the upper extremities and upper trunk area can be active or resistive exercises. Exercises for the lower extremities will be passive and active assistive exercises. A physician must approve any exercise program. The following exercises will serve as a guide when approval has been received.

Appendix A
1. Exercises for the upper back
   Exercises 1 through 7, 9, 10, 11, 15, 16, 17
2. Exercises for abdominal muscles
   Exercises 37, 38, 39
3. Exercises for the hip
   Exercises 43 through 48, 50 through 53
4. Exercises for the knee
   Exercises 65, 66, 68, 69, 71, 72
5. Exercises for the ankle and foot
   Exercises 81 through 86
6. Exercises for deep breathing
   Exercises 142 through 146
7. Exercises for the wrist
   Exercises 111 through 117
8. Exercises for the elbow
   Exercises 118 through 124
9. Exercises for the shoulders
   Exercises 125, 126, 128, 133, 136, 137, 138
10. Exercises for head and neck
    Exercises 139, 140, 141

Initial physical re-education can include mat exercises to mobilize the trunk as preliminary training for other functional activities. Weights and pulleys and other resistance exercises are also useful.

General Exercises

Weight training, flexibility exercises, and cardiovascular endurance activities (long distance track, lap swimming, etc.) should be encouraged whenever possible.

Crutches. Paraplegics can use the following crutch gaits:

Appendix D
No. 4
No. 5
No. 6

Therapeutic and General Exercises for Quadriplegia.

Therapeutic exercises for the quadriplegic are the same as those for the paraplegic. Most will be passive exercises; some active assistive exercises can be used when the patient can assist. There may be some active motion in the upper shoulder, head, and neck areas.

The therapeutic exercises that can be used depend upon the level of spinal cord involvement. All exercises must be approved by a physician.

Weight training is gaining in popularity with quadriplegics, although the element of safety remains a debatable issue when using free weights. Attachment gloves (Action Life Glove, First Grip Cuff) with overlapping velcro fasteners are available which enable low-level quadriplegics to grip dumbbells and barbells. Many prefer to exercise on Universal and Nautilus machines or other weight training machines that require no manual dexterity.

Competitive Sports

The National Wheelchair Athletic Association (NWAA)

One criteria for allowance to compete in NWAA events is that the participant must have a permanent musculoskeletal disability (spinal cord injury, spina bifida, postpolio, and other spinal neuromuscular conditions). Such sports as air weapons, archery, track and field, fencing, swimming, slalom, table tennis, and weight lifting are sanctioned events governed by the NWAA. Athletes compete on a regional basis to qualify for national competition. From there, a United States team is picked to compete internationally. A junior division is available for children from ages 8 through 15.

All athletes must undergo special examinations so that their level of muscular function can be determined. On the basis of these examinations, athletes are placed into one of 7 classes (8 classes for swimming) containing persons judged to be similar in degree of disability (Fig. 4–63). This classification process allows for fair competition.

The U.S. Les Autres Sports Association also serves a limited number of spinal cord injured athletes who are not currently served by the National Wheelchair Athletic Association. These are the athletes who are cord-injured who prefer to ambulate with crutches or other assistive devices, and the very high level cord-injured athletes whose level of disability necessitates the use of an electric wheelchair.

CLASSIFICATIONS

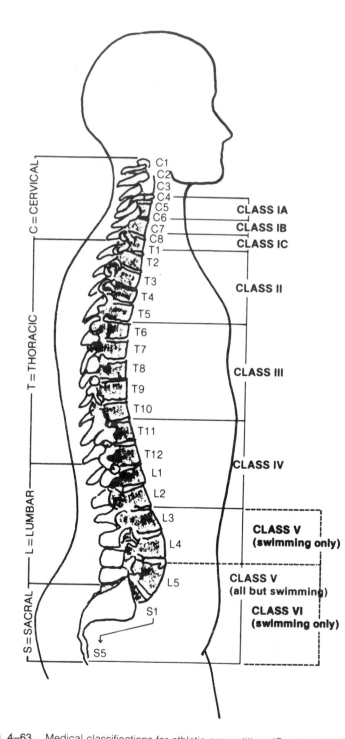

CLASS IA

All cervical lesions with complete or incomplete quadriplegia who have involvement of both hands, weakness of triceps (up to and including grade 3 on testing scale) and with severe weakness of the trunk and lower extremities interfering significantly with trunk balance and the ability to walk.

CLASS IB

All cervical lesions with complete or incomplete quadriplegia who have involvement of upper extremities but less than IA with preservation of normal or good triceps (4 or 5 on testing scale) and with a generalized weakness of the trunk and lower extremities interfering significantly with trunk balance and the ability to walk.

CLASS IC

All cervical lesions with complete or incomplete quadriplegia who have involvement of upper extremities but less than IB with preservation of normal or good triceps (4 or 5 on testing scale) and normal or good finger flexion and extension (grasp and release) but without intrinsic hand function and with a generalized weakness of the trunk and lower extremities interfering significantly with trunk balance and the ability to walk.

CLASS II

Complete or incomplete paraplegia below T1 down to and including T5 or comparable disability with total abdominal paralysis or poor abdominal muscle strength (0–2 on testing scale) and no useful trunk sitting balance.

CLASS III

Complete or incomplete paraplegia or comparable disability below T5 down to and including T10 with upper abdominal and spinal extensor musculature sufficient to provide some element of trunk sitting balance but not normal.

CLASS IV

Complete or incomplete paraplegia or comparable disability below T10 down to and including L2 without quadriceps or very weak quadriceps with a value up to and including 2 on the testing scale and gluteal paralysis.

CLASS V

Complete or incomplete paraplegia or comparable disability below L2 with quadriceps in grades 3–5.

Fig. 4–63.   Medical classifications for athletic competition. (Courtesy of the National Wheelchair Athletic Association.)

Competitive wheelchair athletes are now more conscious of using training techniques and good conditioning habits to improve performance levels. Ten years ago, because of relatively short period of training, many athletes did not attain a high level of fitness. Now, with the advent of the sophisticated sport wheelchair, athletes are able to measure personal and performance goals in more detail and appreciate the outcome of year round training programs.

Hard dedicated work is the only way to success for any athlete. However, for the disabled athlete, the wheelchair is an extension of one's body! Unlike an able bodied athlete, the wheelchair athlete must concern himself about not only his own physical well-being, but the wheelchair as well. If two athletes possess similar competency levels, the one with the superior wheelchair could win the competition.

HEAD TRAUMA

The brain is divided into the cerebrum, the cerebellum, and the brain stem. The cerebrum performs the thinking processes, the cerebellum controls skilled muscular coordination, and the brain stem controls the body's vital function (see Fig. 4–23). An injury to a specific part of the brain can be expected to produce a corresponding problem within a specific part of the body. Since most diseases of the brain, such as stroke or brain tumor, tend to affect primarily one area of the brain, they tend to produce predictable problems. Unlike these diseases of the brain, traumatic head injuries can produce multiple sites of brain injury.[78]

Nature of Head Trauma

The National Head Injury Foundation has defined *traumatic head injury*. It is an insult to the brain, not of a degenerative or congenital nature but caused by an external physical force, that may produce a diminished or altered state of consciousness, which results in impairment of cognitive abilities or physical functioning. It can also result in the disturbance of behavioral or emotional functioning. These impairments may be either temporary or permanent and cause partial or total functional disability or psychologic impairment.

To be more specific, a hard blow to the head can cause damage in a number of ways. Head injury can result in both focal (a bruise that causes tissue damage and bleeding) and diffuse (severe injury to the brain itself) damage that can affect performance ability. Contusions (bruising of brain tissue) tend to be more focal, while white matter injury tends to be more diffuse and, thus, less predictable. The physical manifestations, while they may be severe, may subside long before the behavioral and cognitive problems.[79] The term closed-head injury (CHI) refers to the fact that the patient has sustained a diffuse rather than a focal brain injury.

The initial structural damage of a head injury can include bleeding inside the skull. If bleeding occurs

between the skull and covering of the brain, it is called Epidural Hematoma (Fig. 4–64B). This most often occurs after a skull fracture. If bleeding occurs between the membrane covering the brain and the brain, it is called a Subdural Hematoma (Fig. 4–64C). This frequently accompanies a contusion. If bleeding occurs within the brain tissue, it is termed Intracerebral Hematoma (Fig. 4–64D). This most frequently accompanies contusions of the brain.

Complications such as intracranial bleeding, in addition to representing a neurosurgical emergency, in many instances further worsens the eventual prognosis.

Incidence

According to the National Head Injury Foundation between 30,000 to 50,000 persons each year sustain head trauma that results in impairments severely affecting wellness levels.

Motor vehicle accidents are the primary cause of the most serious of these injuries, and the majority of these victims are teenagers and young adults. 25% of these injuries are considered serious. The number of persons with residual deficits following head injury is unknown.

Head injuries in children is a common occurrence. Those with severe injuries will have economic and personal problems that will persist for a lifetime. Males have tended to have head injuries at a rate of 2 to 1 over females. Head injuries to school age children are most commonly caused by motor vehicle accidents, followed by falls, sports injuries and assaults.[80]

Treatment

The mildly affected person may not need intensive hospitalization unless there is reason for orthopedic intervention. For the more severely involved, once the CHI patient's condition has stabilized, it is then possible to start an aggressive rehabilitation program. Initially, safety becomes a major issue as the patient struggles to overcome problems with confusion, agitation, and inappropriate behavior. Clinical team members strive to coordinate services to overcome the patient's communication, judgment, and perception problems. It is important to coordinate an ongoing assessment tool to measure patient progress during the rehabilitation period. One useful tool is the Rancho Los Amigos level of consciousness scale. The assessment measures the patient's behavior through eight levels of cognitive functioning.

I, II, III—coma and emergence from coma
IV, V—confused, agitated state
VI—advent of appropriate behavior
VII, VIII—focus on high level skill development

As changes occur, various clinical team members act as examiners and match the description of each level to the patient while monitoring progress at periodic intervals. The most rapid recovery usually oc-

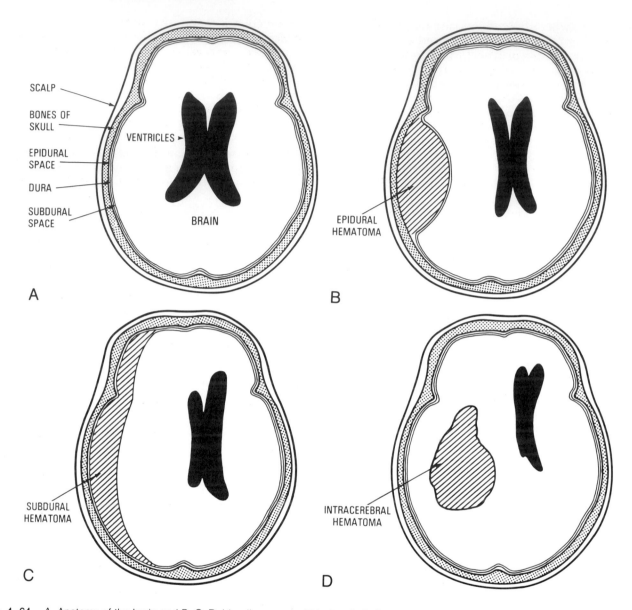

Fig. 4–64. A, Anatomy of the brain and B, C, D, bleeding areas within the skull. (Illustrations courtesy of the Central Nervous System Injury Foundation, 4050 Front St., San Diego, CA 92103.)

curs in the first 6 months, largely due to the brain's ability to heal.[81] However, significant recovery will be variable; many will be independent in ambulation and self-care. Some will demonstrate partial independence, but limited by movement disorders such as spasticity and/or ataxia. The more severely involved will remain totally dependent and need continual nursing care throughout the duration of their life span.

Program Implications

Recreational activities can be introduced once the patient demonstrates appropriate signs of recovery. During therapy, the patient will be involved in figuring out how to cope with new problems and new situations. In addition, program selection may reflect

on "team therapy concepts." This is to work on ambulation skills to complement physical therapy, to improve fine motor coordination to assist occupational therapy, or to increase speed and accuracy in understanding speech and language to aid speech therapy.

It is virtually impossible to discuss the many different intervention strategies, however, a few basic guidelines are discussed below.

Guidelines for Therapeutic Modalities

Rancho Levels 2–3: Sensory stimulation, nature walks, tactic stimulation and experimentation with implements such as in Art Therapy; creative movement with or without background music for psychomotor stimulation.

Rancho Levels 4–6: Creative dramatics, music and art therapy to elicit expressive reactions. Group socialization experiences including community outings. Horticulture therapy, stretching/flexibility exercises, hydrotherapy, and various cognitive games.

Rancho Levels 6–8: Higher order skill progression tasks including sports. Arts and crafts to elicit goal oriented behavior, creative writing, computer games, and horticulture. Leisure counseling with patient and family members including referral to community based recreation agencies.

After return to a regular school program, the CHI student will often need direction and guidance in following a daily schedule. Although the student may look alert and oriented, it is often necessary to find support from others to plan and organize daily routines. Many times, a memory impairment or personality disorder will affect social habits. Memory problems may have lessened, but still persist requiring guidance and understanding from teachers and fellow students alike. It should be understood that the CHI student may be able to give appropriate answers to questions, but demonstrate difficulty with problem solving skills. If such problems are evident, then most likely the student should be enrolled in an adapted physical education program.

Some CHI students will be sensitive to irrelevant stimuli which disrupt their processing skills and attention to task. The frequent noise and distractions associated with a gymnasium is often a disrupting factor. Such adverse conditions frequently heighten emotional responses and affect thought processing skills. Under such circumstances, the student should be placed in a setting where stimuli are controlled in a distraction free environment.

The CHI student will present a variety of deficits. Because of this, the physical education instructor will need to know the extent of the student cognitive and behavior characteristics so as to implement specific learning strategies. For example, a student who demonstrates problems with auditory discrimination and short-term memory recall will need to focus on visual cues to obtain goal-directed behavior. Organizational habits can be facilitated by using a blackboard to record scores or floor markers to direct travel routes in a game situation.

One main objective in an adapted physical education program is to monitor auditory and visual feedback. This is done through a demonstration system and by giving verbal hints that lead to a course of action. Because response time is often delayed, it is important to give the CHI student sufficient time to process and respond to basic instructions. Over time, the instructor tries to eliminate constant concurrent feedback (information during the performance of a skill). Instead, after a demonstration period, the student is required to become more responsible in making his own decisions during the course of a motor sequence. Still, a few subtle hints may be required to keep the student on task, but the purpose is to lessen continual information feedback. As the student becomes more responsive to using self-analysis, then the instructor can focus attention on giving terminal feedback (information given at the end of a performance).

Frequently it is necessary to use organizational landmarks for CHI students who exhibit marked perceptual-motor deficits. An example would be placing numbered markers on the floor to define position changes in the basketball game, Around the World. Effort should focus on direction to location of self and objects in space. Position play activities are useful where the student is required to follow left-right progressions such as in Newcomb, volleyball, and other net games.

Implementation of an obstacle course routine is an excellent activity choice to focus on retention of visual cues while processing verbal commands. After a demonstration period, the instructor can reinforce organizational strategy by using a few key words to define directions. An example would be to use key action words such as "Up", "Over", "Under", etc. The student can repeat directions or the action words at each station. For example, Stand *Up* from the chair, Step *Over* the pole, Crawl *Under* the table, etc. It is best to start obstacle course routines in one direction before adding circle and more complex travel routes.

It should be pointed out that fatigue often accompanies head injury. For this reason, the physical education teacher should be receptive to this problem, if it occurs. No undue pressure should be applied as frustration and anxiety related to CHI can only compound additional psycho-emotional problems. This is especially true if expectation levels are too high as frequently seen in competitive motor drills and sport events.

The organization and structure of controlling motor behavior is an important component of physical education services. Videotaping in adapted physical education is a new but promising evaluation instrument. Using qualitative standards to measure periodic spurts in cognitive and motor behavior will substantiate levels of progress that can be shared with family members, as well as with the student.

Therapeutic Exercises

The exercises prescribed by a physician will depend upon the degree of involvement. For example, some patients will only demonstrate a minimal disability requiring general strengthening exercises, while others may be in a persistent nonresponsive state requiring passive range of motion exercises to overcome severe muscle contractions.

Refer to section on Cerebrovascular Accidents for additional details and suggestions.

General Exercises

All exercises should be approached gradually with slow, but progressive increments. General balance, coordination and fitness related exercises may be useful depending upon the rate of recovery status and/or physical condition of the individual. Weight training may be recommended in some cases.

Appendices B and C

SICKLE CELL ANEMIA

Sickle cell disease is an inherited blood disorder. The gene may be inherited from one or both parents. The parents themselves may not actually have any symptoms of the disease but may be carriers of the defective trait. The carrier can pass this trait on to his children.

Sickle cell anemia exists in 2 forms. In the mild form known as sickle cell trait, a person will have a small portion of sickle cell hemoglobin in his red blood cells, but the cells will function normally. In the severe form the disease can affect all the tissues and organs of the body.

This form of anemia is classified as a molecular disease because of the change that occurs in the molecular structure of the cells. Red blood cells, or erythrocytes, are normally biconcave shaped disks. The red blood cells of a child with sickle cell anemia appear twisted into the shape of a sickle. This twisting usually occurs after the erythrocyte has been deoxygenated, and the rigidity and flexibility of the red cells appears to have decreased. Any slight force produced by movement of the surrounding fluid results in a gross deformity of the red blood cells. Normal erythrocytes would resist such deformity and retain their shapes. Some of the red blood cells of the child with sickle cell anemia undergo a thinning process, break down at a point on the edge of the cell, and assume the shape of a sickle or a crescent moon.

The symptoms of sickle cell anemia, as in most anemias, are weakness, pallor, and fatigue. In addition, one or more of the following signs may appear: painful swelling of the dorsal area of the hands and feet, involvement of the joints and extremities causing limitations of motion, abdominal pain lasting 3 to 4 days, central nervous system involvement causing possible monoplegia or hemiplegia, and at times blood clots that block the flow of blood to local tissue.

Incidence

Statistics on the incidence of sickle cell anemia vary with different reports. The most recent figures indicate that 1 in every 10 American blacks is a carrier of the sickle cell trait. But, only 1 American white in 200 is a sickle cell trait carrier. It is important to note that about 1 in 500 American blacks actually has sickle cell anemia. When both the mother and the father carry the sickle cell trait, it is likely that 1 of 4 children will be born with sickle cell anemia and that 1 child in 4 will be born neither diseased nor a carrier.

Treatment

No specific drug therapy for sickle cell anemia has proven successful. Treatment consists of hospitaliza-tion, medication to relieve pain, intravenous fluids and, occasionally, oxygen. Blood transfusions may be used in critical situations. Preventative medicine is the best solution. This is, avoid situations that produce sickling.

Patients are advised against high altitudes and unpressurized airplanes, or any situation that may cause a moderate lack of oxygen. A lowered amount of oxygen may lead to a crisis with nausea, vomiting, and abdominal pain.

The degree of anemia in patients may increase and decrease, but the anemia rarely disappears. Death in sickle cell anemia patients can result from many medical problems or from damage to vital organs because of lack of oxygen. Today, the life span of patients has been increased through treatment of infections with antibiotic drugs.

Routine screening for sickle cell disease should be done in prenatal clinics. Every black child admitted to a pediatric unit of a hospital should routinely have the test for sickle cell anemia. Men inducted into the Armed Forces could be screened as part of their physical examinations. When the trait is found, genetic counseling should be given to the affected person, particularly if he is a young adult or a parent.

Program Implications

Blacks with sickle cell trait play professional football and baseball. Usually there is no need to restrict activities (Fig. 4–65); however, occasionally an individual will have poor exercise tolerance and need special consideration.

Children with sickle cell disease have a more serious problem. The frequency of crises may keep the child in a hospital for long periods of time. A child hospitalized in a sickle cell crisis requires special considerations from the therapist. These include:

1. Care of the skin, good hygiene, and precauto avoid bruises and cuts that may lead to infection.
2. Proper rest periods.
3. Encouragement of normal exercises and activities after the crisis state has subsided.

During the crisis episode, the child needs emotional support. Young patients may feel a sense of resentment or react in a manner of total uselessness. The therapist should treat the child as normally as possible but set and enforce limits for him. It is best to stay within the framework of safety and suggest only those activities that are recommended by the physician.

Between episodes, the child who has sickle cell disease requires a carefully planned program of sports, games, and physical education. It is not uncommon for children to have a poor self-image and delayed motor development skills. Many children have lacked natural childhood experiences because of their inability to compete physically with their peers. Many parents tend to overprotect the child and stifle his natural instinct for challenging new play experiences.

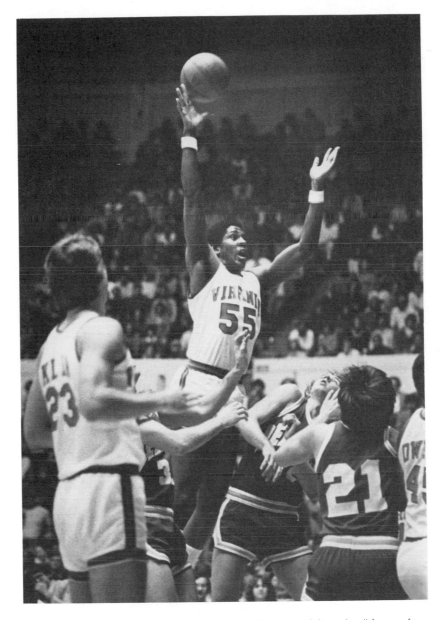

Fig. 4–65. Athletes with sickle cell trait usually have no symptoms and are free to participate in all forms of competitive sports.

It is important to provide children with improved muscle tone through regular exercise and, most important of all, to help children learn to use their muscle power to meet their daily problems.

Many physicians hold different opinions about the types and level of exercise intensity that a child with sickle cell disease may safely engage in. In most cases, physical activities that avoid fatigue, weakness, or body contact are recommended. Swimming should be encouraged. This activity can be done at a leisurely pace without fatigue or stress.

One of the major contributions of recreational sports and physical education to the child with sickle cell disease is the development of a healthy mental attitude. It is important not to overlook this factor.

The NCAA Committee on Competitive Safeguards and Medical Aspects of Sports has issued a statement on the athlete with sickle cell trait. It concludes that the remote chance of a sickling crisis "does not justify any restriction or other policy that places limitation on the healthy athlete with sickle cell trait"; that "all black athletes with the trait (Hb AS) should be informed of the early symptoms of a sickling crisis" and should "seek medical attention promptly if ever experienced," and that "particular attention should be given by team physicians and athletic trainers to preventing dehydration of an athlete with sickle cell trait, whether at high altitude or in early season football practice."

Precautions. Patients who carry the sickle cell trait but do not have the disease are far less prone to sickling phenomenon than those in whom the disease is active, since their red cells contain normal hemoglobin which does not stack or interact with sickle hemoglobin. Therefore, a severe depletion of oxygen or very severe acidosis must be involved before any significant sickling will occur. These patients should avoid:

1. Mountain climbing in high altitudes (above 6,500 feet).
2. Flying in airplanes that do not have pressurized cabins.
3. Swimming underwater and holding breath for long intervals.

Therapeutic Exercises

Specific therapeutic exercises are of little value unless there is a particular weakness or specific condition involved. The specific therapeutic exercises for a particular condition should be indicated by a physician.

General Exercises

General exercises are beneficial in assisting the child to regain strength and muscle tone after crisis periods. These exercises should be carefully regulated to avoid undue fatigue or weakness.

Appendix B

UNDERNUTRITION/EATING DISORDERS

The term *undernutrition* is used to describe a condition in which there is a deficiency of calories but not of a single dominant nutrient. Undernutrition is the most commonly found metabolic abnormality among hospital patients—and in entire populations of many countries of the world.

Almost every serious illness or injury tends to produce general undernutrition by interfering with appetite or assimilation of food. Patients who are seriously ill for a week or more are undernourished for this reason. Poor health habits, such as insufficient sleep and rest, may be secondary factors. Also undernutrition may result from socioeconomic problems—an inability to purchase proper foods in sufficient amounts or lack of knowledge in choosing nutrious foods.

Other common factors that can produce undernutrition are impaired appetite due to surgery, gastrointestinal disease, and traumatic and neurologic disorders interfering with self-feeding. Interference with food consumption can also occur as the result of oral disease, pregnancy anorexia and vomiting, and food allergy. Another common factor is weight gain deprivation secondary to therapy (drugs which cause anorexia and diets which restrict essential foods). For example, a patient may be anemic because of chemotherapy. With prolonged nutritional restriction, loss of muscle mass becomes a major issue with subsequent deterioration in strength and physical stamina.

Grouped under eating disorders, anorexia nervosa and bulimia need particular attention. An anorectic demonstrates a severe appetite failure without a discoverable physical basis. A typical bulimic consumes a large amount of high calorie food within a short period of time and this is followed by purging behavior such as vomiting and use of laxatives.

Serious states of undernutrition are easily recognized. Some of the characteristics are prominent cheekbones and ribs, protruding scapulae, a sharply outlined pelvis, and a generally "bony" appearance. Other recognized symptoms include poor coordination, generalized weakness, hypotension, apathy, and depression.

Incidence

Undernutrition is not confined to any sex, age, or ethnic group; however, there are more reported cases in infants, young children, and adults over 60 than in other age groups.

Anorexia nervosa is most frequently seen in female adolescents, and only about 10% of the patients are boys. Bulimia is often seen in late adolescence. Some studies report that 5 to 10% of adolescent girls and young women are affected by these eating disorders.

Treatment

Individuals who are hospitalized for assessment of undernutrition or unexplained weight loss will need to have an initial team evaluation. Team members frequently include a physician, a social worker, nutritionist, nurse, and various specialized therapists. Other services including psychiatry, and at times psychology, guide other members in coordinating efforts to manage the patient. Principal findings often reflect on an emotional component that complicates undernutrition, especially if weight loss is rapid and suspicious.

Proper and effective treatment is dependent upon accurate diagnosis of the degree and type of undernutrition and an understanding of its cause. Factors that gauge progress include weight gain, involvement in therapy, and attention to nutritional habits. Also, it is important to analyze the circumstances surrounding the patient's ability to attend and socialize freely during social encounters. Changes in symptom behaviors are evaluated closely. This is often done in psychotherapy, and during group recreational activities. We emphatically agree that early treatment and success often depends upon the type, variety, and frequency of social experiences that are available on the hospital unit. Attention and participation in group recreational outlets allows the patient to assume responsibility and make decisions, and at the same time rivet attention away from their fragile medical conditions.

Primary hospitalization on a medical unit is usually recommended in both anorexia nervosa and bulimia. A transfer to a psychiatric setting may be necessary in some cases. Bulimia is widely associated with affective disorders or borderline personality disorder, both of which require somewhat different long-term treatment. The aim should always be early discharge and return to family and community. There are, unfortunately, a number of patients who require changes in their premorbid environment for long-term improvement. This, too, may be an appropriate goal of hospital treatment.[82]

Some hospitalized patients who are treated for undernutrition will need to use nasogastric (NG) tubes for administration of medication and feedings. Surgical procedures may be required, for example in certain gastrointestinal disorders, to relieve obstruction or correct bowel perforation, bleeding, or fistulas.

Program Implications

Therapists should be alert to signs of stress that can aggravate a physical ailment such as seen frequently in Crohn's disease (inflammation of the GI tract that extends through layers of intestinal wall). To add further, many long-term chronic illnesses can place an extra burden on family members. Coping behavior and stress is often shifted to the patient, only complicating issues related to an already low self-esteem. For patients using NG tubes, stress factors are often heightened by changes in physical appearance. This can be both an aggravating physical and emotional concern. When possible, it is important to eliminate environmental isolation by engaging the patient in recreational activities in an area away from the hospital room environment. Freedom of travel outside the patient's room rivets attention away from needless seclusion, promotes independence and sense of freedom from physical restraints.

Frequently a hospitalized patient is undernourished because of enforced passivity during the diagnostic period and later on if there is no guided effort toward restoration of physical well-being. Preoccupation of concern for one's questionable physical status becomes an issue for intervention. A therapeutic recreation specialist often attempts to intervene by using materials such as art to provide an avenue for self-expression. Younger patients are generally more amenable to intervention than adults.

Regardless of the environment, many undernourished children sense a feeling of inferiority and withdraw from vigorous activities. The fragility of an undernourished body reflects on social attitudes and concerns. For example, team sports such as basketball and football can contribute to social problems because the individual must expose his undernourished body to the view of his teammates. In addition, his physical contribution to the group will be limited, and accentuate his feelings of inadequacy. This type of physical activity involvement is not a common occurrence, unless participation is enforced such as in physical education class. Depending upon the cause of undernutrition, before participating in active sports and games most individuals will need to participate in a general conditioning program of graded exercises to strengthen weak and unused muscles.

Concerns of compulsive exercising should be addressed. It appears that many eating disorder patients (especially a person with anorexia nervosa) need to satisfy the fact that their emaciated body is desirable. To expand upon this, exercise then becomes the outlet through which this is expressed. The cycle of uncontrolled exercise (sometimes referred to as "secret exercise") needs to be broken. A therapist is often required to introduce and implement exercise education sessions. It should be proposed that a gradual introduction to exercise would be best served through a session of warm-up, exercise and cool-down. This systematic approach is done to allow the patients to promote better control over their body. In addition, if done jointly or in a group, often socialization and interpersonal relationships are improved.

Since running is a manifestation of compulsive exercise, there has been some debate recently over the relationship of anorexia nervosa and female distance runners, especially those who are programmed to exercise through a training cycle for competitive events. The rationale is based upon the comparison features (psychologic and physical) of anorexia nervosa and those of long distance runners. Weight and Noakes studied 125 competitive female distance runners who were administered the Eating Attitudes Test (EAT) and the Eating Disorder Inventory (EDI) screening tests. A high incidence of anorexia nervosa is shown when EAT and EDI scores are elevated. Research findings indicated 14% of the runners had high EAT scores, only 4% had a history of amenorrhea and low body weight, and only one had a history of anorexia nervosa. The study showed that abnormal eating attitudes and the incidence of anorexia nervosa is no more common among competitive female runners than it is among the general population.[83]

Exercise

Moderate weight-bearing exercise is advisable for patients with low body weights as exercise is one of the protective factors against osteoporosis. Women with low weight and amenorrhea for at least 1 year's duration are at risk for osteoporosis. Since anorexic patients often do not know what a reasonable amount of exercise is, and since bulimic patients often do not get enough exercise, supervised periods of exercise will be of significant benefit to almost all eating disorders patients.[84]

Therapeutic Exercises

No specific therapeutic exercises are recommended unless indicated by a physician. Postural exercises may prove to be valuable. Low balance beam exercises are encouraged in some situations. The use of the beam has a direct influence on the balance muscles (particularly the abdominal muscles which are stabilizers of the trunk and pelvis) and improves self-awareness of general body alignment in motor movements.

Appendix E

General Exercises

General exercises and weight training are beneficial to the undernourished individual. After 1 or 2 weeks of treatment, a cautious program of mild exercise can be started. Feeding alone will not restore strength, and wasted muscles are not rebuilt without exercise. Mild exercises in the supine position should be first, then gradual introduction to those in the standing position, and later to progressive resistive exercises.

Appendices B, C, and F

As per physician orders, aerobic training can begin once body weight returns to normal.

VISUAL IMPAIRMENTS AND BLINDNESS

Anyone with visual acuity in the better eye of 20/200 or less after correction is considered blind. The figure 20/200 means that an individual is able to see at 20 feet what one with normal vision sees at 200 feet. Someone is classified as partially sighted if he can perceive movement, light, and form. The partially blind have a visual acuity between 20/70 and 20/200 in the better eye after correction.

Blindness may be present at birth or may be acquired. Retrolental fibroplasia is the leading cause of blindness of newborn infants. This disorder is caused by oxygen poisoning and results in spasm of the retinal vessels. Both eyes are affected, and it may produce complete or nearly complete blindness.

Other causes of blindness are trauma, rubella of the mother during pregnancy, congenital syphilis, and infection during delivery.

Many children who are blind or have extremely poor vision lack skills in body control, static balance, coordination, and agility. Many of these children are overprotected by their parents, friends, and teachers. As a result, they are not given opportunities for active movement during early childhood. Blind children need to explore as much of their environment as possible and build up concepts that normal children acquire through sight.

Poor posture is another characteristic of the blind, as many adopt a faulty carriage because of their inability to see. They have a tendency to lean forward with their arms stretched out to avoid hitting objects. Some blind children are very tense and walk rigidly with their heads tilted backward.

It is understandable that persons with partial vision are less disadvantaged than those who are totally blind. For example, they are more responsive to various social encounters because of independent mobility. Not surprisingly, individuals with partial vision can control external space without concern for overcoming physical restraints. Social learning skills are often learned through imitation of others. The totally blind cannot examine or perceive nonverbal communication experiences (physical gestures and manual expression). Because of these contributing factors, the blind person adapts much slower to the many varying conditions related to socially oriented behavior.

Incidence

The prevalence of legal blindness in the United States is estimated as almost 600,000 persons. Estimates for school aged population (ages 5 to 19) is 32,000. Rates increase sharply with age. For example, nearly 58% of the legally blind population is 65 years or older.

The U.S. prevalence of "severe visual impairment" (noninstitutional population) is estimated as almost 2 million persons in 1987. The prevalence estimate is 38,000 under age 18 or 1% of the general population. About 78% of the severely visually impaired population is 65 years or older.[85]

Treatment

Early detection of blindness or impaired vision is essential for the treatment and education of the person. The main objectives are to restore or improve sight and to prevent further impairment of vision.

Special care is required in many instances. The totally blind child is often enrolled in a school for the blind, or in special education classes in private or public schools. Auditory instruction and reading by touch perception with the Braille system are emphasized. Children with partial vision may attend regular school providing that the teacher is trained in the methods of teaching the visually impaired. Parents must also be instructed about the needs of their blind and visually impaired children.

Program Implications

Blind children need to become sensitive to auditory and tactile sensations. A common theory among practitioners is that the tactile-kinesthetic sense is the dominant spatial sense in blind persons. This basic need can be facilitated through involvement in therapeutic recreation or adapted physical education programs.

Some of the more common sports for the blind include goal ball, beep baseball, bowling, wrestling, hiking, swimming, horseback riding, and fishing. Other sports, such as football, baseball, air riflery, and basketball, are not recommended unless the rules and regulations are modified drastically. However, even with the more complex sports, certain adaptations can be made to enable the blind to participate with their normal peers. For example, in an adapted form of softball, the blind player can use a regulation bat to hit a soccer ball placed on a batting tee. To score a run, the blind player can run to first base with a sighted person and back to home plate before the ball reaches the catcher. Many other such adaptations can be devised by the instructor and the student.

In addition to developmental needs, a physical education teacher, recreation leader, or therapist should determine the blind person's physical needs, such as development of skeletal muscles, improvement of balance, development of an even gait, the ability to run and perform locomotor skills freely, and correction of posture. In physical education class, some sighted children will share some of these needs with the blind

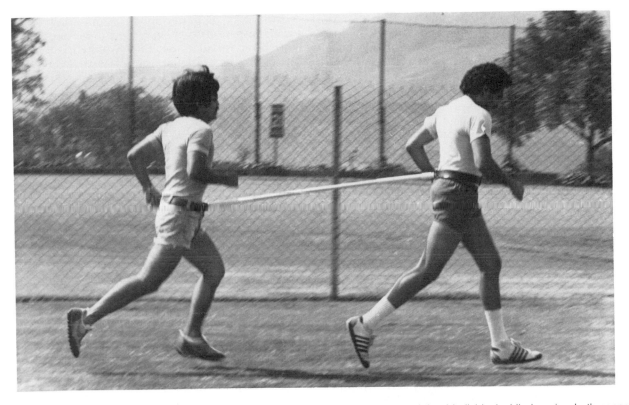

Fig. 4–66. The Freedom Leader—a unique device that joins a trained guide and a nonsighted individual while keeping both separated, thus permitting free movement. (Courtesy of Freedom Leader, P.O. Box 5347, San Pedro, Calif. 90733.)

children. These children may have their physical education together using playground and gymnastic apparatuses such as rings, trapezes, ladders, horizontal bars, balancing boards, jungle gyms, and gym horses, and doing tumbling, and team stunts such as building pyramids and lifting weights. Roller skating, ice skating, downhill skiing, and cross-country skiing (Fig. 4–66) are favorable forms of recreational exercise and sports in which blind and sighted persons can participate together.

Visually handicapped children attending public schools are often not given vigorous physical education, even though their physical fitness should be developed. Common physical fitness tests, such as pull-ups, sit-ups and squat-thrusts, need no modifications for blind participants. Visually handicapped boys and girls can compete fairly with sighted children when Buell's achievement scales are used.[86] These scales are based upon evidence that blind children perform as well as sighted peers in some events and somewhat below normal in others, such as running.

Based on a review of Project Unique data, Winnick reports on muscular strength and endurance test items that only 26 to 41% of the visually impaired group were able to surpass the medium value (50th percentile) of the non-impaired group.[87]

Cardiovascular endurance activities should be encouraged. A Freedom Leader (training bar with shock absorbers) joins a trained guide to a nonsighted part-ner while keeping both separated and permitting free movement and good running posture (Fig. 4–67). This eliminates the holding onto or "human appendage" syndrome and provides a great degree of independence for travel (jogging and hiking) in an outdoor setting.

Ski touring, or cross-country skiing, is a widespread and popular activity among visually impaired people. It is attracting a growing number of blind

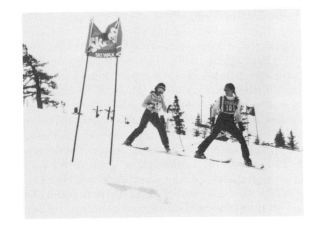

Fig. 4–67. Class B1 athlete being guided by sighted partner at the 1988 USABA Winter National Championships (Alpine Skiing) in Vail, Colorado. (Courtesy of USABA.)

skiers because it provides vigorous exercise combined with social interaction. Obviously, blind skiers prefer to maintain close contact with a sighted partner. Frequently, ski touring takes place on prepared trails that have good tracks. This helps give the blind person a feeling of freedom, security, and joy of movement (refer to section on Cross-country skiing for further information).

The National Federation of State High School Associations has clarified issues pertinent to visually impaired track and field participants to the degree of assistance allowed by a sighted companion.

Any assistance that may be allowed is at the discretion of the meet director or games committee and is not provided "carte blanche" by rule. A situational ruling (situation 33) which has appeared in the rule book since 1961 indicates that track competition is an individual effort and each contestant is expected to run his own race without any help. Bodily contact, such as assistance by another competitor by taking his arm or by some similar action, is subject for disqualification. Situation—ruling of 4.5 8D of the current case book emphasizes that track and field is an individual sport and no advantages should be supplied by a teammate or a nonparticipant. Giving direction to a visually impaired runner is not giving that runner any advantage over a sighted runner.

For the totally blind, visual demonstrations are of no value, and in many instances verbal descriptions have little meaning. It is important to understand that the totally blind can only understand the meaning of complex motor skills through "feel" of the movement. Manual guidance is often necessary. Because demonstration must be on an individual basis, it is slow; however, the instructor must have patience and give the learner needed inspiration and confidence.

During mass group instruction, line formation relays in which balls are passed backward and forward to teammates are popular. Players do not need to make rapid movements or shift their positions in various directions. An example is to have each team line up in single file. At a signal, the first player starts the ball toward the rear, and the last man brings it forward. The first team to finish wins. The method of passing the ball can be varied—once back around the right hip, the next time the left, a third through the legs, and a fourth over the head.

Verbal communication has particular meaning to the performance of the blind players. One interesting game involves the catching of a volleyball or basketball. The instructor stands in the center of a circle of students—the circle having a radius of about 15 feet. Before he throws the ball to a student, he calls his name so that the student can poise himself to receive the ball. Catching it after one bounce, in the case of a drop, does not constitute a miss. Some catches and recoveries are exciting, and the game is very good for developing coordination and improving reflexes.

Swimming is generally recommended for the visually impaired; however, care must be taken to ensure safety regulations. The visually handicapped individual must be receptive to all messages from any of the senses and cultivate memory. During instruction periods, the swimming pool should be equipped with ropes and floating corks to separate the shallow and deep areas. Diving should not be allowed in the general swimming area. Tandem boating (canoeing and sailing) with sighted persons is usually permitted. Crew with a sighted coxswain is an excellent team sport for the blind.

A number of adapted or special devices to aid in solving or reducing the problems arising from blindness can be ordered from the American Foundation for the Blind. Some of the games which can be purchased include dominoes (with prominent raised black dots on white background), brailled cards, and Chinese checkers (with differently shaped wooden men). An audible ball which can be used in the game of kickball can also be purchased. The totally blind batter places the ball on home plate, kicks it, and runs with a sighted partner as in softball.

There are many group games with low organization that need no modification, such as tug of war or crows and cranes (Chapter 8). It is important, however, that games include sounds, so that the player can locate opponents by the sounds of their voices.

Precautions

Children who wear glasses to correct their vision should use glass guards for protection during vigorous physical activities. If this is impractical, then it may be necessary to make appropriate modifications.

Indoor and Outdoor Orientation

Orientation is the process of utilizing the remaining senses to establish one's position and relationship to all other significant objects in one's environment. The blind person must develop a mental image of his environment in order to move safely and efficiently. If this is to be done in a public school setting, then it obviously needs to be done during the first few days of the school year. The physical education teacher must make the environment conducive to learning by following a few guidelines:

1. The blind person must have a course or line of direction from the classroom to the locker room and gymnasium. He needs to become familiar with landmarks on the walls or doorways to facilitate his travel toward his objective. A buddy can be assigned to the blind student for the first few days. However, the blind person should gain independence and be free to travel independently as soon as possible.
2. The blind student should become self-sufficient in caring for daily needs, and he can do this after be becomes familiar with his surroundings. The student should know the direction and position

of the windows, doors, lockers, sink, toilet, water fountain, and shower facilities.

3. Orientation to the gymnasium should begin by a verbal introduction to the surroundings. The blind student should walk around the border or edge of the gymnasium. It is best to allow the student an opportunity to move at his own pace so that he can establish landmarks and clues to determine his position in the environment. It is important, however, to remember that not all landmarks can be identified by touch, for example, basketball standards that are attached to a wall. Eventually the student will use sound discrimination to determine where the standards are located. Listening to sounds in the gymnasium—voices of other children and bouncing balls—will enable the student to discriminate distance and number of children.

4. Basic outdoor orientation should point out clues that may be used in travel. For example, grass, cement, and gravel can serve as travel clues for determining one's position, line of direction, or boundary lines for playing courts or fields. Landmarks such as trees and fences are helpful outside on a playground. The child should be made aware that he must listen and pay attention to travel clues more carefully on a windy day because of the added sounds.

Competitive Sports

United States Association for Blind Athletes (USABA)

The USABA is the national governing body for legally blind athletes who compete on regional, national, and international levels. Blind athletes are given the opportunity to compete through USABA in the following national sports: goalball, gymnastics, judo, powerlifting, tandem cycling, track and field, wrestling, alpine skiing, Nordic skiing, speed skating, and marathon running.

Classification System

B1—Totally blind, may possess light perception but unable to recognize hand shapes at any distance.

B2—Recognize hand shapes up to and including 20/600 or field limited to less than 5 degrees.

B3—Visual acuity greater than 20/600 up to 20/200. Field limitation from 5 to 20 degrees.

The USABA modifies sports only to the extent necessary to encourage participation by athletes with varying degrees of impaired vision. For example, totally blind downhill skiers compete on certified slalom courses by following the shouted, rapid instructions of sighted guides who generally precede them down the course (physical contact and assistance are forbidden) (Fig. 4–67). Totally blind marathon runners follow verbal instructions of sighted companions and are allowed to touch their arm for guidance; totally blind speed skaters follow the verbal instructions of guides who skate ahead of them; and blind sprinters follow either a tightly stretched guide wire or the shouts of a caller.

Therapeutic Exercises

Common postural defects among those with visual impairments are kyphosis, protruding stomach with corresponding lordosis, and head tilting (up or down). This is often referred to as common fatigue-slump posture. The head tilting often results from the fact that the individual has, or once had, some light perception or a small amount of sight in one of his eyes and is trying to focus this eye on the sidewalk or the sky.

Suggested exercises are: Walk and stand tall; stretch the back of the top of the head toward the ceiling; and tuck the stomach in and roll the hips under (this is for the thin as well as the obese). These exercises serve to thrust the shoulders back, not to an exaggerated position, but enough to elevate the chest so that body alignment is exactly as it should be.[88]

General Exercises

General exercises and weight training are beneficial to the blind. Weight training activities are particularly popular with blind boys and young men.

Appendices B and C

Note: It is important to demonstrate all exercises by placing the blind person in the required starting position and guiding him through the prescribed movements. When using the barbell, it is important to begin without weights, as the participant must have a clear understanding of lifting techniques and safety precautions before starting a program of progressive resistive exercises.

Balance beam and self-testing activities provide each person with opportunities to develop agility, balance, and coordination. A sequence of body balance activities aids mobility training. Start with the low balance beam, and place it close to a wall so that the individual will feel confident that he will not get hurt.

Appendix E

Climbing poles or ropes helps develop strength of arms, shoulders, and abdomen. However, safety regulations must be enforced. Children may practice coming down poles or ropes before being allowed to climb. To do this, the child should stand on a chair or ladder and grasp the pole or rope so that it is securely squeezed by his inner thighs and feet. The child then releases the top hand, places it below the bottom hand, and repeats the process until he reaches the floor. Pole and rope climbing is especially helpful because it gives blind children a feeling of moving in space.[89]

REFERENCES

1. Schatzinger, L., et al.: The Patient with Scoliosis. Am J Nurs.
2. Francis, R.: Scoliosis screening of 3,000 college-aged women: The Utah Study-Phase 2, Phys Ther, 68:1513, 1988.
3. Zuega, R., Blount, W., and Discus, W.: Indications for operative treatment of spinal deformities. Wis Med J, 74:33, 1975.

4. Blount, W.P., and Moe, J.H.: The Non-Operative Treatment of Scoliosis and Round Back with the Milwaukee Brace and Exercises in the Brace. Privately published.

5. Hall, J. (Children's Hospital, Boston, Massachusetts): Private correspondence, 1979.

6. Benson, D., Wolf, A., and Shoji, H.: Can the Milwaukee brace patient participate in competitive athletics? Am Sports Med, 5:7, 1977.

7. Ferguson, A.B.: Roentgen of Extremities and Spine. New York, Hoeber, 1949.

8. Crenshaw, A.H.: Cambell's Orthopaedic Surgery. 7th Ed. St. Louis, C.V. Mosby Co., 1987, pp. 32–45.

9. Jackson, D.: Low back pain in young athletes: evaluation of stress reaction and discogenic problems. Am J Sports Med, 7:364, 1979.

10. American Academy of Orthopaedic Surgeons, Low Back Pain (brochure) no publication data.

11. Denton, J.: Lower Back Pain: Coping with A Common Problem. McCall's Magazine, August, 1987, p. 84.

12. Bricklin, M.: The Practical Encyclopedia of Natural Healing. Emmaus, PA, Rodale Press, 1983.

13. Finneson, B.E.: Low Back Pain. Philadelphia, J.B. Lippincott Co, 1973.

13a.Sabolich, J.: The O.K.C. above-knee running system. Clin Prost Orthot, 11:169, 1987.

14. Michael, J.: Prosthetic feet for the amputee athlete. Palaestra, 2:37, 1986.

15. Radocy, B.: Hands for all seasons: upper-extremity sports prosthetics. Palaestra, Winter, 1988.

16. Winnick, J.: Early Movement Experiences and Development Habilitation and Remediation. Philadelphia, W.B. Saunders Co., 1979.

17. Butterworth, M.: Deaf children in physical education. Palaestra, 4:28, 1988.

18. Stewart, D.: Social factors influencing participation in sport for the deaf. Palaestra, 3:23, 1987.

19. Hoekelman, R.A.: Acute Otitis Media in Children; Up-dated International, February, 1974.

20. Olmstead, R.W., et al.: Pattern of hearing following acute otitis media. J Pediatr, 65:252, 1964.

20a.Hoekelman, R.A.: Private correspondence, 1974.

21. American Heart Association, Heart Facts, 1988.

22. Schaeffer, T.E., and Rose, K.D.: Cardiac evaluation for participation in school sports. JAMA, 228:398, 1974.

23. Diamond, E.F.: Children and sports. J Contng Ed in Pediatr, 19:24, 1978.

24. National Heart Institute: Cardiovascular Surgery. U.S. Dept. of Health, Education, and Welfare, Public Health Service Publication No. 1701, 1968.

25. Cooper, K.H.: Aerobics. New York, Bantam Books, Inc., 1969.

26. Cancer Facts and Figures. American Cancer Society, Atlanta, GA, 1988.

26a.Leukemia Society of America: Leukemia, The Nature of the Disease, New York.

27. Arnheim, D., and Sinclair, W.: The Clumsy Child, A Program of Motor Therapy. 2nd Ed. St. Louis, C.V. Mosby Co., 1979.

28. Zimmerman, J.: Goals and Objectives for Developing Normal Movement Patterns. Rockville, MD, Aspen Publishers, 1988.

29. Finnie, N.: Handling the Young Cerebral Palsied Child at Home. 2nd Edition. New York, E.D. Dutton and Company, 1975.

30. Jones, J.: Training Guide to Cerebral Palsy Sports. 3rd Ed., Champaign, IL, Human Kinetics Books, 1988.

31. Gay, L.N.: The Diagnosis and Treatment of Bronchial Asthma. Baltimore, Williams & Wilkins, 1946.

32. Itkin, I.H.: Exercise for the asthmatic patient. J Phys Ther, 44:817, 1964.

33. Verma, S., and Hyde, J.: Physical Education Programs and Exercise-Induced Asthma. Clin Pediatr: 697, 1976.

34. American Medical Association: The Asthmatic Athlete, 1977.

35. Ninety-fourth Ross Conference on Pediatric Research, Ross Laboratories, Columbus, Ohio, 1988.

36. Adams, R.C., and Adamson, E.: Trampoline tumbling for children with chronic lung disease. JOHPER, 44:86, 1973.

37. Orenstein, D., et al.: Exercise and cystic fibrosis. Phys Sports Med, 11:57, 1983.

38. Engerbretson, D.: The Diabetic in Physical Education, Recreation, and Athletics. JOPHER, 48:18, 1977.

39. Drash, A.: Diabetes Mellitus in Childhood: A Review. J Pediatr, 78:919, 1971.

40. Etkind, E., and Cunningham, L.: "Physical Abilities of Diabetic Boys." Paper read at the International Symposium Commemorating the 50th Anniversary of Insulin in Israel, October, 1971. Mimeographed.

41. Armstrong, N., and Wakat, D.: The energetic diabetic: a personal fitness guide. Bowie, MD, Brady Communications Co., Inc., 1986.

42. Campaigne, B., et al.: Effects of a physical activity program on metabolic control and cardiovascular fitness in children with JDDM. Diabetes Care, 7:57, 1984.

43. Canu, R.: Diabetes and Exercise. New York, E.P. Dutton, Inc., 1982.

44. Forsche, C.: The child with epilepsy. JOHPER, 44:84, 1973.

45. Livingston, S., and Berman, W.: Participation of Epileptic Patients in Sports. JAMA, 224:236, 1973.

46. Boone, D.: Physical Activity for the Child with Hemophilia. Inter-Clinic Information Bull, 13:7, 1974.

47. The National Hemophilia Foundation, Hemophilia and Sports, 1984, p. 9.

48. Boone, D., and Spence, C.: Physical Therapy in Hemophilia, The National Hemophilia Foundation, 1976, p. 7.

49. Hancock, C.: How I manage hernias in the athlete. Phys Sports Med, 11:, 1983.

50. Edmunds, L.H.: The clinical picture in Perthes disease. Braces Today Newsletter, Chicago, Pope Foundation, December, 1966.

51. Puthoff, M.: The Physician-Physical Educator Approach to Children with Musculoskeletal Disorder. Postgraduate course lecture, University of Virginia, June, 1973.

52. Bowen, J., and Foster, B.: Perthes disease: Returning children to sports. The Phys and Sports Med, 10:69, 1982.

53. Crowe, W., et al.: Principles and Methods of Adapted Physical Education. 4th Ed. St. Louis, C.V. Mosby Co., 1981.

54. Salter, R.E.: Slipped upper femoral epiphysis. In Textbook of Disorders and Injuries of the Musculoskeletal System. Baltimore, Williams & Wilkins, 1973.

55. Kelsey, J., and Southwick, W.O.: Etiology, Mechanism, and Incidence of Slipped Capital Femoral Epiphysis. AAOS Instructional Course Lectures. Vol. 21. St. Louis, C.V. Mosby Co., 1972.

56. Southwick, W.O. (Section of Orthopedic Surgery, Yale University, New Haven, Connecticut): Private correspondence, 1973.

57. Mital, M., and Matza, R.: Osgood-Schlatter Disease: The Painful Puzzler. The Physician and Sportsmedicine, 5:60, 1977.

58. Crowe, W., Auxter, D., and Pyfer, J.: Principles and Methods of Adapted Physical Education and Recreation. 4th Ed. St. Louis, C.V. Mosby Co., 1981.
59. Simmons, R.: Reach for Fitness. Richard Simmons Reach Foundation. New York, Warner Books, 1986.
60. Seltzer, C.C., and Mayer, J.: An effective weight control program in a public school system. Am J Public Health, National Health, 60:679, 1970.
61. Brownell, K., and Kaye, F.: A school-based behavior modification, nutrition education, and physical activity program for obese children. Am J Clin Nutr, 35:277, 1982.
62. The Skinfold Test, A Clinical Method in Management of Obesity. Cambridge, Maryland, Cambridge Scientific Industries (undated).
63. Vodola, T.M.: Individualized Physical Education Program for the Handicapped Child. Englewood Cliffs, N.J., Prentice-Hall, Inc., 1973.
64. Brownell, K.: Obesity: Understanding and treating a serious prevalent and refractory disorder. J Consult Clin Psychol, 50:820, 1982.
65. Blundell, J.E.: Behavior modification and exercise in the treatment of obesity. Postgrad Med J, 60:37, 1984.
66. Varni, N., and Joffe, M.: Osteogenesis Imperfecta: The basics. Pediatr Nurs, 10:29, 1984.
67. Millar, E.: Chief of Staff, Shriners Hospital for Crippled Children, private correspondence, 1987.
68. Charash, L.: Private correspondence, 1979.
69. Croce, R.: Exercise and physical activity in managing progressive muscular dystrophy: A review for practitioners. Palaestra, 3:9, 1987.
70. Arthritis In Children, Arthritis Medical Information Series. Arthritis Foundation, 1983.
71. Bleck, E., and Nagel, D.: Physically Handicapped Children: A Medical Atlas for Teachers, 2nd Ed. New York, Grune & Stratton, 1981.
72. Anderson, M., and Spain, B.: The Child with Spina Bifida. Denver, Lowe Publishing Co., 1977.
73. Gressang, J.: Perceptual processes of children with myelomeningocele and hydrocephalus. Am J Occup Ther, 28:226, 1974.
74. Spinal Network, Boulder, CO 80306.
75. Ceccotti, F.: Getting started right: introducing sports to the junior athlete. Sports-n-Spokes, Nov.–Dec., 1985, pgs. 7–9.
76. Batavia, A.: Needed: active therapeutic recreation for high level quadriplegics. Ther Rec J, 22:8, 1988.
77. DiCarlo, S.E.: Effect of arm ergometry training on wheelchair propulsion endurance of individuals with quadriplegia. Phys Ther, 68:40, 1988.
78. Marshall, L., Sadler, G., and Marshall, S.: Head Injury. The Central Nervous System Injury Foundation, San Diego, CA 1981.
79. Baggerty, J.: Rehabilitation of the adult with head trauma. Nurs Clin North Am, 21:577, 1986.
80. Gaspard, N., and Boyce, B.: Effects of minor and major head injury in children. Article distributed by National Head Injury Foundation, Framington, MA, 1984.
81. Rehabilitation Brief: Working with brain injured clients. Office of Special Education and Rehabilitation Services, Dept. of Education, 5, Number 5, May, 1982, Washington, D.C.
82. Shenaker, I., and Shaw, H.: Diagnosis and early management of anorexia nervosa and bulimia. Sem Adolescent Med, 2:21, 1986.
83. Weight, L., and Noakes, T.: Is running an analog of anorexia? A survey of the incidence of eating disorders in female distance runners. Med Sci Sports Exerc, 19:213, 1987.
84. Ohlrich, E., and Stephenson, J.: Pitfalls in the care of patients with anorexia nervosa and bulimia. Sem Adol Med, 2:8, 1986.
85. Yearbook of the Association for Education and Rehabilitation of Blind and Visually Impaired. 5, 1987.
86. Buell, C.: Physical Education and Recreation for the Visually Handicapped, 2nd ed., Washington, D.C., AAHPERD, 1982.
87. Winnick, J., and Short, F.: Physical Fitness Testing of the Disabled. Champaign, IL, Human Kinetics Publishers, 1985.
88. Russo, R.: Gym classes for the blind important for many reasons. Information Center: Recreation for the Handicapped, Vo. 4, No. 1, 1969.
89. Johansen, G.: Integrating visually handicapped children into a public elementary school physical education program. JOHPER, 41: 1970.

BIBLIOGRAPHY

Adams, R., et al.: Physical Activity for Patients Wearing Spinal Orthoses. The Phys & Sportsmedicine, 11:75–83, 1983.
American Cancer Society: Facts and Figures. New York, The Society, 1988.
American Heart Association: Prevention of Rheumatic Fever (professional education material), 1985.
Armstrong, N., and Wakat, D.: The Energetic Diabetic, A Personal Fitness Guide. Bowie, MD, Brady Communications Co., Inc., 1985.
Aronson, S.M., Hartman, E.D., and Sahs, A.L., Eds: Guidelines for Stroke Care; U.S. Dept. of Health, Education, and Welfare, DHEW Pub #(HRA) 76–14017, Superintendent of Documents, U.S. Govt. Printing Office, Wash., D.C., 1976.
Barrow, H.M., McGee, R., and Tritschler, K.A.: A Practical Approach to Measurement in Physical Education. 4th Ed. Philadelphia, Lea & Febiger, 1989.
Bondy, P.K., ed.: Duncan's Diseases of Metabolism. 6th Ed. Philadelphia, W.B. Saunders Co., 1969.
Brooke, M.: A Clinician's View of Neuromuscular Diseases. Baltimore, Williams & Wilkins, 1977.
Brunner, L.S., and Suddarth, D.S.: Textbook of Medical-Surgical Nursing. Philadelphia, J.B. Lippincott Co., 1975.
Campbell, A.L.: Tube Feeding: Parental Perspective. Exceptional Parent, April, 1988, pgs. 36–40.
Clifton, M.: A developmental approach to perceptual-motor experiences. JOHPER, 11:34, 1970.
Cratty, B.J.: Developmental Sequences of Perceptual Motor Tasks. Freeport, L.I., N.Y., Educational Activities, Inc., 1967.
Crile, G., Jr.: What Women Should Know about the Breast Cancer Controversy. New York, Macmillan, 1973.
Crile, G., Jr.: Partial mastectomy for carcinoma of breast. Surg Gyn Obs, 136:929, June 1973.
Crowe, W. et al.: Principles and Methods of Adapted Phy. Ed. & Rec. 4th Ed. St. Louis, C.V. Mosby Co., 1981.
Department of Public Instruction: Guidelines for Adapted Physical Education. Harrisburg, Pa., Commonwealth of Pennsylvania, 1966.
Duckett, C.L.: Caring for children with sickle cell anemia. Children, 18 (No. 6): 227, 1971.
Farmer, T.W., ed.: Pediatric Neurology. New York, Harper & Row, 1964.
Fensterman-Normansell, K.: Simple Ways to Modify Exercises for the Disabled. Handicapped Sport Report, 7:no. 1, 1987–88.
Fowler, Roy S., and Fordyce, W.E.: Stroke: Why Do They Behave That Way? American Heart Assn. (Originally published by the Washington State Heart Assn., 1974.)
Gallahue, D.: Understanding Motor Development in Children. New York, John Wiley & Sons, 1982.

Gering, R.L.: The sickle cell anemia story: what a difference a valine makes. Ward's Bull, *13* (No. 92): 1 & 5, 1973.

Gillis, L.: Diagnosis in Orthopaedics. London, Butterworths, 1969.

Griffin, P. et al.: Legg-Calve-Perthes Disease: Treatment and Prognosis. Ortho Clin N Am, *11,* no. 1, Jan. 1980.

Hatfield, E.M.: Causes of blindness in school children. The Sight Saving Review, *33*:9, 1963.

Herkowitz, J.: A perceptual motor training program to improve the gross motor abilities of preschoolers. JOHPER, *41*:38, April 1970.

Illingworth, R.S.: Common Symptoms of Disease in Children. 3rd Edition. Oxford & Edinburgh, Blackwell Scientific Publications, 1971.

Ireland, J., Wray, D., and Fiexer, C.: Hearing for Success in the Classroom. Teaching Exceptional Children, Winter, 1988.

Kalakian, L. and Eichstaedt, C.: Developmental/Adapted Phy. Ed., Making Ability Count. Minneapolis, Burgess Pub. Co., 1982.

Kaplan, S.A.: Growth Disorders in Children & Adolescents. Springfield, Charles C Thomas, 1964.

Kegel, B.: Sports and Rec for Those with Lower Limb Amputation or Impairment. J. Rehab. Res. Develop. Clin. Supplement No. 1, Washington, D.C., 1985.

Kelly, E.D.: Adapted and Corrective Physical Education. New York, Ronald Press Company, 1968.

Kephard, E.J.: Behavioral integration of problem children through remedial physical education. JOHPER, *41*:45, 1970.

Kephart, N.C.: The Slow Learner in the Classroom. Columbus, Charles E. Merrill, 1960.

Kendall, H.O., Kendall, F.P., and Boynton, D.: Posture and Pain. Baltimore, Williams & Wilkins, 1952.

Krusen, F.H.: Physical Medicine. Philadelphia, W.B. Saunders Co., 1941.

LeMars, T., and Lebanowich, S.: The History of Sport Wheelchairs—Part III. Sports-n-Spokes, July–Aug., 1984, pgs. 12–16.

Licht, S., Ed.: Stroke and Its Rehabilitation, Physical Medicine Library, Volume XII. Baltimore, Waverly Press, Inc., 1975.

Licht, S.: Therapeutic Exercise. Baltimore, Waverly Press, Inc., 1965.

Mamaril, A.P.: Preventing complications after radical mastectomy. Am J Nurs, *74*:2000, 1974.

Mathews, D.K., Krause, R., and Shaw, V.: The Science of Physical Education for Handicapped Children. New York, Harper Brothers, 1962.

Michele, A.A.: Iliopsoas. Springfield, Charles C Thomas, 1962.

Milligan, G.: Fitness is Free, But You Have to Work for It. A Physical Fitness Program for Spinal Cord Injured Persons. Arkansas Rec. and Training Ctr., U. Arkansas, June, 1979.

Nash, C.: Current Concepts Review: Scoliosis Bracing. J Bone Joint Surg, *62*-A:848–852, 1980.

National Tuberculosis Association: Bronchial Asthma, A Booklet for Patients. New York, National Tuberculosis Association, 1966.

National Tuberculosis Association: Asthma. New York, National Tuberculosis Association, 1968.

Oliver, J.N.: Blindness and the child's sequence of development. JOHPER, *41*:37, 1970.

Purtilo, D.T.: A Survey of Human Diseases. California, Addison-Wesley, 1978.

Radler, D.H., and Kephart, N.C.: Success Through Play. New York, Harper & Row, 1960.

Radocy, B.: Hands for All Seasons: Upper-Extremity Sports Prosthetics. Palaestra, *4*:24–46, 1988.

Respiratory Disease Association of Hennepin County: Physical Conditioning Course for Children with Asthma. Minneapolis, 1965.

Sherril, C.: Adapted Physical Education and Recreation. 3rd Ed. Dubuque, Iowa, Wm. C. Brown, 1986.

Siegel, I.M., and Turner, M.: Postural training for the blind. Am Phys Ther Assoc, *45*:683, 1965.

Smith, C.A.: The Critically Ill Child, Diagnosis and Management. Philadelphia, W.B. Saunders Co., 1972.

Smith, H.M.: Implications for movement education experiences drawn from perceptual-motor research. JOHPER, *41*:30, 1970.

Song, J.: Pathology of Sickle Cell Disease. Springfield, Charles C Thomas, 1971.

Thompson, G., Rubin, I., and Bilenker, R.: Comprehensive Management of Cerebral Palsy. New York, Grune & Stratton, 1983.

———: Scoliosis, A Handbook for Patients. Scoliosis Research Society, Chicago, IL (no publication date).

Travis, L.: An Instructional Aid in Insulin-Dependent Diabetes Mellitus. 7th ed., Austin, TX, American Diabetes Assoc., Texas Affiliate, 1985.

Tronzo, R.G.: Surgery of the Hip Joint. Philadelphia, Lea & Febiger, 1973.

Turek, S.L.: Orthopaedics. Philadelphia, J.B. Lippincott Co., 1967.

Ubell, E.: Cure for Diabetes. Parade Magazine, April, 1985, pgs 12–14.

United States Department of Health, Education and Welfare—Public Health Service: Sickle Cell Anemia. Washington, D.C., U.S. Government Printing Office, 1965.

Weil, U.: Osteogenesis Imperfecta, Historical Background. Clin. Orthopaedics Related Research no. 159, Sept. 1981, pgs. 6–10.

Wiseman, D.: A Practical Approach to Adapted Physical Education. Reading, Mass., Addison-Wesley Pub. Co., 1982.

5 *Posture Evaluation*

Posture is the relative arrangement of the parts of the body. The Posture Committee of the American Academy of Orthopaedic Surgeons describes good posture as that state of muscular and skeletal balance which protects the supporting structures of the body against injury or progressive deformity irrespective of the attitude (erect, lying, squatting, stooping) in which these structures are working or resting. Under such conditions, the muscles function most efficiently, and the thoracic and abdominal organs are afforded the optimum positions. Poor posture is a faulty relationship between the various parts of the body which produces increased strain on the supporting structures and in which there is less efficient balance of the body over its base of support.

The human body is made up of approximately 200 bones and 700 muscles. If all the bones and muscles are functioning properly, the body is in proper alignment. However, individual differences—gravitational pull, stress, strains, and physical handicaps—must be considered. These factors result in deviations from an "ideal" posture.

Every school system should provide a thorough posture evaluation sometime during the elementary school years. Early detection of posture problems may aid in preventing medical problems later in life. The sixth grade would be an excellent time to test each child, because of the accelerated growth beginning approximately at this age level. However, individual school systems could devise their own programs based on a child's grade level or on individual referral or a combination of both.

POSTURE GRID

One successful method of evaluation uses a posture grid (Fig. 5–1). The grid is constructed by mounting a sheet of plywood (½ inch thick, 6 feet 6 inches high, 3 feet wide) on a frame. This grid can be fastened to a wall or mounted so that it stands alone and is portable. A metal arm is attached perpendicularly to the top of the frame so that it extends approximately 2 feet forward. A plumb bob is suspended from this arm by a line bisecting the length of the grid. Horizontal and vertical lines, forming 3-inch squares over the entire board are painted on the plywood. These squares are used to locate and record posture problems. A board, 21 inches square, is placed on the floor between the grid and the plumb line. Footprints are painted on the board as a guide for proper position-

ing, and a heel rest is placed on the footboard for alignment.

Several other preliminary procedures should precede evaluation after construction of the grid. One step is parent notification; a form letter is sent to parents a week or two before the evaluation.

The letter could read as follows:

Dear Parents:
During the present school year it is our plan to conduct a posture screening evaluation of pupils in the schools. The purpose of this screening is to identify those individuals having problems of faulty posture. This evaluation will be conducted under the supervision of a member of our staff. All girls will be screened by a female instructor, and all boys by a male instructor.

Each pupil will be advised in advance of the exact date of his evaluation.

If for any reason you have objections to or questions about this posture evaluation of your child, please notify us in writing at your earliest convenience.

Evaluators must be selected and trained. The training can be accomplished at a workshop or inservice day and should include familiarization with all aspects of the evaluation procedure. Booklets should be made up which discuss the specific points to be evaluated, and the entire process should be explained in a step-by-step manner so that all evaluators will conduct screenings according to the same standards.

The evaluator should be of the same sex as the children being examined. Since children will be evaluated in their underclothes, the area to be used must afford privacy. The examination should be conducted in a closed room with a screen in front of a lockable door. A sign should be posted on the outside of the door. In addition to the evaluation area, a separate dressing area should be set aside in which the child can wait until it is time for his evaluation. Weight and height measurements can be taken in the dressing area.

A printed form containing the student's name, grade, and age (in years and months) is used by the evaluator (Fig. 5–2). The form has horizontal and vertical lines (like those on the grid) over which there is a silhouette of a body viewed from the rear. The form also contains space for pertinent medical information, such as histories of fractures, dislocations, surgery, or specific medical problems which might have influenced the individual's posture. Each anatomic point is evaluated and given a rating between

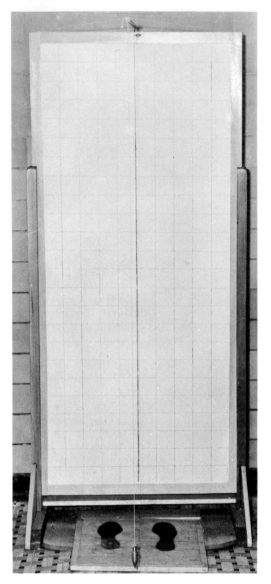

Fig. 5–1.   The posture grid used for evaluation. Note the plumb line and the painted footprints for positioning.

1 and 4: 1 indicates that there is no problem; 2, a questionable problem; 3, a mild problem; and 4, a serious problem.

Procedure

Positioning the Child and Obtaining Medical Data
The child stands on the footboard facing the grid with the plumb line behind him (Fig. 5–3). The evaluator sits 10 to 12 feet away with the printed form. The medical history should be taken first (Fig. 5–4). This brief period will allow the child to relax and assume his usual standing position.

Evaluating the Rear View
The evaluator should note 5 points in reference to the plumb line. The plumb line should:

1. Coincide with the midline of the body;
2. Pass behind the center of the head and the spinous processes of the vertebrae;
3. Bisect the gluteal folds;
4. Be equidistant from the lower extremities.

Anatomic points to observe from the rear view are as follows:

1. Position of the Head
   a. Is the head tilted left or right? (Use vertical grid lines to judge angle of tilt; indicate angles on the silhouette and evaluate severity from 1 to 4.)
   b. Is the head rotated to the left or right? (Use vertical grid lines.)
2. Shoulder Level
   a. Is one shoulder higher or lower than the other? (Use horizontal grid lines as the standard.) The right shoulder will be a little lower if individual is right-handed; the left, if individual is left-handed.
3. Scapula
   a. Is the scapula winged? (Is the vertebral border pulled away from the posterior aspect of the spinal processes of the vertebrae?) Is the inferior angle of the scapula normal at the level of the seventh thoracic vertebra? The inferior angle of the scapula will be slightly lower on the side of the dominant hand.
4. Ribs
   a. Are the ribs more prominent on one side than on the other side?
5. Hip Level
   a. Is one hip higher or lower? (Use horizontal grid lines. If the evaluator cannot observe hip level, he should place his hands on the crest of the ilium, and observe any difference in the level of the hands.) Unequal hip level may be indicative of unequal leg length or a curve in the lumbar spine.
6. Upper and Lower Spine
   a. Does the spine have a lateral C-curve? (Use plumb line; mark direction of convexity of the curve on the silhouette; evaluate its severity.) Low shoulder and high hip on the same side of the body may indicate a C-curve. If there is doubt, have student bend at waist with his hands toward his toes; rub spinous processes of the vertebrae briskly with fingertips until a hyperemia of the skin appears. When the student stands up, the outline of the spine will be visible.
7. Gluteal Fold
   a. Are the folds on the buttocks uneven? (Use horizontal grid lines.) Uneven gluteal folds may be indicative of unequal leg length or uneven hip level.
8. Lower Extremities
   a. Are the knees "knocked," or are the legs "bowed"?

Screening Form

School _____ Teacher _____

Name _____ Date _____ Grade _____ M __ F __

Age _____ Wt. _____ Ht. _____
     Years   Months   Lbs.   Inches

Handedness L _____ R _____
Leg Length   L _____ R _____
Thigh Girth   L _____ R _____
Calf Girth   L _____ R _____
Biceps Girth L _____ R _____

	1	2	3	4
Head Tilt (R)	_____	_____	_____	_____
(L)	_____	_____	_____	_____
Shoulder Level				
Higher (R) Lower	_____	_____	_____	_____
Higher (L) Lower	_____	_____	_____	_____
Upper Spine (Dorsal)				
(R) Curve	_____	_____	_____	_____
(L) Curve	_____	_____	_____	_____
Scapula				
Higher (R) Lower	_____	_____	_____	_____
Higher (L) Lower	_____	_____	_____	_____
Ribs				
(R) Prominent	_____	_____	_____	_____
(L) Prominent	_____	_____	_____	_____
Lower Spine (Lumbar)				
(R) Curve	_____	_____	_____	_____
(L) Curve	_____	_____	_____	_____
Hip Level				
Higher (R) Lower	_____	_____	_____	_____
Higher (L) Lower	_____	_____	_____	_____
Gluteal Cleft				
Higher (R) Lower	_____	_____	_____	_____
Higher (L) Lower	_____	_____	_____	_____
Legs - Knockknee	_____	_____	_____	_____
Bowed	_____	_____	_____	_____
Popliteal Line				
Higher (R) Lower	_____	_____	_____	_____
Higher (L) Lower	_____	_____	_____	_____
Pronation of Feet				
(R)	_____	_____	_____	_____
(L)	_____	_____	_____	_____

Fig. 5–2. Screening form for use in posture evaluation.

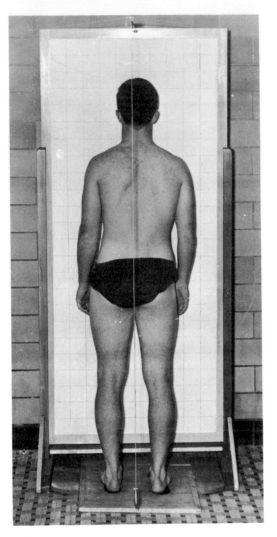

Fig. 5–3. Boy in position for evaluation at the posture grid.

9. Popliteal Line
   a. Are the lines on the posterior aspect of the knee uneven? (Use horizontal grid lines.) Uneven lines may be indicative of unequal leg length.
10. Ankles
   a. Is the position of the Achilles tendon normal? (Indicate any irregularity on the silhouette.)
11. Feet
   a. Is the placement of the feet normal? (Indicate any internal or external rotation.)

Evaluating the Side View
The evaluator should turn the footboard before examining the side view.
   The plumb line should:
1. Pass through the lobe of the ear;
2. Pass through the shoulder joint (if the arm hangs normally);
3. Bisect distance between front and back of the chest;
4. Pass midway between the small of the back and the abdomen;
5. Traverse the greater trochanter of the femur;
6. Pass slightly in front (anterior) of the midline of the knee;
7. Terminate slightly in front (anterior) of the lateral malleolus of the ankle.
Anatomic points to observe in the side view are as follows:
1. Position of the Head
   a. Does the head lean forward or backward? (Use the plumb line and the vertical grid lines.)
   b. Are the cervical vertebrae curved or flattened?
2. Shoulders
   a. Is there kyphosis? Is the dorsal curve (upper back) of the spine exaggerated?
   b. Is the scapula winged? Is there a prominence of the inferior angle of the scapula or the entire vertebral border?
3. Upper Spine
   a. Is the convexity of the thoracic vertebrae exaggerated?
4. Lower Back
   a. Is the concavity of the lumbar curve exaggerated? (Use vertical grid lines on the silhouette.)
5. Abdominal Area
   a. Is there abdominal muscle weakness?
6. Hips
   a. Is there flexion of the hip joint, either with knees straight or flexed? Tightness of the iliopsoas muscles may be the cause. The iliopsoas muscles originate above the hip joint, at the site of the transverse processes of all lumbar vertebrae and the upper two thirds of the iliac fossa; they insert into the lesser trochanter of the femur. The contracting action or tightness of this muscle group may cause the knee or lower leg to be flexed on the pelvis.
7. Knees
   a. Is there flexion or hyperextension?

Anthropometric Data
For this test, the student lies down on his back (supine position). The evaluator uses a *metal* tape measure to ensure accuracy.
1. Leg Length
   a. Locate the crest of the anterior superior spine of the ilium.
   b. Place one end of metal tape on the crest of the anterior superior spine.
   c. Measure down to the internal malleolus of the ankle of the same leg. (Measurements must be accurate to ¼ inch.)
   d. Record information on form.
   e. Repeat the procedure on the other leg.

Previous Medical History:

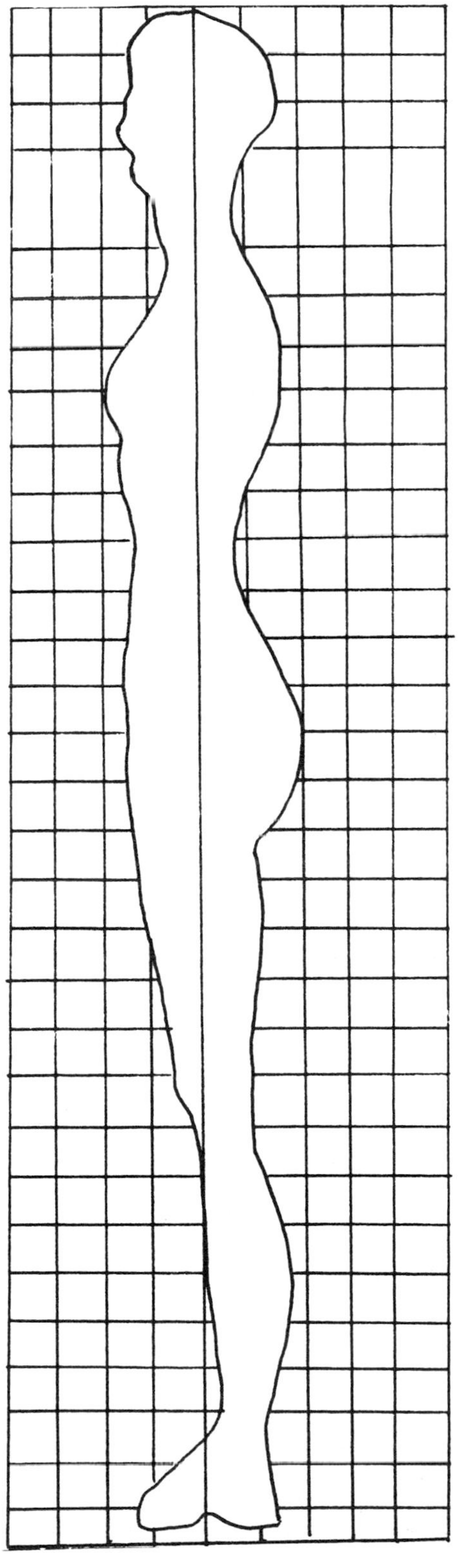

		1	2	3	4
Head	Forward	___	___	___	___
	Backward	___	___	___	___
Shoulder	Cupping	___	___	___	___
Kyphosis		___	___	___	___
Scapula	Winging	___	___	___	___
Lordosis		___	___	___	___
Hip Flexion		___	___	___	___
Body	Forward	___	___	___	___
	Backward	___	___	___	___
Knee	Flexion	___	___	___	___
	Hyper-Extension	___	___	___	___
Arch	Depression	___	___	___	___

Examiner's Remarks:

_____

_____

_____

_____

_____

_____

Fig. 5–4. Reverse of form for use in posture evaluation (Fig. 5–2). Note space for pertinent medical history at top.

Screening Form

Smith _____ Murphy _____
School   Teacher

Name __Jones, John_____

Age __11__ __3__ Wt. __90__ Ht. __58__
Years Months   Lbs.   Inches

Date _____ Grade __6__ M _X_ F __

Handedness	L ____	R _X_	
Leg Length	L _26_	R _26_	
Thigh Girth	L _14_	R _14_	4" above patella
Calf Girth	L _9_	R _9_	4" below patella
Biceps Girth	L _6_	R _6_	5"

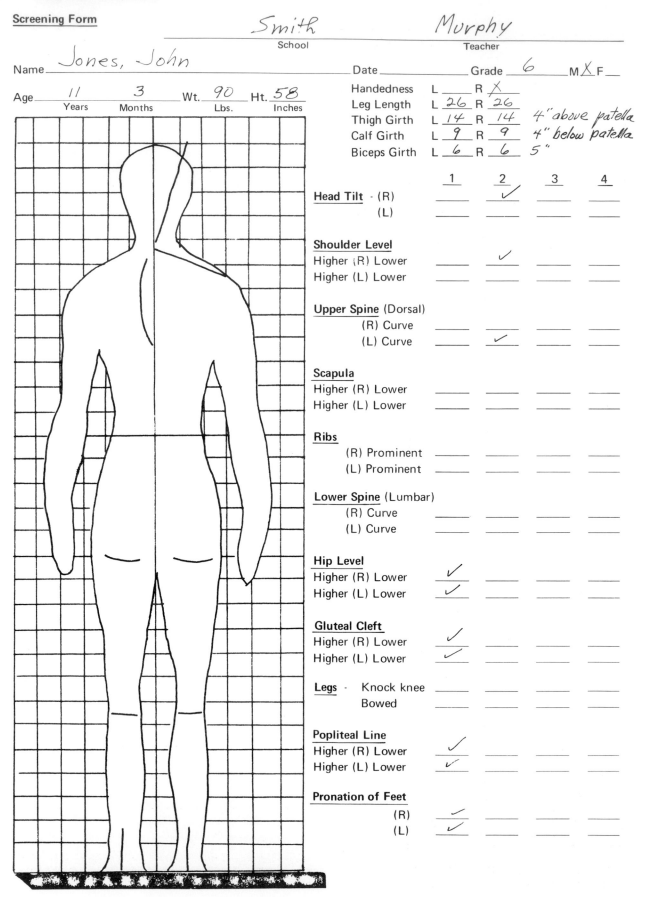

	1	2	3	4
Head Tilt - (R)	____	✓	____	____
(L)	____	____	____	____
Shoulder Level				
Higher (R) Lower	____	✓	____	____
Higher (L) Lower	____	____	____	____
Upper Spine (Dorsal)				
(R) Curve	____	____	____	____
(L) Curve	____	✓	____	____
Scapula				
Higher (R) Lower	____	____	____	____
Higher (L) Lower	____	____	____	____
Ribs				
(R) Prominent	____	____	____	____
(L) Prominent	____	____	____	____
Lower Spine (Lumbar)				
(R) Curve	____	____	____	____
(L) Curve	____	____	____	____
Hip Level				
Higher (R) Lower	✓	____	____	____
Higher (L) Lower	✓	____	____	____
Gluteal Cleft				
Higher (R) Lower	✓	____	____	____
Higher (L) Lower	✓	____	____	____
Legs - Knock knee	____	____	____	____
Bowed	____	____	____	____
Popliteal Line				
Higher (R) Lower	✓	____	____	____
Higher (L) Lower	✓	____	____	____
Pronation of Feet				
(R)	✓	____	____	____
(L)	✓	____	____	____

Previous Medical History: *F/. (L) Femur 2 years ago (1969) ...l.*

o/f ladder

(Try to obtain accurate information—exact dates and how injury occurred or why surgery performed.)

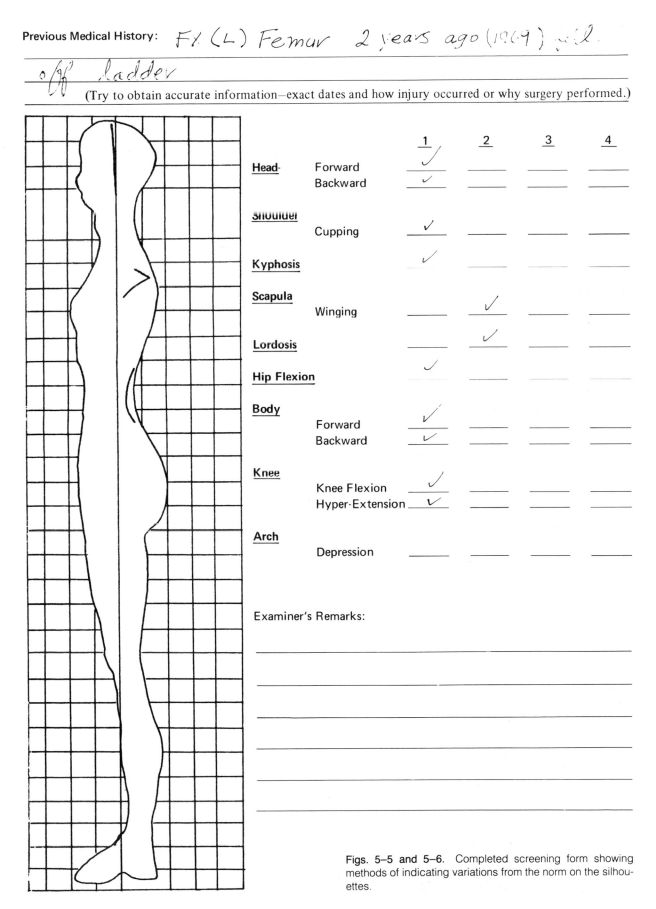

		1	2	3	4
Head	Forward	✓			
	Backward	✓			
Shoulder					
	Cupping	✓			
Kyphosis		✓			
Scapula					
	Winging		✓		
Lordosis			✓		
Hip Flexion		✓			
Body					
	Forward	✓			
	Backward	✓			
Knee					
	Knee Flexion	✓			
	Hyper-Extension	✓			
Arch					
	Depression				

Examiner's Remarks:

_____

_____

_____

_____

_____

_____

Figs. 5–5 and 5–6. Completed screening form showing methods of indicating variations from the norm on the silhouettes.

2. Thigh Girth
   a. Take measurement approximately 4 to 6 inches above (superior to) the tip of the patella. (Use greater distance for taller individuals.)
   b. Record the exact distance above the patella on the form.
   c. Measure around the thigh at point indicated with metal tape.
   d. Record measurement.
   e. Measure the other thigh the same distance above (superior to) the patella; record measurement.
3. Calf Girth
   a. Take measurement approximately 4 to 6 inches below (inferior to) the tip of the patella.
   b. Record the exact distance below the patella on the form.
   c. Measure around calf with metal tape at point indicated.
   d. Record measurement.
   e. Measure the other calf the same distance below (inferior to) the patella; record measurement.
4. Biceps Girth
   a. Flex elbow to approximately 30°.
   b. Take measurement 4 to 6 inches above (superior to) the flexed elbow.
   c. Record the exact distance above the elbow on the form.
   d. Measure around biceps with *metal tape* at point indicated.
   e. Record measurement
   f. Measure the other arm the same distance above the flexed elbow; record measurement.

The maximum score under this procedure is 65. A single item score of 1 or a composite score of 39 or below would be indicative of posture problems. In addition to the scoring, the evaluator should also make specific comments that he can consider when making recommendations for further examination by a physician.

The following is the procedure that may be used when rating children with the New York Posture Test:
1. Record child's name and grade level on his form prior to evaluation.
2. Construct a posture grid or purchase a Symmetrigraf or other type of commercially produced grid to evaluate students.
3. Obtain a metal or plastic tray with a foam rubber or other absorbent insert filled with a foot disinfectant solution.
4. Have the child stand in front of the constructed posture grid or behind the Symmetrigraf.
5. Note the following 5 points in reference to the plumb line or midline reference point. The plumb line or midline reference point should:

a. Coincide with the midline of the body.
b. Pass behind the center of the head.
c. Pass behind the spinous processes of the vertebrae.
d. Bisect the gluteal folds.
e. Be equidistant between the lower extremities.
6. The evaluator observes the child and records the proper scores as indicated by the chart.
7. When the child has been evaluated in the rear view, he steps into the metal or plastic tray and then onto a white sheet of paper to check for foot problems. The scores are recorded on the rating chart.
8. The child then assumes a side view position either in front of the constructed posture grid or behind the Symmetrigraf.
9. The evaluator observes the child and records the proper scores as indicated by the chart.
10. Upon completion of the evaluation, the scores on each item are totaled and recorded in the proper block.

The New York Posture Rating Form can be utilized from grades 4 to 12 or ages can be substituted over the grade level blocks. The same form can be utilized for the same student over many years.

A letter should be sent to the parents of children who need medical attention (Figs. 5–7 and 5–8). This letter should indicate that the findings are not a medical diagnosis and request that the parents take the child to a physician for a follow-up.

SCOLIOSIS EVALUATION

Scoliosis is a postural defect that can be identified during routine posture evaluations such as the programs discussed previously in this section. However, we would be remiss if we did not call special attention to this serious problem and provide a method of evaluating all adolescent children for it. For background information on scoliosis, see Chapter 4, "Survey of Prevalent Defects."

Scoliosis usually occurs between the ages of 10 and 16, occurring 6 to 10 times more often in girls than in boys. It is during this adolescent age period and beyond that most parents/guardians do not observe their child undressed. Early changes are subtle and insidious but can lead to very serious problems. Early diagnosis of scoliosis allows the use of conservative and effective methods of treatment. If the scoliosis is undetected and progresses to the advanced deformity stage, then major surgical procedures, with higher risks and less satisfactory results, may be necessary. Many states, such as Delaware, Minnesota, California, and, recently, New Jersey have laws requiring scoliosis evaluations. In 1974, The American Academy of Orthopaedic Surgeons issued the following statement:

The American Academy of Orthopaedic Surgeons hereby gives its official recommendation to any program of routine evaluation of school children for the detection of scoliosis

Student's Name	Grade

School

Dear Parents:

The Department of Physical Education conducts a posture screening evaluation of all students. This evaluation is conducted under the supervision of a staff member.

It should be clearly understood that THE FINDINGS ARE NOT MEDICAL DIAGNOSES. We recommend that you discuss with your family physician the item or items that we have checked in the list below concerning your child's posture. If you or your physician would like further information, contact

Mr. Alfred N. Daniel, Phone 123·4567

To meet the special needs of students with postural deviations, the Physical Education Department provides a program of Developmental or Adapted Physical Education which may be substituted in part for the regular program. In order to be included in this program a student must have the approval of his parents.

We will attempt to meet the needs of as many of the students selected for this program as possible. Therefore, in making his decision, the student with parental guidance would evaluate the importance of the program as prescribed to help improve his particular posture problem.

Below is the check list. The items checked show postural deviations which pertain to your child.

1. Forward head
2. Head tilt
3. Unequal shoulder level
4. Kyphosis (round shoulder)
5. Winging of scapula (shoulder blade protrusion)

6. Spine curvature
7. Lordosis (hollow back)
8. Unequal hip level
9. Knee flexion
10. Unequal leg length

COMMENTS:_____

_____

Sincerely yours,

Fig. 5–7. Sample letter sent to parents whose children need consultation with a physician.

Dear Parents:

It is necessary to have the permission of the parents before the student may participate in the Developmental or Adapted Physical Education Program. Please indicate any past illnesses or injuries that may be of value to your child's program.

Sincerely,

I understand that these findings are NOT medical diagnosis.

I hereby grant permission for_____to participate in
Developmental or Adapted Physical Education.   Name

_____   _____
Date   (Parent or Guardian)

I hereby DO NOT grant permission for_____to participate in
Developmental Physical Education.   Name

_____   _____
Date   (Parent or Guardian)

REMARKS:_____

_____

_____

_____

Fig. 5–8. Sample form letter for acknowledgement of receipt of posture evaluation report and for granting of permission for the child to participate in the Developmental or Adapted Physical Education Program.

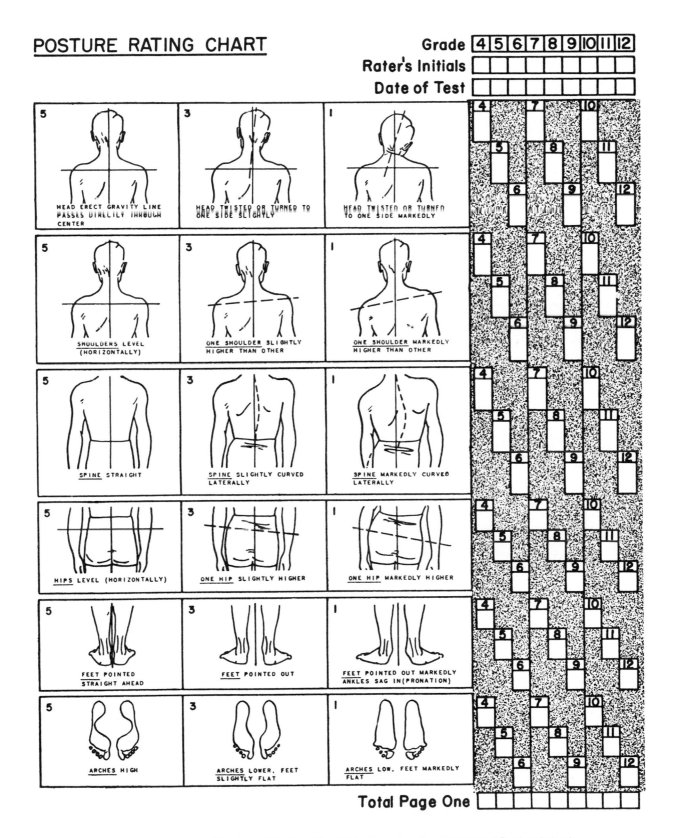

Fig. 5–9. New York posture rating chart. (Courtesy of the New York State Education Department and Bardeen's Inc.)

Fig. 5—9 continued.

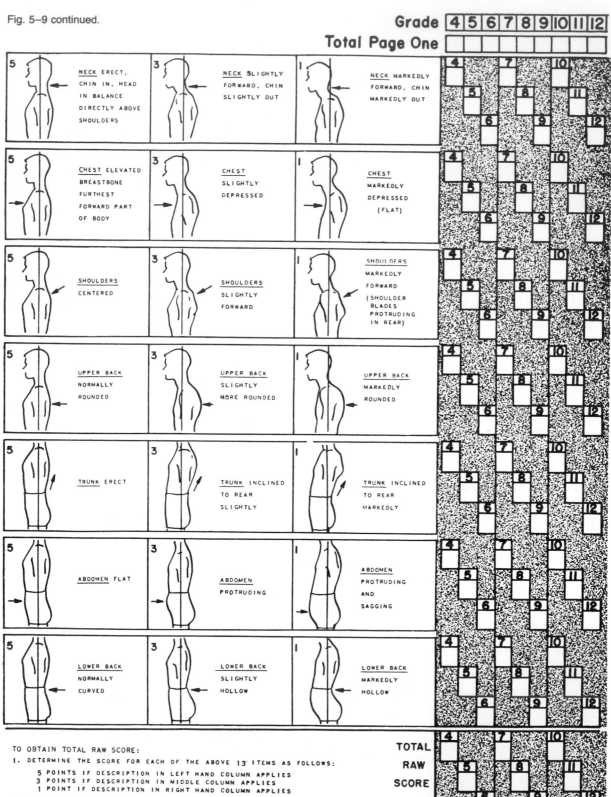

TO OBTAIN TOTAL RAW SCORE:

1. DETERMINE THE SCORE FOR EACH OF THE ABOVE 13 ITEMS AS FOLLOWS:

    5 POINTS IF DESCRIPTION IN LEFT HAND COLUMN APPLIES
    3 POINTS IF DESCRIPTION IN MIDDLE COLUMN APPLIES
    1 POINT IF DESCRIPTION IN RIGHT HAND COLUMN APPLIES

2. ENTER SCORE FOR EACH ITEM UNDER PROPER GRADE IN THE SCORING COLUMN

3. ADD ALL 13 SCORES AND PLACE TOTAL IN APPROPRIATE SPACE

and other crippling spine deformities. The Academy recognizes that by early detection, more appropriate treatment can be given and better total treatment of this disability health problem can be carried out.

Results from the California, Delaware, and Minnesota programs indicate that 8% to 13% of school age children have a detectable degree of scoliosis.

An initial evaluation can be conducted on a group basis. One method of approach is to conduct the evaluation during the physical education class; another is to have the school nurse conduct the evaluations. The parents/guardians should be given a letter or notice (Fig. 5–10) regarding the evaluation.

The evaluator should be of the same sex as the children being evaluated. This is especially true for adolescent girls because they are self-conscious at this age and may not discuss such symptoms as an uneven hemline, waist that is not the same on both sides, or uneven breast sizes with a male evaluator. Female school nurses should be able to evaluate both male and female children. The initial evaluation can be done in the physical education locker room or in a classroom; the children can be seen in classes or groups. Children should be evaluated in 2-piece bathing suits, shorts and halters, or even bras and pants for the girls and bathing suits, gym shorts, or underclothing for the boys.

For the initial group screening, the children line up and come forward one at a time to the evaluator. The evaluator observes the child from the rear, paying attention to the following areas:

    shoulder level (equal?)
    hip level (equal?)
    waistline (equal?)
    spine (curved to one side?)
    shoulder blades (is one more prominent?)
    distance between the arms (equal?)

Still with his back to the evaluator, the child should place his palms together, his feet together, straighten his knees, and bend over at the waist to approximately 90°. His arms should be relaxed and hanging freely. The following points should be observed in the child's lower back to upper back/neck areas:

    Is there a hump on one side of the back?
    Is there a compensating hump on the other side of the back?
    Is there a difference in levels between the sides of the back?
    Feel vertebrae by running finger down the spine
    Are the sides of the back symmetric?

Then the child should return to a standing position, turn around and face the evaluator. Again the child should place his palms and feet together, straighten his knees and bend over at the waist to approximately

Dear Parents/Guardians:

There will be a screening program for scoliosis for all pupils ages   through

Scoliosis is defined as a condition of the spine in which the spine may curve to the left or right. It is most commonly found during the time of rapid growth and may progress if not treated. The purpose of the screening program is to recognize scoliosis in its earliest stages.

Your son/daughter will be advised in advance of the exact date of his/her screening by the school nurse or physical educator.

Female pupils are requested to wear a two piece bathing suit or a halter and shorts. Male pupils will be evaluated in shorts.

If your child is suspected of a possible scoliosis, you will be given written notice with a recommendation for further evaluation by your family physician or specialist.

If you, for any reason, have objections to this scoliosis screening of your child, please notify the school your child attends, in writing, at your earliest convenience.

Thank you for your cooperation.

                                        Sincerely,

Fig. 5–10.   Sample letter informing parents of screening program for scoliosis.

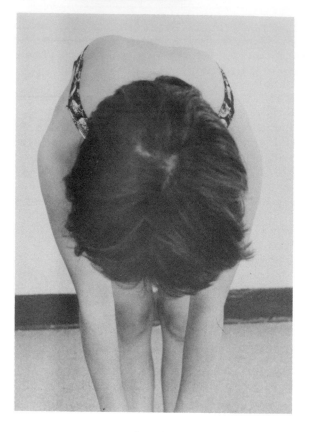

Fig. 5–11. Child being evaluated for scoliosis. Note "hump" on child's upper back.

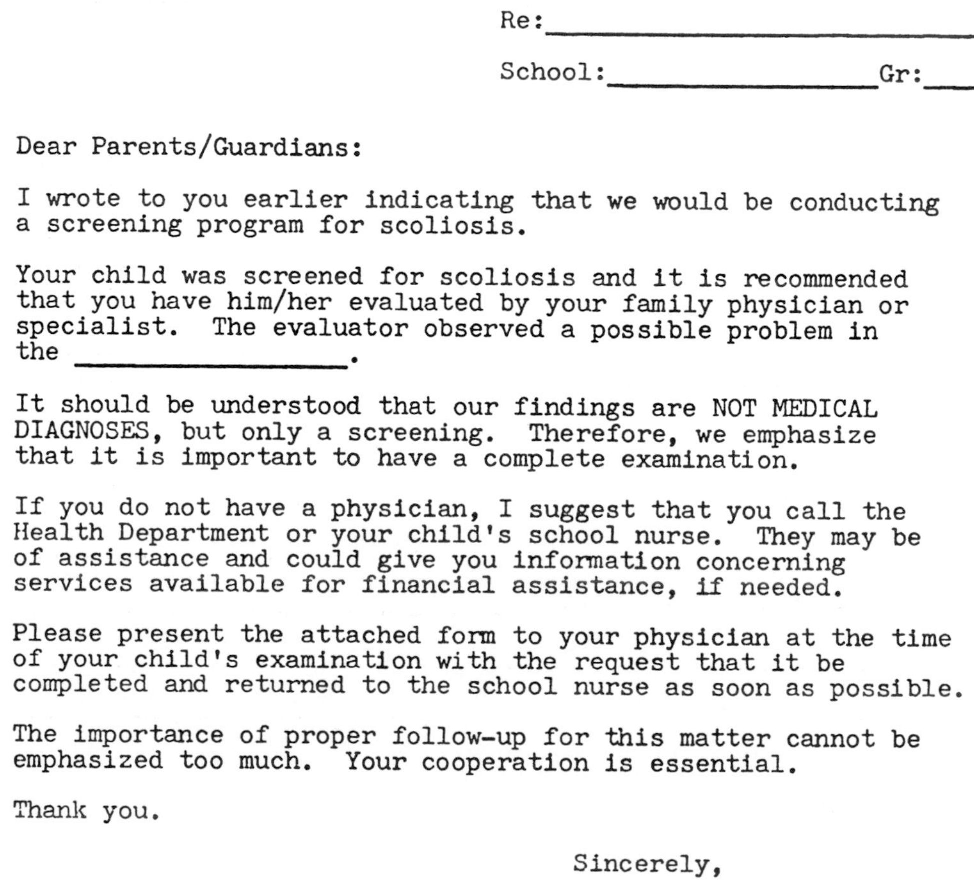

Re:_____

School:_____Gr:_____

Dear Parents/Guardians:

I wrote to you earlier indicating that we would be conducting a screening program for scoliosis.

Your child was screened for scoliosis and it is recommended that you have him/her evaluated by your family physician or specialist. The evaluator observed a possible problem in the _____.

It should be understood that our findings are NOT MEDICAL DIAGNOSES, but only a screening. Therefore, we emphasize that it is important to have a complete examination.

If you do not have a physician, I suggest that you call the Health Department or your child's school nurse. They may be of assistance and could give you information concerning services available for financial assistance, if needed.

Please present the attached form to your physician at the time of your child's examination with the request that it be completed and returned to the school nurse as soon as possible.

The importance of proper follow-up for this matter cannot be emphasized too much. Your cooperation is essential.

Thank you.

Sincerely,

Fig. 5–12. Sample letter sent to parents whose children need consultation with a physician.

SCOLIOSIS SCREENING REPORT 19___ - 19___

Name_____Birth Date _____Age_____Sex M___F___

Parents_____Address_____

School_____Grade_____Family Physician_____

_____
HISTORY
_____
Prior Awareness: No ___ Yes ___ How long_____
Symptoms, Complaints _____

Family History of Scoliosis (state relationship to student) No ___ Yes ___

_____

_____

Remarks_____

_____
| | Under Care | Other Reason X-Ray |
| X-Ray Refused _____ | Prior to Screening_____ | Not Taken _____ |

_____

SCREENING X-RAY REPORT

X-Ray Taken at _____Read by_____
X-Ray Results: 1. Negative ___
                2. Scoliosis ___   Degree of Curve: Type of Curve:
                                    1. Less than 10° ___   1. Thoracic _____
                                    2. 10° to 20° ___   2. Double Major ____
                                    3. 20° to 40° ___   3. Thoracolumbar ___
                                    4. 40° to 55° ___   4. Lumbar _____
                                    5. More than 55° ___   5. Other _____
                3. Kyphosis/Lordosis ___
                4. Other _____

_____
RECOMMENDATIONS

1. Discharge _____   2. Rescreen next year _____

Repeat AP Standing X-Ray: 3. 6 months _____

4. 12 months _____   5. Other _____

6. Refer for Orthopedic Evaluation _____

7. Other _____

_____   _____
      Date   Physician Signature

Fig. 5-13. Scoliosis screening report.

Table 5–1.
EXERCISES FOR LOWER BACK

Instructions

1. Do the exercises marked by the *therapist* or *instructor*.
2. All exercises should be done at home as well as during Developmental Physical Education classes.
3. Each exercise to be done___repetitions___times per day.

Exercises

1. Lie on back: knees bent, feet flat on floor. Try to roll pelvis by forcing lower back to ground and abdomen in.
2. Repeat No. 1; then lift head and shoulders upward and touch knees with fingertips.
3. Repeat No. 1; slide one leg down until the knee is straight on the ground, raise the leg upward, bend the knee and then straighten and lower to starting position; repeat on opposite side.
4. Lie on back:
   a. Draw one knee to chest with hands and hold.
   b. Draw both knees toward chest, grasp with hands and pull.
5. Lie on back:
   a. Draw both knees to chest.
   b. Roll forward and up to a sitting position.
6. Sit with legs spread and toes turned in, arms raised at the sides, shoulder high:
   a. Swing right hand to left foot, left arm behind.
   b. Return and swing left hand to the right foot.
7. Stand against wall, heels 4 inches from wall, head, shoulders and hips touching the wall: pull in abdomen and push lower back against wall.
8. Stand with back flattened against wall: raise heels, bend knees and squat, stand up, keeping back flat against wall.
9. Sit on a stool placed against the wall: bend forward at the hips until back is arched; slowly straighten up until the lower back, shoulders, and head touch wall.
10. Repeat number 8, but stand 4 inches away from wall.
11. Keep knee straight.
    a. Raise one leg at a time.
    b. Raise both legs together.
12. Lie on abdomen, arms extended overhead:
    a. Lift opposite arm and leg.
    b. Lift same arm and leg.

Table 5–2.
EXERCISES FOR UPPER BACK

Instructions

1. Only do exercises marked by the *therapist* or *instructor*.
2. Each exercise to be done___repetitions___times per day.

Exercises

1. Lie on abdomen, arms down by sides: pinch shoulder blades together.
2. Lie on abdomen, arms down by sides, elbows straight, palms up toward ceiling: raise arms upward.
3. Lie on abdomen, place back of hands in the small of the back: raise elbows and shoulders up.
4. Lie on abdomen, arms down by sides: raise head, shoulders, and chest up.
5. Lie on abdomen, arms stretched out at shoulder level, elbows straight, palms forward or downward: raise arms upward.
6. Lie on abdomen, arms halfway between shoulders and head, elbows straight, palms down: raise arms upward.
7. Lie on abdomen, arms straight out over head, elbows straight, palms down: raise arms upward.
8. Sit on a stool, back flat against wall, arms up at shoulder level, backs of hands against wall: raise arms upward and out; keep hands against wall.
9. Stand in front of wall pulleys, arms up at shoulder level, elbows bent to 90°, pull weights back.
10. Stand in front of wall pulleys; keep arms and elbows up at shoulder level and elbows straight: pull weights back
11. Stand in front of wall pulleys, arms straight out at shoulder level, elbows straight: pull weight downward and then arms backward.
12. Stand in front of wall pulleys: pull weight and arms upward over head.
13. Sit on a stool, back flat against wall, arms up at shoulder level, back of hands against wall: touch hands over head keeping hands against wall.
14. Lie on abdomen: hold a wand or weighted bar behind back and raise it toward ceiling, hold for 3 counts; return to prone position.

90°. The child should now be observed from upper back/neck areas to low back areas (Fig. 5–11). The areas listed above in the rear view should be observed again from the front view.

Finally, the child turns sideways to the evaluator and repeats the procedure for bending forward and the body positions indicated above. The same body areas are observed from the side. In this position, the child can also be evaluated for kyphosis. If a child is suspected of having scoliosis, his name should be placed on a list for recheck or indicated by a code in a roll book or master check sheet.

The child should be rechecked later by the evaluator to be certain of the possibility of scoliosis. If a child is suspected of having a problem, a letter or memo (Fig. 5–12) should be sent to the parent/guardian. A follow-up report (Fig. 5–13) may be attached to the letter or memo sent home. This may afford statistical data and future follow-up studies on children in whom scoliosis is suspected.

INITIATING THE PROGRAM

The identification of specific problems is one benefit of a posture evaluation program. Many handicaps can be improved if early diagnosis is combined with training; for this reason it is important for all school systems to have posture evaluation and training programs for all students.

In a school program, a letter is forwarded to the parents of the students who need attention (Figs. 5–7 and 5–8). The letter states that the findings are *not* a medical diagnosis and urges the parents to take the child to a physician for a follow-up. If there are any questions, the parents or the physician may contact the evaluator. It is requested that parents acknowledge the letter, whether they approve or refuse the program. Refusal statements should be kept on file for reference in case of future questions.

**Table 5–3.
EXERCISES FOR STRENGTHENING
ABDOMINAL MUSCLES**

Instructions

1. Only do the exercises marked by the *therapist* or *instructor*.
2. Each exercise to be done___repetitions___times per day.

Exercises

1. Pelvic tilt.
2. Lie on back with knees bent, arms stretched forward: raise head, pull in abdomen and raise to a sitting position.
3. Lie on back with knees bent, arms folded across chest:
   a. Pull in abdomen and raise to a sitting position.
   b. Return to starting position, relax, then repeat.
4. Lie on back with knees bent:
   a. With hands touching sides of head, pull in abdomen and raise the body to a sitting position.
   b. Return to a starting position, relax, then repeat.
5. Sit erect on a chair with feet apart and hands behind head; bend from side to side; pull elbows back and keep back arched.
6. Lie on back with hips and knees flexed, and feet under bottom rung of stall bars; clasp hands behind head, elbows back:
   a. Slowly raise head and shoulders until they are 6 inches off the mat. Return slowly.
   b. Repeat a. As you come up, twist to the left and return slowly.
   c. Repeat a. As you come up, twist to the right and return slowly.
7. Lie on back, legs straight, with arms stretched forward:
   a. Raise head and sit up, twisting the trunk repeat the sit-up, twisting the trunk to the right so that the left hand touches the toes of the right foot.
   c. Return to starting position, relax, then repeat the series of 2 sit-ups.

Scheduling Classes

The scheduling of rehabilitation classes for students or patients is the next major consideration. Patients in a rehabilitation center can be treated during sessions of physical therapy or developmental or adapted physical education. Scheduling classes for students in a public school will require consultation with the guidance department and the administration in order to establish procedures.

One method is to schedule students for special treatment during the time their regular physical education sessions meet. If the time allotted for physical education is less than 2 or 3 sessions each week, perhaps students can be excused from a study hall for posture classes. If time during the school day is unavailable, after-school programs, lunchtime programs, or even Saturday or evening programs can be initiated. Scheduling may be difficult, but the need warrants the effort.

Students should have one or 2 sessions each week if classes are scheduled for an entire school year or a semester. The 6-week, or "block period," system would call for daily sessions. Extracurricular classes require a strong supplemental home program because of the limited time spent at school sessions.

A class of 6 to 8 students is desirable in a school program, as larger classes lead to confusion. The instructor must be able to spend time with each student in order to assist, encourage, and adjust routines properly.

Student or Patient Information

Children in a posture program must understand their problems. Printed information and individual demonstrations are valuable. Slides, movies, and transparencies can be used to illustrate the causes of a problem, the bones and muscles involved, and the necessary corrective exercises. Pictures, drawings, bulletin board displays, and other visual aids should be used.

Exercise Forms

Once the individual is aware of his needs, a specific exercise program can be initiated. These exercises should be printed and given to both the parents/guardians and the child (Tables 5–1, 5–2, and 5–3). Additional exercises can be added as needed. Complete exercise programs for all anticipated conditions or problems should be planned before the program begins so that the instructors can follow an orderly schedule. For additional exercises see Appendix A, Therapeutic Exercises.

Records

A folder for each individual in the program should include the evaluation form, parental permission slip, exercise procedures, and other information. Progress notes should be written periodically, noting changes or other information of value. As the folders contain confidential material, they should be kept in a locked file cabinet when not in use.

SUMMARY

The evaluation of posture is an important link in the total process of physical education or rehabilitation. It is often overlooked or neglected, although good posture is the basis of all healthy growth and development.

The rehabilitation center owes the patient a chance to regain the maximum use of his body. The school system owes its youngsters a commitment to their physical problems by providing early diagnosis and a planned program for intervention.

BIBLIOGRAPHY

Adair, I.V., et al.: Moire topography in scoliosis screening. Clin Orthop, *129*:165, 1974.

Alexander, M.M. and Brown, M.S.: Pediatric Physical Diagnosis for Nurses. New York, McGraw-Hill Book Co., 1974.

Banta, J.V.: Early recognition of orthopedic problems in childhood. J School Health, *44*:39, 1974.

Barness, L.A.: Manual of Pediatric Physical Diagnosis. 4th Edition. Chicago, Year Book Publishers, Inc., 1972.

Barrow, H.M. and McGee, R.: A Practical Approach to Measurement in Physical Education. 2nd Edition. Philadelphia, Lea & Febiger, 1971.

Bates, B.: A Guide to Physical Examination. Philadelphia, J.B. Lippincott Co., 1974.

Clarke, H.H. and Clarke, D.H.: Developmental and Adapted Physical Education. Englewood Cliffs, N.J., Prentice-Hall, Inc., 1963.

Colwell, H.R.: Genetic aspects of orthopedic diseases. Am J Nurs, 70:763, 1970.

Daniels, A.S. and Davis, E.A.: Adapted Physical Education. New York, Harper & Row, 1965.

Daniels, L., Williams, M., and Worthingham, C.: Muscles Testing Techniques of Manual Examination. 2nd Edition. Philadelphia, W.B. Saunders Company, 1956.

Department of Public Instruction: Guidelines for Adapted Physical Education. Harrisburg, Commonwealth of Pennsylvania, 1966.

Dunn, B., et al: Scoliosis Screening. Pediatrics, 61:794, 1978.

Dwyer, A.P. and Slinger, B.S.: School Screening for Scoliosis: Our Challenging Responsibility. Aust NZ J Surg, 48:439, 1978.

Frost, J., et al.: Scoliosis screening pilot project—A preliminary report to development of a statewide school program. Hawaii Med J, 37:361, 1978.

Frost, L.: Posture and Body Mechanics. University of Iowa Extension Bulletin, State University of Iowa, 1955.

Gaines, R.W.: Scoliosis and Kyphosis. Missouri Medicine, March, 1980, pgs. 124–134.

Gray, A.: Screening for scoliosis—A threatening curve. The School Nurse, Winter 1977—78, pgs. 5, 8.

Harlin, V.K.: How We Do It. J School Health, 47:483, 1977.

Hensinger, R., et al.: Orthopedic screening of school age children. Orthop Rev, 4:23, 1975.

Keim, H.A.: Scoliosis Clinical Symposia, Summit, CIBA, 30(No. 1):1, 1978.

Kelly, E.D.: Adapted and Corrective Physical Education. 4th Edition. New York, Ronald Press Company, 1968.

Kendall, H.O. and Kendall, F.P.: Muscles Testing and Function. Baltimore, Williams & Wilkins Company, 1949.

Mathews, D.K., et al.: The Science of Physical Education for Handicapped Children. New York, Harper Brothers, 1962.

Posture Committee of the American Academy of Orthopaedic Surgeons: Posture and its relationship to orthpaedic disabilities. 1947.

Renshaw, T.S., et al.: School screening for the early detection of scoliosis in children. Conn Med, 43:139, 1979.

Scott, M.G. and French, E.: Measurement and Evaluation in Physical Education. Dubuque, Iowa, William C. Brown, 1959.

Sells, C.J. and May, E.A.: Scoliosis screening in public schools. Am J Nurs, 74:60, 1974.

Shifrin, L.A.: Scoliosis: current concepts. Clin Pediatr, 11:594, 1972.

State of New York: The New York State Physical Fitness Test: A Manual for Teachers of Physical Education. Albany, Division of Health, Physical Education, and Recreation, New York State Department of Education, 1958.

Sullivan, J.A. and Tompkins, S.F.: Development of a scoliosis screening program in Oklahoma schools. J Okla State Med Assoc, 71:52, 1978.

Vodola, T.M.: Individualized Physical Education Programs for the Handicapped Child. Englewood Cliffs, N.J., Prentice-Hall, Inc., 1973.

Wallace, A.P.: A scoliosis screening program. J Sch Health, 47:619, 1977.

Wallace, R.B. and Moe, J.H.: A plea for the routine school examination of children for spinal deformity. Minn Med, 57:419, 1974.

Writer, D.: Scoliosis screening. J Sch Health, 44:563, 1974.

Winter, R.B.: How to find a spinal deformity—look for it. Mod Med, 43:38, 1975.

Winter, R.B.: Idiopathic Scoliosis. Minn Med, 55:529, 1972.

FILMS

Scoliosis Research Society
P.O. Box 2001
Park Ridge, Illinois 60068
Spinal Screening Program Training Film or VHS Videotape.

6 *Organization Practices and Strategies*

With the current trend toward increasing challenging experiences for disabled persons, it is obvious that there exists a wide variation of programs and services to meet individual needs. Because the scope of organizational and administrative practices is so diverse, readers are encouraged to review other books on the subject.

Recreation services for the disabled are typically coordinated by professionals with degrees in therapeutic recreation or community recreation. In the traditional medical model, a therapeutic recreation specialist will often be part of an interdisciplinary team and report to a physician either directly in team meetings and/or indirectly through progress notes in a medical chart.

An adapted physical education specialist is usually linked to a public school setting, although a few professionals are engaged in medical and clinical programs. Some adapted specialists work with other related service personnel (O.T. and P.T.) in coordinating intervention strategies.

Both adapted physical educators and therapeutic recreation specialists attempt to provide purposive intervention strategies to accomplish stated objectives. The term activity analysis, often associated with the discipline of therapeutic recreation, can also apply to adapted physical education. Essentially activity analysis means the identification of basic inherent qualities of an activity through which goal attainment can be achieved. To accomplish this, the program leader must evaluate the tool (choice of activity, equipment, etc.) and the procedure (physical requirements, interaction pattern, etc.). Simply stated, it is important to make choices dependent upon the participant's abilities, interests, and needs. Various models for activity analysis have been developed, but will not be discussed here.

INSTRUCTIONAL MODIFICATION

Program modifications often include changing a traditional unit or activity to accommodate a physically disabled (Pd) student. This can be done by reducing the size of the playing area, using stations in teaching, alternating the number of players on a team, etc. By defining the many components that make up a game or sport, one is able to adapt and make appropriate program decisions. Variations in one or more of the following six categories should aid the instructor or therapist in making adaptations:

1. Players
2. Equipment
3. Movement Pattern (locomotor or non-locomotor)
4. Organizational Pattern (playing area configuration)
5. Rules
6. Purpose of Desired Outcome

Before a traditional activity is changed it is imperative to determine what social, emotional, or physical behaviors are planned from the experience and what are the desired objectives. As with traditional activities, it is helpful to start with lead-up skill progression units and/or practice sessions to assess the proficiency level of each participant. Review of activity components should focus on individual needs if participation values are to be used. However, it is possible to change one or more of the components to reach desired objectives. For example, in a school soccer unit if a physical education instructor is emphasizing visual intensity skills for a shy and distractible pupil, then a circle formation drill rather than a file formation would be best suited to meet individual needs. Eye contact could be enhanced as the individual focuses on the whole group as opposed to only a few members. In this situation a change in the organization pattern is done to focus attention to individual needs. Another example pertains to a therapeutic recreation session. In a low organized game situation, if a severely spastic cerebral palsied patient is unable to grasp a ball for throwing at a ground target then the therapist can substitute a ramp to compensate for functional deficiencies. The game would then emphasize pushing rather than throwing a ball, consequently the movement pattern is changed to "fit" the capabilities of the patient.

Application of skills learned during stationary practice and moving skill drills comprises the bulk of any team game or sport unit. The program leader needs to assess each physically disabled (Pd) player to determine in what manner each will contribute to the group activity. If for some reason the (Pd) player is unable to engage in regular play, then alternatives must be planned. For example, use less skilled players for specialty skills, such as a designated hitter in softball, and have them concentrate on developing just those special skills.

In general, the six categories (players, equipment, movement pattern, organization pattern, rules and

COMMON ADAPTATIONS FOR TEAM GAMES AND SPORTS

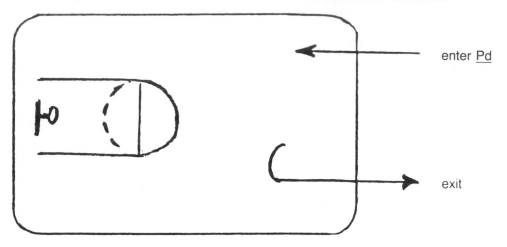

enter Pd

exit

Fig. 6–1. Enter-exit play.

purpose) should be changed as little as possible when modifying for a (Pd) player. If too much diversity is used in any one of the six categories, then a traditional unit takes on a new meaning. The focus of attention then shifts to the less skilled player which disrupts the intention of the mainstreaming process. The purpose is to integrate, but at a level that does not affect the participation skills of regular group members.

Some team activities allow for varying degrees of mobility and a player with a functional limitation can play in a position that requires limited movement. For example, in Floor Hockey, a (Pd) player can team up with an able bodied teammate and play goalie.

The following section discusses techniques for adapting activities commonly included in physical education curricula. These adaptations can also be used in recreation programs and other learning environments where the mainstreaming process is used. This

is not an exhaustive source of current concepts, but only a sampling of general strategies and guidelines. It should be pointed out that these modifications are not likely to impede the performance skills for other non-disabled participants enrolled in the class or activity program.

A. Enter-Exit Play (Fig. 6–1). *Description:* The (Pd) student makes one play within regular court or field situation and then leaves playing area. Example—Allow (Pd) player to shoot foul shots in basketball and then immediately leave game situation.

The (Pd) player contributes directly to team play action by performing a specialty skill inside the playing area, but not interfered with by other players. Safety considerations are fulfilled as the player is out of the main flow of activity. Regular play continues after the (Pd) player leaves the court or field area.

B. Out-Of-Bounds Play (Fig. 6–2). *Description:* The (Pd) player stays outside of regular court or field,

Pd

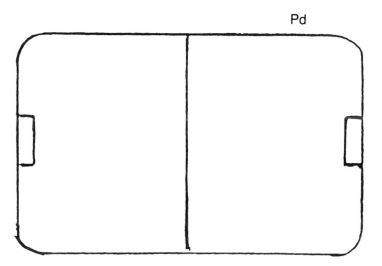

Fig. 6–2. Out-of-bounds play.

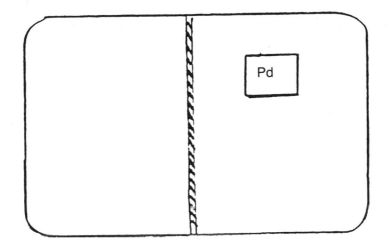

Fig. 6–3.   Safety zone play.

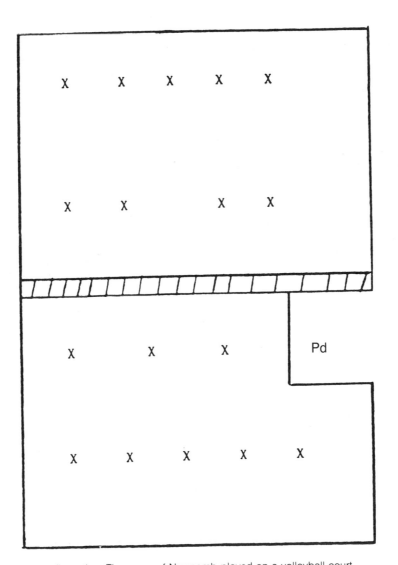

Fig. 6–4.   Alternative playing area configuration. The game of Newcomb played on a volleyball court.

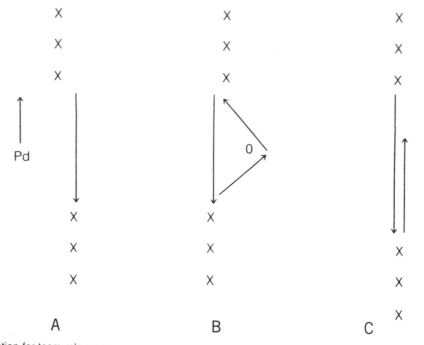

Fig. 6–5. Travel route option for team relay race.

but has responsibilities for special play situations. Example—Allow (Pd) player to throw all out-of-bounds balls to teammates in soccer.

Instead of remaining in a stationary position the (Pd) player can act as a "rover" and move along a portion of the side line to follow the flow of action. When there is a stop in action or delay caused by an out-of-bounds play then the (Pd) player can perform the specialty skill. This should be done without interference from an opposing player. After the play the normal flow of activity can continue without disruption and regular rules can apply. Safety issues are not a main concern because the (Pd) player is positioned outside the playing area.

C. Safety Zone Play (Fig. 6–3). *Description:* The (Pd) player stays within playing court or field, but is confined to safety zone area (marked by lines). This is primarily done for *safety* reasons. No teammates or opponents are allowed to go into the zone. If safety zone is entered by another play then an infraction or penalty is usually called. Example—Allow (Pd) player to act as server within zone on every play or alternate plays in game of volleyball.

The (Pd) player is positioned inside the playing area which provides a more normal approach to team play. However, the player is at risk for injury to self or others when involved in a fast paced activity. Unconscious or uncontrolled entry into the safety zone by a teammate or opposing player may have disastrous re-

sults if bodily contact is made. However, the (Pd) player is not in a position to affect the performance skills of the other players.

D. Alternative Playing Court Configuration (Fig. 6–4). As an example, this game of Newcomb, the (Pd) player always starts play at the beginning of the game and after every score by using a serve throw over the net. Play continues as all other players catch and throw the ball by following regular rules. The (Pd) player remains in a stationary position outside the boundary line.

Changing the configuration of a court or playing area diverts attention away from normalcy. All players can be accommodated, but skill levels can be suppressed in team activities if space provisions are essentially designed for inclusion of the (Pd) player. Space modifications are easier to use in individual and dual games/sports because the (Pd) player's pursuit of independence is more readily achieved.

E. Travel Route Option (Fig. 6–5). A single file formation is used as the organizational pattern. The line of travel can be shortened for the (Pd) player (#A). The course can have an alternate route (#B) and/or longer travel line (#C) for regular players. The purpose is to equalize competition where teams are essentially even in terms of performance skills. By going first, the (Pd) player is not likely to lag behind or fail to "keep up" with the more highly talented players. Travel route options are useful in speed drills and relays.

COMMON ADAPTATIONS FOR ELEMENTARY SCHOOL GAMES/ACTIVITIES

Vary distance to move by shortening it for physically disabled player or lengthening it for normal player. For example, in a relay race have the disabled player travel a shorter route to reach his teammate (Fig. 6–5).

Organizational Patterns or positions on playing field. (Circular movement, exchange position, move to center and back, move across center line and back, squad formation, etc.)

Play with partner, join hands or have "normal" player push wheelchair and act as a single person. (Consider appliance as extension of body.)

For example,

In goal ball relay, wheelchair player is pushed by normal player. Once players reach basket, each player alternates shooting at basket. All other players play regular rules.

Vary the boundaries. Make the formation larger for normal players, shorter for physically disabled players.

In game of individual balloon volleyball, normal player plays in widened court area opposite net. The physically disabled player plays in narrowed court area on opposite side where confined positioning will enhance a more accurate approach to striking the balloon.

COMMON ADAPTATIONS FOR ELEMENTARY SCHOOL GAMES/ACTIVITIES

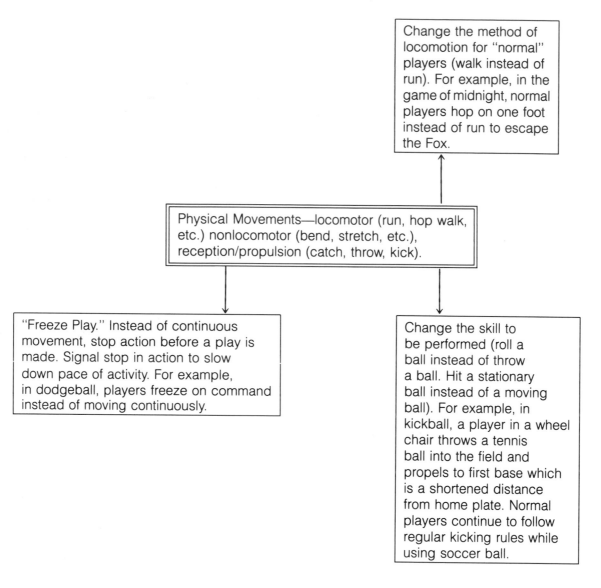

Change the method of locomotion for "normal" players (walk instead of run). For example, in the game of midnight, normal players hop on one foot instead of run to escape the Fox.

Physical Movements—locomotor (run, hop walk, etc.) nonlocomotor (bend, stretch, etc.), reception/propulsion (catch, throw, kick).

"Freeze Play." Instead of continuous movement, stop action before a play is made. Signal stop in action to slow down pace of activity. For example, in dodgeball, players freeze on command instead of moving continuously.

Change the skill to be performed (roll a ball instead of throw a ball. Hit a stationary ball instead of a moving ball). For example, in kickball, a player in a wheel chair throws a tennis ball into the field and propels to first base which is a shortened distance from home plate. Normal players continue to follow regular kicking rules while using soccer ball.

7 *Adapted Sports, Games, and Activities*

The origin of sports, games, and activities adapted to the needs of the physically disabled can be traced to the end of World War II. Thousands of disabled veterans then joined the already existing group of people with congenital and traumatic handicaps.

The enthusiasm and concern originally displayed for these returning heroes was rapidly displaced by apathy from most of the public, some of the Veterans Hospitals, a few private rehabilitation agencies, and most importantly, the veterans and their families.

The returning veterans required not only physical rebuilding, but also emotional, psychologic, and social rebuilding. The physical treatment of wounds and residual problems was not enough. The veterans had even greater drives for sports, games, and activities after the war than they had before their injuries.

From the outset, it was apparent that adaptations were going to be necessary for the program. Many of the early adaptations were the result of the imaginative efforts of the participants. When they saw a need for a change in equipment to fit a prosthesis or a change in rules to accommodate wheelchairs, they made it. In addition, they gathered together with others who needed the same adaptations; as a result, groups were formed for the sole purpose of providing activities for the disabled. In this manner, veterans and those working with them began to explore the possibilities of sports, games, and activities for the physically challenged.

Participating in adapted sports and games gives an individual the opportunity to become physically fit, develop hobbies, become more active, learn leisure time skills, and undergo positive social and group experiences.

OBJECTIVES OF ADAPTED SPORTS

Sports for the physically disabled are increasing in scope and interest throughout the world. Various sports associations are being organized nationally in many countries, and other organizations coordinate the international activities. However, the meaning of sports needs to be clarified before further discussion. For some persons, competitive wheelchair sports fulfill certain basic needs. If competition is important to the individual, that is fine, but it should not be the only goal. For example, in some situations, the aim of sports is to meet therapeutic needs for the purpose of physical and psychologic rehabilitation or habilitation. Still, for some individuals the objective of involvement in sports is to fulfill leisure time pursuits. Regardless of the type of program (competitive, therapeutic, or leisure), the goal of the program leader is to help physically disabled persons compensate for their specific problem by mastering and finding personal achievement in selected activities.

Participation in sports, games, and activities fulfills certain objectives. However, it is important to determine the objectives before the activity starts. For example, an activity may focus on physical development to improve weakened and affected muscles. In such cases, the objective is to aid in restoration of function to disabled parts. Sports, games, and activities can also fulfill social and emotional objectives. The ability to have fun and to elicit positive reactions from participation may improve a person's social development and self-concept.

Modification of sport and game rules should not be discouraged and should be regulated to meet the needs of the group. Utilization of individual differences must be suited to the developmental level of the person. Frequently, rules are designed to slow down or sustain the pace of an activity to compensate for the movement limitations of the participant. Such an example is tennis, which is one of the popular wheelchair sports. The rules and regulations of wheelchair tennis are the same as in regular tennis except that the player gets two bounces instead of one bounce before the play is called dead. The first bounce must be in the court, but the second bounce can land anywhere. The reason for the two bounces is that it makes drop shorts, or short balls, easier to hit and the game is more fun if players stay behind the baseline and rally the ball back and forth across the net.[1] Under such circumstances, as in wheelchair tennis, adaptations of the normal routine are often necessary to free the player from any imposed constraints.

There has been some controversy among professional recreators regarding the use of adapted devices in various situations and the ramifications of such as they relate to the person undergoing the recreational experience. Needless to say, certain considerations need to be determined before utilizing adapted devices for special population groups. In many situations, adapted devices are designed for the physically disabled to compensate or substitute for loss of muscle strength or function. However, certain situations may dictate the use of devices for other handicapping conditions, such as blindness, and severely or profoundly mentally retarded groups. In such situations, the objective, of course, is to assist in general motor control and independent functioning.

Cowart states that a program leader should think about adapting equipment when a participant is unable to initiate an activity independently with existing supplies.[2] In therapeutic recreation programs, especially when active treatment is taking place, emphasis should not be on the adapted device, but on the person and therapeutic/rehabilitation efforts built on its use. Obviously, for some individuals, achievement will be limited unless the device is used. It is necessary to remember, however, that the independent participation should be encouraged for some participants. This is based on the assumption that a normal outcome is the major goal. In such cases, elimination of the device is necessary to encourage progress in terms of measurable achievement without external support. An adapted device could be used the wrong way if no specific objectives are identified prior to introducing the device to a patient in a therapeutic program. Individual appraisal, including possible detrimental effects of using the device, must always be considered.

Another consideration is the person's attitude toward the adapted device. Not every individual will approve of using the device for independent functioning. Individual acceptance must be gained through the cooperative efforts of the program leader and the participant. The main concern is that the individual not feel self-conscious about using the device.

Some professionals involved in therapeutic recreation programs assume that adapted devices are "gadgets" or "gimmicks" and only benefit those who design, manufacture, or distribute them. Needless to say, a few so-called "therapeutic devices" are expensive and of questionable importance as recreational tools. It is immature, however, to say that devices are "gadgets." When studying factors that limit performance skills, the well-meaning designer has only one purpose in mind: to promote physical and psychologic mobility toward independence for the consumer. Others feel that devices distract from "normalcy" and only make disabled persons more dependent upon external support. This is not the case if proper judgment is used by the program leader prior to introducing the device. Each person should have the opportunity to develop and utilize his abilities and interests. As stated earlier, the use of adapted devices provides varied opportunities for involvement, thus creating more expanded use of activities. Physically disabled persons are encouraged to participate with their normal peers as much as possible. With this in mind, activities must be planned with possible adaptations that allow for this type of participation. Once a skill is refined, regardless of whether a device is used, certain desirable behaviors are frequently created, such as heightened self-esteem and cooperative social interaction.

Disabled persons have varied interests and different needs. Not all program leaders utilize the same principles, psychology, philosophy, and modalities in assisting the atypical individual to adjust to various situations. It is important, however, to determine the responses or changes that are desired as the result of the recreation experience. Frequently, to achieve this goal, the individual participating in the experience must master certain skills, either through independent functioning or with the aid of an adapted device that helps compensate for a handicap.

When we talk about normalization, the emphasis is frequently directed at combining non-disabled and disabled persons in group activities. This is not to imply that physical classification or homogeneous grouping is unimportant in discussing competitive sports. Direct involvement with persons with similar disabilities is a fair and direct approach to equalizing competition, as evidenced by the wheelchair sports movement in this country. However, this is not always possible in leisure or therapeutic recreation and physical education programs. For example, the imaginative program leader is often confronted with obstacles such as programming for one physically limited person and ten, or more, able-bodied individuals. Frequently, there is no way for the normalization process to take place unless rules are modified or adapted equipment is used. Personal satisfaction is gratifying when the disabled person feels a sense of belonging. Remember, each disabled individual must successfully meet challenges that lead to continued growth in self-identification. For some, the answer is competitive sports. For others, alternatives can only be developed through the leadership of a creative program leader. It is obvious that many individuals with physically limiting conditions would be unable to participate with their normal peers unless alternative measures were used to compensate for functional deficiencies.

SPORT PARTICIPATION GUIDELINES

Almost all sports can be adapted for persons with physical disabilities. The American Academy of Orthopedic Surgeons has developed a "participation possibility chart" which includes some of the major physical disabilities and major sporting activities. To clarify further, when "Individualized" is noted, it means, while the activity may be clearly inappropriate for some people with certain disabilities, it may well be possible for others in the same category. "Adapted" means that in almost all cases adaptation of equipment or rules will be necessary.

Obviously when assessing a patient and a sport there are numerous concerns to take into account as mentioned frequently in other sections of the book. The "participation possibility chart" (Table 7–1) will guide the reader in preparing for more detailed information on adapted sports later in the chapter.

PARTICIPATION POSSIBILITY CHART	Archery	Bicycling	Tricycling	Bowling	Canoeing/kayaking	Diving	Fencing	Field events*	Fishing	Golf	Horseback riding	Rifle shooting	Sailing	Scuba diving	Skating (roller & ice)	Skiing (downhill)	Skiing (cross-country)	Swimming	Table tennis	Tennis	Tennis (wheelchair)	Track	Track (wheelchair)	Weight lifting	Wheelchair poling	Baseball	Softball	Basketball	Basketball (wheelchair)	Football (tackle)	Football (touch)	Football (wheelchair)	Ice hockey	Sledge hockey	Soccer	Soccer (wheelchair)	Volleyball
AMPUTATIONS																																					
Upper Extremity	RA	R	R	R	RA	R	R	R	R	RA	R	RA	R	R	R	R	R	R	R	R	R		R		R	R	R	R		R	R		R		R		R
Lower Extremity (AK)	R	R	R	R	R	R	I		R	R	R	R	R	R	R	I	RA	RA	R	R	I	R		R	R	RA	RA		R	I	I	R			R	I	R	R
Lower Extremity (BK)	R	R	R	R	R	R	R	R	R	R	R	R	R	R	R	R	R	R	R	R	R	R		R	I	R	R	I	R	R	I	I	I		R	I	R
CEREBRAL PALSY																																					
Ambulatory	R	R	R	R	R	R	I		R	R	R	R	R	R	I	R	RA	RA	R	R	R		R		R	R	R	I		I	I		I		R		R
Wheelchair	R	I	I	R	R	I	I		I	R	I	I	R	R			I	R		R		R	R	R		I	I	R		R	I		R	I			
SPINAL CORD DISRUPTION																																					
Cervical	RA		RA	RA	IA			I	R	X	RA	R			IA	IA	R	RA		IA		R		I			I			I		I			I		IA
High-thoracic (T1–T5)	R		R	R	R		RA	R	R	RA	I	R	R	R		IA	IA	R	R		R		R	R	R	HA	HA		R		R		R		R	RA
Low thoracolumbar (T6–L3)	R		R	R	R		RA	R	R	RA	R	R	R	R		RA	RA	R	R		R		R	R	R	RA	RA		R		R		R		R	RA
Lumbosacral (L4 sacral)	R	R	R	R	R	R	R	R	R	R	R	R	R	R	R	I	R	R	R	R	R	R		R		R	R	R	I	I	R	I	I		R		R
NEUROMUSCULAR DISORDERS																																					
Muscular dystrophy	RA	I	R	R	I	I		R	R	R	I	RA	R	I	I	I	I	R	R	I	I	I	I		R	I	I	I	I		I	I	I	I	I	I	I
Spinal muscular atrophy	RA	I	R	R	I	I		R	R	R	I	RA	R	I	I	I	I	R	R	I	I	I	I		R	I	I	I	I		I	I	I	I	I	I	I
Charcot-Marie-Tooth	R	R	R	R	R	R	R	R	R	R	R	R	R	R	R	R	R	R	R	R	R	R		R		R	R	R		R	R		I		R		R
Ataxias	R	I	I	R	I	I		R	R	I	I	R	R	I	I	I	R	R	R	R	R	I	R	I	R	I	I	I	R		I	I	I	I	I	R	I
OTHERS																																					
Osteogenesis imperfecta	R	I	R	R	R	I	R	R	R	I	I	R	R	I	I	I	R	R	R	R	R	R	R	I	R	I	I	I	R	X	I	I	X	X	X	R	I
Arthrogryposis	R	I	I	R	R	I	I	R	R	I	R	R	R	I	I	I	R	R	R	R	R		R		I	R	R	R	X	R	I	I		I		R
Juvenile rheumatoid arthritis	RA	I	I	RA	R	I	I	I	R	I	I	R	R	I	I	I	R	R	I	I	I	I	I	I	I	I	I	I	I	I	I	I	I	I	I	I
Hemophilia	RA	R	R	R	R	R	R	R	R	R	R	R	R	R	R	I	R	R	R	R	I		R		I	I	R	R	X	I	X		I		R
Skeletal dysplasias	R	R	R	R	R	R	R	R	R	R	R	R	R	R	R	R	RA	R	R	R	R		R		I	R	R	R		I	R		R		R		R

*clubthrow, discus, javelin, shotput

R = Recommended
I = Individualized
A = Adapted
X = Not Recommended
Blank = No information or not applicable

TABLE TENNIS

The first known mention of a game resembling table tennis is a "miniature lawn tennis game" in a London catalog from 1884. It has been recorded that the first person to originate a game similar to our modern game was Charles Barter, who took out a British patent in 1891 for cork balls, clamp posts, and rectangular millboard rackets.[3] The game became popular in the United States in the late 1920s, and today it is recognized as one of our most popular indoor recreational activities.

Adapted for the Physically Disabled

Surface Table Tennis

Surface table tennis, an adapted version of the regular game, is played on a special table with paddles and a small ball. The object of the game is to hit the ball through an open space in the net so that it cannot be returned by the opponent. The game is won by the first player who scores 15 points, unless both players have scored 14 points, in which case the winner of the game is the first who scores 2 points in succession.

The modified game can be used in physical education and recreational programs for young children, the poorly coordinated, those with poor vision, and those with poor reactions. It can be a low-organization activity or serve as a preliminary to regular table tennis. Two or 4 people can play this modified version of the game by hitting a regulation table tennis ball so that it moves on the surface of the table instead of in the air as in regular table tennis (Fig. 7–1).

Equipment

The following equipment is necessary:
1. a regular table tennis paddle and ball can be used.

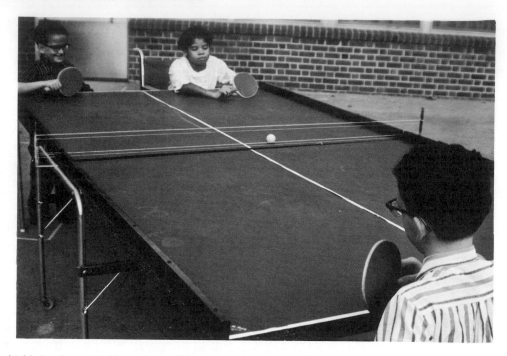

Fig. 7–1.   Adapted table tennis match. Note adapted net and side rails.

2. Table: a regular table can be used with wooden rails (1½ inches in height) attached to the sides.
3. Net: the adapted net should be made from string or cord, and attached to the standards with a 2″ opening in the middle (Fig. 7–1).

NOTE: Another alternative is to raise a regular net about 3 to 3½ inches from the playing surface to allow the passage of the ball under the net.

Techniques and Rules

The tennis grip is the recommended grip for beginners and is used by most players. The paddle is grasped with the thumb and forefinger on opposite sides of the blade, and the other fingers are placed around the handle.

Basic Strokes

1. Forehand (for right-handers): The forehand stroke should be used when the ball approaches the player's right. The paddle is brought to the right side of the body as it makes contact with the ball on the "thumb side" of the paddle.
2. Backhand (for right-handers): The backhand stroke is used when the ball comes toward the left side or the front of the body. The paddle is turned so that the "forefinger face" is used. The arm is held in front or crosses the body for this stroke.

   Left-handers use the forehand stroke for balls on their left side and the backhand for balls on their right.

Choice of Ends and Service. The choice of ends and the right to be server should be decided by a coin toss.

The Serve. The server should place the ball on the surface of the table. The ball should then be struck so that it rolls through the open space in the net to the opponent's court.

The following 4 rules apply to the serve:

1. If the player is severely disabled, the referee may place the ball on the playing surface in a favorable position for the player to hit the ball.
2. If a player misses the ball when attempting to serve, he is allowed to serve again.
3. Only one direct paddle hit is allowed to serve the ball through the open space in the net. If the server fails on his first attempt, his opponent becomes the server.
4. The serve changes hands after every dead ball and every point.

The Return. A ball, having been served or returned in play, should be struck so that it passes directly through the open space in the net and touches the opponent's court. Play continues even if the ball passes through the strands of cord in the upper and lower parts of the net.

Scoring. One point is made by a player if:

1. The ball is hit *over* the net by the opponent, either on the bounce or in the air.
2. The opponent hits the ball into the string on raised net, or not with enough force so that it fails to go into the opposite side of the court, either on the serve or return.
3. The opponent hits the ball twice in succession. Only one direct hit is allowed.
4. A player purposely makes no attempt to hit the ball.

Dead Ball. A stop or rest in the action occurs if:

1. The ball is hit by the server or receiver so that it goes over the side rail and off the table.

2. The ball is hit by the server or receiver but fails to roll on the playing surface as far as the net; that is, if the ball stops on the surface of the table between the player and net, a dead ball is called.

3. The ball is hit through the open space on a good service or good return, but the receiver is unable to reach the ball with his paddle because of his physical limitations.

4. The ball hits the receiver's hand, arm, or wheelchair without touching his paddle.

5. The ball splits or fractures during play.

Doubles. The surface of the table is divided into 2 equal parts by a white line ⅛ inch wide running parallel to the side lines (as on the table in Fig. 7–1). This allows doubles, or team, play.

Each team has both players stationed beside one another at one end of the table, and each player is responsible for his half of the court. At no time can a player hit a ball that is in his teammate's half of the court. If a player commits this violation, a point is scored for the opposing team. The teammates alternate the serve after dead balls and points.

All other rules and regulations for singles play apply to doubles play.

Assistive Devices

Many severely disabled individuals can play adapted or regular table tennis by using assistive devices.

Ball Bearing Feeder. This device (Fig. 7–2) provides assistance for shoulder and elbow motion by using gravity to substitute for a loss of power, supporting the weight of the arm so that even the weak muscles can move it, and reducing friction as the arm is moved.

Bi-handled Paddle. This special paddle (Fig. 7–3) is designed to assist players with upper-extremity involvement in making broader and freer movements with both hands while playing adapted table tennis. The paddle acts as an assistive device for increasing

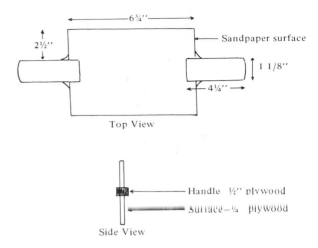

Fig. 7–3. Bi-handled paddle.

limited joint movements through proper positioning of the hand and fingers. The bi-handled paddle is not usually recommended for playing regular table tennis.

Adapted (Strap-on) Table Tennis Paddle. The regular table tennis paddle can be easily adapted for individuals who have no functional finger flexion or ability to grasp. The original adaptation was designed for a person with C-6 quadriplegia as a result of a traumatic spinal cord injury. This individual had the ability to strike, thereby using deltoid muscles to flex and abduct the shoulder, and biceps to control the positioning of the paddle. The strap-on paddle is used frequently in regular table tennis matches.

The device is attached to the back of the handle via Velcro straps. When securely fastened, the paddle enables the person to strike the ball with the backhand motion. Unfortunately, when the paddle is attached in this manner the person is unable to use a forehand motion.

The adaptation of the paddle is quite simple (Fig. 7–4). A webbed strap is securely attached (nailed or screwed) to the front portion of the handle. The strap must be long enough to go around the wrist. Velcro material is sewn into the strap in proper position to keep the paddle tight. The other strap is secured with two flathead screws, short enough not to penetrate completely through the blade of the paddle. The screws are placed approximately 3 inches apart, with additional strapping available to cross over the metacarpophalangeal joint. Velcro is also used on this strap to ensure adjustable but secure placement.

Table Tennis Cuff.* This device (Fig. 7–5) secures firmly to the hand with a clip that is attached to a metal clamp on the paddle. An overlapping velcro strap secures the cuff in a functional position. Another design feature is a wing nut that can be adjusted to maintain the paddle in any position. The device is

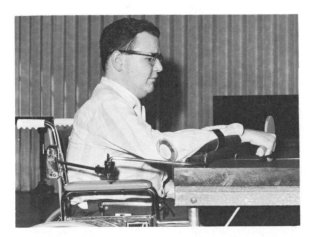

Fig. 7–2. Player with muscular dystrophy using the ball bearing feeder in a match.

*For further information, contact Maddox Inc., Pequannock, NJ 07440.

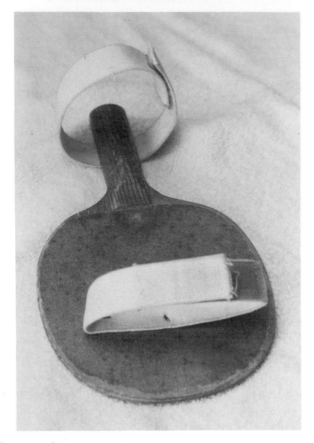

Fig. 7–4.   Strap-on paddle.

useful for any player who has limited finger movement and grip strength. It can be used in regular or surface table tennis.

Regular Table Tennis

Regular table tennis involves eye-hand coordination, good balance, and instinctive reactions. Many of the fundamentals are similar to the adapted version, but the player must respond more quickly to game situations, because the ball is constantly in flight. The sport can be adapted for almost everyone, including high-level quadriplegics who have no grip strength and even persons who have lost manipulative control of their fingers (Fig. 7–6). Game skills include accuracy for hitting the ball over, but close to, the net, putting English (spin) on the ball, and varying the game plan by using hard smashes, lob shots, and other strokes in order to keep the opponent off stride.

The game may be played by 2 or 4 people. A game is won by the first player to score 21 points unless both players have scored 20 points, in which case the winner of the game is the first player who wins 2 more points than his opponent.

Case History: J.L. was a normal and athletic young man until tragedy struck. While helping a neighbor with farming chores, he fell into a moving hay binder and suffered severe lacerations, partial amputation of his right forearm, complete amputation of his left arm (above the elbow), and complete amputation of his right leg (below the knee). Implantation surgery was performed on all three extremities at the University of Virginia Hospital. J.L. subsequently lost his entire right lower leg, however, both arms are healing properly.

After months of intensive surgery and hospitalization, J.L. was transferred to the Kluge Children's Rehabilitation Center for prosthetic fitting and rehabilitation. An important part of his life (sports and recreation) had been void during his hospitalization. Upon first approach, J.L. was hesitant to attempt any type of recreation. The functions J.L. was able to perform with his right arm included slight supination and pronation of forearm, flexion of the forearm, and abduction and flexion of the shoulder. He had no ability to use finger flexors or intrinsic muscles of the hand.

Initially, J.L. was able to participate in simple striking activities when an object was thrown in his range of movement. This was done with an adapted badminton racquet and a table tennis paddle (Fig. 7–6). Eventually, his ability to manipulate the racquets improved to a point at which he was able to participate in target games (e.g., target badminton). Eventually, he was able to participate in regular table tennis, badminton, miniature golf, riflery, bowling (with the use of an adapted-pusher), and billiards.

Wheelchair Table Tennis

Wheelchair table tennis is played according to rules of the United States Table Tennis Association with a few adaptations to accommodate the physically disabled participant. For example, in NWAA sanctioned play Class 1A, 1B and 1C players can tape or otherwise secure the racket to the hand (Fig. 7–7). In sanctioned USAAA events, only Class A1 competitors (bilateral above-knee amputees) are allowed to play from a wheelchair.

Because of poor finger and hand control, the 3 quadriplegic classes (1A, 1B, and 1C) are given special considerations for serving. First, they are not required to project the ball upward from the palm of the free hand. Second, the player has the option of holding the ball and projecting it upward in any manner, or he may bounce the ball on the table rather than project it upward. No spin is allowed on the ball during service.

Ajustments for Specific Disabilities

Amputations

Unilateral Upper-Extremity. Generally, the loss of one limb does not prevent a person from learning regular game skills. The player can use a regular paddle with the unaffected arm. He can also wear his prosthesis while playing to assist in the development of balance. One hand serving skills will need to be perfected, but most amputees can learn to execute the basic fundamentals with sufficient practice.

Bilateral Upper-Extremity. Loss of a functional paddle hand is a major problem. Some below-elbow amputees have experimented with bi-handled paddles modified to fit the terminal device of the prosthesis; however, this has been found too clumsy. It is better if a regular paddle is modified so that the amputee can control

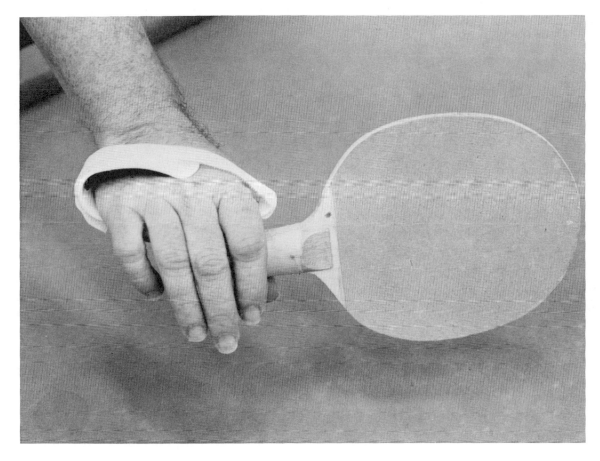

Fig. 7–5. Table tennis cuff.

the single handle with his terminal device, thus freeing the remaining artificial limb for balance.

Unilateral Lower-Extremity. After receiving their prosthesis, most unilateral lower-limb amputees can adjust to regular table tennis. In some situations, beginners have problems shifting their body weight when attempting to return a fast-moving ball hit to their involved side.

Bilateral Lower-Extremity. The major problem, the inability to shift body weight rapidly, is usually overcome with sufficient practice. Play from the upright position should be encouraged after the player feels comfortable wearing his artificial limbs.

Chronic Obstructive Lung Disease. Most individuals with chronic obstructive lung disease can participate in regular table tennis.

Blindness. Blind players have a distinct disadvantage; however, modifications can overcome their inability to see the ball. Surface table tennis is recommended. Totally blind players can use a bi-handled paddle held so the edge of the blade is resting on the surface of the table. The player should feel the top edge of the blade before each serve to make sure it is upright. The therapist, instructor, or referee can assist the blind player by giving a verbal signal as soon as the ball passes through the open space in the net.

The game should be played in a room that is free from noise and distraction.

Therapeutic Note: Auditory sensitivity skills can be developed. The blind player should learn to follow the path of the ball by following the sound it makes as it moves over the surface of the table.

Cardiovascular Disorders. Many persons with a cardiac disturbance can play the regular game of table tennis. However, the adapted version can be used to increase exercise tolerance and reduce fatigue thresholds for players who lack physical stamina. Energy consumption can be controlled in table tennis lending its importance to a low level training activity during cardiac rehabilitation.

Cerebral Palsy. Persons with cerebral palsy need slow and patient training if they are to attain purposeful motor movements. The instructor should teach the fundamental skills to each individual before putting him into game situations. Since the antagonistic muscle groups contract simultaneously with the protagonists, it is impossible for some spastic players to use the proper stroke in every situation and to control the forehand stroke motion. Adapted table tennis is usually not recommended for athetoid patients because of their purposeless contractions and marked inco-

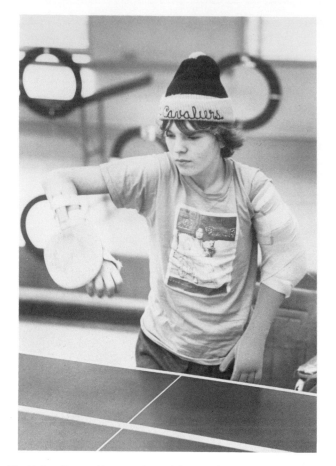

Fig. 7–6.   Competitive match participant using strap-on paddle.

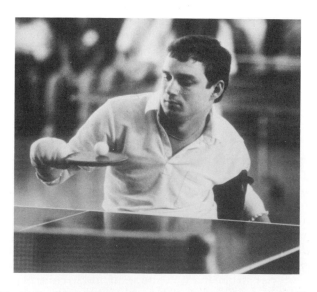

Fig. 7–7.   Quadriplegic using adapted serve during competitive match. (Courtesy of Paralyzed Veterans Administration, 801 18th Street, NW, Washington, DC 20006.)

ordination. The player with spastic diplegia can often learn to play the regular game.

Head Trauma. The ability to play will obviously depend upon the physical and mental status of the player. The adapted game is useful during the early recovery period for some players to facilitate making automatic motor responses to following and striking a moving object. With some players, processing skills can be challenged. Table tennis (regular or adapted) is a safe game which fosters the processing of basic input. Problem solving can be improved through judgment of using either a backhand or forehand stroke in game situations. Ball placement strategy is another important factor in improving motor planning skills.

Players with severe mobility problems can play the ball suspension game (refer to chapter on Low Organization Games).

Hemiplegia. Program adjustments for the hemiplegic depend upon the degree of involvement. The therapeutic values of using the bi-handled paddle are active exercise of the affected extremity, muscle re-education, prevention of contractures, and coordination exercise.

Many hemiplegics can play the regular game, and some recreational players prefer to bounce the ball on the table during service.

Hip Joint Disorders. The ability to play depends upon the treatment procedures prescribed by the orthopedic surgeon. Nonweight-bearing restrictions are recommended during a portion of the treatment period; thus, some players must play surface table tennis from a bed or stretcher.

Players using abduction appliances can play the adapted game from a standing position but will have difficulty shifting their body weight laterally to cover the designated playing area. In such cases, adapted or regular doubles play is more desirable than singles play. The player who is starting a gait-training program after surgical correction can support his body weight against the table with the aid of the nondominant upper limb. This relieves the affected lower extremity from bearing weight. Close supervision is required so weight is not shifted to the affected side.

Osteogenesis Imperfecta. The adapted or regular game can be used depending upon the physical capabilities of the player. Those using a wheelchair with reduced function in the playing arm and/or balance problems can play the adapted version, or in some cases play the regular game with some restriction in ability to cover the whole playing area. Many ambulatory players can play the regular game. Joint mobility will need to be assessed to assure that the player will be capable of reaching serves and engaging in rallies.

Overweight and Obesity. Vigorous physical activity is often part of a weight control program. Morbidly obese persons are not usually agile and cannot maneuver easily. Adapted table tennis is recommended for the poorly coordinated, because it can be played with a minimum amount of footwork in a small area. The adapted version should be used to lead up to regular table tennis.

Paraplegia. Beginners can play the adapted version as a lead up to regular table tennis. However, after sufficient practice, most paraplegics can compete in regular table tennis with their peers. Sufficient time will be needed to perfect the forehand stroke, and some players due to poor trunk mobility may not be able to cover large areas of the table. Players with lesions below T10 should learn to play with the brakes off, provided the wheelchair can be maneuvered by the free hand.[4]

Therapeutic Note: Trunk rotation and agility skills are influenced by the constant shifting of position in a wheelchair.

Progressive Muscular Disorders. The ability to play from a standing or sitting position depends on the stage of involvement. Players with moderate to severe muscle weakness will be required to play the adapted version. Use of a ball bearing feeder is useful for those with pronounced weakness in the shoulder girdle. Doubles play is often recommended especially for the wheelchairbound player who has limited arm control and range of motion. The ball suspension game is another alternative for the more severely involved player (refer to Low Organization Games chapter).

Quadriplegia. The adapted version can be used to learn the basic game techniques. Those with high cervical lesions cannot play because of their inability to control their upper extremities. Whenever possible, the regular game should be encouraged for players who have functional skills.

Various grip adaptations will be required for quadriplegics with midcervical lesions. These include wrist cuffs, special gloves, and various strapping techniques (Fig. 7–7). Poor sitting balance may be a problem, and if it occurs will limit the players in leaning over to control backhand strokes. Players without tricep muscles use outward rotation of the shoulders to play backhand shots. Quadriplegics may serve without upward projection of the ball. This can be done, for example, from back of the free hand or on the paddle. Some players have used a tenodesis splint to play, but it frequently tires the wrist extensors, and applies excessive pressure to the hands. In view of the adaptations, many quadriplegics can play regular table tennis with a high degree of success.

Rheumatoid Arthritis. Most players can compete in regular table tennis. Enlargement of the interphalangeal joints may prevent the player from securing a firm handle grip. To compensate, experimentation with various adapted paddles may be necessary for competition in either the regular or adapted games.

Therapeutic Note. The bi-handled paddle may be recommended for players needing active extension exercise of both hands and arms. Similarly, during active treatment, hand splints may be used to align the involved fingers in a rigid, but more extended position.

Allowance is usually made to remove the splints during game situations.

Abnormal Posture. Regular table tennis is encouraged for this group. Wearing of a spinal orthosis should not impede the learning of game skills. Postspinal fusion patients may need to alternate standing and sitting time depending upon their tolerance level.

Undernutrition. In most cases, this group should be able to play regular table tennis. The therapist or instructor may need to control the intensity of the game situation to overcome effects of reduced stamina and or emotional lability.

AIR RIFLERY

The history of the air gun parallels that of firearms, as it started back in prehistory with the blowing of pebbles through hollow reeds with enough force to stun or kill game. Historic evidence of the air gun dates from the fifteenth century, when the principle of using air or gas to drive a ball or pellet was applied. Air guns were made in one form or another in Europe as early as 1600 and in the United States around the mid-1880s. The Daisy, one of the best known of the spring-and-plunger air guns, was developed in 1888. In 1890, a break type of cocking device was introduced. About 1913, another design, which was adapted from the slide, or trombone, cocking action in use on shotguns at that time, became known as the "pump gun."

There are 3 basic types of air guns: spring, pneumatic, and gas (CO_2).

In a spring air gun, a spring is compressed when the rifle is cocked. A plunger compresses air through the barrel when the trigger is squeezed, and the air activates the projectile toward the target. The velocity of the projectile is always the same.

In a pneumatic air rifle, a pump builds up air pressure in a reservoir. Air is released when the trigger is squeezed, and this drives the projectile out of the barrel toward the target. Unlike the spring-type air rifle, the amount of compressed air is determined by the number of pumps, and the velocity of the projectile can be changed.

A gas (CO_2) rifle uses liquid gas which is stored in a tiny metal bottle. When the bottle is placed in the rifle, the seal is punctured; this lets the liquid turn to a gas. A quantity of gas is released into the bore after every trigger squeeze, and the released gas activates the projectile toward the target. Recharging is generally required after 30 to 60 shots.

Modern air guns vary greatly in velocity, which in turn determines injury risk. A velocity of 180 ft./second can penetrate the eye, and an impact velocity of 370 ft./s. can penetrate skin and bone[5] (note Fig. 7–8).

Adapted for the Physically Disabled

The first formal shooting therapy for the physically disabled was introduced at Gillette State Hospital, St.

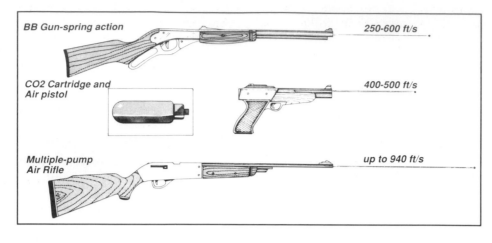

Fig. 7–8. Pictured above are the three types of air-guns including velocity range. (Courtesy of For Kids' Sake publication, Box 484 Medical Center University of VA, Charlottesville, VA 22908.)

Paul, Minnesota, in 1954. The original site was a .22 rimfire-based 50-foot range, formed and endowed by American Legion Post #5 of St. Paul. Daisy spring and piston-powered air rifles were chosen for use, because they pose less hazard to beginning shooters; they have a low but consistent power from shot to shot; and it is as difficult for the marksman to achieve a perfect score on the 15-foot range with an air rifle as on the 50-foot range with .22 Short rimfires.[6]

The National Rifle Association (NRA) has actively supported air riflery as a therapeutic activity. Various research applications have focused on the therapeutic implications of the sport for physical restoration and rehabilitation. Competitive shooting is gaining in popularity. The USCPAA has 10 meter events in Target Special BB gun or .177 (4.5mm) rifle. Shooters are grouped according to functional ability in 8 different classes. No assistance is permitted in the physical aiming of the rifle, other than the mounting onto a tripod or similar device and loading the firearm. The NWAA sanctions air gun competition for spinal cord injured shooters. The competition is comprised of three positions; prone, kneeling, and standing. The position names are actually in respect to the placement of the elbows or arms. In the standing position, arms and legs cannot be touching any support, such as a shooting table. The prone position requires that both elbows be resting on a table or support board. Only one elbow is allowed in the kneeling position. Quadriplegics, however, are allowed a support stand for the rifle barrel in all three positions.

Precision Air Riflery

Precision air riflery is becoming a popular target shooting sport for the physically disabled. In contrast to BB gun shooting, a .177 caliber pellet air gun is more efficient and more reliable. Unquestionably good performance is the result of a detailed and complex engineering design that offers the utmost in shooting accuracy. All of the precision air rifles de-

velop power from a single cocking stroke of the barrel or a sidelever system as seen in the Feinwerkbau model. As for accuracy, many models could consistently hit a pin head at 33 feet.

Most precision air rifles weigh between 6 and 7 pounds. The weight of the rifle can be a problem for some shooters, but this can be compensated for in most cases by using barrel rests (tripods or shooting tables). However, because of the gun's construction, there is no recoil and the internal mainspring system fires silently. Another positive feature is the light trigger action. This is especially important for shooters with limited use of the trigger hand. Quadriplegics with no finger flexion movements have become superb shooters by using pencils attached to the hand to substitute for loss of a trigger finger.

NRA sanctioned .177 caliber air rifle or pistol matches can only be conducted at 33 feet (10 meters). .177 caliber air rifles are grouped into 4 categories (economy, intermediate all-purpose arms, sporters, and match). Differences are especially related to degree of refinement and suitability of need. Obviously, cost depends upon the degree of technical perfection and workmanship. Further information regarding source lists can be obtained from local gun shops, sporting goods dealers, or by writing to the NRA.

Equipment

The equipment and materials for air riflery are relatively simple and inexpensive:
1. Air rifles: with lever cocking actions (Daisy model 499 is recommended).* There should be at least one rifle for every 3 students in the group.
2. BBs: These are available in case quantities.
3. Targets: official National Rifle Association 15-foot targets.
4. Range: A 15-foot range with a safe backstop makes both indoor and outdoor shooting pos-

*Daisy Manufacturing Co., Inc., Rogers, Arkansas 72757-0220.

sible. The backstop may be made from cardboard boxes, 12 inches or more in depth, with at least 2 square feet of front surface, to serve as a backstop, target holder and BB trap.

Training

Jaycee Shooting Education Program
The Daisy Manufacturing Company, Inc. with the help of the United States Jaycees and many other organizations, has taught gun safety and shooting fundamentals to millions of youngsters in the last 20 years. Today more than 2,000 Jaycee chapters conduct Daisy-sponsored shooting education programs.

While the youngsters learn gun safety in the Daisy/ Jaycees programs, they also enter into the arena of international competition. Participating Jaycee chapters sponsor teams of five of their best shooters, and those teams compete for statewide championships. The state champions then compete against other state champions, as well as some foreign teams, in the annual Daisy/U.S. Jaycees International BB Gun Championship Match (Fig. 7–9).

How to Shoot
Ambulatory Shooters. In aiming properly, correct alignment of the sights is the first requirement. The second is to keep the rifle from tipping right or left (called "canting"). The rifle should be held firmly (not rigidly) at the grip with just enough pressure to stabilize the butt of the stock against the shoulder. The opposite hand should hold the rifle even more gently;

it merely steadies the aim and aids in swinging the rifle right or left, up or down. The cheek should rest against the stock for steadiness, in such a position that the eye comes naturally and consistently into the correct line of aim. The thumb should be across the top of the grip to gain better control without tautness. This type of hold will also help trigger squeeze.

When the sights are closely aligned with the target, place the forefinger on the trigger. (Either the first or second joint may be used, depending on which is more comfortable; however, the first joint is generally preferred and recommended.) Just before commencing the squeeze off, take a deep breath, let out about half of it, and do not breathe against while pinpointing aim and squeezing the trigger. Squeeze slowly.

Wheelchair-User Shooters. Shooters in wheelchairs can shoot either facing the target directly or on a 45-degree angle. Usually a participant will shoot facing the target when a lapboard tripod or table is used as an assist.

Shooting Positions
Air riflery is one of the few sports that offers alternative body positions that can compensate for functional limitations. The following illustrations point out various adapted shooting positions and compare them to approved normal shooting positions.

The directions below are for a right-handed shooter; a left-hander should reverse the directions.

Prone Position. The body is at an angle of 45 degrees with the line of aim; the spine is straight; the

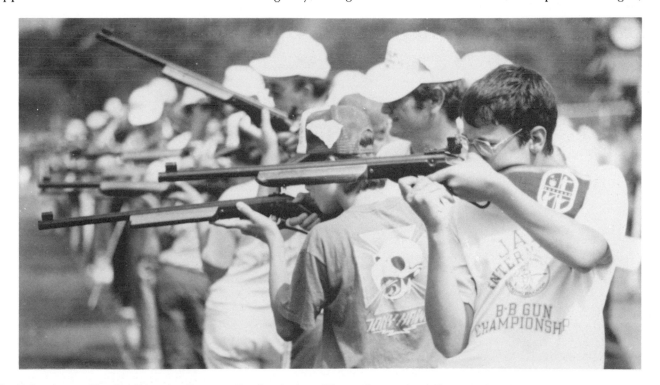

Fig. 7–9. Jaycee Shooting Education Program. Drawing the best BB gun shooters from all across America and England, the Daisy/U.S. Jaycees International BB Gun Championship Match tests the 8- through 14-year-old competitors' marksmanship abilities.

legs are well spread; and the insides of both feet are as nearly flat on the ground as possible without strain. Both elbows are well under the body. The rifle is not gripped tightly, and the entire body remains relaxed. This position can also be assumed on a bed. The prone position is the one most frequently used because it is the steadiest of all shooting positions and affords the greatest accuracy in firing.

Patients confined to litters for postoperative managment or for treatment of decubitus ulcers can generally shoot comfortably from the prone position, provided that the weight of the gun is not overwhelming (Fig. 7–10). Marksmen limited by lower-extremity bracing, but who have good upper-extremity strength can assume a prone position to overcome limitations imposed by poor standing balance and tolerance.

Sitting Position. The marksman sits half-faced to the right; feet are well apart and well braced on the heels, which are dug slightly into the ground; body leans forward; both arms rest inside the legs and are well braced. Wheelchair shooters can use the lapboard aid or tripod assist in this position.

Depending upon the strength of the wheelchair marksman, the placement of the chair can be at a 90-degree angle with the target. Marksmen with involvement of the upper extremities can use a lapboard or tripod while facing the target. Patients who are confined to a bed but have medical permission to sit can use an overbed table for support (Fig. 7–11).

Kneeling Position. The marksman kneels on the right knee, half-faced to the right, and sits on the right heel; the left knee is bent so that the left lower leg is vertical; the left arm is well under the rifle and rests on the left knee with the point of the elbow beyond the kneecap; the right elbow is approximately at the

height of the shoulder. Sitting on the side of the foot instead of the heel is permissible.

The physically disabled marksman who is unable to assume a kneeling position often has to rely on a sitting position with a backrest to compensate for poor balance and/or involvement of the lower extremities. The elbow of the arm supporting the gun rests on the knee or leg (Fig. 7–12).

Standing Position. The marksman stands half-faced to the right, with his feet between 1 and 2 feet apart; the body is erect and well balanced; the left elbow is well under the rifle; the rifle rests on the palm of the left hand which grasps the rifle in front of the point of balance; the butt of the gun is held high and firm against the right shoulder. The right elbow should be at about the same height as the shoulder.

Functional limitations prohibit some physically disabled marksmen from shooting from standing positions without some kind of support. To compensate, a tripod system or similar device can be used as a reliable support system (Fig. 7–13). Another method by which a wheelchair-bound shooter can simulate a standing position is by shooting from the chair while restricting both of the upper extremities from touching a support system, including the arm rests of the wheelchair.

Range Procedures

Only when the instructor is sure that the shooters know how the air gun functions should he take them onto the range to learn shooting skills. The younger they are, the longer it will take them to accustom themselves to handling guns. To instruct students:
1. Lay out air guns, one for each firing position, with the muzzle facing backstops.

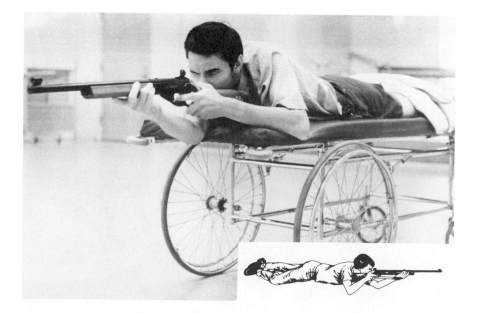

Fig. 7–10.   Marksman who had reconstructive surgery of his ankles shooting a Daisy Model 99 BB gun from the prone position on a litter. Illustration of normal prone shooting position courtesy of the National Rifle Association, 1600 Rhode Island Ave. NW, Washington, DC 20036.

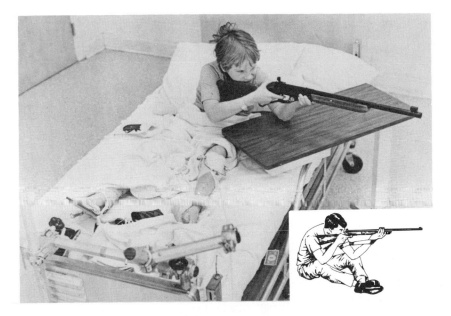

Fig. 7–11. Preoperative patient confined to traction participating in air-riflery from sitting position. Illustration of normal sitting shooting position courtesy of the National Rifle Association, 1600 Rhode Island Ave. NW, Washington, DC 20036.

2. Attach targets, which can be identified by shooter's name, to face of backstops.

After shooters take their positions on the firing line, firing commands are as follows:

1. At the command, "Ready on right, ready on left," shooters call out if not ready.
2. At the command, "Cock the gun," shooter picks up gun, hands it to coach to cock or in some cases cocks his own gun.
3. At the command, "Ready on the firing line," shooter places gun in shooting position.
4. At the command, "Commence firing," shooter fires one round at target and then places gun on the floor. This procedure will be continued until 5 rounds have been completed.
5. At the command, "Cease firing," everyone stops immediately and presses safety button.

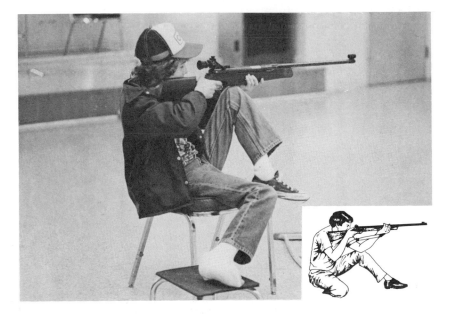

Fig. 7–12. A 15-year-old boy whose diagnosis is Charcot-Marie-Tooth disease (progressive peroneal muscular atrophy) using sitting position with back and knee rests to maintain functional sight alignment with Model 300 Feinwerkbau air rifle. As a recent postoperative patient, he had to elevate the affected limb to eliminate any problems related to weight bearing on the recently applied cast. Illustration of normal kneeling shooting position courtesy of the National Rifle Association, 1600 Rhode Island Ave. NW, Washington, DC 20036.

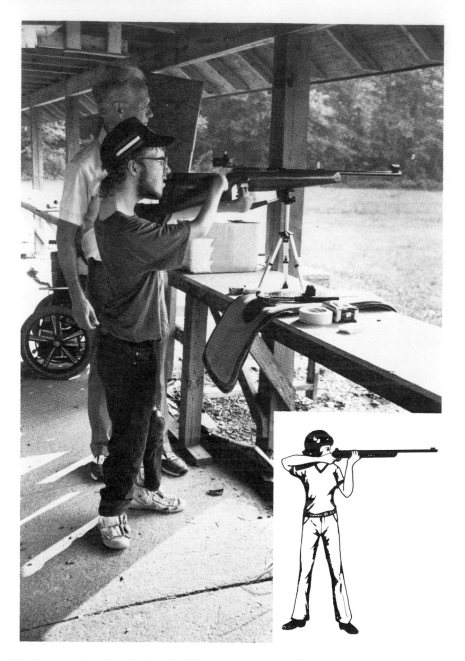

Fig. 7–13. Marksman with arthrogryposis using tripod assist. Illustration of normal shooting position courtesy of the National Rifle Association, 1600 Rhode Island Ave. NW, Washington, DC 20036.

When the sitting, kneeling, or standing position is used, the shooter will hold the gun with the stock resting on the floor until the command to cock is announced

Program Note: In a section pertaining to physically handicapped shooters, the Official Rulebook of the Daisy/U.S. Jaycee State and International BB Gun Matches, Section 4.5 indicates the following:

4.5 Physically Handicapped Shooters—A shooter who because of physical handicap cannot fire from one or more of the prescribed shooting positions outlined in these Rules, or who must use special equipment when firing, is privileged to petition the Protest Committee for permission to assume a special position or to use modified equipment or both. This petition will be in the form of a written request from the person concerned to the Committee outlining in detail the reasons why the special position must be assumed or the special equipment must be used. The petition will be accompanied by pictures of the shooter in the position he desires approved and, if special equipment is required, the picture will show how this equipment is used. The petition and all pictures must be furnished in exact duplicate. The petition must be accompanied by a doctor's statement if the physical handicap is not completely evident in the pictures submitted.

The rulebook contains more information regarding Protest Committee details, and the reader is referred to it for further information.

Assistive Devices

Lapboard. A lapboard attaches to the wheelchair with strips of velcro or mounting brackets. The lapboard is a support system to rest one or both elbows for stability. Some shooters use their lapboard to mount a spotting scope and for placement of their ammunition. One concern for the shooter is that the lapboard can be unsettling and possibly move if not tightly secured to the wheelchair.

W/C SR-77 Shooting Rest.* The Rest is designed for high level quadriplegics who have limited or no functional use of their arms. The rifle stock has to be shortened and once mounted, it is operated by two 12 volt DC motors, and uses the wheelchair's batteries for support. A joystick is used to control the motors, which moves the Rest left and right or up and down. Once on target, a sip on the vacuum tube will fire the rifle. The joystick can be chin or hand operated, depending on the ability of the user. No firearm larger than a 6MM should be used on the Rest, and it should be an automatic for less recoil.

Forearm Adapter.† The original design was for an amputee equipped with a GRIP Terminal Device. The device is designed to substitute for a loss of a grip hand and is especially useful to B/E amputees (Fig. 7–14). It is constructed of aluminum and ABS plastic to custom mount to the shotgun forearm. The aircraft aluminum provides the needed structural support, while the plastic provides the proper curvatures for mounting to the forearm and for the pistol grip itself. Similar modifications can be made by consulting a local gunsmith.

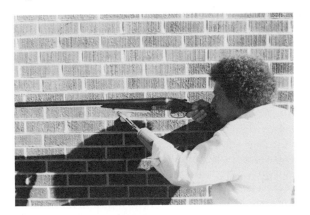

Fig. 7–14. Amputee Forearm Adapter. (Courtesy of Therapeutic Recreation Systems.)

---

*For further information write to R.W. Bowen, SR-77 Enterprises, 363 Maple St., Chadron, NE 69337.

†For further information write to Therapeutic Recreation Systems, 1280 28th St., Suite 3, Boulder, CO 80303

Hand Substitutes (Hooks). Various plastic hook devices can be used to substitute for the loss of a trigger finger or grip hand. Most are designed so the hook is affixed to the palm of the hand with a restraining strap that encircles the wrist. Hook devices are primarily used with quadriplegics who have wrist extension and good elbow flexion (C-6 and C-7). With this consideration, the shooter is completely capable of mastering an independent trigger pull.

Shoulder Harness with Butt Placement Attachment. The harness was originally designed for a C5 quadriplegic who had difficulty stabilizing the butt of the rifle against his shoulder during target shooting (Fig. 7–15A and B). The system works well for shooters who lack arm strength and functional ability to control the alignment of the rifle. A leather harness has a butt attachment secured to the chest plate with rivets. The lower part of the harness is designed like a belt system, and customized to fit the user. The side flap has velcro straps attached with rivets which stabilizes the stock to the harness. Consult a leather or saddle dealer for similar modifications.

Tripod. The tripod assist enables the shooter with upper-limb involvement (cerebral palsy, progressive muscle disorders, etc.) to participate in target shooting (Fig. 7–13). An adjustable camera tripod can be modified by securing a U-shaped barrel holder for stable placement of the rifle. Another concept is to drill holes in the forearm to insert the U-section. This provides more of a challenge because the shooter has some margin of error to overcome when aiming because there is no rigid support system for the barrel.

Various compact shooting scopes have been modified for use as tripod holders. By removing the scope and adding a barrel mount or similar stabilizer, the shooter has an ideal support system. The compact tripod is best utilized when placed on a shooting table or when shooting from the prone position.

Adjustments for Specific Disabilities

Amputations

Unilateral Upper-Extremity. Prior to receiving his prosthesis, a below-elbow amputee is encouraged to use the residual limb to balance the gun barrel when shooting from the standing position. The terminal device is not a good substitute for the missing grip hand; however, it is conceivable that certain modifications could be made to the forearm of the gun to accommodate the hook fingers. If the shooter intends to use the terminal device as a substitute for the missing trigger finger, then it is recommended that he shoot from the kneeling position. This position braces the left elbow (of right-handers) and keeps the gun reasonably steady. The unaffected grip hand can be used to push the butt of the stock securely against the shoulder.

The amputee can also shoot from other positions depending upon the ability to achieve a stable sight picture. Some unilateral A/E amputees use other

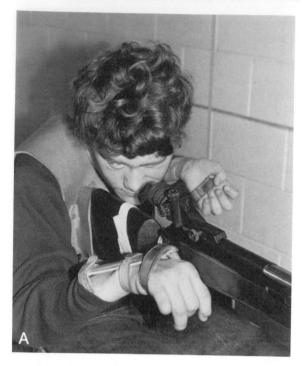

Fig. 7–15. *A*, Shoulder harness system for stabilization of rifle butt. Note velcro straps which secure rifle into sleeve. *B*, Shoulder harness with butt placement sleeve.

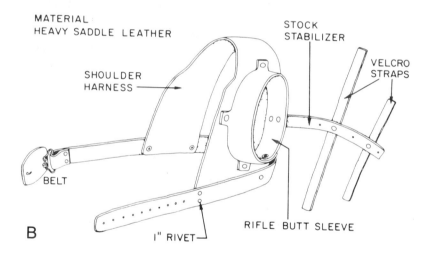

modifications (shortened barrel and stock) to lighten and balance the firearm.

NOTE: Some amputees feel that a prosthesis is a detriment in shooting sports. The reason is that a prosthesis lacks the sensory feedback as in a normal extremity which affects weight distribution, feel, and sense of controlling the firearm.

Bilateral Upper-Extremity. This group needs considerable assistance because of their inability to control the movement of the gun. The tripod assistive device will usually be needed to brace the barrel of the gun while the amputee pulls the trigger with his terminal device. A shoulder harness system may be useful in some cases. No standard pattern of shooting has been designed for this group, because an individual style should be worked out to take full advantage of the remaining potential of the particular patient.

Unilateral Lower-Extremity. The recent lower-extremity amputee can shoot from the prone position, but the standing position is encouraged once the prosthesis is fitted because it helps the shooter to develop stationary balance skills. Major problems usually are not encountered after the amputee learns to distribute his weight evenly. The B/K amputee who wears a prosthesis should be able to assume the four traditional shooting positions without difficulty.

Bilateral Lower-Extremity. The loss of both lower limbs does not interfere with learning target shooting skills. Many amputees prefer not to wear their prosthesis and shoot from a wheelchair or prone position.

Chronic Obstructive Lung Disease. Riflery is beneficial to this group because it develops the breath control needed for holding the gun in firing position and pulling the trigger. The sport has been used as a means of relaxation and as a prescription for safe exercise conditioning.

Therapeutic Note: Individuals with chronic lung disease are often shallow breathers, and the ability to use the diaphragm to control breathing (as in the partial breath exhalation prior to the trigger squeeze motion) can improve conscious breathing habits.

Blindness. Air riflery is unsuitable for the totally blind unless a sighted assistant aids the shooter by sighting the target (preferably tin cans); however, the partially sighted can use telescope sights to magnify the target. Any shooting position can be used, but the prone is popular.

Cardiovascular Disorders. Air riflery is a low intensity activity which can be used to prevent the clinical complications of inactivity. Also, since target shooting is performed from a static position requiring little body movement, the sport can make a significant contribution at the beginning of an exercise program for hospitalized patients. The choice of shooting position often depends upon the physical condition of the individual. The work capacity of the patient can be increased by graduating him from a prone or sitting position to a standing position.

Cerebral Palsy. Most persons with cerebral palsy can learn to shoot a BB gun with some degree of accuracy. Depending upon the type and severity of the condition, modifications can be made in shooting techniques, and the tripod assistive device can be used. For some shooters, the assistant will need to sight the target and aid these patients in holding the stock of the gun steady. Competition must be controlled, and the activity discontinued upon any signs of frustration. The cerebral palsied constitute a large percentage of shooters in air rifle programs, so the instructor should be aware of the two basic problems which are characteristic of these shooters:

1. Many shooters, including those with mild spasticity, have a natural tendency to close their eyes prior to the trigger squeeze.
2. Most beginners are unable to relax during the trigger squeeze motion. This causes "flinching," which means the shooter jerks the trigger and braces against the kick.

Some shooters will have problems holding a static sitting position, especially those limited by athetosis. In some cases, on an experimental basis, the rifle could be locked to a rigid mounting system. Even with this type of adaption, shooting sports should not be recommended if there are noticeable severe deviations in postural control, balance, and stability. Head control is another issue of concern. The shooter with spastic diplegia is usually not affected and is able to maintain a consistent sight picture. However, shooters with spastic quadriparesis often have difficulty and demonstrate body alignment problems. If good head control is unattainable for independent sight alignment, then target shooting should not be recommended.

Head Trauma. Air riflery as a clinical sport should not be recommended if the post-trauma patient has significant residual problems with memory and personal social adjustment. However, once the patient reacts consistently to stimuli, the cognitive demands (following safety rules and range commands, altering sight picture to improve consistency of grouping shots, etc.) may encourage expression to situational demands. This would obviously relate to the patient who demonstrates good directed behavior (Rancho Level 6–8).

Adapted equipment may be needed, but most often used with shooters who have residual effects of right- or left-side involvement (refer to section on Hemiplegia).

Hemiplegia. The loss of a grip hand will cause problems. Some hemiplegics will have a disturbance of hand sensation, and many will have only slight shoulder motion, but essentially no functional limb. To compensate, in rifle target shooting, it may be necessary to insert the forearm or barrel in a support system (tripod or similar device). Success has been reported with the Thompson Center Carbine using the Choote pistol grip buttstock. It is lightweight, well-balanced and perfect for "one handed" shooting.* Various calibers are available, depending upon choice. Some customized adaptations have been designed to allow for one armed control. The marksman may prefer to use a pistol, because it is essentially a one-arm shooting sport.

The hemiplegic who is interested in recreational target shooting is generally comfortable using the sitting position (wheelchair or straightback chair). However, due to the degree of involvement, concerns for proper posture particularly shoulder and symmetrical alignment are important factors to consider. Also, pronation of the hand is often a natural position, for hemiplegics supination of the hand is difficult to assume. As already noted, this causes problems with the loss of a grip hand. In addition, to eliminate sagging of the shoulder it may be necessary to elevate the nonfunctioning upper-limb on a table when shooting with the aid of a mounting system. When standing, some hemiplegics prefer to support their motionless arm in a sling. Standing balance skills will vary depending upon degree of involvement. For this reason it might not be practical to use the standing position when shooters demonstrate severe knee flexion deformities.

Therapeutic Note: The tripod should not be used as a standard piece of equipment. With some shooters in rehabilitation programs if the involved upper limb is used in active exercise, then the primary goals are

---

*Write to Stuart's Sports Specialties, 7081 Chad St., Anchorage, AL 99518 for further information.

to stretch muscle contractures and increase limited joint movement without assistive devices.

Hip Joint Disorders. Treatment often includes reduced activity and weight-bearing restrictions on the affected hip for a portion of the rehabilitation period. For the bedridden patient, the sitting or prone shooting positions can be used. The wheelchair-bound shooter should not encounter any major problems when adjusting to the sport.

The prone position is recommended for shooters wearing abduction appliances and for those who had recent surgical correction. Precision of movement through concentration is best established when the shooter is placed in a position that will not affect his equilibrium. Another advantage of the prone position is that it reduces muscular tension, enhances relaxation, and increases awareness of the proper positioning of the upper limbs.

Osteogenesis Imperfecta. Wheelchair shooters will generally need a rigid support system to rest the rifle. To compensate for limitations in arm extension and strength, shooters often prefer to shorten the stock and/or use various barrel mounts. Some shooters with short stature place the butt over the shoulder while turning the entire rifle counter-clockwise until a sight picture is achieved. Ambulatory shooters will need to be assessed on an individual basis to determine the most effective shooting position based on functional ability.

Overweight and Obesity. No special adaptations are needed for this group. Faulty distribution of weight does cause clumsiness, particularly if the shooter has large deposits of adipose tissue in the upper arm which interfere with positioning of the gun stock.

Paraplegia. Air riflery for the wheelchair-bound paraplegic can be used to increase muscle strength, sitting balance, and endurance, because several muscles are used when aiming the gun. The slow lifting motion used to bring the gun to the shoulder exercises the muscles of both arms and shoulders. To assist with balance, many high level paraplegics prefer to rest one or both elbows on a support system.

Athletes involved in competitive shooting will need a similar lapboard system to participate in kneeling (one elbow rest) or prone (two elbow rest) firing position from a wheelchair.

Assistive devices should be kept to a minimum, because feelings of inferiority are more frequent if the paraplegic relies on them to aid upper-extremity movements. Weakened muscles must not, however, be overused; in some situations, the wheelchair lapboard must be used to assist the shooter in making coordinated movements.

Progressive Muscular Disorders. This group usually needs assistance when participating in air riflery. Development of shooting skills will depend upon the degree of muscle involvement. Patients in the advanced stages of muscular dystrophy will have trouble mastering the trigger squeeze motion, and as a result, the instructor will need to assist them.

Those who ambulate with aid of long leg braces may participate from the standing position, but the shooter should support his elbows on a shooting table.

Note of Caution: The severely involved have poor trunk balance. In such cases, the shooter is at a disadvantage, since his shooting posture is affected. Watch for signs of early fatigue. Various support systems (arm suspension slings, barrel mounts, etc.) may be required to compensate for generalized muscle weakness.

Quadriplegia. The degree of motor functioning will influence the ease and speed with which independence can be achieved from the sitting position. C2, C3, and C4 shooters will need to use a chin, mouth, or breath control device to operate a cable or pressure switch, or similar system to activate the trigger. Once equipment is applied, the shooter will need an assistant to load and unload the firearm. C5, C6, and some C7 shooters (varies in individual cases) will need lightweight hook systems to act as a trigger finger. A pencil inserted into a cock-up splint is another alternative. Barrel mounts will be needed to support the weight of the forearm, and various harness systems can be used to position the rifle butt. Independent trigger squeeze motion is generally present in C6 and C7 shooters. As a rule, the wheelchairbound shooter will be able to fully utilize his remaining power by facing directly at the target.

In competitive NWAA events, the quadriplegic is allowed a support stand for the rifle barrel in all three positions.

Rheumatoid Arthritis. The degree of joint involvement determines which shooting position is best suited for the patient. Air riflery can provide digital exercises by requiring movement of the fingers through various ranges of motion and with differing degrees of intensity. The various movements associated with gun handling can also provide joint and muscle-stretching exercises.

Hand grip strength and finger action control needs to be evaluated before enlisting the person with arthritis in a shooting program. Adapted equipment may be needed to avoid joint stress.

Abnormal Posture. The principles of treatment for structural scoliosis are directed at straightening the spine and stabilizing it in the corrected position. Air riflery is easily adaptable to patients using corrective casts and braces. Patients wearing Milwaukee braces or orthoplast jackets have considerably more freedom of movement. The sitting and standing positions are recommended for this group.

Undernutrition. Participation depends upon the strength and endurance of the shooter. Air riflery can be used in general conditioning programs in hospitals to increase the patient's tolerance for upright activities, and to prevent psychologic consequences of inactivity. Naturally, participation is contraindicated in cases of undernutrition so severe that wasted muscles are strained by bearing the weight of the gun.

ANGLING

Fishing has been referred to in the literature and portrayed in the art of every civilization. Four-thousand-year-old Egyptian art depicts figures fishing with a rod and line, with a hand line, and with a net. There are references to fishing in ancient Greek, Roman, Hebrew, and Chinese writings. In the twentieth century, sport fishing, or angling, came to mean fishing with a rod, reel, line, and hook. It is still a growing sport, particularly in industrialized countries, and it is practiced with pleasure in many nations.

The skills used in angling are casting and fishing. In teaching casting skills, emphasis is given to learning the easy fundamentals and to the continued use of the activity as a leisure-time recreational sport. Competitive games such as skish (a casting game) and tournament casting offer opportunities to create more interest and cooperation.

Adapted for the Physically Disabled

Today, whether it's trout fishing at a small Colorado stream, dock fishing at a mountain lake in Maine, or surf fishing off the Outer Banks in North Carolina there is a place for the mobility impaired angler. Typically individualistic and adventuresome, the sport of fishing is easily adaptable to most disabled sportsmen. Sometimes finding a "nibble" seems like a lifetime, but just being outside in a quiet and natural environment provides a relaxing, sometimes non-intrusive peace of mind. Disabled fishing tournaments are now becoming popular and there is speculation that a national circuit could become a reality in the near future. One of the premier tournaments is the Bass Tournament for the Physically Disabled in Texas. In 1988 the tournament featured fishing from Kayaks with more than 80 participants.

Although not widely used in clinical recreation or public school physical education classes, angling can provide therapy as well as fun in special classes for physically disabled patients/students. An important feature of the sport is that it can be practiced either indoors or outdoors.

Indoor or outdoor swimming pools are excellent places for instruction and practice in casting. Angling can be challenging and satisfying, particularly to the disabled person who is unable to take part in strenuous sports.

Equipment

A beginning program should have enough equipment to serve at least three persons. The size of the class can be doubled by assigning two persons to each set of equipment. When one is casting, the other acts as coach; the "coach" also learns by pointing out the mistakes of the caster. Formal lectures should be kept to a minimum, with practice sessions occupying most of the time.

The basic equipment for one individual includes rod, reel, line, and practice plug.

1. Rod: The fishing rod must be tough and must bend easily without breaking. All rods are thick at the handle and taper to a slender tip, but they vary in length, weight, material, and style. The bait-casting rod is between 3½ and 6 feet long, and the fly rod is usually between 6 and 9 feet. Graphite rods are recommended because they require little care, yet are strong and flexible.
2. Reel: A reel is a spool that is turned by a crank and attached to the handle of the rod. By means of a reel, a long line can be cast out or played out to a running fish. The spincast reel is most popular with beginners.
3. Line: Lines are usually made of nylon or silk. For spinning, a special kind of casting, the nylon is often a single strand, called *monofilament*. Lines are made to bear a certain weight; this weight is called the line's *test strength*. The test strength chosen depends on the kind of fish to be caught, the type of lure, and the nature of the water; 50 to 100 yards of nylon monofilament line 6 to 8 pound test are recommended for target casting.
4. Leader: The leader is a length of nylon or wire tied between the lure and the line. It provides strength and can be from 12 inches to 12 feet or more in length.
5. Plugs: Plugs, or lures, are made of wood, metal, or plastic in a form to imitate some natural food of the fish. Practice casting plugs are usually made of rubber.
6. Sinker: The sinker is a metal weight attached to the line near the hook. It is used to lower a baited hook below the surface of the water where the fish are feeding.
7. Float, or Bobber: The accessory is used by still fishermen. The float is made of cork, ordinary wood, or plastic and shows by its movements when a fish is nibbling at the bait or has been hooked.

Techniques

How to Cast. In target casting, which is casting for accuracy, the caster may stand directly facing the target or slightly sideways, with his right foot slightly advanced (for right-handers). The target is sighted by looking at it through the top of the tip of the rod. The left arm should be held to the side of the body in a relaxed position.

After the rod is lined up with the target, the tip of the rod is brought slowly and smoothly to a vertical position and stopped. A forward motion is then made by sharply flicking the wrist and extending the forearm; the wrist action is very important.

During the forward motion, the line is held in place by the thumb on the reel button or by varying the pressure of the thumb on the spool. When the rod is on approximately a 45-degree angle, the pressure should be released, allowing the line and plug to run toward the target.

Accurate casting requires practice. Sidearm casting is usually easier for the beginner, but overhead casting is preferred because it is more accurate (Fig. 7–16).

The introduction of casting games can add an interesting dimension to instructional classes (Figs. 7–17 and 7–18).

Assistive Devices*

Ampo Fisher I.† This device enables the unilateral upper-extremity amputee to independently operate a fishing reel with a prosthesis. A turning arm which weighs only 4 oz. is used in place of the hook fingers. A nylon bearing replaces a standard reel handle. To retrieve the line, the amputee inserts the turning arm over the nylon bearing and cranks. The turning arm can be changed to a hook in a few seconds by loosening the thumb screw on the quick change unit. The device works well with a Shimano MLX-200 Fast Cast System.

Van's EZ Cast. This device is especially useful to quadriplegics and other anglers limited by restricted arm movement (Fig. 7–19). The rod and assembly unit is attached to the arm rest of a wheelchair so the rod is pointed behind the angler (as in a normal cast-

---

*For a complete line of the many listed products write to J.L. Pachner, Ltd., P.O. Box 164, Trabuco Cyn, CA 92678.

†Write to Bassmatic, 2512 Columbus Rd., NE P.O. Box 2017, Canton, OH 44705 for additional information.

ing position). The rod is pushed forward automatically releasing the line holder. A special splint (detailed drawing enclosed with device) is needed for anglers who need assistance in reeling in the line. The angler must have limited use of one arm to control the device.

Batick Bracket. Designed by Philip Batick, a quadriplegic, the device can be used by anglers with limited use of their hands. The bracket is designed to lock the angler's casting hand in position between two foam sections while bypassing the actual need to grasp the slender rod handle (Fig. 7–20). The bracket has also been used successfully with post-burn anglers with no or minimal use of their fingers.

The product can be purchased from Zebro‡ for a $2.00 handling charge.

Pole Lock. This unique device can be mounted to a boat, dock, or any other desirable location. The Pole Lock holds the rod, not the handle. This relieves the angler who is unable to continuously manipulate the rod and reel, such as those with muscular weakness and fine motor coordination problems. The Pole Lock can be used when trolling, drift, or still fishing.

Rod Holders. Various tubular rod holders are commercially available which attach to the arm rest of a wheelchair with mounting brackets. Most can be adjusted to the desired angle and designed to fit baitcast, spin, and spincast rods.

A number of rod holders with suspender like harness systems are available for one-armed anglers

---

‡For further information write to Zebco Division, Brunswick Corp., Box 270P, Tulsa, OK 74101.

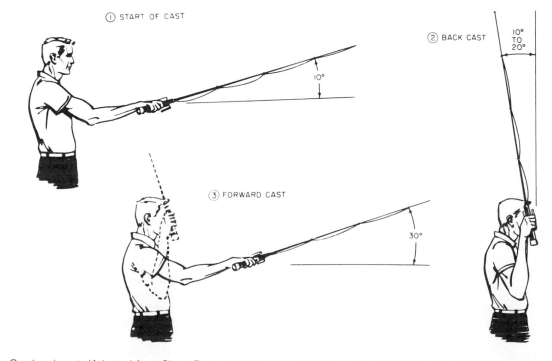

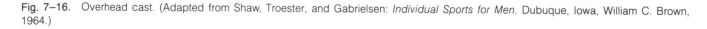

Fig. 7–16. Overhead cast. (Adapted from Shaw, Troester, and Gabrielsen: *Individual Sports for Men*. Dubuque, Iowa, William C. Brown, 1964.)

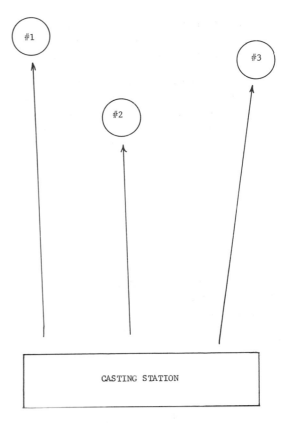

Fig. 7–17. Skish, a casting game involving accuracy in target casting at various distances. The name of the game is a combination of the words *skill* and *fish*.

Scoring: Each participant casts 20 times at each target. One point is awarded for each direct hit (plug landing inside target or a similar goal). All three targets can be used simultaneously to speed up the game, with the players changing position after each has had 20 casts at a target. Player with the greatest number of hits at the end of 60 casts is the winner.

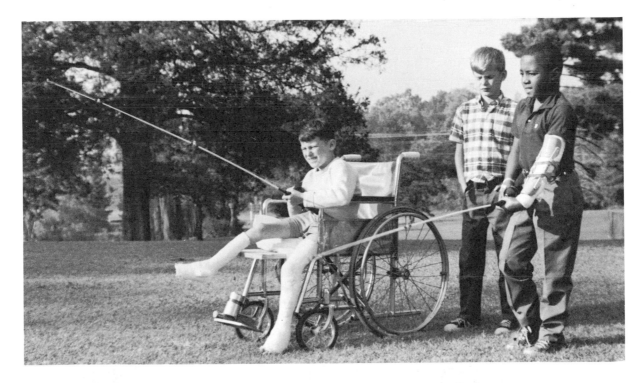

Fig. 7–18. Speed-casting match. The boy in the wheelchair is a postoperative patient with congenital clubfeet. Angling can increase upper-extremity muscle strength, coordination, and balance. The tin can on the front pedal contains an assortment of casting plugs.

Speed casting is a variation of skish. Each player casts for 5 minutes at each target. The player with the high score at the end of 15 minutes is the winner.

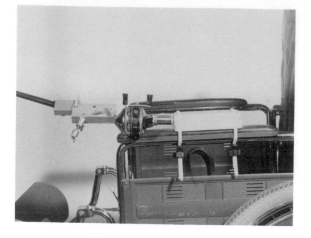

Fig. 7–19. Van's EZ Cast. Illustration of rod position after being pushed forward to release line. Note clamps holding device to chair arm. (Courtesy of The Creative Shop, P.O. Box 7, Leona, TN 38468.)

(hemiplegics and amputees). The FreeHanderson Recreation Belt (Fig. 7–21) is a harness system (weighs approximately 3 pounds) which includes a sturdy extension plate that securely locks a rod in place. Another unique feature is a line holding device that allows the user to bait the hook with one hand. The Handi-Gear* is another popular harness system which is made of aluminum and weighs approximately 14 oz (Fig. 7–22). The one-armed angler casts and then inserts the rod butt into the holding tube. By pushing down and twisting, the rod is locked in place. To cast again, the user simply pushes down on the rod and with a quick twist releases it from the tube. Rods and reels capable of handling 15-pound test line work well with the Handi-Gear.

Electronic Fishing Reels. Miya Epoch features a complete line of electronic reels. The reels have various programming features. The electric reel cranks itself and the angler sets the drag according to the conditions at hand. Similar to a conventional reel, the drag is held on the up-stroke, and then lets the reel wind automatically on the down-stroke. The ME 350 is a good starter reel and operates from a small 12 volt D.C. power pack. It is operated with a light touch on the micro switch and drag lever. The reel is especially useful for anglers who lack muscular strength and endurance in the arms.

Individual constructed electronic fishing reels are custom made for the more severely involved angler (high level quadriplegic, those with progressive muscle disorders, etc.). By using mouth control, the sipping action initiates the reeling mechanism while the puffing stops the gears (Fig. 7–23).

The construction design consists of 5 major components; the rod, reel, drive train, control system and chair mounting. At the base of the rod is an 18-inch aluminum section. This section includes; the motor,

*Write to Shellee Industries, 678 Berriman St., Brooklyn, NY 12208.

transmission box and reel which are attached in one unit. The rod is connected to the aluminum base by a 2-inch male-female ferrule fitting. The reel is a Zebco 404 closed-faced spinning reel. The motor is a 3150 R.P.M., high torque, reversible, 12-volt field motor. To conserve torque and decrease R.P.M.s, the gears of the motor are reduced to one-inch and 3.5-inch gears. Two bearing sets allow the gears to fit inside the transmission case. At this point the device is fully operational for a sip-n-puff control system and can be custom fitted for electric wheelchair function.

The Royal Bee Corporation is another popular source for electric retrieve fishing reels. Special features include push button control, rapid retrieve, 12 volt battery operation, and one hand operation (Fig. 7–24) in casting, trolling, or any type fishing required.

Adjustments for Specific Disabilities

Amputations
Unilateral Upper-Extremity. Electronic fishing reels are often recommended for this group of amputees which can be used with or without the aid of the prosthesis. Body awareness exercise through the operation of the rod and reel is a major therapeutic goal in clinical programs.

Some anglers hold the rod in the terminal device, and wind the reel as well as cast with the non-affected limb. The Ampo Fisher I is another alternative for the angler who prefers to wear his prosthesis.

Bilateral Upper-Extremity. The loss of a grip hand for the rod is a major problem. However, some bilateral below-elbow amputees have used electronic reels. This group of amputees is often encouraged to use cane poles. A special terminal device can be made that connects the rod directly to the wrist unit of the prosthesis. Rod holders may be helpful in some situations.

Unilateral Lower-Extremity. Amputees in this group will be able to perform the overhead cast from either a sitting or a standing position. No problems should be encountered with this group.

Bilateral Lower-Extremity. This group of anglers, especially A/K amputees, usually prefer to cast from a sitting position. When standing, newly acquired amputees who are adjusting to their prostheses will often have difficulty maintaining balance during the forward motion of the overhead cast.

Chronic Obstructive Lung Disease. Angling is a sport universally enjoyed by adults, including emphysema patients. On rare occasions, asthmatics have difficulty fishing on wet and rainy days when dampness can precipitate breathing problems. Most participants with chronic lung disease are able to learn the fundamentals of casting without difficulty.

Visual Impairments. Angling is recommended for partially and totally blind persons. However, the learning process is slow until the individual familiarizes himself with the mechanics of the rod and reel. The instructor will need to assist the blind angler verbally to enable him to aim the cast. The assistant must

THE BATICK BRACKET from ZEBCO

Figure 1

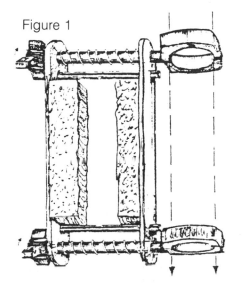

.. Bracket will fit most straight-handled fishing rods

.. Knobs on bracket are for increasing or decreasing tension between the two foam pieces

Hand fits between the two foam pieces as shown in Figure 2

.. Bracket may be mounted for either right-handed or left-handed use

.. Figure 2 shows a double-knob handle, but, single-knob handle may be preferred

Figure 2

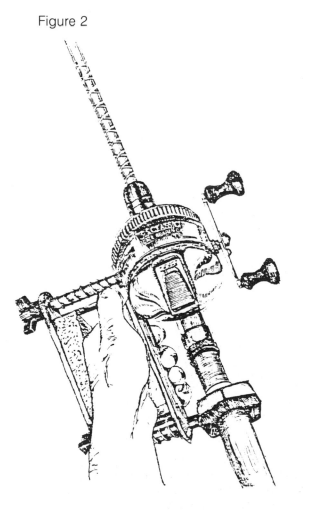

Fig. 7–20.   Batick Bracket. (Courtesy of Zebco.)

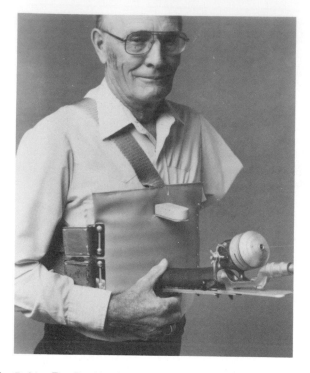

Fig. 7–21.   The FreeHanderson Recreation Belt. (Courtesy of The FreeHanderson Co., P.O. Box 4543, Helena, MT 59604.)

also watch for overhead obstructions. Improved body control will help develop feelings of self-confidence and self-reliance.

Cardiovascular Disorders. Physical limitations of patients with cardiac conditions vary, depending upon the degree and amount of malfunction of the heart. Many individuals will be able to participate without restrictions, since angling is not strenuous. The activity is also encouraged because it is self-directed.

Cerebral Palsy. The cerebral-palsied individual lacks normal muscle control and balance. The beginner should master repetitive dry casting movements before he casts with the line. It is important to improve rhythm and to exercise the involved parts in normal movements. Athetoid patients have a distinct disadvantage because their unpurposeful movements interfere with motor patterns. Excitement, tension, and nervousness increase the amount of involuntary movement. Successful participation is important for the cerebral palsied; therefore, the individual may gain confidence in his ability just by reeling in the line. The therapeutic value of angling results from the purposeful use of certain muscle groups in controlling directional movements. Muscle relaxation is a prerequisite for successful casting.

Use of adapted equipment will need to be assessed on an individual basis.

Hemiplegia. Two basic therapeutic objectives of this type of disability are achieving maximum return of neuromuscular function to the affected side and maintaining strength and endurance in the unaffected

side. An exercise program can include angling as a supplementary activity. The hemiplegic can experiment with his affected hand by reeling in the line while bracing the rod against his body with the unaffected arm. Finger and wrist exercise such as this can help the therapist or instructor measure range of motion and strength. Those with severe contractures of the involved upper extremity will need to use rod holders or in some cases, electronic reels. Standing tolerance must be sufficient before the patient is allowed to cast from an upright position.

Head Trauma. Angling is a quiet and safe outdoor sport that is performed in a calm environment. Because of this reason it is a popular therapeutic modality for head trauma patients during the rehabilitation recovery period. The angler should demonstrate good judgment and reliability in using a rod and reel, however, those with cognitive deficits may demonstrate periods of distraction and impatience. The program leader may need to stay within close proximity, provide reassurance, and emphasize attention to detail: controlling placement of rod, providing verbal cues to reel in line, etc. Depending upon degree of involvement, adapted devices especially one armed harness or belt systems will be needed (refer to paragraph on Hemiplegia). Other devices especially those for wheelchair-user anglers will need to be assessed on an individual basis.

Hip Joint Disorders. Depending on early treatment procedures, it is possible for an individual to learn the techniques of angling from a wheelchair or from a sitting position in bed. If he is ambulatory with weight-bearing restrictions, then care should be taken to see that he is capable of independent standing with the aid of crutches or a special brace.

Standing balance will be a problem for children wearing abduction appliances especially during the early phases of ambulation. The angler may need to support his body weight with one crutch and cast with his free, dominant upper extremity.

Osteogenesis Imperfecta. Angling is a safe and popular sport for younger OI participants because it does not stress the skeletal system. For some, restricted elbow joint and arm movement may cause problems, but this is often overcome by using a 2-handed casting motion. Use of adapted devices will vary depending upon the degree of physical involvement.

Overweight and Obesity. Angling may be used successfully with the obese because weight is not a handicap to performance. The casting motion is a single response movement that requires minimal arm and shoulder action. The overweight individual should be able to learn casting skills without too much difficulty. Angling is not a physically challenging sport, but the extremely obese person may have difficulty developing rhythm during the forward motion of the rod.

Paraplegia. The sport of angling is frequently prescribed for paraplegics. In addition to promoting tolerance for sitting in a wheelchair, the sport provides

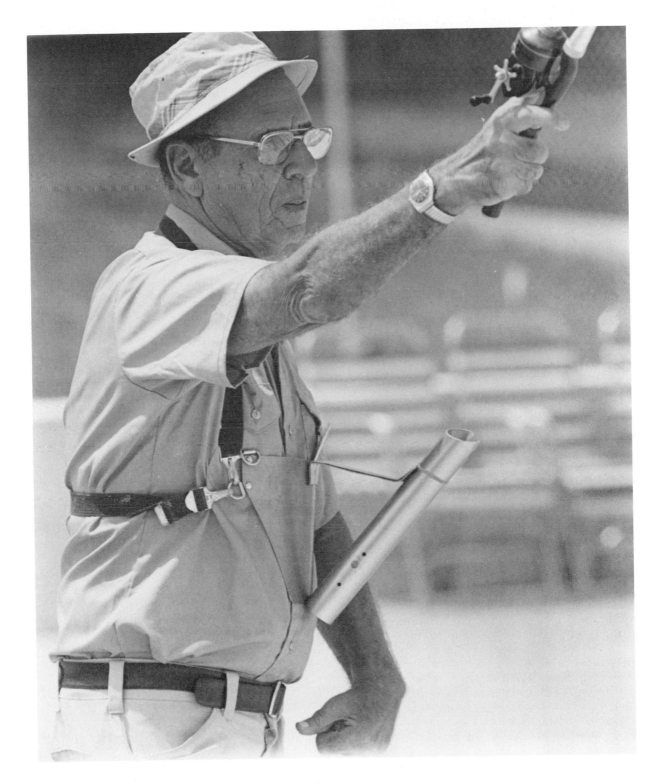

Fig. 7–22. Handi-Gear. (Courtesy of Shellee Industries.)

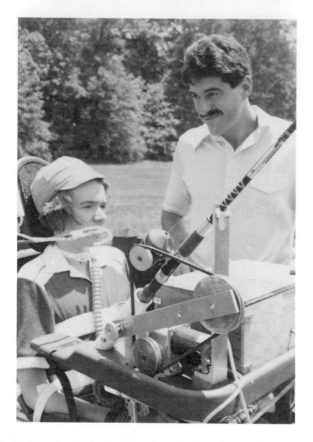

Fig. 7–23. Customized electronic reel with sip and puff control. A pond with a flat bank area or dock is ideal for anglers with pneumatic control systems. (Courtesy of Frederico Ceccotti.)

social adjustment and a life-long hobby. Those with a complete spinal paraplegia at T-9 generally or above should use a seat belt when casting. Most paraplegics have sufficient arm and shoulder strength to complete the casting motion.

The wheelchair-user paraplegic has a distinct advantage, because the firm base provided by the wheelchair can aid the caster in performing the required casting skills. Beginners, particularly those with high thoracic lesions, have a tendency to shift their weight forward during the casting motion. A seat belt should be provided to correct this problem. No major problems are likely to occur after the caster develops the smooth motion associated with the overhead cast. Middle-aged and older paraplegics will find angling an enjoyable sport and many engage in fishing from boats and kayaks.

Progressive Muscular Disorders. Program adjustments for this group vary because of the progressive nature of the disease. Muscle weakness interferes with controlling the rod and reel when casting for distance and accuracy. Some participants can place both hands on the rod handle to cast, but those with more advanced forms of muscle disease will be unable to lift their arms to perform the desired movement. Although casting is a simple movement, it is important

to realize its psychologic implications: failure to control the distance of the plug can be frustrating. The patient should avoid unnecessary discouragement and overfatigue. Arm fatigue is often overcome by using pole holders.

The weight of the rod and reel, though seemingly light, may pose problems for this group. Some anglers are able to compensate for their muscle weakness by keeping both hands on the handle or using a pole lock to mount the reel when fishing. During casting games, targets must be moved close to the caster. Evaluation of shoulder girdle strength is important before introducing the sport. The forward motion of the overhead cast may cause the caster to lose his balance unless a seat belt is used to correct this problem. Electronic reels or Van's EZ Cast may be recommended in some cases.

Quadriplegia. Functional loss of varying degrees of the upper-limbs poses a problem especially in performing the casting motion. Some low level quadriplegics use grasping gloves or splints to hold and manipulate the rod, and others prefer to use the Batick Bracket. Mid-level quadriplegics with some shoulder function and elbow flexion but minimal hand function often use Van's EZ Cast, especially when dock fishing. Electronic fishing reels can be purchased or customized for the individual angler depending upon functional skills and choice of equipment (Fig. 7–25).

Rheumatoid Arthritis. The instructor should evaluate each individual including hand function and thumb mobility to determine the acceptability of angling for

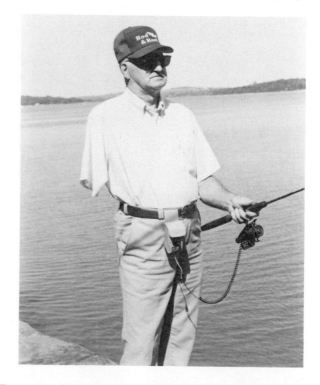

Fig. 7–24. Royal Bee electric retrieve fishing reel. (Courtesy of Royal Bee Corp., P.O. Box 2000, Powhusca, OK 74056.)

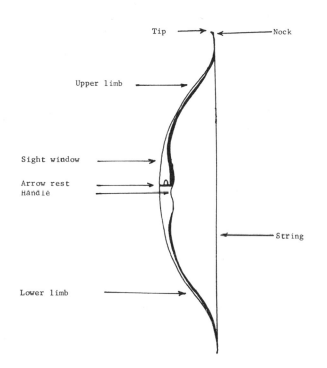

Fig. 7–25. The parts of a bow.

his condition. In some situations, the range of motion of the joints may be improved by enlisting the patient in a casting program; however, in other cases, angling may be contraindicated since the required joint motion may cause pain and stiffness. Assistive devices may be needed in some situations.

NOTE: Wrist motion is critical when casting for accuracy as well as coordination of grip and thumb action. It is important to point out that effective use of the hands often depends on the range of motion at the shoulders, elbows, and wrists.

Abnormal Posture. Sports such as angling which call for poise and balance are highly desirable for the individuals with structural spinal deformities. Those ambulating with a Milwaukee brace, orthoplast jacket or postoperative cast will find little anatomic restriction in performing the casting motion.

Undernutrition. When prescribing sports for the underweight person, it is important to select activities that will not embarrass the person. Lack of upper-arm and shoulder strength may interfere with the development of casting skills, but usually, sufficient practice will bring success. Social approval for the group generally comes first from single response activities such as angling rather than from active team sports. The beginner with a weak grip and poor wrist control may be encouraged to start by learning side-arm casting.

ARCHERY

Historically, the bow has been a close friend of man in his search for food, for protection from invaders,

and in his pursuit of enjoyment. Its use dates far back beyond recorded history for more than 5,000 years. The National Archery Association (NAA) was organized in 1879 and is the oldest national archery organization in the United States. The Federation Internationale de Tir à l'Arc, founded in 1931, is the international governing body of archery. In 1972 archery became an official Olympic sport.

Target courses for this sport are laid out on level terrain, and shooting positions are laid out along straight lines parallel to the targets at carefully measured distances. Any type of hand-held bow is allowed in target archery, and any kind of sight, point-of-aim or other type of aiming device, may be used. Arrows are shot in groups of 6; on a given signal, the contestants advance to the targets to score the results.

Adapted for the Physically Disabled

Archery is one of the oldest sports for the physically disabled; during the last 20 years it has become one of the most important rehabilitation activities of the paraplegic. The fact that using a bow requires coordination of the muscles of the individual's back, shoulders, arms, and eyes lends much to its popularity among therapists and physical educators who work with the physically disabled.

Target archery is also a popular competitive sport. However, particular rulings apply to archers during competition. For example, shooting releases are allowed for Class I and II athletes in USCPAA competition. In NWAA competition, a release can be used only by Class 1A, 1B or 1C archers.

Archery has evolved into a year-round multimillion-dollar business, since people are now able to shoot year round, indoors and out, and most can afford the relatively small expenditure for a backyard range. Its appeal to all age groups makes it a significant skill activity which should be taught to the physically disabled.

Equipment

The cardinal rule when selecting archery equipment is *get the most for your money; buy and use good equipment.* Properly fitted equipment is essential, and the beginner should rely on a qualified expert to match the various components and tackle items properly.

1. Bow (Fig. 7–26): There are 3 types of bows: the straight bow, recurve bow, and compound bow. A laminated fiberglass recurve bow is by far the best selection for target shooting. This type of bow combines stability, reliability, and durability.

   Following is a general draw-weight guide to be used as a starting point for fitting an individual with a bow:

Small children	10 to 15 lbs.
10 to 12-year-olds	15 to 20 lbs.
Teen-age girls and women	20 to 30 lbs.
Teen-age boys and men	30 to 40 lbs.

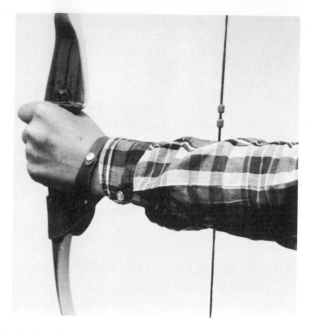

Fig. 7–26.   A bow sling, an assist for archers.

Beginning hunting bows for men 40 to 55 lbs.

Bows vary in length from 4 to 6 feet or more. A 48-inch bow is recommended for children confined to wheelchairs.

2. Arrows: Since the arrow receives more abuse than any other part of the equipment, it should be sturdy, but relatively inexpensive. The aluminum arrow fits these qualifications, although beginners usually use wooden arrows because they are less expensive. However, aluminum arrows are much more rugged; they will stand a lot of abuse, and will remain straight.

The length of the arrow is important. The correct length is determined by the arm span of the archer. Most archery shops can provide assistance in selecting arrow weight and length.

3. Arm Guard: The arm guard, usually made of leather, protects the arm and wrist from the sting of the bowstring. The arm guard is worn on the inside of the forearm that holds the bow.

4. Finger Tab and Glove: The finger tab and glove protect the hand that draws the bowstring. Nock locks (rubber stoppers), which fit over the string to protect the fingers, are also popular.

5. Quiver: This accessory is used to hold the arrows. The belt quiver is popular; however, the ground quiver is recommended for the wheelchair-bound shooter, since the arrows can be conveniently placed at the side of the chair.

6. Target Face: The face is generally 48 inches in diameter and is attached to the target butt. The center gold spot (bull's-eye) is 9.6 inches in diameter and is surrounded by four concentric bands of red, blue, black, and white.

7. Target Backstop: The shooting area must be safe, and it must confine any stray arrows. The use of an earth or sand backstop is encouraged; however, commercially available nylon-mesh backstops make excellent indoor-outdoor arrow stops.

How to Shoot the Longbow

Ambulatory Archers. The instructions given are for a right-handed archer; for a left-handed archer, the procedures should be reversed.

1. Stance: The archer should stand at a right angle to the target with his left side toward it. The body should be erect, but relaxed; the feet should be spread slightly apart for good balance.

2. Nocking: Hold the bow firmly, but not tightly, in a horizontal position with the back of the hand up. Place the nock of the arrow in the bowstring with the cock feather up so the shaft rests on the arrow rest. Hook the first 3 fingers of the right hand around the string with the arrow nock between the first and second fingers. Then turn the bow to a vertical position.

3. Draw: In one continuous motion, the shooting hand draws the string and arrow back to the side of the face. This is called the *anchor point* and is a definite spot on the face to which either the index finger or middle finger of the drawing hand is brought on every draw. The right arm should be level with the shoulder as the draw is made. Do not bend the elbow of the bow arm.

4. Aim: In the point-of-aim method, a spot above or below the target is sighted. Aim over the tip of the arrow at a predetermined spot. Most archers develop their own sighting styles with practice.

5. Release: Relax the fingers that are drawing the line and release the string smoothly. Do not move the shooting arm; the draw fingers should straighten slightly after the arrow is released.

6. Follow-through: Remain in a relatively fixed position until the arrow makes contact with the target.

Wheelchair Archers. A wheelchair archer shoots the bow the same as the ambulatory archer except that he uses a different stance. Archery requires the shooter to have a wide solid base from which to shoot; wheelchairs are the ready-made answer to the best possible solid base. With the chair positioned at a 90-degree angle with the target, the archer enjoys a firm and stable base instead of the normal bobbing and weaving associated with beginners who shoot from the standing position.

Wheelchair archers with strong spinal extensor muscles should find a relaxed shooting position while resting comfortably against the back of their chair. Most coaches advise against shooting while sitting up straight.

To prepare for a smooth draw motion, the wheelchair archer frequently removes his armrest. This allows him to draw the bowstring back farther to an anchor point.

Scoring
Scoring values for the standard target face are gold, 9; red, 7; blue, 5; black, 3; white, 1. Thus, a perfect round of 6 arrows in the gold bull's-eye earns 54 points.

An arrow that either rebounds from the scoring face or passes through the scoring face so that it is not visible from the front can be counted as 7 points at 60 years or less, or as 5 points on ranges longer than 60 yards.

Assistive Devices
Various kinds of commercially available assistive devices are used in archery. These range from detachable stabilizers that are screwed into the bow to aid balance to an assortment of bow straps and finger slings which correct bow hand errors. A few popular types of archery assists are discussed here.

Bow Sling. This assist (Fig. 7–26) is recommended for archers who have loose bow grips. The bow sling has been used by many shooters with mild spastic cerebral palsy, since they have a natural tendency to drop the bow at the instant when the string is released. The sling helps stabilize the wrist and hand for positive bow control. Another feature is that the bow sling prevents the bow from dropping upon release of the bowstring. The bow sling can be purchased from most sport shops or archery equipment companies.

Below-Elbow Amputee Adapter Device. This archery assist (Figs. 7–27 and 7–28) is held by the terminal device with the hook fingers fitted into the grooves of the assist. The bowstring is held by the small tip of the device while the archer draws the bow. The archer keeps his arm at a right angle to the body; when full draw is reached a slight rotation of the prosthesis releases the string and the arrow.

It is advisable for the amputee archer to use a pair of commercially available small rubber stoppers (arrow-nocks) to hold the arrow on the string.

The adapter device has an advantage over other devices for below-elbow amputees, because it requires active use of the prosthesis.

Wheelchair Bowstringer. This device (Fig. 7–29) is not absolutely necessary, but it is extremely useful. Wheelchair archers can be more independent with the aid of this accessory because the bowstringer discourages the shooter from relying on an able-bodied person to assist. The bowstringer is recommended only for archers with good upper-extremity strength.

Adapted Archery Bow. This device (Fig. 7–30) was designed by Jim Cowart, Alameda Schools, Alameda, California, for use by the more severely involved archer. The bow and support system are mounted on a camera tripod. The bow is constructed so that an assistant draws the string into the release aid. The archer then applies slight finger pressure on the trigger of the release aid to activate the arrow toward the target. Vertical and horizontal adjustments are made by the assistant in response to the commands of the archer.

Construction details will not be discussed at length. The support system, which is bolted to the belly of the bow, should be made of aluminum ($1/16$ inch thick). The support arm, which is attached to the tripod, can be made of wood ($1\frac{1}{2}'' \times 1\frac{1}{2}''$). This will correspond with the approximate length of the draw for a 12 to 20 pound pull bow using a 26" arrow. The trade name of this release device is Hot Shot Release, manufactured by the Stuart Manufacturing Company, Rockwell, Texas.

An archery wrist support, long arm brace, release cuff* and mechanical release (Fig. 7–31)† are examples of equipment that can be used in a total shooting system. Equipment design is for archers with limited upper extremity function.

*Write to Access to Recreation, 2509 E. Thousand Oaks Blvd., Suite 430, Thousand Oaks, CA 91362, for further information on specialized archery equipment.

†For information on mechanical releases, write to Tru-Fire Corp., 732 State St., N. Fond Du Lac, WI 54935.

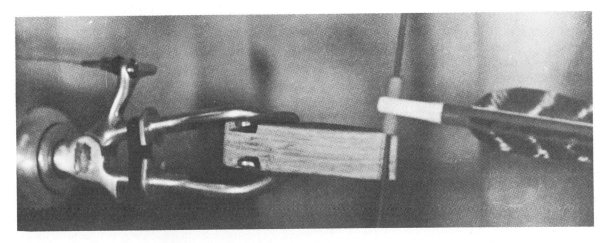

Fig. 7–27. An adapter device for the below-elbow amputee.

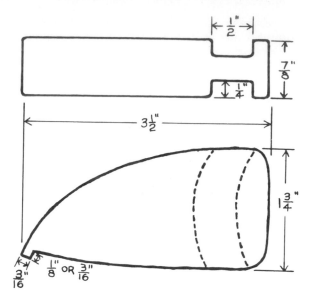

Fig. 7–28. Design of the amputee archery assist. The assist can be made from any available hard wood, but white oak is recommended. The amputee grasps the block of wood (3″ × 4″ × 1″), and the outline of his hook fingers is drawn on the block with a soft pencil. A router is then used to cut a track (¼″ deep × ½″ wide) in the block. If a drill is used instead of a router, the track must be smoothed.

Elbow Brace. A brace can be used to avoid excessive bending of the elbow. Different custom made braces are available and designed to be used with hemiplegics and quadriplegics. The illustration shown (Fig. 7–32) is a brace that provides a rigid link from the bow to the chest wall, thus bypassing the elbow, wrist, and hand in transferring the force of the draw motion to the trunk. Made of aluminum, it has a telescoping joint to allow proper adjustment of bow length. Two wooden clamps attach the bow to the brace above and below the hand grip. No modification in the bow is required. Various strapping techniques can be used to stabilize the brace to the bow arm.

Program Adjustments for Specific Disabilities

The therapist or instructor should evaluate each individual, particularly those with upper-extremity involvement, to determine if the recurve bow is the logical choice of equipment. If not, then shooting with a crossbow may be recommended. Certain disabilities not discussed here are possible candidates for crossbow shooting.

Amputations

Unilateral Upper-Extremity. The below-elbow amputee can learn proper shooting techniques with the aid of the below-elbow amputee adapter device. The shooter must have sufficient strength in the unaffected extremity to hold the bow properly. Beginners will usually have problems releasing the bowstring with the prosthesis.

Some amputees make adaptations (rubber, foam, etc.) to the grip portion of the bow for secure attachment of the terminal device.

Bilateral Upper-Extremity. Loss of both hands poses major problems. The crossbow with the aid of the tripod assistive device is generally recommended for this group of amputees.

Unilateral Lower-Extremity. Beginners will have problems maintaining a comfortable base for an indefinite period of time; however, no major problems should occur with this group of amputees if the shooter has sufficient upper-extremity strength. Therapeutically, archery can be used for balance training and as preparation for independent ambulation. Once the prosthesis is fitted, the erect position can be adopted.

Bilateral Lower-Extremity. The problem of balance is present with many above-knee amputees; however, if the shooter can spread his feet properly for good balance, then the major concern becomes that of standing tolerance. Prosthetic awareness skills are greatly enhanced through practicing lower-extremity positioning to secure a relaxed and stable shooting base.

Chronic Obstructive Lung Disease. Archery is not a vigorous sport, so it is often encouraged for patients with asthma, bronchiectasis, and emphysema. Therapeutically, the sport provides for increase in chest expansion, breath control, and good posture. Since breath control is important to proper shooting, archery is a natural sport for patients with chronic lung disease. Breath control should be emphasized after the full draw is reached, during the holding period when the aiming is done.

Blindness. Various types of telescopic sights can be purchased which will aid the partially sighted archer. The Glassboro[7] method for teaching the totally blind is as follows:

1. Arrows must be carefully selected, and the archer's arm and shoulder strength carefully evaluated.
2. Teach the shooter how to nock the bow to the arrow. Teach the difference between the feel of the cock feather and the hen feather. The archer should also be able to feel the nock indention.
3. Place the arrows in a quiver strapped around the shooter's waist. The archer should now be able to manipulate the arrows as a sighted person could.
4. Foot Position. Construct a foot board to enable the archer to position his feet properly on a right angle to the target.
5. After the feet and body are in proper alignment, the arrow is nocked to the bow. Draw the bow until the string touches the lips and the thumb is anchored to the jaw bone. These movements are done continuously until the archer feels confident. At the start, the draw arm may need to be held in place. Also, the bow arm may need

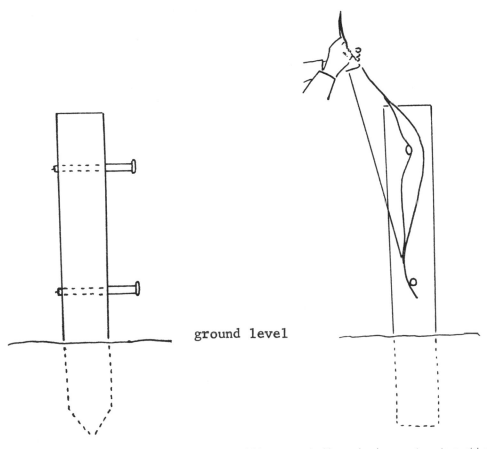

ground level

Fig. 7–29. Wheelchair bowstringer. The bolt on the bowstringer should be covered with garden hose or tape to avoid damage to the finish of the bow.

to be guided in a straight up-and-down relationship to the floor or ground.

6. Devise a towline. A rope is suspended from the middle of the top of the target to a nail that is attached to the foot board. This has a twofold purpose. The archer is able to walk to the target by himself and is able to keep the bow in a horizontal position by placing it against the rope.

7. To create more independence, a system of self-scoring is encouraged. This is done by covering each color of the target with an unusual texture of material. The materials that can be used are sandpaper for gold, satin for red, terry cloth for blue, cotton for black, and nothing for the white portion.

8. The blind archer is now able to approach the target, know how many arrows hit the target, and how many points are made. He can return to the foot board, record the score in braille, and be ready to begin the whole process again.

Cardiovascular Disorders. There should be no apparent problems associated with this group, provided that care is taken not to exceed the level of activity prescribed by the physician. Participation in archery can assist recovery by strengthening the superficial back muscles, trunk, and upper limbs. The sport can also be used as a method of teaching breath control.

Therapeutic Note: Some physical education authorities do not recommend archery for patients with cardiac conditions because of the Valsalva effect. (After breath is held, the chest is stabilized, causing elevation of the arterial blood pressure as a result of the increased pressure in the thoracic region, which prevents blood from returning to the heart. If the effort is prolonged, the blood pressure falls after its initial rise.)

We advocate the early use of lightweight bows. Experiences with rheumatic heart and postcardiac-surgery archers using lightweight bows have shown that the shooter never holds his breath long enough during the draw motion to endanger blood flow to the heart. Naturally, the chest should be stabilized after the draw motion is completed, but there is no need to consciously expand the rib cage in anticipation of strain during the expiratory phase of breathing, which occurs after the arrow is released. We do not mean to imply, however, that archery should be the first activity participated in after the patient obtains medical permission to enter into the program of sports. Upper-limb and shoulder-girdle strengthening with pulley weights would be excellent lead-up exercises.

Cerebral Palsy. Participation in archery is difficult for persons with cerebral palsy in which neuromus-

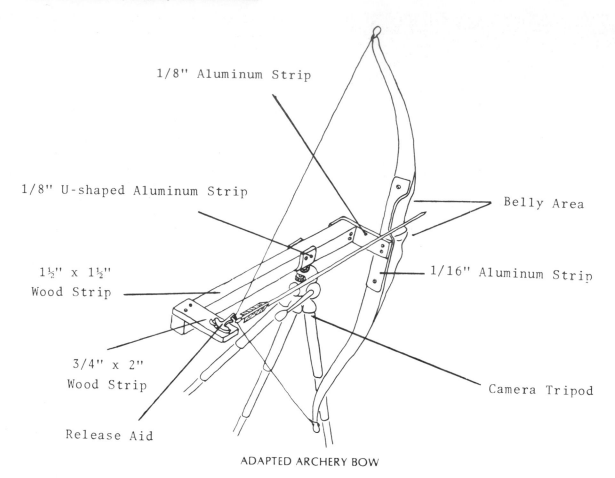

1/8" Aluminum Strip

1/8" U-shaped Aluminum Strip

Belly Area

1½" x 1½"
Wood Strip

1/16" Aluminum Strip

3/4" x 2"
Wood Strip

Camera Tripod

Release Aid

ADAPTED ARCHERY BOW

Fig. 7–30.   Adapted archery bow. (Courtesy of American Alliance for Health, Physical Education, Recreation and Dance.)

cular disorders, such as tactile or proprioceptive disturbances, spasticity, tremor, or other extraneous movements (especially of the upper limbs), are a predominate feature. Each person with cerebral palsy must be evaluated on an individual basis. For those with mild involvement, archery can be used to promote muscle awareness and relaxation skills. An elbow brace may be needed for archers with reduced arm and wrist function. An adapted archery bow may be utilized in some circumstances.

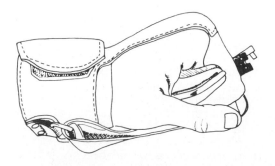

Fig. 7–31.   Archery release cuff and mechanical release. (Courtesy of Applied Technology for Independent Living, 2008 Lowry Ave., N.E. Minneapolis, MN 55418.)

Hemiplegia. The major difficulty with this group is their inability to draw the bow properly with the affected limb. The shooter with mild hemiplegia needs a lightweight bow, and the instructor must spend a considerable amount of time in teaching him the fundamentals of good shooting. Therapeutic benefits include exercise of the affected arm in grasp, release, supination, and pronation with associated movements from the elbow and shoulder.

An adapted archery bow may be recommended to substitute for loss of function, or a splint designed to maintain the affected bow arm in full extension (Fig. 7–32).

Hip Joint Disorders. During the early postoperative stage, the archer must shoot from a sitting position. If the wheelchair is used in non-weight-bearing treatment, then the shooter's sitting tolerance must be carefully evaluated. Problems of standing balance develop after partial weight-bearing therapy is introduced for crutch users. Consequently, the sitting position may be preferred during this phase of treatment also.

Archers wearing abduction appliances may need some kind of support to develop a stable shooting base (Fig. 7–33). The pulling forces of the bow and bow arm or strong anchor point, and as a result will not be able to engage in target archery without adapted equipment. Some OI archers have used the adapted archery bow to compensate for a weak draw motion. Crossbow target shooting is another alternative.

Head Trauma. Archery is a sport involving extreme concentration. To participate, the recovery head trauma participant will need to be alert and oriented to the environment. If the archer demonstrates an inability to process and sequence the teaching steps involved or has problems concentrating on the target, then the sport is not recommended. Persistence of fine motor problems and visual spatial deficits may be other issues of concern. (Refer to section on Hemiplegia for additional information.)

Therapeutic Note: During the recovery stage, some persons can benefit from the deliberate attention to detail associated with archery. For example, it is a sport that emphasizes controlled touch, vision, and position sense. Patients who are not limited by moderate-severe motor deficits can often benefit from the physical and mental challenges associated with the sport.

Progressive Muscle Disorders. The muscle strength required to participate in archery is a major factor for this group. Generally, some compensation has to be made and this can be accomplished by using an

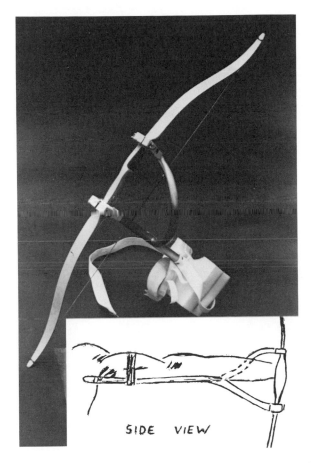

Fig. 7–32. Elbow brace assistive device which was designed for a hemiplegic who had normal strength at the shoulder, but minimal strength and flexion contracture of the arm.

string can affect equilibrium; thus, balance and stability are essential points that need immediate attention.

Overweight and Obesity. Lack of flexibility and poor range of motion of the joints are two major problems that may interfere with learning good shooting techniques. Many beginners tend to rely on their arms to do all the work and fail to recognize the value of good posture and balance. Often overweight shooters grip the bow too tightly, causing the arrows to slap the bow on release. Archery may be encouraged to compensate for lack of organic efficiency.

Paraplegia. Archery will help strengthen the shoulder and arm muscles. It is an excellent sport to improve sitting balance because the shooter's center of gravity is altered once the bow arm is lifted. Weakened muscles should not, however, be strained or overworked; therefore, completion of a medically prescribed physical therapy program of upper-extremity strengthening exercises is usually recommended before the paraplegic is enlisted in an archery program. A seat belt is often used for archers with lesions above the T-9 level (Fig. 7–34).

Osteogenesis Imperfecta. Archers with decreased function of the elbow joint cannot fixate a straight

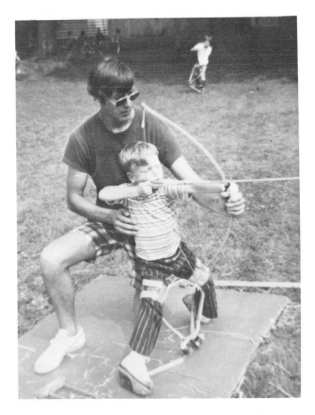

Fig. 7–33. Young archer wearing an abduction appliance.

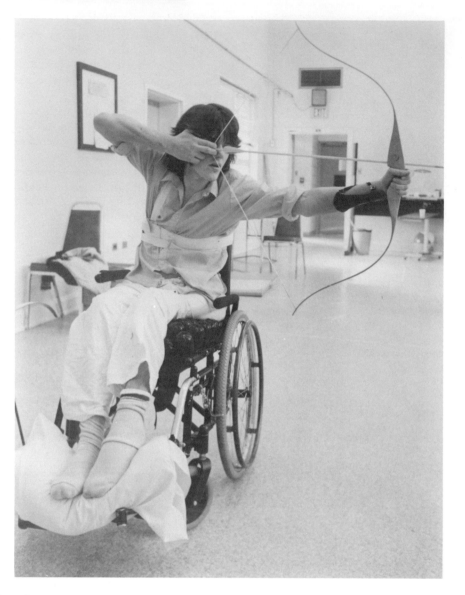

Fig. 7–34. Paraplegic archer.

adapted archery bow or engaging in crossbow target shooting.

Rheumatoid Arthritis. The ability to participate in archery will naturally depend upon the degree of joint involvement. If medical permission is granted, then the sport can be used to increase joint range of motion and shoulder and arm strength. Under no circumstances should a patient with inflamed joints attempt to shoot a longbow.

Assessment of hand function is critical, especially for archers who have permanent joint changes in the digits. The shooting hand must be functional on the draw motion; usage of the first three fingers is necessary. The role of the thumb is not vital and finger abduction/adduction is not essential. It should be pointed out that persons with finger involvement often have digits that become fusiform in shape. How-

ever, the joint furthest toward the tip (which is responsible for controlling the draw motion) is rarely involved. Rubber nock locks are often helpful to relieve tension on the fingers when drawing the bowstring. Shooting releases can also be used in some situations.

Elbow bracing may be required for shooters with involvement of the bow arm. For the severely involved, the crossbow may be the logical choice of equipment.

Abnormal Posture. Since the primary aims of treatment of scoliosis, lordosis, and kyphosis are to overcome rigidity of the spine, to secure correction of the deformity, and to develop muscle strength, archery is sometimes beneficial for these persons. However, there must be medical permission to participate. Strengthening of the superficial back muscles and the development of good relaxed posture are the therapeutic goals of archery for this group of patients.

Therapeutic Note: Archery has great therapeutic value for postural improvement. The pulling aspects of the sport enhance balance and control because they require the archer to readjust his center of gravity in relation to a stationary base and the opposing forces of the bow and string. The primary draw is a pushing and pulling action that uses the upper arm, shoulder, and back muscles. The secondary draw keeps the bowstring at full draw until the archer has completed his aim and released the arrow. In this activity the shoulders move backward, the shoulder blades approach each other, and the upper back muscles "oppose" the pull of the bow being drawn. Correct body alignment is required throughout, thus enhancing the therapeutic value of archery for persons with scoliosis, kyphosis, and other spinal deformities.

Undernutrition. The sport of archery is performed from a stationary position and can be used to increase the work tolerance of undernourished patients. In such situations, medical permission must be granted, since the patient's unused muscles must not be overworked. The major problem associated with this group is lack of strength. Beginners will usually have difficulty in drawing the string because of the lack of shoulder strength.

Quadriplegia (Hook) Archery. Quadriplegics who have wrist extension and good elbow flexion (C-6 and C-7) can participate in archery if a hook is affixed to the palm of their hand. The TSS SYG III shooting releases are utilized by archers who do not have finger function to draw the bowstring[8] (see section on assistive devices). This enables the quadriplegic to pull the bow with the biceps and deltoids. In this method, the bow hand is fixed to the grip portion of the bow by a leather appliance or other support system. The arrow is released by extension of the wrist (Fig. 7–35).

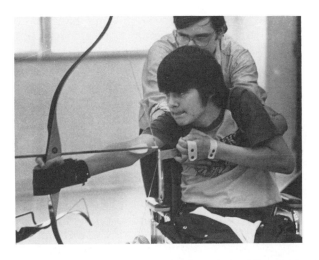

Fig. 7–35. Quadriplegic participating in archery while using hook appliance.

The archer without triceps needs a splint to maintain the elbow in extension.

Special considerations are provided for quadriplegics during events sanctioned by the National Wheelchair Athletic Association. Special aids such as hooks are permitted in place of finger tabs or gloves. Also, quadriplegic archers may be tied or otherwise strapped into their wheelchairs to maintain balance and support. However, archers are not permitted to rest their arm or shoulders on any part of the chair for stability.

Readers are encouraged to read the NWAA Official Rulebook for further information on specific wheelchair archery rules.

WHEELCHAIR CROSSBOW TARGET SHOOTING

Crossbow shooting provides a unique and challenging activity for the disabled population who are unable to engage in regular archery programs. The archer using the longbow must have good muscle strength in his arms and shoulders, as well as a strong back, before the mastery of the proper shooting techniques can be achieved. The crossbow thus makes it possible for the more physically limited groups such as those with general muscle weakness and upper-extremity involvement to engage in archery programs. These handicapping conditions may include shooters with upper-extremity amputations, hemiplegia, progressive muscle disorders, and quadriplegia.

The crossbow is a short, powerful bow attached to a modified gun stock. It can be a dangerous weapon if handled improperly and for this reason the element of safety becomes a major issue especially if used in clinical sports and rehabilitation programs. The crossbow should always be used under the supervision of an adult. Like a rifle, sighting and trigger squeeze movements are done by the shooter. Loading the bolt (arrow) is done by an able-bodied assistant. Suggested draw weights for target crossbows are 30 to 35 pounds for children between 9 and 12 years of age and somewhat higher weights for older children and beginning adults. Equipment can be purchased at most sporting goods stores.

Wheelchair shooters who are right handed will either shoot on an angle (with foot rests pointing just to the right of the target and shoulders turned slightly more to the left) or facing the target directly if using a tripod assist. A tripod or similar adjustable support system can be used with the more severely involved shooter to balance and hold the forepart of the crossbow securely (Fig. 7–36). We firmly believe that if the participant is unable to sight and fire correctly by himself, he should not participate in the sport.

Adjustments for Specific Disabilities

Amputations
Upper-Extremity. The tripod assistive device is particularly helpful for the unilateral upper-extremity

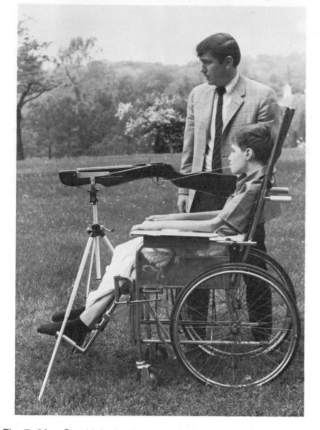

Fig. 7–36. Quadriplegic shooting crossbow with a mouthpiece.

amputee because it can serve as a substitute for the missing limb; but some amputee archers prefer to use the terminal device of the prosthesis as the grip hand. However, unless the shoulder stock is securely held in position, the crossbow will tend to tilt. Shortening the shoulder stock is recommended by many crossbow experts as one possible solution to this problem. Another solution is to use a chest strap, or harness. In some situations with the upper-extremity amputee, the terminal device will be used as the shooting hand. Under these circumstances, the instructor occasionally will need to guide the hook fingers around the trigger. Some bilateral above-elbow amputees have become excellent crossbow shooters.

Hemiplegia. Although this type of disability may be congenital or acquired, it is most often associated with cerebral palsy; the arm is usually more affected than the leg. The ability to participate in the sport will depend upon the degree of affliction. In most situations, the tripod assistive device can compensate for weakness of the affected arm. Standing tolerance must be thoroughly evaluated; if necessary, the participant can shoot from a sitting position. Before teaching the basic shooting techniques, the instructor should secure the crossbow in the stabilizer and, if possible, let the shooter use the affected arm as the guide for the crossbow. Poor hand-eye coordination

is another common difficulty; although crossbow shooting is primarily a single-response activity (simple one-act movement, generally in one plane), directionality, coordination, and balance are all necessary for successful participation.

Progressive Muscular Disorders. Program adjustments will naturally depend upon the severity of the involvement and the functional ability of the participant. The tripod assistive device is particularly helpful for those disabled by progressive muscular weakness, because it can compensate for the lack of arm and shoulder girdle strength. In most situations, an individual who ambulates with a severe waddling gait and lordosis will need to shoot the crossbow from a sitting position with the aid of the tripod. It is essential that the therapist evaluate trunk balance and sitting posture, as the more severely involved shooter may require a back support or seat belt in order to obtain a good shooting position. In these situations, the assistant will usually need to guide the shoulder stock of the crossbow while the shooter releases the trigger with both hands.

Quadriplegia. The quadriplegic will require a great deal of assistance from the instructor. Sitting tolerance and balance must be thoroughly evaluated before enlisting the patient in a crossbow program. It has been suggested that a harness be used to hold the stock of the crossbow against the shooter's shoulder to allow for complete independence in shooting, but it is our opinion that an assistant should help the quadriplegic, because a strap or harness can put undesirable pressure on the shoulder, particularly if a kick accompanies the trigger release. Safety must also be considered, and the quadriplegic must have close personal attention when shooting. The quadriplegic may also need assistance in maintaining good body alignment after each shot, and a seat belt should be used to maintain proper shooting posture.

Special considerations must be made to compensate for the lack of finger flexion movements. Pencils or similar devices attached to the shooting hand can substitute for the natural movements of a trigger finger.

Case History: The patient was 14 years old with quadriplegia due to a spinal cord injury at the C-3 level. He could tolerate a maximum of 30 minutes of crossbow shooting each day, which allowed time for shooting 15 to 20 bolts each session.

A mouthpiece connected by a wire attached to the trigger was used to release the bolt, since the shooter had no voluntary control of his arms (Fig. 7–36). Supportive strength from the upper trapezius and neck musculature permitted the archer to jerk his head backward to pull the trigger. An attendant had to load the bolts and hold the stock against the shooter's right shoulder. The shooter was completely independent in sighting, and the attendant guided the crossbow only upon verbal orders from the shooter.

This boy became an excellent crossbow archer at distances of 20 to 30 yards; he won 19 dual competitive matches while losing only 3 against less severely disabled wheelchair-bound shooters. He also holds the best accuracy record ever recorded in bull's-eye shooting at the Kluge Children's Rehabilitation Center by scoring 5 consecutive hits in a ¾-inch bull's-eye at 20 yards. The sport of crossbow shooting helped develop self-confidence, provided a hobby, and was a tremendous morale builder during this boy's hospitalization. In addition, the strength of his neck and trapezius muscles increased by being actively used in the sport.

Rheumatoid Arthritis. Since most arthritics have periods of exacerbation, the instructor should be aware of the problems of actively inflamed joints. The tripod assistive device is extremely helpful for those individuals with severe involvement of the wrists, elbows, or fingers. Two primary therapeutic benefits from nonstrenuous physical activities are to elicit upper extremity and shoulder girdle mobility and increase exercise tolerance. Crossbow shooting with the necessary adaptations is an excellent choice of activity that places little stress on the affected joints.

RACQUET SPORTS

The growth in the opportunities for racquet sports (badminton, racquetball, and tennis) in recent years is astounding. One important aspect to consider is the ease in which disabled participants can be integrated into play as doubles partners with able-bodied friends. In addition, numerous competitive opportunities are available through local, state, regional, national and international competition.

Because of its adaptability to small areas, limited requirements for skill development, and flexibility for use in clinical settings, badminton will be discussed in more detail in comparison to the other racquet sports.

BADMINTON

The name *badminton* was adopted by a group of English army officers home on leave from India in 1873, who played the game at Badminton, the country estate of the Duke of Beaufort, in Gloucestershire, England. The game was developed in India by the English military in the early 1870s and was called *poona* at that time. The International Badminton Federation (IBF), founded in 1934, is the world governing body of the game.

The game consists entirely of volleying, meaning that the shuttlecock must be struck in midair before it touches the floor or ground.

The game is played indoors or out, with 2 players on each side (called *doubles* if players are of the same sex or *mixed doubles* if one player is woman and the other a man) or with one player on each side (called *singles*). The modified doubles and triples versions are designed for the physically disabled.

The game is won by the first side to score 15 points; a match is 3 games, the winners to have won 2 of the 3.

Adapted for the Physically Disabled

In various forms, badminton has been played by the physically disabled for many years. One of the more successful adaptations of badminton is a game called *balloon badminton,* in which a balloon is substituted for the shuttlecock, table tennis paddles are used instead of rackets, and no limitations are placed on the number of players. This popular backyard racket game can be modified for the physically disabled in a number of different ways, lending to its popularity for therapy and general recreation. Box badminton is becoming popular in clinical settings.

Equipment
The following equipment is needed:
1. Badminton shuttlecock (shuttle or bird): Made of cork and feathers, this is the object that is struck. Plastic shuttles are acceptable for general play.
2. Racquet: The racquet is usually strung with high-test nylon and weighs approximately 5 oz. when strung; it has no specific size.
3. Net: The net is 30 inches deep; the top line of the net should be 5 feet 1 inch high at the posts and 5 feet high in the middle. The supporting posts are set just outside the lines. (Adjustments in height can be made in adapted games.)

Techniques and Rules

How to Play
The instructor should teach the basic fundamentals before the players compete in an actual game.
1. Grip: The racquet handle is grasped with the hand in a V-shape as if one were shaking hands with the racquet.
2. Beginners should first practice keeping the shuttlecock aloft as long as possible. This allows them to learn the movements of the wrist and elbow in relation to the movements of the racquet. The players should practice this drill in an open area.
3. Underhand lift stroke: This stroke is used to serve the shuttlecock. The left foot is placed forward (for right-handed players), and the left hand holds the shuttlecock by the feathers, waist high to the right of the body. The racquet is swung back in a straight plane and then brought forward to make contact with the shuttlecock. The left hand releases the shuttlecock just before it is hit.

   Beginners should practice the underhand lift stroke or overhead stroke for players with motor problems by serving the shuttlecock over the net from behind the short service line. Targets (hoops) can be placed on the ground at various intervals within the opposite back court, and the beginner can practice accuracy in serving by trying to hit the shuttlecock into the hoops.
4. Other strokes: In addition to the underhand lift stroke, there are four other basic strokes.
   Clear: The high clear shot is made toward the opposite back line. It can be made with either an overhead or underhand stroke and is pri-

marily a defensive stroke that can be used anywhere on the court.

Smash: The smash stroke is executed from the overhead position and is a fast, hard-hit, downward-angled shot made close to the net.

Drop shot: The drop shot is a light upward stroke that causes the shuttlecock to drop immediately upon crossing the net. The wrist is held rigid.

Drive: The drive is a fast, flat, shot hit horizontally about net height. Just before contact, the wrist is snapped forward.

Deception is employed by using varying combinations of these basic shots so that the opponent cannot anticipate which one is coming. The velocity of the shuttle in flight reaches 110 mph, but it slows down rapidly. Badminton is a game of fast action and judgment, and great accuracy; the ability to use different strokes will vary according to the nature of the player's disability.

Laws of Badminton (Regular Rules)

Choice of Ends and Service. The choice of ends and the right to be server are decided by a coin toss.

The Serve. The side that is serving is called the "IN" side, and the receiving side the "OUT" side. The server and receiver must be in their proper courts (Fig. 7–37). The other two players in doubles may stand anywhere, provided that they do not block the sight or otherwise obstruct an opponent. In singles, the server starts from the right service court and serves to the receiver in the opposite service court. If the server wins the rally, he scores a point. The next serve is from the left service court to the receiver in opposite left service court. This process of alternating courts continues as long as the server wins points. Players win points only when on the IN side, that is, when serving. When a server loses a rally, he loses the serve (but not a point), and his opponent serves and alternates courts in the same manner. In doubles, service starts with the player in the right service court. He continues to serve from alternate courts as long as his side wins.

Faults. A fault is a playing violation that ends a rally. A fault made by a player of the IN side puts the server out; if made by a player whose side is OUT, a fault counts as a point for the IN side.

It is a fault:

1. If, in serving, the shuttlecock at the instant of being struck is higher than the server's waist. (Unless adapted rules indicate otherwise. For example, using an overhead serve.)
2. If, in serving, the shuttlecock falls outside the service court lines.
3. If, either in service or play, the shuttlecock falls outside the boundaries of the court, or passes through or under the net, or fails to pass the net, or touches the roof or side walls, or touches the person or dress of a player on the same side.

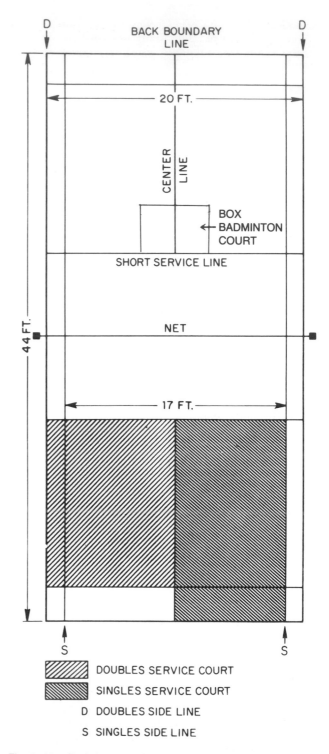

Fig. 7–37. Badminton playing courts. (From Seaton, D.C., et al.: *Physical Education Handbook,* 5th Ed. Englewood Cliffs, Prentice-Hall, 1969.)

4. If the shuttlecock in play is struck before it crosses to the striker's side of the net.
5. If, when the shuttlecock is in play, a player touches the net or its support with racquet, person, or dress.
6. If, in play, a player strikes the shuttlecock (unless he thereby makes a good return) or is struck by it, whether he is standing within or outside the boundaries of the court.
7. If a player obstructs an opponent or invades an opponent's court.

A "let" means that the play in question is invalidated and, therefore, played over without penalties. If in service the shuttle touches the net, it is a "let" provided the service is otherwise good. (If in the course of a rally the shuttle touches and passes over the net, it does not invalidate the stroke.) A "let" may be called for any unforeseen or accidental hindrance.

Modified Doubles and Triples Play (Handicap Rules)

In the modified doubles and triples play of badminton, all rules are the same as those for the regular game except:

Players
1. Players do not alternate courts. In doubles, one player is responsible for the back court and one for the front court. In triples, two players are responsible for the back court and one for the front court.

   Players who are restricted in movement, such as those playing from wheelchairs or crutches, should be positioned in the front court. Players with little or no disability in their lower limbs should be responsible for the back court.
2. A wheelchair-user player in the front court is permitted to have the back wheels of his wheelchair extended beyond the short service line (Fig. 7–38).
3. It is a fault if in serving or volleying, a front-court player moves into the back court or a back-court player moves into the front court. Players must respect the short service line and stay within their respective courts. At no time during a game is a player allowed to cross the line except as noted in rule 2.

   In triples play, a similar rule can be used to forbid the back-court players from crossing the center line. Before commencing play, the rule should be discussed and voted upon. It is an optional rule which will vary according to the physical ability of the players.

Serving
1. The server has two opportunities to strike the shuttlecock over the net. No fault is scored after the first serve if the shuttlecock falls outside the boundaries of the court (server's side) or passes through or under the net or fails to pass the net.
2. The server is allowed to serve again if he misses the shuttlecock in his first attempt to serve.

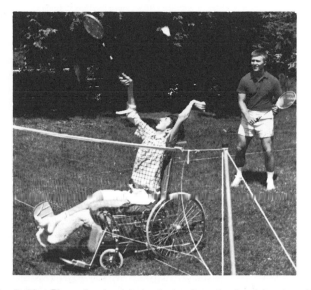

Fig. 7–38. Player in wheelchair playing from the front-court position. Notice that he is using an extension-handle racquet. His able-bodied teammate is playing the back court.

3. The player can serve the shuttlecock to any player on the opposing team.
4. Players assigned to the front court have the option of serving either from the front or back court. (Wheelchair players prefer the front court; crutch players prefer the back court.)

Box Badminton

Box badminton is an adapted game (Fig. 7–37) that shortens the court area for the mobility impaired player. The game is designed to pair an able-bodied player against a disabled competitor who is restricted in movement (wheelchair-user, crutch-user, or those positioned in a standing platform.)

In singles action, the disabled player is positioned in the box court, and is only responsible for returning the shuttlecock if it is hit in that area. The opponent who is mobile is responsible for covering his court (without alterations in dimensions). A fault is called if the player fails to hit the shuttlecock in his opponent's box court. All other regular rules apply to the game.

Assistive Devices

When properly played, badminton requires a great deal of speed, power, and endurance. Some players who are limited by lower- or upper-extremity involvement may be aided by 2 assistive devices.

Amputee Serving Tray. The serving tray enables the unilateral above- or below-elbow amputee to actively use his prosthesis when serving the shuttlecock. The shaft of the tray is grasped firmly with the terminal device; additional support is provided by a forearm control cuff that is molded from thermoplastic to fit the prosthesis. The shuttlecock is placed in the serving tray with the feathers resting in the tray. After adjusting the terminal device so the tray is on a slight angle, the player can release the bird by lifting and rotating his artificial arm. The player uses his unaffected arm to execute the underhand serve stroke.

To make a serving tray, bend a wire coat hanger into the shape of the tray (Fig. 7–39). The wire should be long enough to extend from the control cuff to the tray. Cut off a soup or vegetable can to make a base about 3-inches in diameter with a 1-inch rim. Bend edges of can over wire frame, and solder. An orthotist should then complete the device by fitting the thermoplastic around the wire shaft and control cuff.

Extension-Handle Racquet. In some cases, an extension-handle racquet is helpful for a wheelchair player in the front court. The added length allows the player to reach higher and farther behind his head to return overhead shots (Fig. 7–38).

The device is easy to make: just cut off the handle from an old badminton racquet at the end of the grip and attach it to a regular racquet. The next step is to screw the added handle into the shaft of the regular racquet.

Adjustments for Specific Disabilities

Amputations

Unilateral Upper-Extremity. There are no major problems with this group of amputees. The serving tray assistive device can be worn throughout the game to promote prosthetic awareness skills, and the artificial limb can assist in the development of balance and coordination, particularly when volleying.

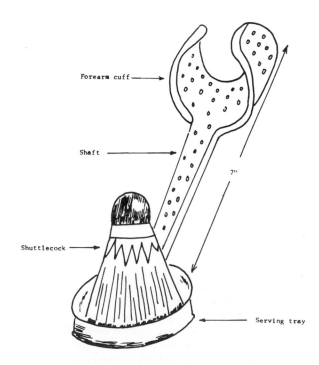

Fig. 7–39. Design of amputee serving tray.

Some amputees can play without their prosthesis while manipulating the shuttlecock and racquet with the non-affected upper-extremity.

Bilateral Upper-Extremity. The main difficulty with players limited by loss of both limbs is their inability to grasp a racquet properly. This and the loss of the serving hand usually rule out participation in badminton. In some situations, however, strapped-on racquets have been used successfully with below-elbow amputees; the racquet is taped or strapped to the residual limb, and the player must build his game plan around his ability to use drop shots.

Unilateral Lower-Extremity. Many below-knee amputees have become proficient badminton players, but above-knee amputees have considerably more difficulty in making the necessary movements. The modified doubles or triples version is recommended for beginners to compensate for their lack of standing balance and tolerance. Box badminton is another alternative. Both groups of amputees (AK and BK) often have difficulty moving backward and using smash and drive strokes when volleying.

Bilateral Lower-Extremity. As mentioned previously, the major problem with players limited by lower-limb amputations is their inability to coordinate footwork and to move rapidly in various directions. Some amputees may prefer to play from a wheelchair. To promote confidence, the instructor should encourage the modified versions of regular badminton, or box badminton.

Chronic Obstructive Lung Disease. Most individuals with chronic lung disease can participate in badminton with minimal difficulty. It is important to watch carefully for signs of early fatigue, particularly outdoors in warm weather. Badminton can be used as a physical conditioning sport and as a means of improving lung ventilation.

Blindness. The blind are unable to play badminton since the shuttlecock travels fast and is noiseless. They can, however, play an adapted version of balloon badminton with a bell inside the balloon. The deficient neuromuscular control of some players causes problems with forward and backward movements.

Cardiovascular Disorders. Medical permission must be obtained before badminton is introduced to cardiac patients. Depending upon the extent of involvement, the game can be used to promote organic efficiency and increase exercise tolerance. Rest periods should be enforced, and, if necessary, the game should be shortened to avoid fatigue. If there are restrictions on ambulation, then the player may play box badminton to prevent fatigue. Doubles or triples play may be recommended to reduce the intensity of the exercise.

Cerebral Palsy. Persons with cerebral palsy have numerous limitations; therefore, the instructor should evaluate the functional skills of each individual before introducing him to the sport of badminton. If he is unable to learn the basic serve strokes, then the game

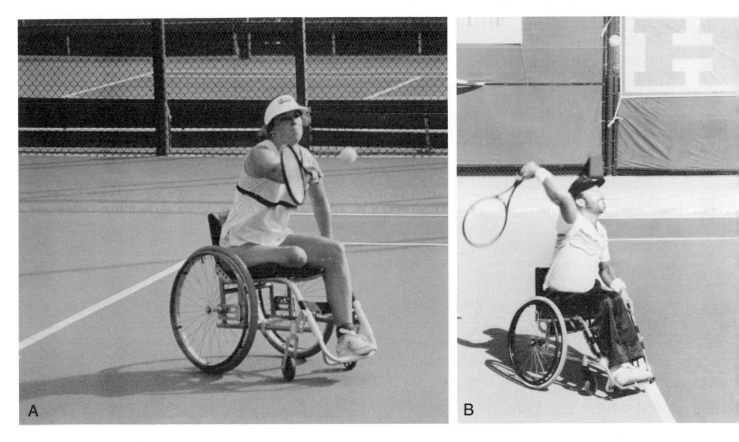

Fig. 7–40.   Two national wheelchair tennis stars demonstrating basic techniques. A. Valerie Wallace using forehand stroke. Note forward weight shift while holding onto the chair for balance. (Photo by Chuck Rorabaugh.) B. Brad Parks (T-11 paraplegic) currently #1 ranked player preparing to serve ball in front of hitting shoulder. (Photo by Wendy Parks.) (Courtesy of National Foundation of Wheelchair Tennis.)

should not be encouraged. Since badminton is a game of concentrated movements, most persons with cerebral palsy will be unable to play because of poor coordination. Instead of playing the regular badminton, low organization serving games may be substituted to allow the player to learn repetitive single response motor skills.

The minimally involved player can usually adapt to regular or modified game situations. Ambulatory players with mild to moderate spasticity will have difficulty shifting weight and rotating the body on the backswing motion.

Head Trauma. The regular game of badminton is fast paced, oftentimes requiring the player to make quick decisions. For some head trauma patients, the game is too fast especially if the player is unable to react spontaneously. Players with visual motor deficits often have difficulty tracking the moving shuttlecock and using proper stroke techniques. In this situation, regular play is not recommended, but adapted serving games such as target badminton (refer to Low Organization Games chapter) may be used. Positional sense in the court area can often be guided by an able-bodied teammate during doubles or triples play. Box badminton is another alternative, especially for the player who has mobility problems, but no major cog-

nitive deficits (refer to Hemiplegia for additional guidelines).

Hemiplegia. Independent ambulation is the ultimate objective of treatment for many hemiplegics. Elevation activities are taught as the patient progresses; therefore, program adjustments will depend upon the degree of involvement. Badminton can be used to help maintain strength in the unaffected side and to contribute to muscle re-education procedures in the affected side. The obvious difficulties in participation are the inability to coordinate footwork and difficulty in the development of serving skills; however, many hemiplegics can use the racquet hand to toss the shuttlecock in the air for serving. The instructor should encourage the player to use his affected arm to serve, provided of course that he can position it properly. Beginners should start with box badminton, or doubles play.

Hip Joint Disorders. The wheelchair-user can play box badminton with an extension-handle racquet. For ambulatory players using an abduction appliance or crutches, safety becomes an important factor. The player must be reminded to play within a specified zone; consequently, he must restrict his movements and the resultant poor balance may interfere with his game skills. To lessen the possibility of falling, modified triples play should be encouraged, and the player should play only in the front court area. Box badminton is another alternative.

Osteogenesis Imperfecta. The ability to execute game skills will depend upon the player's upper-extremity functioning. Limited joint mobility may affect the player's ability to control and manipulate the racquet while attempting to execute various strokes. Some ambulatory players may be able to play without adaptions in equipment or rules.

Overweight and Obesity. Badminton is recommended for obese persons because the energy expenditure in the sport is approximately 400 calories per hour if played vigorously. Many obese players are slow and clumsy in learning the basic badminton strokes and have difficulty bending forward to execute the underhand serve stroke. At the same time they often try to overpower the shuttlecock by using an extended backswing with the racquet. The instructor will usually need to spend a great deal of time teaching obese players the fundamentals of a soft, even, underhand stroke.

Paraplegia. Sitting balance must be carefully evaluated, since the use of various strokes in badminton depends on the ability of the player to shift his weight in the wheelchair. Badminton can help the paraplegic maneuver his wheelchair, strengthen his upper limbs and shoulders. A seat belt or other restraining device around the chest is recommended for players with lesions above the T-9 level. Box badminton is an alternative for some beginners.

Note: Myelomeningocele players (L-4 level with orthotic aids, L-5 and S-1 levels) can often perform adequately from the upright position, provided that their range of mobility is limited to a specified area.

Progressive Muscular Disorders. Badminton is usually not recommended for wheelchair patients with progressive muscle disease. Even ambulatory players with mild involvement have limited range of motion and poor balance, and this interferes with learning the game skills. In most cases, the player will only be able to execute the forehand overhead shot. Relatively independent individuals who ambulate with a mild waddling gait and have lordosis will be able to play low organization serving games, provided that shoulder girdle strength is sufficient. The instructor should watch for signs of early fatigue.

Rheumatoid Arthritis. Considerable wrist and elbow motion is required in the game of badminton; therefore, each individual with rheumatoid arthritis must be evaluated. The sport requires quick reversal movements, so it is imperative that the instructor take precautions to prevent further pain or damage to the involved joints. A patient requiring minimal medical management should be able to play the game without adaptations, provided that he knows his tolerance for uninterrupted activity.

Quadriplegia. Involvement of all 4 limbs limits high level SCI players, however, badminton may be played by low level quads using grip gloves or other racquet adaptations similar to tennis.

Abnormal Posture. Treatment for structural scoliosis is directed toward straightening the spine and stabilizing it in the corrected position. Because of the rigidity of the back and limitation in neck motion, players wearing Milwaukee braces have problems executing the underhand serve and drop shots. Players wearing orthoplast jackets should have no difficulty playing badminton. Badminton is recommended for balance training and stretching of the muscles of the upper torso. Postspinal fusion patients can play box badminton during the early rehabilitation period.

WHEELCHAIR TENNIS

There has been tremendous growth in the sport of wheelchair tennis since its inception in 1976. Today more than 6,000 competitors from many states and countries have actively participated in the sport. The National Foundation of Wheelchair Tennis was founded in 1980 with the purpose of educating, promoting, fostering and developing the sport of wheelchair tennis. This has been accomplished through instructional clinics, exhibitions and competitive tournaments for disabled adults and children and sports camps for disabled children 7 to 18 years of age. Now there are five divisions of competition (from Open for the most talented players to "D" division for novice players for men, and three divisions for women). There are also junior divisions for under 18 years and a Quad division for persons with impairments in the upper extremities.

Wheelchair mobility is an important aspect of the sport. The player should maintain the grip on the racquet while moving the chair into position for a shot. Practice in wheelchair mobility is essential, even for the novice player. Mobility practice should encourage starting from the ready position. This is the position you should assume just before your opponent strikes the ball. In wheelchair tennis, this position is facing the net, with the hands on the wheels and ready to propel the chair in the desired direction.

Wheelchair positioning is learned through practice. The player must predict the flight and bounce of the ball and then move the wheelchair in the right position as well as getting the racquet back to stroke the ball (Fig. 7–40A). This is complicated even further by the fact that lateral movement is difficult. The player needs to judge angles to which the wheelchair must be positioned to compensate for reduced mobility. The ability to perform quick turns is also important. This skill is often necessary after hitting a backhand stroke, and then turning to position toward center court.

Equipment

Regular tennis equipment (racquet and balls) can be used. A hard surface court with regular dimensions is recommended. Mobility is enhanced with a wheelchair that is lightweight with a low or adjustable center of gravity.

Quadriplegics and others with limited grip strength may use The Sport Grip: Orthotic Racquet Holder.* It must be custom molded by an orthotist for each individual, and molding instructions are obtainable from the distributing company.

Rule Modifications. There are only a few modifications from the standard rules of tennis. One major change is the allowance for two bounces of the tennis ball prior to its return over the net. As in the United States Tennis Association Rules Book, following a serve the ball must land in the service court initially, on the return the second bounce can be inside or outside the basic court markings. The reason for the two bounce rule is on short shots and drop shots the player must be able to have a realistic chance to return the ball. Except for during the serve, the player has the option of playing the ball in the air (volley), on one bounce or following the second bounce. During the service, the server must keep the back wheels of the wheelchair behind the service line until contact with the ball has been made. Otherwise it is a wheel fault. Quadriplegic players may have someone bounce the ball for them to initiate the bounce serve.

Balance is an important tehnique to learn especially on the serve because recovery from the forward thrust is difficult. Drill exercises in ball tossing are especially helpful to establish a neuromuscular pattern. Players who demonstrate balance problems can start the serving motion with the racquet back in the strike position. This will allow the player to grasp the side of the chair before hitting the ball (Fig. 7–40B). When playing tennis from a wheelchair, there should be a weight shift in the trunk from back to front during the contact portion of the swing. During the weight shift stage, if balance is a problem, the player should maintain body control by holding onto the knee or side of the wheelchair.

Fundamental skills and techniques regarding the grips, service, strokes, and strategy will not be discussed and readers are encouraged to contact the National Foundation of Wheelchair Tennis for further information.

QUAD TENNIS

Low level quads (C-6, C-7, and C-8) have the potential to play tennis. The main concern is how to grip the racquet. Some players use an elastic bandage and others simply tape the hand to the racquet. Another alternative is to use the Sport Grip orthosis. It provides for a firm grip on the racquet, and there is a rubber pad for added traction to propel the wheelchair. However, it is impossible to alternate forehand and backhand strokes once the assistive device is ap-

*Contact Access to Recreation, 2509 E. Thousand Oaks Blvd., Suite 430, Thousand Oaks, CA 91362 for further information.

plied. Consequently the attachment must be positioned for either a backhand or forehand stroke.

Quad tennis is somewhat slower than the game that is played by those with good upper-body strength, but it still involves using strategy and is just as competitive. An overhand serve is difficult to perform, thus most players use a bounce-drop serve.

BOWLING

In various forms, games like bowling have been played for thousands of years. One of the first countries to introduce a sport similar to modern bowling was Germany in the early 1300s. The Germans rolled or threw stones at wooden clubs called *kegels*, and bowlers today are still often called keglers. The Dutch introduced bowling to America when they founded New Amsterdam in the 1600s. The American Bowling Congress (ABC), which was organized in 1895, is still the major governing body of the sport.

The object of the game is to roll a ball down a lane so that it knocks down 10 wooden pins. A game consists of 10 frames. Each bowler rolls his ball twice in each frame, unless he scores a strike (knocks down all 10 pins on the first ball). The bowler who has the highest score at the end of 10 frames is declared the winner.

Tenpin bowling is the standard and most popular version of the game in the United States. Duckpin bowling, a variation using smaller pins and balls, is played mainly in the eastern United States.

Adapted for the Physically Disabled

Bowling for the physically disabled began soon after World War II in Veterans Administration hospitals; at first, the sport was particularly popular with paraplegics and amputees. Bowling for the more severely disabled was not widely accepted until the late 1950s when certain assistive devices were introduced for those with muscle weakness and upper-extremity involvement. Wheelchair bowling, conducted in accordance with American Bowling Congress rules, was formally introduced in the National Wheelchair Games in New York in 1957. It is no longer an event in the National Wheelchair Games, but is recommended for regional or invitational meets. The American Wheelchair Bowling Association, Inc. (AWBA), which was formed in 1962, has established uniform rules and regulations to govern wheelchair bowling. The AWBA holds National Wheelchair Bowling Tournaments in various areas of the country each year. Bowling for the blind originated in the New York and Philadelphia areas; the first tournament was held in 1948. The American Blind Bowling Association, which was organized in 1951, is the official sanctioning organization for blind bowling leagues in the United States and Canada.

Today bowling is one of the most popular indoor sports for the disabled because it can be enjoyed by almost everyone, regardless of the extent of physical disability. The sport is a lifetime sport with great therapeutic potential. It is also widely accepted as a clinical sport (Fig. 7–41). It requires poise, balance, accuracy, synchronization of movements of the upper and lower parts of the body, and maximization of gravity utilized to produce force. It can be an interesting way to develop body awareness; to strengthen muscles in the arms, legs, and trunk; and to improve coordination and body control.

Equipment

All ambulatory bowlers should wear special bowling shoes and loose, nonconfining clothing.

The following specifications of the ABC govern bowling equipment:

1. Ball: Bowling balls range in weight from 8 to 16 pounds. Each has 3 holes in which the bowler places the 2 middle fingers and thumb. The thumb hole should be comfortably loose; the finger holes comfortably snug.
2. Pins: The height is 15 inches; the diameter at the base, 2¼ inches. The pins are set in a 3-foot triangle; each is 12 inches from the nearest pins measuring from center to center.

Techniques

Ambulatory Bowlers

The instructions given are for a right-handed bowler; for a left-handed bowler, the procedures should be reversed.

1. Pendulum swing: The fundamental movement of bowling is the pendulum swing. The bowler stands behind the foul line with the left foot slightly ahead of the right; both feet are straight and about 4 to 6 inches apart. The player stoops over, his feet in position, and fully extends the arm, with the ball hanging like a pendulum. He leans forward, bends his knees slightly, and starts the pendulum motion by swinging the arm slightly and down straight, then far back, then forward.
2. Release: The ball should be released on the forward swing, just over the foul line. The bowler concentrates on keeping the thumb pointed forward. If the ball curves left or right into the gutter, the next ball should be directed at an angle which compensates for the curve.
3. Delivery: Methods for stepping up to the foul line before rolling the ball down the alley vary, but most bowlers use the 4 step delivery or approach. The starting point is usually about 12 feet behind the foul line, but this will vary considerably for ambulatory bowlers who have lower-extremity involvement. A relaxed stance is taken at the starting point with the ball held slightly above the waist. The approach rhythm is right-left-right-slide. On the first step (right foot), the ball is carried forward and down to the side. As the left foot comes forward the ball

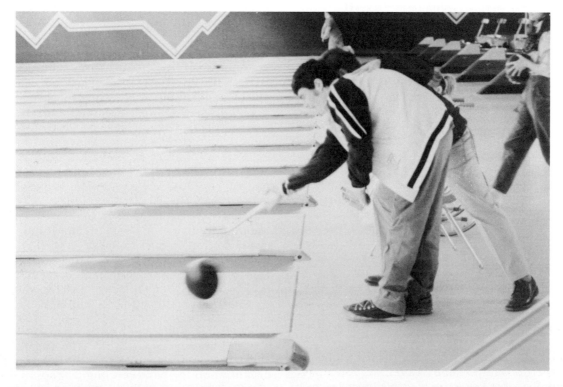

Fig. 7–41. This 17-year-old bowler with left hemiplegia secondary to a cerebrovascular accident is in a position of guarded assistance with the instructor. Although the bowler was able to release the ball independently, he was unable to take a step approach due to balance problems. In this situation, the therapist was required to assist by giving tactile and proprioceptive cues to aid positional sense. (Note wrist lock, and arm position on bowler's back.)

is swung back, and as the right foot comes forward the ball reaches the top of the backswing. The bowler then goes into a slide on the left foot and starts the forward downswing and release.

Guarded Assistance and Ambulatory Bowlers with Balance Problems

With guarded assistance, the bowler releases the ball independently but with questionable safety so that someone is present and ready to give support. In some situations, an able-bodied assistant may need to stand next to the ambulatory bowler and assist with balance. Other support measures can include giving proprioceptive input (compressing the spine so the bowler remains in crouch position) and/or assist with the arm swing motion (apply pressure to the bowler's wrist to prevent it from turning) (Fig. 7–41).

Poor stability forces caused by ataxia, muscle weakness, hemiplegia, etc. will often interfere with the bowler making weight shifts and performing the arm swing motion. This can occur even though the bowler may be wearing a lower-limb orthotic device. Some bowlers will be able to take a step, and release the ball with the opposite side throwing arm. Others, with more pronounced balance problems, will be unable to bear stable weight on the affected side. For example, right-handed bowlers with left-side involvement will prefer to bowl while stepping off the right leg. Some bowlers because of instability problems will be unable to use a step approach, consequently motion and swing control will be limited.

Wheelchair Bowlers

Most wheelchair bowlers prefer to use balls that weigh approximately 10 pounds.

The way in which a wheelchair-user rolls the ball is the same as the way the ambulatory bowler does, except that the step approach is eliminated. Bowlers who use a wheelchair but have good upper-extremity strength will follow the procedures for the pendulum swing and release already described.

If the wheelchair is not equipped with a removable arm rest, then a seat cushion should be used to raise the bowler and enable him to swing his arm comfortably when delivering the ball. The wheelchair should be positioned so that the front pedals are 2 to 4 inches behind the foul line. Either the brakes must be applied before bowling or an assistant must hold the wheelchair steady so that it does not move as the bowler releases the ball. The bowler must lean over the side of the wheelchair to permit his arm to swing freely when delivering the ball. A preliminary swing often helps him balance himself and aim the ball before the actual throw.

The wheelchair bowler can sometimes retrieve the ball from the ball-return rack without assistance and carry the ball on his lap when returning to position at the foul line. In some instances, an assistant may be required to retrieve the ball. The bowler can also use a ball holder to carry the ball from the return rack back to the foul line.

Ramp "Chute" Bowling

The ramp has become an integral part of the specialized bowling equipment used by those with severe limitations. The ramps are designed so that the bowler has the advantage of remaining in a stationary position and has only to push the ball down the ramp for delivery (Fig. 7–42). An able-bodied assistant, however, is usually needed to retrieve the bowling ball

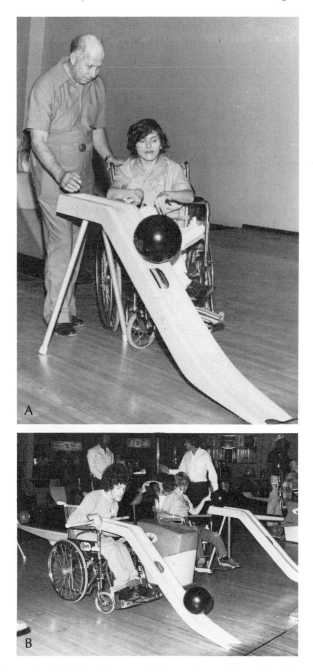

Fig. 7–42. Bowling Booster. *A,* Conventional side position lineup; *B,* Ramp modified for support on the wheelchair arms. (Photograph courtesy of R & B Products.)

from the ball return rack. Some bowlers can move the ramp when aiming at certain pins, but others will need to give verbal directions to the assistant during this phase of the game. The AWBA does not allow ramp bowling in national tournament competition, because the rules maintain that a bowler must apply his own force and direction when delivering the ball. However, ramp bowling is a popular and enjoyable recreation activity for persons who are severely limited by upper- and lower-extremity involvement.

Heavier balls work best on ramps. Balls with finger holes need to be carefully positioned (usually so the holes are slightly off center). The bowler should push from behind the ball (not on top) to achieve a true roll down the ramp. Trial and error with different balls is usually necessary until a desirable and consistent roll is achieved.

Chute bowlers, like stick bowlers, have the advantage of using an undrilled bowling ball. With the proper understanding and control of the ball's weight block, the smooth, unblemished surface makes for an especially true roll. As is also the case with stick bowling, chute bowling requires more time on the part of the bowler, and more tolerance from other bowlers on the same lanes.*

Stick Bowling

This form of bowling is designed for persons with upper-extremity involvement who have difficulty gripping a ball. The bowling stick, a device similar to a shuffleboard stick, is usually made from rigid alu-

---

*Lane, J. and Schoof, D.: Wheelchair Bowling, Huntington Beach, CA: Wheelchair Bowlers of Southern California.

minum (Fig. 7–43). The bowler fully controls the device, but an able-bodied assistant usually must lift the ball from the ball return rack. The AWBA does approve stick bowling in AWBA sanctioned national tournament competition because the bowler applies his own force and direction when delivering the ball.

Assistive Devices

Obviously, many physically disabled persons, particularly those with upper-limb involvement, would not be able to bowl without assistive devices. Various types of adapted equipment have been developed in recent years.

Bowling Ball Holder-Ring.† This device provides a third hand for the wheelchair-user. The holder-ring is made of $\frac{3}{8}$-inch diameter steel and is easily attached to the arm of most wheelchairs (Fig. 7–44). The device holds the ball while the bowler pushes up to the foul line to bowl. The result is added safety, because the wheelchair-user need no longer place the ball in his lap while maneuvering his wheelchair up the approach lane.

Bowling Booster.‡ The booster is 30 inches high, and can be placed in front of, or alongside, a bowler (see Fig. 7–42). This device has a number of positive features: it is made of lightweight fiberglass (weighing approximately 15 lbs.) which makes it easy to carry from place to place, and the legs can be removed and inserted into clips inside the ramp, which also makes

---

†Available from George Snyder, 5809 N.E. 21st Avenue, Fort Lauderdale, Florida 33308.

‡Available from R & B Products, 6943 Bittersweet Drive, Pensacola, Florida 32506.

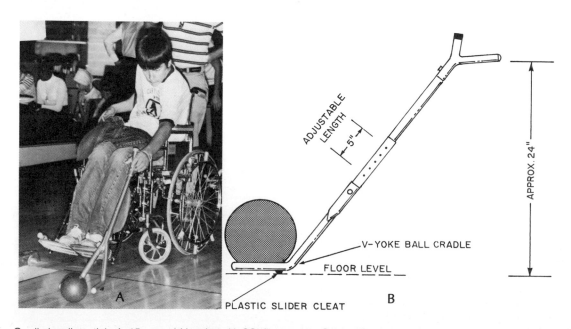

Fig. 7–43.   Cradle bowling stick. A, 15-year-old bowler with SCI (incomplete C-6 level) using bowling stick made from rigid aluminum tubing to push duckpin ball down the lane. The bowler had wrist extensor function, but no finger or thumb motion of the right hand, and only some finger flexors and extensors on the left. (Note the Velcro strap encircling the hand to stabilize the stick.) Essentially, the bowler applied his own force and direction when delivering the ball. B, Schematic drawing.

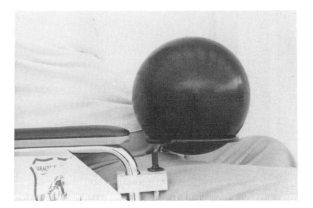

Fig. 7–44.   Bowling ball holder-ring.

for easy carrying. In addition, the central groove is designed to accommodate both tenpin and duckpin balls. The mechanics for using the device are the same as those for the Bowling Frame Unit.

Bowling Frame Unit. * This device was developed for persons with little or no use of their arms. With the bowling frame centered in front of the lane, a severely disabled person can bowl without lifting the ball. An assistant places the ball on the highest point of the frame. The bowler need only push the ball slightly for it to roll down the frame toward the bowling pins. The unit is not commercially available, but it may be duplicated by anyone who wishes to do so (Fig. 7–45).

Smaller tubular ramps can be purchased that can be disassembled for easy storage and transportation.

Bowling Attachment for Amputees. † This device has a neoprene expansion sleeve at the end which is compressed by a spring and can be caused to expand. When the control cable pulls on the "thumb," the sleeve is stretched and becomes thinner. The firm grip inside the bowling ball finger hole is released by the same action used to open a conventional hook and is almost a natural action in bowling.

Bowling Cues (Stick/Pushers). Various types of bowling cues, sometimes called "sticks" or "pushers," are available from distributors or can be custom made by each bowler to suit his own needs. Some have plastic or Teflon non-skid skis on the bottom while other models have wheels. This device provides compensation for the bowler who has upper-extremity involvement and/or loss of grip strength. Other adjustable cues easily adjust in length for use by either sitting or standing bowlers. However, a tenpin ball will not fit firmly into the "belly" of some devices. Therefore, an assistant often must hold the ball in position until the bowler starts the push-off phase or delivery motion. Strap-on pushers are used mostly by persons who have weak grip strength and lost finger flexion move-

ments. The important thing to remember is that the bowler must apply his own force and direction when delivering the ball.

The Cradle Bowling Stick‡ (Fig. 7–43B) is used by bowlers with insufficient tricep muscle strength and weak shoulder girdle muscles. Two motions are required to propel the ball with the stick: first, a forward push, then a lifting motion. The stick can be used for duckpin or tenpin bowling.

Adapter-Pusher Device. The adapter-pusher device was originally designed for the wheelchair-user bowling with upper extremity strength insufficient for lifting the ball (Fig. 7–46). The adapter-pusher can be used in two positions. In the front position, the device is positioned directly in front of the wheelchair, and the bowler uses both hands on the handle to push the ball down the lane. In the side position, which is preferred, the device is used with one hand at the side of the wheelchair.

The instructor will need to assist the bowler by retrieving the ball from the return rack and placing it in the "face" (front) of the pusher. He must then steady it until the bowler gives the command, "Let go." At this instant, the bowler pushes the ball down the lane by extending his arm forward, remembering to keep a firm grip on the handle when completing the follow through motion.

Handlebar-Extension Accessory. The handlebar-extension accessory (Fig. 7–46C) is used with the adapter-pusher device by ambulatory bowlers who are unable to lift the ball. It can be attached to the handle of the adapter-pusher device by fitting a piece of wood into the aluminum shaft. The accessory can be removed to allow wheelchair-users to bowl with the same pusher. The device has been used most frequently by bowlers with limited hand function such as arthritics and post-burn patients.

The device is made from ⅜-inch pipe. An L-shaped pipe fitting is used to attach the stabilizer to the shaft, and a T-shaped pipe fitting is used to attach the handlebar to the shaft. The wooden handlebar is made from a 1-inch dowel with holes drilled to fit the ⅜-inch pipe.

Handle Grip Bowling Ball. § This unique bowling ball has a built-in handle that snaps back instantly upon release (Fig. 7–47). It is ideal for bowlers who have upper-extremity involvement and for those who have difficulty with digital control (e.g., spasticity and ataxia). It is available in 10, 12, 14, or 16 pound models, and is approved by the ABC for competitive play (apply in writing to the ABC).

---

*Designed by Abilitics, Inc., Human Resources Center, Albertson, Long Island, New York.

†A Hosmer Dorrance product that is available from any certified prosthetic facility.

‡The Cradle Bowling Stick can be purchased from P & Q Lifts, Inc., 1457 63 Circle North, Pinellas Park, Florida 33565.

§M.L. Betric Co., P.O. Box 690, South Orange, N.J. 07079 and Flaghouse, Inc., 150 No. MacQuesten Pkwy., Mt. Vernon, NY 10550.

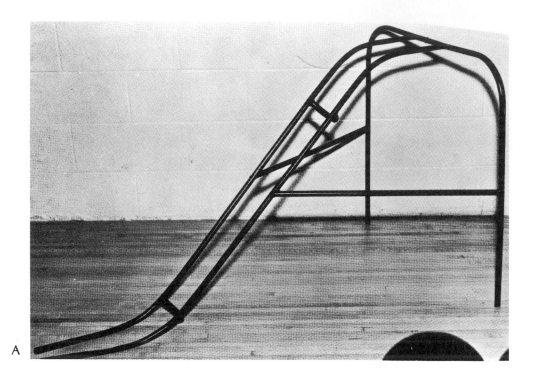

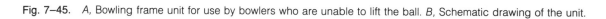

Fig. 7–45.   *A*, Bowling frame unit for use by bowlers who are unable to lift the ball. *B*, Schematic drawing of the unit.

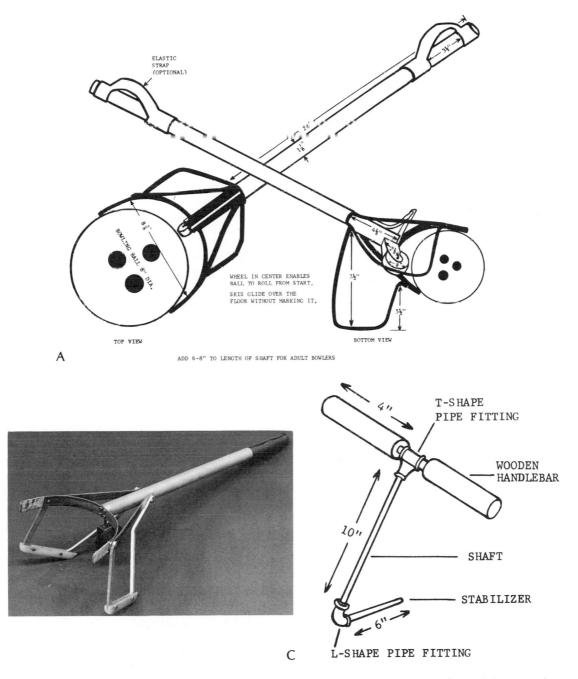

Fig. 7–46.   Adapter-pusher device for the bowler in a wheelchair. *A*, Schematic diagram. *B*, Photograph. *C*, Handlebar-extension accessory.

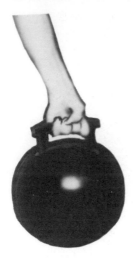

Fig. 7–47. Handle-grip bowling ball.

Adjustments for Specific Disabilities

Amputations

Unilateral Upper-Extremity. Generally, this group of amputees can bowl with little or no difficulty. The bowler can use the terminal device for help in holding the ball above his waist at the starting position. This position is recommended because it promotes concentration and relaxation prior to starting the approach. It is suggested that the bowler wear his prosthesis while bowling because it can assist in the development of balance and coordination during the approach and delivery. Amputee bowlers can also use the Hosmer/Dorrance attachment if they prefer to use their prosthetic limb when throwing the ball.

Unilateral Lower-Extremity. Some unilateral lower-extremity amputees prefer to bowl from a stationary position at the foul line, while others prefer to use a 2- or 4-step approach. In most instances, the steps they take are shorter than those taken by the normal bowler. This group tends to turn their left foot perpendicular to the line of approach when releasing the ball, thus causing an incorrect swing and follow-through to the right. Another common problem, particularly with above-knee amputees, is difficulty in achieving a smooth approach. The first 2 steps are often too fast and followed by an abrupt stop at the foul line and a jerky back-swing.

Bilateral Upper-Extremity. Those with standard, bilateral above-elbow amputations can possibly use the handlebar-extension bowling ball pusher. The bowler naturally needs to grasp the handlebar firmly in order to control the movement of the ball properly. The instructor will have to evaluate shoulder strength to determine the possible benefits and problems from the flexion-extension movements required to use the device. The Hosmer/Dorrance bowling attachment is another device recommended for bilateral upper-extremity amputees.

The more severely involved, particularly those using shoulder-disarticulation prostheses, can bowl with the assistance of bowling ramps.

Bilateral Lower-Extremity. As mentioned previously, the major problem with bowlers who are limited by lower-limb amputations is the inability to achieve rhythm during the approach. This difficulty is often caused by a tendency to hesitate after one of the steps. Usually, bilateral lower-extremity bowlers prefer to use the stationary position, although some bowl from wheelchairs to compensate for their inability to coordinate footwork and arm swing.

Chronic Obstructive Lung Disease. Many individuals with chronic obstructive lung disease have a low exercise tolerance level and cannot participate in uninterrupted exercise. Bowling is a sport that provides intermittent exercise and rest periods. Furthermore, in most cases it does not impede normal ventilation. Its therapeutic values include improvement in ventilation by increasing the rate and depth of respiration to meet the increased oxygen consumption. Special adaptations are generally not needed for this group.

Therapeutic Note: Some children and adolescents with chronic obstructive lung disease show poor growth increments and are unable to perform in strength related sports. However, body size and muscle strength are not imposing factors in bowling. For this reason, the sport is often recommended for persons with restricted energy outputs.

Blindness. Members of the American Blind Bowlers Association are eligible to belong to Area Blind Bowling Associations. An ABBA league definition is one that has four or more teams, blind and sighted, that bowl on a regular schedule, and maintain averages for each bowler.

The beginning blind bowler should first learn the pendulum swing from a stationary position at the foul line. A guide rail (Fig. 7–48) is often used to help the bowler locate the proper starting point by crooking his elbow over the rail.* The guide rail is positioned so that as the ball hangs at the side of the bowler in his delivery hand it is in direct line with the center of the lane. Once the guide rail has been positioned at that point, it should not be moved for the remainder of the game. Blind bowlers usually use a 2- or 3-step approach followed by a straight ball delivery. In the ABBA National Blind Bowling Championship Tournament, 15-foot guide rails are the standard rails with the option of using a 12-foot rail.

The totally blind bowler is dependent upon a sighted assistant to tell him which pins are still standing after the first ball. Once he knows, he can adjust his starting point in relation to the guide rail. The distance of the sidestep to the proper starting position for the second ball is learned through practice with the aid of an assistant.

---

*Further information may be obtained from the American Foundation for the Blind, 15 W. 16th St., New York, New York 10011.

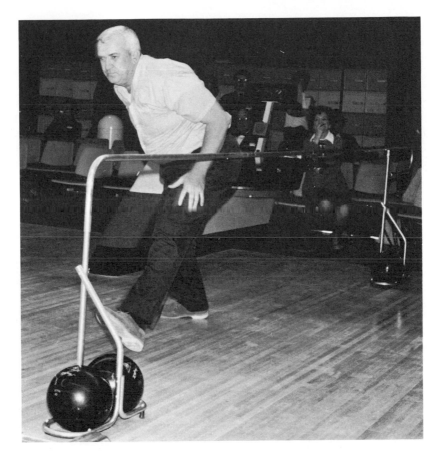

Fig. 7–48.   Blind bowler using a guide rail.

Cardiovascular Disorders. Permission should be obtained from the physician before a cardiac patient participates in bowling. If the sport is part of a graded exercise regimen, then the major objectives would be (1) to increase general physical and heart-muscle strength and (2) to obtain the psychologic benefits of participation in a lifetime sport. Individuals whose physical activity is markedly restricted may bowl from a sitting position. Careful watch should be kept for signs of fatigue and dyspnea, and all activity should be stopped at the onset of any symptoms of circulatory embarrassment.

The cardiac rehabilitation patient needs to achieve attainable goals. From a physical fitness viewpoint, bowling is a sport that offers short bursts of energy followed by a brief rest period, thus cardiorespiratory endurance is low. Because of this, the sport is safe and work tolerance levels can be monitored closely by the participant.

Cerebral Palsy. As most persons with cerebral palsy have numerous limitations, the program leader should evaluate the total intellectual and motor capacities of the patient before introducing him to bowling. Spastic patients will have exaggerated stretch-reflex movements which will cause problems in learning the basic maneuvers. Repetitive practice of the bowling fundamentals is helpful. If the individual is severely affected and unable to develop the initial pendulum-swing skill, it may be necessary to provide an assistive device. Those with athetosis will naturally be limited in their participation; however, bowling ramps can be used to compensate for their involuntary jerky movements. An assistant will need to lift the ball from the ball-return rack and adjust the bowling ramp according to the verbal instructions of the bowler.

Therapeutic Note: The handle grip bowling ball is useful to some spastic bowlers, because the device minimizes the motions of the contracted flexor muscles, and digital placement is less important than with a regular ball. However, the weight of the ball coupled with the excessive leaning away from midline can produce excessive muscle tone in some bowlers, and is obviously contraindicated.

Ambulatory bowlers with balance problems such as those with moderate-severe involvement of one or both legs may need to sit and bowl from a standard chair. Others prefer to stand while holding onto a support system (straightback chair, guide rail) with the non-throwing hand.

Head Trauma. The ability to bowl will be dependent on a number of factors. Some head trauma bowlers will be wheelchair-users while others will be ambulatory. Most important, however, the bowler should be capable of goal directed behavior with some basic problem solving skills. Bowling is somewhat repetitious. There is not a lot of shifting from one concept to another, or unpredictable changes, and from this standpoint is often suggested for some head trauma patients who need to develop basic motor planning skills. Balance and equilibrium reactions will need to be assessed for some ambulatory bowlers. Adapted devices may be needed depending upon the degree of motor involvement.

Visual perceptual deficits may cause problems for bowlers limited by right hemisphere damage. Those with visual field disturbances and visual spatial deficits may not be suitable candidates for bowling.

Hemiplegia. Program adjustments for hemiplegics will depend upon the degree of affliction. The usual problem is the inability to coordinate footwork with swing. The handlebar-extension bowling accessory is recommended in clinical bowling as a means of providing the bowler with body-awareness exercise. He can develop bimanual skills by using the affected arm as an assist, while using the unaffected arm as the main force. Assistive devices should be kept to a minimum because most hemiplegics can adapt to the sport of bowling from a stationary position. In fact, many hemiplegics prefer to bowl from the stationary position, because it eliminates the effects of a jerky and unbalanced moving approach. Guarded assistance bowling from the standing position is another alternative (Fig. 7–42).

Hip Joint Disorders. Treatment procedures within this group will vary somewhat, although restriction of weight-bearing is recommended during a portion of the treatment period. Some patients using crutches can bowl from a standing position, using only one crutch for support while freeing the dominant throwing hand. Bowlers with precarious standing balance skills should obviously bowl from a sitting position. Those with medical permission to bowl from a wheelchair will experience fewer problems: however, before they begin bowling, the therapist should evaluate sitting tolerance, realize the anatomic limitations, and then remain within the bounds of safety.

Note of Caution: Bowlers using abduction appliances will have considerably more difficulty because of their problems in establishing the relationship between weight transfer and balance in a synchronized fashion. The bowler must stabilize his position so that the pendulum swing is smooth and in a straight line with the desired direction of force.

Some bowlers using the Scottish Rite orthosis have used a 2-hand, between-the-leg release. Other bowlers who use this type of appliance prefer to stand, but use a ramp to substitute for their inability to coordinate a smooth release motion.

Osteogenesis Imperfecta. Wheelchair bowlers will frequently compete in ramp bowling due to generalized weakness and involvement of the throwing arm. Ambulatory bowlers will need to be assessed on an individual basis regarding basic techniques, although many prefer to use regular 8 or 10 pound balls or the handle grip ball. Bowlers with moderately reduced function in the throwing arm will need to use a short pendulum swing on the delivery motion.

Overweight and Obesity. Energy expenditure in bowling is approximately 350 calories per hour; consequently, it is a recommended physical activity for obese persons, provided that they do it consistently, without continual rest periods. Bowlers limited by morbid obesity often lack rhythmic approaches, because they lack joint flexibility. Most beginners prefer to use a 6- or 8-step approach to compensate for their inability to take long strides, but this approach usually increases the jerkiness of the delivery.

Also, this group has a tendency to use excessive power while forcing the delivery of a lightweight ball. For this reason, heavier balls are often suggested to overcome this problem.

Paraplegia. Sitting balance must be evaluated carefully, since the bowler must develop a comfortable arm-swing motion while leaning over the side of the wheelchair. Some beginners tend to use a high backswing and this causes the ball to hit the hand rim of the wheelchair during the forward swing. If the ball is swung too high, the momentum of the forward swing can throw the bowler off balance and cause an improper follow-through. With sufficient practice, bowling is an excellent sport to develop stability and body balance. In some situations, assistive devices may be needed. The bowling ball holder-ring is a useful piece of equipment for this group of bowlers.

Progressive Muscular Disorders. In most instances, this group of patients will be unable to throw an 8- to 10-pound bowling ball because of the lack of arm and shoulder strength. Bowling pushers are not usually recommended, because wheelchair patients cannot generate enough force to push the ball down the lane with any degree of speed or accuracy. This problem is also prevalent among those who ambulate with a waddling gait and who have lordosis. In the majority of these cases, the bowling ramp is the most suitable device to use.

Quadriplegia. In order to participate in bowling, persons with high cervical lesions may need to use a bowling ramp. Many patients with lesions at the C-6 or C-7 level have used various types of assistive appliances and bowling-pusher devices. Different kinds of straps have also been used to attach the bowler's hand firmly to the handle of the adapter-pusher. The program leader should evaluate the sitting balance of each participant and use a seat belt for those persons with nonfunctioning trunk muscles. The handle grip bowling ball is recommended for bowlers with low cervical lesions. The cradle bowling stick is another useful assistive device.

Rheumatoid Arthritis. The ability of the arthritic to bowl depends upon the severity of the disease and the joints affected. Those with fingers joint involvement may not be able to assume a conventional grip or tolerate the external pressure imposed by the weight of a bowling ball. Some arthritics have used special drilled balls with 5 fingers holes, but they are not recommended unless approved by a physician. The handle grip ball is an alternative is some cases. In addition to arm strength, the ability to learn basic bowling techniques will depend upon the available range of motion at the shoulder, elbow, and wrist joints. Persons with more serious forms of arthritis will need to use a handlebar-extension pusher or ramp.

Abnormal Posture. Bowlers wearing a spinal orthosis often have difficulty bending at the waist and making a comfortable knee bend to achieve the full swing motion of the arm and shoulder. It is important to create a low center of gravity to compensate for a lack of a flexible back. Because of this, maintenance of good body control has excellent therapeutic implications for brace/jacket wearers.

Postspinal fusion patients will demonstrate similar problems and need to be evaluated on an individual basis. The person undergoing treatment for kyphosis may be allowed to bowl with his friends if he chooses to do so, but he should be made aware of and encouraged to participate in sports and recreational activities that have greater therapeutic value for his particular condition. This is especially important if the individual is not wearing a brace or jacket for treatment.

Undernutrition. It is important to review the therapeutic values that can be derived for each case before enrolling the individual in the sport of bowling. If the cause of the undernutrition is psychogenic, then participation in group activities may be a useful social stimulant. In general, the major problem will be the inability of the bowler to throw an 8- to 10-pound ball because of lack of strength. The handlebar-extension adapter-pusher device or adjustable length cue can be used for ambulatory participants in this category, but this sometimes only magnifies a fragile self-image as the device can be interpreted as a physical aid.

Therapeutic Note: Frequently, bowling has been used as a stimulus for good postural control and to increase endurance in the upright position. This often has specific relevance for those with undernutrition, who are limited in their ability to sustain minimal amounts of low to moderate intensity exercise.

Duckpin Bowling

Duckpin bowling is often described as the "little pin" game, because a regulation duckpin only measures $9^{13}/_{32}$ inches high. The duckpin ball has no finger holes and weighs slightly more than 3 pounds. The National Duckpin Bowling Congress located in Washington, D.C. is the governing body of the sport.

Unlike tenpin bowling, a player is allowed 3 balls per frame, except when he makes a strike or a spare. If all pins are knocked down with one ball (a strike), the player is finished for that frame. If a spare is made (all pins knocked down with 2 balls), the player does not take his third ball. Strikes and spares are scored the same way they are in tenpin bowling. If all 10 pins are knocked down on the third ball, 10 points are awarded for that frame.

Program Notes

Duckpin bowling is especially attractive to the physically disabled. The main difference between tenpin and duckpin bowling lies in the weight of the bowling ball. The duckpin bowling ball is lightweight and easy to handle, thus the strength of the bowler does not determine the skill of the bowler. The ease and ability to perform the physical requirements of the sport contribute to the security and independence of the participant. This is especially important for players confined to special appliances and mobility aids (wheelchairs, crutches, and standing appliances). For ambulatory players, the lightweight ball is advantageous because it does not overload one side of the body. This is especially important for individuals with unilateral defects (stroke hemiplegia, cerebral palsy hemiplegia, and such temporary orthopedic problems as confinement of a limb in a cast postfracture). Generally, body alignment and support balance are not adversely affected during the execution of throwing from the upright position. As a result, the bowler can analyze the positioning of his body segments in detail without straining or exerting too much force on his lower back, leg, or throwing arm.

Program adjustments for specific disabilities are generally the same as those for tenpin bowling. It is important to point out that not all assistive devices are designed for use in both tenpin bowling and duckpin bowling.

Case History: E.Z. was a likeable, athletically inclined young teenager who excelled in duckpin bowling (106 average, and a high single award winning game of the season with a score of 156). Tragedy struck suddenly when she lost complete control of her left side and her speech and sight were affected. Extensive tests revealed that she had a malformed blood vessel which had ruptured, causing blood to collect in her brain. Two operations were required to remove the blood and repair the ruptured vessel.

A duckpin bowler since the age of 9, E.Z. was determined to overcome adversity and return to the sport she loved so much. A few months after her illness, E.Z. started practicing while using a walker for balance support and a brace on her left leg. Her coach assisted her by handing her balls as required, resetting the pins, and assisting her to and from her seat. E.Z. progressed steadily, eventually dispensing with her walker, but still requiring a leg brace and special shoes (Fig. 7–49). Although the use of her left hand was limited, she returned to league bowling and during the first season following her illness, she averaged a score of 83 and bowled a 302 set in the Connecticut State Junior Tournament.

In her third season, while using a moving approach, despite a leg brace and special shoes, E.Z. earned various "Bowler of the Week" honors while scoring 136 and 146 in

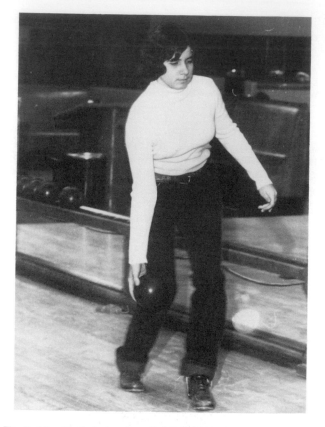

Fig. 7–49. Duckpin bowler with left-side hemiplegia participating in Youth Duckpin Bowling Association League.

games and 332 and 349 in series. It is obvious that her will to overcome her handicap and pursue her love for duckpin bowling are feats of extraordinary determination.

FLOOR (COSOM) HOCKEY

Ice hockey, Canada's national sport, has been traced to games of field hockey that British troops played on frozen lakes and ponds in Ontario and Nova Scotia in the late 1800s. The sport has been an official Olympic game since 1920. Cosom hockey often referred to as floor, or Safe-T-Play Hockey originated in Battle Creek, Michigan, in 1962 and is an adaptation of the original game.

A combination of ice hockey and basketball, floor hockey can be played indoors or outdoors. It is played with lightweight plastic sticks and pucks or balls. Each team attempts to control the puck and hit it past the opponent's goal line to score a point. The team that scores the most points after the end of 3 periods is the winner.

Adapted for the Physically Disabled

Floor hockey as a clinical sport originated at the University of Virginia Kluge Children's Rehabilitation Center. Special rules and regulations were adopted so that the sport would be safe for the disabled, but would enable them to experience the excitement and

competition of strenuous play. The severely disabled can compete on equal terms with their normal peers, provided that they play in positions that compensate for their physical limitations. The game is highly active, yet the possibility of injury is only slight. Because of this reason it is a popular activity for school physical education programs.

The size of the playing court (Fig. 7–50) can be modified according to the space that is available (indoors or outdoors). No court dimensions are prescribed, except for the length of the restricted area.

Equipment

The following equipment* is necessary.
1. Hockey sticks: The sticks are made of flexible polyethylene plastic and weigh approximately 6½ ounces. For league play, 5 extra sticks should be kept on hand. The goalkeeper uses a special stick which weighs 7 ounces.
2. Ball: A softball-sized wiffle ball is used instead of the regular puck.
3. Hockey Goals: Various types of indoor and outdoor hockey goals are available. The elementary goal has an opening 44 by 42 inches high. The official-size hockey goal is 72 inches wide, 54 inches high, and 18 inches deep (Fig. 7–51).

Techniques and Rules

Stick-Handling Techniques for Ambulatory Players
1. The hands are held 8 to 12 inches apart on the stick. Right-handed players keep the right hand lower; left-handed players, the left hand.
2. Shots can be made forehanded or backhanded. The floor hockey stick is made so that shots can be played off either face of the blade. If additional rigidity is desired in the stick, a ½-inch dowel can be inserted the full length of the shaft.
3. The players should concentrate on control and direction of the puck or ball; they should not attempt to hit it a great distance. For accuracy as well as for safety, the stick must not be swung above the waist.
4. The stick should be carried low at all times and held in readiness to intercept shots of opponents, to pass to teammates, and to seize an opening for a goal shot.
5. A player should not make wide swings at the ball, but get in close, control the ball with the stick blade, and pass to a teammate if he is in position to score. Speed, accuracy, and control are the skills for which to strive.
6. Wrist action is important. A "flicking" motion is best for speed and accuracy. Hand, wrist, and forearm action control the stick most effectively.

Stick-Handling Techniques for Wheelchair Players. The techniques used by ambulatory players for stick handling also apply to wheelchair-users, except that

*Cosom Safe-T-Play Hockey Set available from Sportime, One Sportime Way, Atlanta, GA 30360.

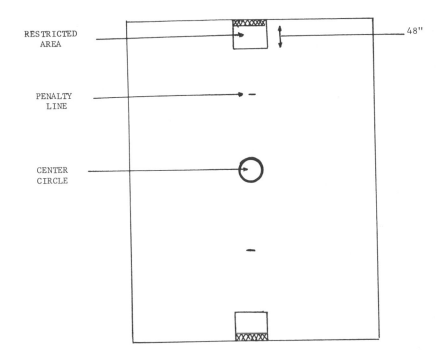

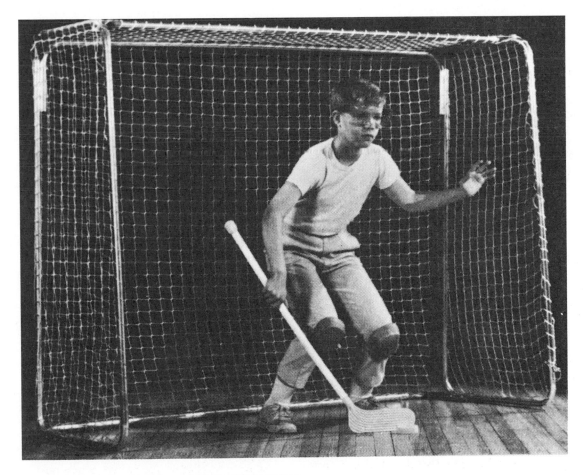

Fig. 7–50. Diagram of court for floor hockey.

Fig. 7–51. Official-size hockey goal. Note protective equipment gear.

they usually control the stick with one hand (Fig. 7–52). The stick is carried on the player's lap or in some cases with one hand when he is maneuvering the wheelchair with both hands.

The Team. Each team usually consists of 4 players: one goalkeeper, who stops shots with his stick or by maneuvering his wheelchair into the path of the moving ball to block it, and 3 forwards, who are allowed to move full court and lead the offensive play. Each forward must play a defensive game when the opposing team has control of the ball.

The number of players can be changed, but it is suggested that a minimum of 3 and a maximum of 5 be used on a team.

The Game. A game has 3 periods of 12 minutes each with a 2-minute rest between periods. The clock starts when the ball is put in play and touched by a member of either team. Play is continuous unless the official calls a time-out.

The Play. A face off at center court is used to start the game. The team that is behind in score at the end of the first and second periods is given possession of the ball to start play in the following periods. The penalty for starting before the whistle is loss of possession. Any forward may start play by hitting the ball (free-in) from the center circle to a teammate.

Scoring. Whenever the ball passes across the goal line on the ground, one point is scored. No point is scored if the ball goes past the goal line in the air. Under no circumstances can a goal be scored on a foul.

Goalkeeping. The goalkeeper has complete freedom of movement inside the restricted area, but he cannot go beyond this area at any time. If the ball becomes lodged underneath the goalie's wheelchair or litter, then play stops; the goalie can make a "free hit" to a teammate.

Out of Bounds. Boundary lines (taped or painted line) should be marked on the playing court. If the ball is hit out of bounds, then a member of the opposing team is allowed a "free pass" to a teammate from the spot where the ball went out.

Fouls
1. Roughing foul: Hacking or striking with the stick, pushing and direct contact with wheelchairs or any other action considered dangerous to other players. Players are to play the ball, not rough-up the opponent. Players charged with a roughing foul must sit out for 5 minutes. During this period, the team must play short-handed.
2. Floor violations:
   a. Entering the goalie's restricted area. Under no circumstances is a forward's wheelchair or hockey stick allowed in the restricted area.
   b. Hitting an opponent's ball on a free pass.
   c. Touching ball with hand.
   d. Using feet to maneuver the wheelchair. The player must keep his feet on the foot pedals at all times.

The penalty for committing a floor violation is a penalty shot for the opposing team. The opposing team (player of choice) receives a free shot from the penalty line (10 feet from the front restricted line).

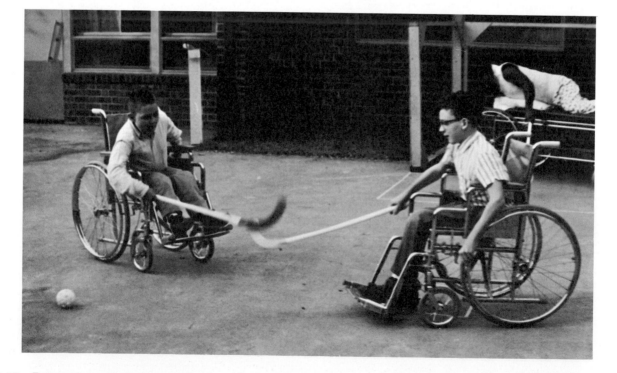

Fig. 7–52.   Fast-moving action is always a part of floor hockey. No other wheelchair sport offers so much activity for the physically disabled.

All players must move behind the penalty line except the goalie, who has the responsibility of trying to stop the ball from going past the goal line. A player charged with 3 fouls (combining roughing and floor violations) shall be removed from the game.

Overtime Games. These shall be "sudden death." The winner is the first team to score. If no change in the score is recorded at the end of 10 minutes, then the game is a tie.

Substitution. Free substitution is allowed. Substitution is allowed only after the ball is ruled dead by the official. No substitution is allowed for a player in penalty box for roughing.

Time-Out. No team time-out is allowed. The official may call time-out if the game is delayed for some reason (misconduct, floor violations, roughing fouls, or injury).

Face Off. The term *face off* is used when 2 players simultaneously attempt to hit the ball from the center circle at the command of the referee. The ball is placed in the middle of the circle until the whistle is blown for play to start. A face off is used under the following situations:

1. To start a game.
2. To start a period if the score is tied.
3. To resume play after questionable decisions (when opposing players simultaneously hit the ball out of bounds).

Special Ruling: Safety Zone Play

This space modification outlines (tape or other markings) the limited area in which a disadvantaged player can move within the regular court area. It is basically designed as a safety feature for the mobility impaired player. The zone can be a large box, or a line drawn across the court from sideline to sideline within close proximity to the restricted goal area. In the box version rules can apply that prevent players from entering the zone.

Adjustments for Specific Disabilities

Amputations

Unilateral Upper-Extremity. Involvement of one arm will not deter participation to any great extent. If use of the dominant hand is lost, this will cause problems at first, but practice at handling the stick with the unaffected extremity will overcome this. A padded mitten should be worn to protect both the hook fingers and the opponent in case of bodily contact. In controlled competition situations as in clinical programs, it may be recommended to make adaptations to the stick handle to accommodate the hook fingers. Balance training and prosthetic awareness skills are important values of the game. An amputee should play the forward position.

Bilateral Upper-Extremity. Those who have lost the use of both arms will have difficulty meeting the physical demands of the forward position, but they can play as goalies. Loss of wrist action will interfere with controlling the stick; however, the amputee can learn to block shots with his feet and legs.

Unilateral Lower-Extremity. Involvement of one lower limb will restrict some players from running at full speed for a whole game. Many below-knee amputees who have learned to play a defensive game at the forward position then lend assistance to the goalie instead of moving into position for playing offense. Wheelchair participation is recommended for the leg amputee who has not learned to use his prosthesis. The forward position is good for the patient needing preprosthetic exercise or prosthetic appliance exercise.

Bilateral Lower-Extremity. Because of poor balance, players who are missing both lower limbs often have difficulty playing the forward position except from a wheelchair. However, some bilateral B/K amputees have played a forward position, but within a designated zone. The suggested position is often that of goalie.

Chronic Obstructive Lung Disease. Vigorous and prolonged activity may be contraindicated, since some individuals with chronic lung disease have low tolerance levels for physical exertion. Floor hockey can be used as a progressive developmental sport; however, the instructor should have a clear understanding of each player's capacity for participation in uninterrupted activity. Activity should be stopped at once if any signs of dyspnea or bronchial spasm are evidenced. The patient may play any position, depending upon his condition.

Therapeutic Note: Players with cystic fibrosis should be encouraged to play the forward position. Intermittent running aids in loosening mucus from the bronchial tree.

Blindness. Floor hockey is not recommended for the blind because the game is very swift. However, modified games with audible balls can be designed for the totally blind.

Cardiovascular Disorders. Those with cardiac conditions must have medical permission, as highly competitive play may be contraindicated. The instructor should know the functional capacity of each player and limit him accordingly. The goalie position is frequently recommended because it is less strenuous.

Therapeutic Note: If a progressive exercise program is one of the treatment objectives, then the work output of the player can be adjusted by altering the range of the playing area. A fullback position can be created and thereby offer more flexibility in a limited participation method by staying within the limits of safety.

Cerebral Palsy. Ambulatory CP players (Class VI, VII, and VIII) can often play the forward position in floor hockey, or modifications of the game requiring zone play. However, some players in class VI may have problems with stick handling due to involvement of the upper-limbs. For example, players with moderate to severe athetosis may be required to play a goalie position to overcome deficiencies in balance and hand control. Players with minimal spasticity are usually not limited to any significant degree.

Wheelchair-users will have more pronounced problems in controlling both the wheelchair and stick at the same time. However, even players who are dependent on a motorized chair can be relegated to a goalie position. Some players may not be able to grip a stick due to lack of hand function, but various strapping techniques can be used to overcome this problem. The forward position is often suggested for players who can propel their wheelchair independently as often seen with the class III athlete.

One of the common problems related to CP players is their inability to control the direction of the puck or ball. If mobility problems persist due to the nature and degree of competition, then the instructor should spend time on teaching the fundamentals and strategy of playing the goalie position. Group stimulation and teamwork are important game values.

Head Trauma. Players (Rancho Level VI) who show goal-directed behavior can often play the game of floor hockey. However, the fast paced action involving directional changes may be confusing to some players. If the player is inconsistently oriented to time and place, then further assessment will be needed before engaging the patient in game situations. The program leader can also use the team game to develop appropriate interaction skills (refer to section on Hemiplegia for other details).

Therapeutic Note: The program leader can use the game to assess selective attention to task. While the CHI player is in the goalie position, the therapist can assess reaction to game responses such as anticipation or prediction of following the puck and player movement.

Hemiplegia. The ambulatory and nonambulatory hemiplegic has a distinct disadvantage because the affected extremity must be properly positioned if he is to control the stick with both hands. The hemiplegic player may prefer to use only the nonaffected limb to hold the stick. The program leader may need to support or discourage such action depending upon the specific objectives involved. Frequently, the main objectives are to provide body awareness skills and maintain strength and endurance in the unaffected body parts. As a goalie, the player can experiment by using his affected upper extremity to assist in controlling the stick movements. This position can also be used to promote balance training. Players with mild to moderate spasticity may be able to run and play the forward position, providing balance and functional skills on the nonaffected side are good.

Hip Joint Disorders. Players wearing containment appliances and postoperative patients using crutches will have mobility problems. The safest position would be goalie where body contact is prohibited. Some Scottish-Rite abduction brace wearers are able to adapt and learn locomotor efficiency skills rather easily. If body checking is controlled, then some players may

be able to play the forward position. Patients confined to Buck's traction are often at a disadvantage because of their inability to shift body weight during the immobilization period. Those confined to spring and slings traction are obviously more versatile with freedom of trunk and leg action (although abducted) which provides independence in controlling the stick. The goalie position is recommended for this group.

Some players using containment appliances have engaged in zone play, but body checking should be absolutely forbidden.

Osteogenesis Imperfecta. Due to the vigorous nature of the game, players with OI are often relegated to the goalie position. Wheelchair players, including those using a motorized chair, can play a defensive posture. For example, the player can roam the backfield to cut off opposing players from the goal, puck, or teammates. When playing goalie, the wheelchair can be placed sideways across the goal. The player can move his chair back and forth to block the puck with the tires or stick blade.

Overweight and Obesity. Overweight persons need to burn up calories through vigorous exercise; consequently, floor hockey is ideal for this purpose. Low physical fitness skills may hinder the player in certain stick movements such as dribbling the ball and making short, rapid taps with the stick. The suggested position for the obese person is forward, in most cases.

The highly unfit, or deconditioned obese player may find the sport too traumatic to the ankle and knee joints unless assigned to a goalie position.

Paraplegia. Depending upon the competitive nature of the game, floor hockey can provide sustained effort in wheelchair maneuverability skills. Fast turns and quick starts are necessary to react to offensive and defensive strategies which results in arm and shoulder exercise. Medical concerns may take precedence for rehabilitation patients and this will require the therapist to regulate the degree of competition, thereby restricting high sticking, body checking, etc. Seat belts may be used to assist with balance. The forward position is generally recommended.

Progressive Muscle Disorders. Ambulatory players limited by lordosis and an unstable gait pattern will have difficulty adjusting to floor hockey due to the fast paced action of the game. This will be complicated by their inability to make postural changes while manipulating the stick. Restricted zone play is a possible solution, but again safety issues are factors to consider due to the possibility of being unable to avoid onrushing opponents. The goalie position is recommended in most cases.

Wheelchair players lack mobility skills, consequently will have difficulty moving over the court area. The suggested position is goalie. Players using a motorized chair can act as "roamers" while moving about and blocking out offensive players and using defensive strategy by moving back and forth in front of the restricted goal area. Watch for signs of early fatigue.

Rheumatoid Arthritis. This group must not be overworked, and the desirable amount of physical exercise depends upon the extent of involvement. The suggested position is goalie if physical limitations prohibit body contact or excessive running.

Quadriplegia. Participation in floor hockey is not usually encouraged, but some low level quadriplegics have used "strap-on" sticks. The goalie position is often recommended. Players using motorized wheelchairs can act as "roamers."

Abnormal Posture. Participation in floor hockey may provide certain gains in muscle and ligament tone. Because of the lack of a flexible back, Milwaukee-brace wearers play with sticks with longer handles; and in most cases they should play the forward position. Since body contact is forbidden, it may be necessary to stop play at the first sign of body checking. The orthoplast jacket wearer should be able to play without difficulty.

Undernutrition. The ability of the undernourished individual to participate in floor hockey depends on the underlying cause of the disorder. Muscle weakness, poor coordination, and lack of vitality are common characteristics of this group. Strenuous, continuous play must be controlled because the undernourished player tends to withdraw from vigorous activity. The suggested position is goalie. The forward position can be introduced to the less severely involved, if there are rest periods.

GOLF

The exact origin of golf is not really known. Written reports indicate that the Romans played a version of golf with a bent stick and a leather ball stuffed with feathers. In 1754, the first rules to govern the sport were established by a committee at the St. Andrew's Golf Club in Scotland. The game was introduced to the United States in the late 1800s. The United States Golf Association was established in 1894.

Adapted for the Physically Disabled

Golf is unique in that it is truly a sport of player against the course. Golf courses have ratings based upon difficulty and length of each hole. Competition can be equalized because the sport incorporates a handicapping score system that enables all players to be rated according to ability. Another feature is that the pace of game is such that most disabled persons can play without undue physical stress. Based upon the functional capacity of the golfer, the individual can use a motorized golf cart for course travel, ride and walk part-time, or walk full-time.

The popularity of golf for disabled adults has grown rapidly during the last decade, and more recently efforts have focused attention to the junior population. This improvement is due, in part, to the

actions of the National Amputee Golf Association (NAGA). This organization, founded in 1954, has been instrumental in promoting the sport. Over the years, NAGA has held *Learn to Golf* clinics for the physically challenged, sponsored tournaments, and lobbied for rulings and improved technology related to the sport of golf. The Professional Golfers Association (PGA) formed a Committee for Liaison with the Physically Limited in 1984. In 1986, the PGA, Junior Golf Foundation published the First Swing Program. The seminars stress using golf as a rehabilitation medium in recreation and therapy, and are designed to provide instruction for rehabilitation professionals. Readers can write to the NAGA for further information on the First Swing Seminars, and Learn to Golf Clinics.

Equipment
1. Course—Generally a level terrain should be encouraged especially if golf carts are to be considered.
2. A regular starter kit of clubs should be considered including a #3 wood, a putter, and #3, #5, #7, and #9 irons. Disabled golfers often use customized clubs. Depending upon the skills of the golfer, the angle of the shaft can be modified to insure the clubhead will rest appropriately on the ground. Shaft dimension and flexibility can also be modified to assist a golfer with a limited swing. A club professional should be consulted about club design and certain specifications prior to purchasing golf clubs. The grip handle can also be changed to accommodate a golfer with limited grip strength. For example, the circumference of the grip can be increased enabling the golfer to grip the club firmly enough to control the club through impact of the ball.

Techniques
An important first step in becoming a successful teacher of golf for the disabled is to acquire the book, *Teaching Golf to Special Populations* by DeDe Owens.* It is an excellent source for giving specific instructional tips for a variety of physical limiting conditions.

The type of golf grip will vary, but one of most popular is the overlapping grip (Fig. 7–53). One of the features of this grip is the placement of the little finger of the right hand which wraps around the crevice formed by the first two fingers of the left hand (for right-handed players).

The stance involves slightly bending the knees with the toes turned slightly outward. Weight is evenly distributed. The knees, hips, and shoulders remain square. Stability of the stance position will need to be carefully assessed by the golf instructor. Poor stability is often associated with range of motion limitations which will affect the golfer's ability to master the swing

*Owens, D. Teaching Golf to Special Populations. West Point, NY, Leisure Press, 1984.

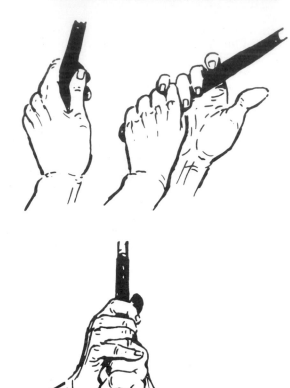

Fig. 7–53.   Overlapping grip. (From *Sports and Recreational Activities for Men and Women,* Courtesy of C.V. Mosby Company.)

motion (refer to section on assistive devices for additional details).

The golfer's swing plane is one that occurs approximately between the shoulder and neck. The sequence starts with the legs and hips, followed by the arms, and finally the wrists. The downswing motion follows the same swing plane sequence. The length of the backswing will vary depending upon the distance of the required shot. The follow-through after impact is with the hands held high.

The standard golf swing technique may not be the model for the swing that is developed by the physically disabled golfer. In some cases, weight distribution and address position will have to be modified in order to maximize the motion potential. Upper body mobility is another factor to consider, and this too is crucial to a free arm swing motion. Trial and error methods are often required to determine the most effective swing style.

Rules

The standard USGA rules of golf also apply to the physically disabled golfer. Through the USGA Handicapping System, everyone who plays is equal. Certain provisions have been made recently. For example, prosthetic devices are no longer considered artificial

aids that would otherwise be a cause for disqualification. Another revision that occurred with lobbying efforts of NAGA referred to the National Collegiate Athletic Association (NCAA) ruling not allowing motorized carts. The ruling now has an exception for permanently disabled persons unable to walk the full course.

Assistive Devices

Balance aids can contribute to stability forces during the arm swing motion. One example is a tripod seat (often designed by the individual) that enables the golfer to swing his club from a seated position. This portable device can be used at most any location on the golf course. Golfers who ambulate with crutches can also use a tripod seating position. For some players, balance may not be a problem when putting, consequently the golfer may be able to balance with one crutch (or in some cases two crutches) while freeing the dominant upper-extremity to swing the putter.

Amputee Golf Grip (A.G.G.).* The upper-limb amputee attaches the A.G.G. by threading a ½″ rod into the wrist socket of the prosthesis. It attaches and locks securely in place on any part of the club head for use during driving, chipping and putting (Fig. 7–54). It also meets the rules requirements of the U.S.G.A. for artificial limbs.

Spring levered golf arms that simulate the characteristics of a natural wrist are popular. One device designed by F.B. Goldman† has a stainless steel ter-

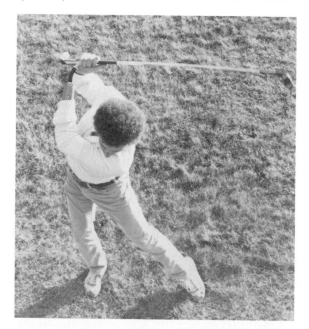

Fig. 7–54.   The AGG device which allows for full rotation during the backswing, squared club face at impact and complete follow-through during the downswing. (Courtesy of Access to Recreation.)

*Write to Access to Recreation.
†Write to Pete Goldman, Transland Management Corp., 2225 One Dallas Center, Dallas TX 75201.

minal insertion for the club which has a clamp to tighten the grip. Another golf arm designed by Wayne Vecellotti‡ uses a two pronged fork that is attached to a slotted steel device. The sleeve is attached to the golf club at a narrow part of the shaft, then slides up to fit tightly to the uppermost part of the golf grip.

Program Adjustment for Specific Disabilities

Golf is a flexible sport, and it can be modified for individual differences. However, there are some problems that can occur for the wheelchair-user when attempting to play the traditional sport as will be discussed in this section.

Since most of the physically challenged golfers are ambulatory, attention will focus on this population while alternative considerations for all groupings will be discussed in the section on golf putting games.

Wheelchair-Users. Golf can be played from a seated position. However, without means to travel other than by wheelchair may make it extremely difficult for the golfer to move about the course. Motorized carts can be modified to enable the nonambulatory golfer to participate. For example, a seat can be modified to swivel into position for each stroke. Some players who can stabilize their lower-limbs, most frequently users of braces, or prosthetic limbs (bilateral A/K amputee), can use a modified tripod seat, or lean against a golf cart.

Unfortunately, problems with accessibility are common concerns. It is impossible to drive a cart on a green to putt. The same holds true with a wheelchair, as the wheels may damage the putting surface. This is not to say the wheelchair user should not try to play on a course, but options may be limited due to course maintenance policies. Some golfers have putted while sitting on the turf.

Lower Extremity Amputations. A/K and B/K amputees who wear their prosthesis should be able to develop an efficient arm swing motion. Oftentimes, however, A/K amputees need to experiment for a longer period of time with their stance position, which will require some motion to support the swing action of the upper body. A weight distribution which is even to forward, with an upper-body posture over the ball, is recommended. Some bilateral A/K golfers with balance problems need to use a support system (golf cart with swivel seat or tripod seat). Many amputee golfers will angle their left foot outward (for righthanders) to provide balance throughout the swing (Fig. 7–55A).

Some lower-extremity amputees who wear a prosthesis also use a rotator (positioned in the shank of the prosthesis which simulates normal body rotation). The rotator provides for some normalcy in the swing, however, it is not an imperative item to have in order to enjoy the sport (as seen in Fig. 7–55B). A Swivel Golf Shoe is another alternative. The swivel can be built into a conventional golf shoe to allow rotation. The golfer should contact a prosthetist technician for details.

One legged golf is another possibility, but swing motion is dependent on balance. Swing action is accelerated once the golfer is able to isolate upper body movement. Longo* suggests addressing the ball in line with the foot. This position forms a straight line that runs directly through the center of the body. The body is centered over its "axis center line," and the knees are slightly bent throughout the swing. Surprisingly, some one legged golfers have been able to hit a ball 250 yards off a tee.

Upper Extremity Amputation. Golf can be played successfully by the unilateral upper limb amputee. The prosthesis is used as a support, while the unaffected arm generates the acceleration in the swing. A decision must be made whether to play with the residual limb towards the ball or away from the ball. Generally, playing with the residual limb to the rear is preferred as it allows for more swinging action of the lower body. In general, rear side A/E and B/E amputees have fewer control problems than the target side A/E and B/E amputee. A top grip position of the target hand is recommended for increased wrist action through impact.

It is suggested that B/E amputees play with a prosthetic device designed specifically for golf to enhance upper limb mobility and control. The A.G.G. is a popular device that simulates wrist-action of the human wrist and facilitates a smooth, fluid swing. It can be used by both A/E and B/E amputees (Fig. 7–54).

One armed golf is possible, but difficult to learn. Clubhead speed is naturally affected, and to compensate it is necessary to use lightweight clubs with highly flexible shafts. Grip control is obviously important, and this depends to some degree upon position stability. On the forward swing, motion is started with the club arm, not the legs. Both knees should be bent to add stability to the swing motion.

Cerebral Palsy. The ambulatory person with spastic diplegia who has good total body balance skills, but only minimal involvement of the legs, often has the physical attributes to play golf. Spasticity, to any degree, in the upper-limbs will generally interfere with the golfer's downswing plane. The golf swing is started from the legs and hips, and players with hip and knee flexion contractures often have difficulty isolating the sequence of body movements while maintaining a firm base of support.

As with any ambulatory CP golfer, including the mild hemiplegic, efforts to assist in developing a comfortable grip on the golf club and to achieve balance support during the swing motion will be helpful. This may include playing from an elevated sitting position or perhaps using a short swing to compensate for the instability.

‡Write to Wayne Vecellotti, 1435 Mason, Joliet, IL 60435.

*Longo, P. Challenge Golf, A Game For Everyone. Amputee Golfer, 1989. Pgs. 22–24.

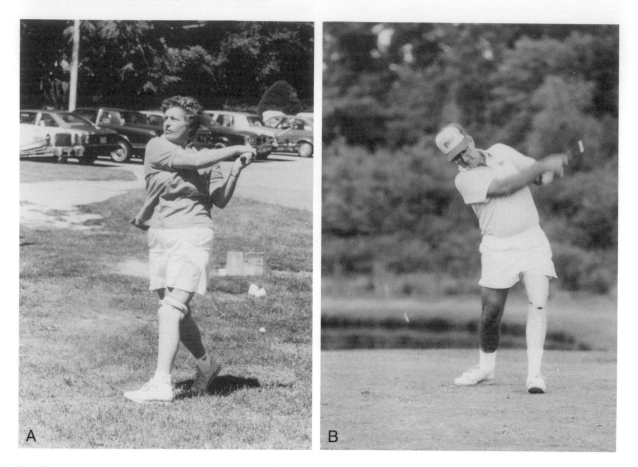

Fig. 7–55.   Amputee golfers demonstrating golf swing motion. (A) Completion of the swing for a left B/K, wearing supercondular suspension and no rotator. In order to overcome the torque forces on the residual limb, the left foot is angled outward to a position that allows balance throughout the swing and a comfortable follow through. (B) A/K golfer wearing standard prosthesis and no ankle rotator which requires the knee to be locked in full extension position. The golfer finishes the swing by spinning on the right heel. (Courtesy of National Amputee Golfers Association.)

For the more severely involved, it would be more appropriate and less frustrating to participate in golf putting games.

Arthritis

Osteoarthritis. This type of arthritis is joint specific and likely painful or limiting in only a few joints. Consequently, the affected joint and amount or trauma dictate the types of modifications that are necessary. Likely, if it is lower extremity related simply utilizing a golf cart to reduce the stress placed on the joint during walking will be sufficient. If it is upper extremity related, maintaining range of motion and strength of the affected joints will enable the golfer to stay active longer. Reducing the stress on the affected joint might occur by modifying the swing. One example might be to shorten the backswing to reduce shoulder stress. As people age, more and more suffer from osteoarthritis due to the gradual wear and tear on the joints. Additionally, many people learn to play golf in their later years thus osteoarthritis does not usually preclude people from participating in the

sport. If the golfer conscientiously works to maintain strength and range of motion in the affected joint, then the likelihood of playing golf longer with less pain is quite possible.

Rheumatoid Arthritis. This systemic type of arthritis again affects people to different degrees and joint locations. However, typically the hands and shoulder joints are affected. Grip modifications and high friction gloves can help the golfer by reducing the tension needed to appropriately grip the club through contact. Maintenance of strength and range of motion is vital to help the golfer maintain a functional swing motion. However, if a full swing is not possible, then the player should attempt to improve on the other aspects of the game such as perfecting chip shots and putting.

Golf Putting Games

Putting a golf ball is a matter of individual choice, providing the player is able to judge the length of the backswing to correspond with the length of the hole. It is a stationary activity and there must be no body movement other than arm swing action. The game has excellent therapeutic implications for patients who are slowly regaining muscle endurance and need specific time alloted trials for increasing standing tolerance and balance (with or without standing appliances, crutches, etc.).

Putt-Putt Golf Courses of America, Inc. was instrumental in designing the first wheelchair accessible course at the Kluge Children's Rehabilitation Center (Fig. 7–56) and similar designs have been built at various medical agencies and summer camps in recent years. Golf-ette, a new indoor/outdoor putting game, is now becoming popular and is being played on a wide scale in various treatment and recreational facilities (Fig. 7–57). It is also a game that can be used in public school adapted physical education programs.

Equipment

Golf equipment includes small, hard balls and a variety of clubs. Each club is designed to play a particular type of stroke or to hit the ball a certain distance. In choosing equipment, it is not always necessary to buy the most expensive golf balls and clubs.

1. Golf Balls: The regulation golf ball is used.
2. Putter: Of the clubs used in regular golf, only the putter is needed for miniature golf. Putters* vary in form and shape, but always have straight faces. Putters are constructed so they will roll the ball along the ground toward the hole. It is important that a putter be balanced and weighted properly so that the golfer can command complete control over the path of the ball.
3. Golf Course: The size of the putting course depends upon a number of factors.† It is recom-

---

*For further information regarding carpet putters, contact Southern Golf Distributors, P.O. Box 35207, Fayetteville, N.C. 28303.

†For assistance in construction of PUTT-PUTT courses, contact PUTT-PUTT Golf Courses of America, Inc., P.O. Box 5237, 3007 Fort Bragg Road, Fayetteville, N.C. 28303.

mended that there be at least 4 holes in order to offer some variation in play. The total cost of a permanent outdoor course depends upon local labor costs and the size of the course.

Various indoor putting games including Golf-ette can be purchased from distributors.

The suggested width of each hole is 3 feet from the tee mat to back bump board. The length from tee mat to each hole should vary from 8 to 14 feet.

Technique

The instructor should always encourage or demonstrate proper game skills. This includes the use of the bump boards for bank shots and the proper placement of the ball on the tee mat. It should be emphasized that a soft, even stroke will usually result in a lower score. The instructions given are for right-handed golfers and must, naturally, be reversed to suit left-handed players.

Ambulatory Players. Concentration and confidence are two primary requirements for good putting. The golfer should face the ball with the weight of his body evenly distributed on both feet. The grip will vary with each individual. The shoulders should be over the ball, and the knees should be slightly bent. The left arm should be close to the body and right forearm close to the right thigh. The backswing should be slow in a pendulum movement, and the forward stroke should be sharp and crisp. Little or no elbow movement is required, as the movement is primarily from the shoulders.

Wheelchair Players. Some wheelchair-users prefer to face the putting hole instead of the ball. This position may be necessary for some severely disabled players if they are to obtain maximum power on the backswing motion. The wheelchair player with poor upper-extremity strength should learn to guide the putter by placing the dominant hand low on the shaft.

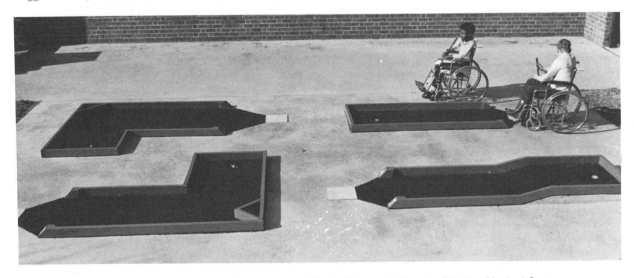

Fig. 7–56.   Four-hole putting course at the Kluge Children's Rehabilitation Center, University of Virgina Medical Center.

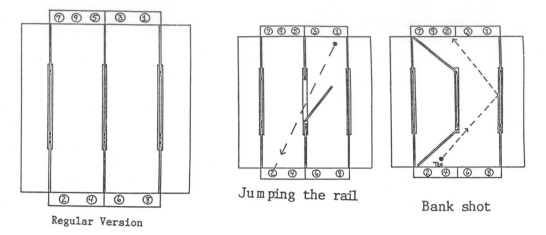

Regular Version   Jumping the rail   Bank shot

Fig. 7–57.   Adaptations of the game, Golf-ette. For further information on Hurt's Golf-ette, write to 131 College Circle, Staunton, VA 24401.

The backward and forward stroke motion will again be a pendulum movement from the shoulders.

Handicap Score. Stroke play is the more exacting method of scoring; however, a handicap score system should be used when competition is very unequal. In handicap play, the player with the lower average score is required to give strokes to the higher average golfer. However, before the handicap system is used, it is necessary to record the average score for each participant. In some instances, two practice rounds must be played before each player's score is averaged. The difference between the players' average scores will be the number of strokes subtracted from the weaker player's score during competitive play.

Assistive Devices

The "Putter Finger"—a soft molded rubber suction cup designed to fit on the grip end of any putter (Fig. 7–58). This device does away with the necessity to bend or stoop down to retrieve the ball. Simply by extending the putter out and placing it on top of the golf ball, the player can recover his ball. Putter Fingers can be obtained from the Southern Golf Distributors, Inc.

Another useful device is a mini-putter. This device eliminates the need to use two hands when putting (Fig. 7–59).

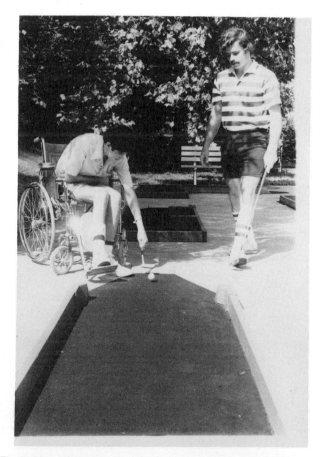

Fig. 7–59.   Mini-putter. Essentially, this adaptation is a regular putter with the handle cut off which enables the player to achieve a more controlled swing motion. The mini-putter is designed primarily for the one-handed putter such as the hemiplegic.

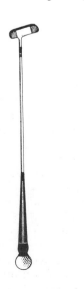

Fig. 7–58.   Putter Finger.

Adjustments for Special Disabilities

Amputations

Unilateral Upper-Extremity. The recent amputee can play by controlling the golf club with one hand. After the prosthesis is fitted, the golfer can experiment by using the artificial limb to guide the putter while the unaffected arm supplies the force for the pendulum swing motion. No major problems should be encountered with this group of amputees.

Bilateral Upper-Extremity. It is possible for this group of amputees to play putting games, provided that the hook fingers can be securely attached to the handle and shaft of the putter. It is important, however, to keep the terminal device of the dominant side low on the shaft to control the movement of the club head on a direct line to the hole.

Unilateral Lower-Extremity. Loss of a lower limb will not pose a major problem and the putting stance will vary with each individual. The above-knee amputee may not be able to secure a comfortable stance; however, he can usually make the necessary adjustment by using a wide base of support.

Bilateral Lower-Extremity. The bilateral lower-extremity amputee will tend to use a rigid putting stance. Most beginners with above-knee amputations will compensate for loss of knee motion by using a wide base. On the other hand, below-knee amputees will have a definite advantage because they will be able to bend their knees and relax during the putting motion. Recent lower-limb amputees or those with balance problems can play from a wheelchair. However, play from an upright position is encouraged once the artificial limbs are properly fitted.

Chronic Obstructive Lung Disease.
Mild exercise encourages the patient not to focus all his attention on his disorder. One of the greatest advantages to putting games lies in the age range of those able to participate. Emphysema patients enjoy playing putting games because they can compete at a leisurely pace without aggravating their condition. Elderly players who experience problems on forward bending (pain, loss of balance) can use the Putter-Finger.

Blindness.
The totally blind player can make certain adjustments which will enable him to participate in putting games. The player can judge the distance from the tee mat to the hole by pacing it off. If the distance of the first putt is accurately judged, the golfer will not be left with a difficult second putt. An assistant will be needed to aid in positional alignment when addressing the ball. The blind golfer will need to spend considerable time in developing a compact grip and proper stroke motion. Beginners may have poor kinesthetic awareness skills and will tend to turn the club face on the forward swing motion. Mini-beepers can also be purchased to provide auditory clues for the position of the putting hole.

Cardiovascular Disorders.
Gradual exercise, both physical and mental, is performed in accordance with the physician's orders as the patient's condition improves. Golf putting games are an excellent sport for patients with cardiac conditions, because it can be played without undue exertion, and the player can control the pace of the game.

Cerebral Palsy.
The ability for this group to play putting games will obviously depend upon a number of factors. Players with incomplete cylindrical or spherical grasp, and limited by moderate to severe spasticity or athetosis will have major problems. If an independent grip (with or without strapping for stabilization of the hand) and a purposeful pendulum swing motion is unattainable, then the game is not recommended. The player with spastic diplegia can usually adapt to game situations, although poor-standing balance may interfere with developing a comfortable stance and swing.

Note: Chutes with speed control adapters for the severely involved player can be used, and such devices are being explored within various recreational and clinical settings.

Head Trauma.
During the rehabilitation period, golf putting games can be introduced to facilitate certain emotional and physical responses. Although players may present variable cognitive disorders, the game is rather simple to learn. Play is done from a stationary position with essentially only arm movement; therefore, players who demonstrate goal-directed behavior, but with mobility and perceptual-motor deficits can even play the game. Ambulatory players with motor planning deficits will need extra practice time to concentrate on learning a comfortable stance, and slow and steady swing motion with the putter. Because of the slow tempo of the game, speed of processing time is not a major issue of concern.

Hemiplegia.
Maximum return of neuromuscular function to the affected extremities is the paramount goal. Positioning the affected arm on the handle of the putter will reeducate the muscles. When assuming the putting stance, the hemiplegic may not be able to distribute his weight equally on both feet because of the weakness of his affected limb. Balance, coordination, and strength can be improved by partial weight-bearing activities. The mini-putter is suggested for the wheelchair user.

Hip Joint Disorders.
Putting games can be introduced to players learning to adapt to their new orthosis for the purpose of improving standing balance and tolerance. Once stability is achieved, minimal assistance will be needed. The game of Golf-ette is recommended because the side rails can be moved to accommodate players wearing abduction appliances or using crutches. Postoperative players using a 3-point gait will prefer to use a crutch in one hand for support while using the free hand to control the putter.

Osteogenesis Imperfecta.
Ambulatory golfers with well-aligned extremities should be able to play putting games without difficulty. Wheelchair players will need

to make alterations in their grip if upper-extremity deformities and contractures interfere with manipulating a putter. Assessment of other equipment needs will often focus attention to weight and length of putter.

Overweight and Obesity. Most obese golfers are able to adjust to game situations. Beginners tend to overpower the ball by using a high backswing. Care must be taken to teach the golfer to follow a simple sequence of motion each time he addresses and swings at the ball.

Paraplegia. No major problems should be encountered with this group. Sitting balance needs to be assessed to determine if a seat or chest belt will be needed to assist in maintaining good trunk control. Most players prefer to face directly at the hole when putting. This position provides for vertical alignment and a more comfortable back swing motion.

Progressive Muscular Disorders. Golf putting games are encouraged for persons with progressive muscle disease because they are unable to engage in vigorous physical activity. Ambulatory players can usually play without adaptations. Grip strength and arm swing motion will need to be assessed on an individual basis, especially with players who are using a wheelchair. It is reasonable to conclude that players with advanced muscle deterioration and trunk instability will be unable to play the game, unless special ball chutes can be secured to the wheelchair. The Putter Finger may be useful for players with sitting balance problems, but who have sufficient strength to manipulate a putter.

Quadriplegia. Low level quadriplegics have the capabilities of playing golf putting games. Foam rubber grip handles can stabilize the hand in a more functional position, and in some cases it is necessary to strap the hand to the putter.

Rheumatoid Arthritis. Most arthritics can participate without difficulty. Golf is contraindicated when the joints of the wrists and fingers are swollen and painful. Therapeutic values may result from joint range of motion exercise.

Abnormal Posture. Ambulatory patients in Milwaukee braces will be unable to bend forward to putt comfortably. Since head movement is restricted, the player will have to stand away from the tee mat so he can make eye contact with the ball. The "putter finger" is a useful device for players confined to a postoperative cast or brace during the early rehabilitation period. Orthoplast jacket wearers should have no problems playing this game.

Undernutrition. Golf putting games are an ideal sport for the underweight patient because they are a single-response activity, and the player's lack of strength does not interfere with learning putting skills. Brief rest periods may be necessary if fatigue seems excessive or prolonged. Some players have a weak grip and tend to use an unsteady backswing causing a poor follow-through.

Therapeutic Note: If the cause of poor putting is faulty posture, a period of waiting until strength is gained may be required. The putting motion will not encourage good posture, since the player must bend forward at the waist to line up the ball with the hole.

Golf-ette*

Golf-ette is a new concept in putting for the physically disabled. Game equipment consists of three sections of 4-foot swinging rails connected to a 4-foot self-supporting base. The swinging rails are attached to the base with wing nuts. Rectangular-shaped frames contain the holes and the greens. The fairway is comprised of a 4′ × 12′ carpet. The game can be assembled and taken apart in a matter of a few minutes, lending support to time saving measures.

A unique feature of the game is the moveable side rails. Wheelchair-users can maneuver freely on the putting surface without concern for negotiating over and around the rails (Fig. 17–58). By swinging the rails away from the surface, the player can easily approach the ball and assume a putting position (Fig. 7–60). After the ball is hit the rail can be swung back to the original position. In effect, the movable side rails offer safe entry and exit points. This feature allows players using various mobility aids such as pick-up walkers and crutches to play the game, as well as those confined to a stretcher in a prone position. The game has also been used successfully with patients confined to a bed in a supine position.

Space is at a premium especially in many hospital units. However, Golf-ette only requires 64 square feet of playing area and can be played indoors or outdoors without disrupting existing structural surroundings.

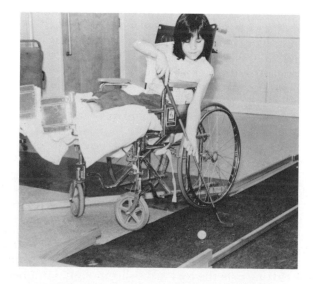

Fig. 7–60. Wheelchair-user playing Golf-ette. Note moveable side rails.

*131 College Circle, Staunton, VA 24401.

HORSEBACK RIDING

The horse has been one of man's most useful animals for thousands of years. Horses brought to Mexico by the Spanish in 1519 were probably the ancestors of wild American horses. The quick and willing obedience of the horse has helped make it one of man's most valuable animals.

Horsemen and horses from many lands compete in international horse shows. Most shows in the United States follow the rules of the American Horse Shows Association. Local horsemen's clubs throughout the country hold shows in which riders compete in many events, such as jumping and performance of various gaits. As many spectators support horse racing and horse shows as attend football and baseball games.

The art of riding on horseback is called *equitation*. There are many types of equitation, but the type described in this section is called the balanced forward hunter seat. This allows full freedom for the horse's natural movement while the rider can aid, direct, and control the horse.

Adapted for the Physically Disabled

The idea of using horseback riding for its therapeutic values is not new. Riding for the disabled began in Scandinavia; shortly thereafter, the Superintendent Physiotherapist at Winford Orthopaedic Hospital, near Bristol, England, initiated a program that proved so successful it encouraged other centers to establish similar programs. By 1965, interest in such projects was so great that the Advisory Council on Riding for the Disabled was set up under the auspices of the British Horse Society. United States therapists have promoted riding less zealously, although beginnings have been made at centers in various parts of the country. The North American Riding for the Handicapped Association, organized in 1969, is the major advisory board on riding for the disabled in the United States and Canada. It guides over 200 centers and 4,000 riders a year.

Equestrian events are included in USCPAA competition. Included are dressage, relay race, equitation, jumping and obstacle course.

Horseback riding requires the involvement of the whole body and utilizes every muscle and joint. The development of muscle strength, as well as body image and total body awareness, is a significant therapeutic contribution. Moreover, the development of balance and coordination is implicit in the activity. Cerebral palsied patients, in particular, must learn adjusted movements to compensate for the inept postures manifest in their handicap; that is, learn to develop compensatory balance and coordination patterns. Horseback riding requires essentially the same thing. The rider aligns his center of balance with that of the horse and learns to maintain his balance by adjusting his body to compensate for the horse's movement. Three basic concepts must be learned if one is to ride properly, and, for the cerebral palsied child, they are directly applicable to the learning of balancing skills on the ground.

The primary aim of using therapeutic exercises is to mobilize the trunk while coordinating the action of various muscle groups. Neuromuscular coordination is enhanced while making postural changes and eliciting equilibrium reactions (Fig. 7–61).

Equipment

Clothing must be comfortable. The rider must protect his legs from the irritation of rubbing against the saddle. Long, tight-fitting breeches are usually worn to provide comfort and protection. Boots, or any shoes with heels, keep the feet from slipping out of the stirrups. Riding helmets (or some kind of protective headgear) are recommended.

1. Saddle: Riders in the United States generally use either an English saddle or a Western saddle. The rider should choose the kind of saddle that suits his riding.

   Many riders prefer the English saddle because it is padded and more comfortable (Fig. 7–62). It is also flatter and weighs less than the Western saddle. Jockeys and exhibition riders who need extra speed use the English saddle. Many beginners, however, prefer the Western saddle (progression to the English saddle may be possible

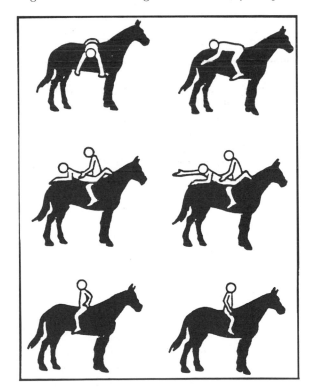

Fig. 7–61. Horseback riding can be specifically therapeutic. Often referred to as hippotherapy (creative means of exercise) it is often conducted by a physical therapist who works jointly with a riding instructor. Shown above are examples of some therapeutic exercise positions. (Reprinted from Physical Therapy, 65:1505, 1988, with permission of the American Physical Therapy Association.)

at a later time), because it has a saddle horn or pommel, which they can hold until they learn to keep their balance. Cowboys and rodeo riders use the Western saddle.

2. Bridle: This is the part of the equipment used to control the horse; it consists of straps and metal pieces that fit on the horse's head and into its mouth (Fig. 7–62). Beginners usually ride with a snaffle bridle, which has a jointed bit (mouth-piece) that is gentle on the horse. The bit of the snaffle bridle pulls on the corners of the horse's lips. The single set of reins can be handled easily by the rider.

Riding Technique

Before anyone can learn to ride properly, he must know something about the parts of the horse, its psychology, and how it is trained. The horse is an animal of low intelligence with little ability to understand strange objects or unfamiliar situations; therefore, it is naturally timid and easily confused and frightened. It does, however, have a marvelous memory which enables it to learn how to obey the rider's commands. It associates the same sensation with a specific command; that is, the rider's heel in his side always means to move his hindquarters away. If both heels go into his sides it means to go forward. Horses are trained with the use of reward and punishment.

Mounting

First, a rider must learn to mount (get on) a horse. The rider always mounts from the horse's left side. He stands near the horse's shoulder and grasps the reins and the horse's mane with the left hand. He

then grasps the cantle with the right hand and places the left foot in the stirrup.

The rider springs up to stand in the left stirrup, taking care not to jerk the reins with his left hand. He moves the right hand to the pommel, swings the right leg over the horse's back, and puts the right foot in the stirrup.

Some individuals with upper-extremity involvement will have difficulty mounting a horse. In some situations, the instructor will need to steady the rider and keep him from falling backward. Riders with hemiplegia, upper-extremity amputations, and cerebral palsy will need considerable assistance in mounting. The assistant will also need to help the rider adjust the length of the stirrup.

A mounting ramp with a sloping ascent can be built for use by the more seriously involved user.

The Sidewalker

The responsibility of the sidewalker is to maintain the sitting balance of the rider (Fig. 7–63). Depending on the degree of difficulty there will be either one or two sidewalkers with each student. If a rider starts to slip, the sidewalker is responsible for trying to right him in the saddle. (The sidewalker's grip control is transferred through the safety belt.)

Position at the Halt

In order for the rider to move in unison with his horse, his body must be positioned along the horse's center of balance which runs straight down from the horse's withers as shown in Figure 7–64. The rider places the point of his knee and toe along this line so that both the horse and he are in balance (Fig. 7–65).

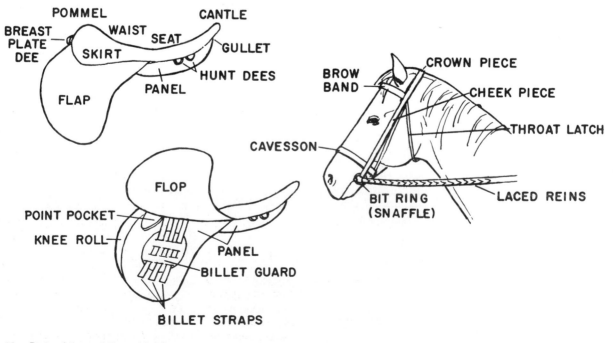

Fig. 7–62. Parts of the saddle and bridle.

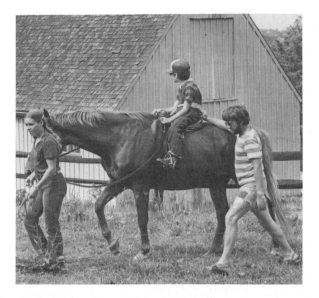

Fig. 7-63. Sidewalker stabilizing rider who is wearing a safety belt.

Position at a Trot

The trot is a 2-beat gait. The horse's diagonally opposite hooves hit the ground at the same time; that is, the right forefoot and the left hindfoot hit the ground at the same time.

1. Posting Trot: Posting is standing up and sitting down in the saddle while the horse is trotting. The rider is in rhythm with the horse's 2 beats: he stands up on the count of 2. The diagram of the rider's position (Fig. 7-66) shows that his shoulders are moved forward into line with the horse's center of balance; the shoulder, knee, and toe are all in the same line. The hands are always stationary because the horse's head does not move while trotting. When posting, the rider does not stand up high; he simply lets the horse's natural bounce push him up. On the second beat he sits down lightly. When he stands up, the knees are thrust into the knee roll of the saddle. The movement should be relaxed and smooth—in harmony with the horse's own movements.

2. Sitting Trot: The rider's position is the same as at the halt. The main things to remember are to keep the hands still and to relax, absorbing the shock of the horse's bounce in the 4 natural springs of the body: the ankles, the knees, the hips, and the back. These natural springs will not work unless they are relaxed.

Posting on Diagonals

The rider must learn to ride in balance with the horse. When the horse is moving around a riding ring, his outside leg has to do more work because it has more distance to cover (Fig. 7-67).

Both of the horse's legs should do the same amount of work; the rider must learn to "post on the diagonal." This means to ride so that when the horse's outside leg goes up the rider stands up out of the saddle so that the leg does not have to carry his weight; he sits down when the inside leg goes up, making it carry the rider's weight. In this way, both the horse's front legs do an equal amount of work, and the horse's balance is equal while moving in a circle.

Grooming

The skin of the horse is a good indicator of its health, as well as its protective covering. If the hair is dull or dry, it indicates the existence of any of the following problems: (1) constipation; (2) parasites; (3) teeth that are too sharp; (4) insufficient grooming; or (5) overwork and fatigue.

A horse should be groomed completely once every day to promote cleanliness, prevent sores and stimulate circulation. He should also be brushed before and after every ride. A half-hour massage with a curry comb now and then is also good for the horse.

Assistive Devices

Adapted Reins. Some disabled riders are unable to use both hands when guiding the horse. Also, beginners will need practice in rein leverage to utilize the subtle movements of the wrists in proper conjunction with their legs to make the horse respond. For riders with disability of one arm, an adaptive rein bar or similar device can be fashioned to fit between the reins at a suitable distance from the horse's mouth (Fig. 7-68). The rider can hold the middle of the bar with his unaffected hand and use wrist movement, which is sufficiently multiplied by the bar to simulate the leverage of two hands on the reins. The rein bar has also been effectively used for some riders who have involvement of both upper limbs. The bar serves as a teaching device which can be eliminated once the rider has learned how to use his legs to do most of the guiding.

The rein bar is 10 to 12 inches long and 1 inch in diameter. At each end, a hole is bored at a right angle

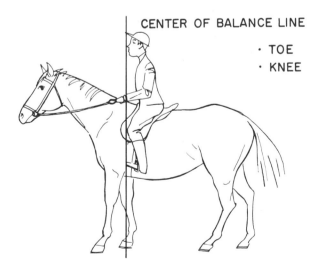

CENTER OF BALANCE LINE

· TOE

· KNEE

Fig. 7-64. Position at the halt.

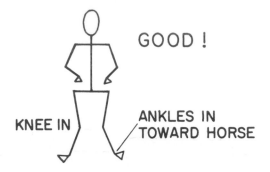
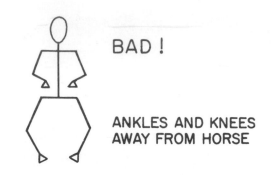

Fig. 7–65.   Good and bad riding techniques.

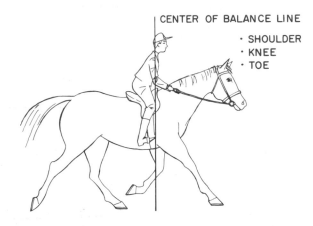

Fig. 7–66.   Sitting position at a trot.

to the long axis of the bar. Through these holes 6-inch leather thongs are inserted; the thongs are then tied to the reins. The center of the bar is wrapped in twine which is glued securely in place.

The Pegasus Riding Program (Darien, Connecticut) has successfully used foam rubber wrapped around the reins to facilitate grip action. The added, cushioned width to the reins makes them easier to grasp, while it strengthens the muscles needed to grip at the same time. A knot has to be tied in the rein directly behind the foam rubber to keep it from sliding towards the rider.

The Humes Rein. The Humes Rein (so named for the boy for whom it was created) was designed by the Wayne DuPage Hunt Pony Club Program for Exceptional Children (Wayne, Illinois). Basically, the Humes Rein is designed for persons who have involvement of their hands (e.g., amputation, arthrogryposis, hemiplegia). The oval handholds are shaped into large loops to permit the hands to slip easily both in and out (Figs. 7–69 and 7–70). The distance between the handholds and the horse's mouth can be adjusted easily at the bit. Even though the force of control is generated by wrist and arm movement, the rider is able to ride confidently and successfully.

Safety Belts. This piece of equipment (a wide web belt) (Fig. 7–71) is especially useful for the insecure rider or the rider who has precarious sitting balance. An able-bodied sidewalker can hold onto the belt handle to help the rider maintain proper sitting posture while on his mount. Essentially, this is more comfortable and easier than trying to position the rider by holding his clothing. A leather or saddle dealer can assist with design and construction.

Peacock Stirrup. This is a specially made safety stirrup (Fig. 7–72). One side of the iron is like a regular stirrup, but the other side is made of "breakaway" material such as elastic or rubber. When pressure is applied to the "breakaway" material, it releases, making it impossible for a foot to get caught in the stirrup in the event of a fall.

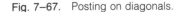

Fig. 7–67.   Posting on diagonals.

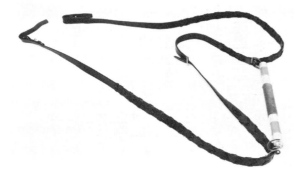

Fig. 7–68. Adaptive rein bar.

Devonshire Boot. The Devonshire boot (Fig. 7–73) is designed to prevent the rider's foot from slipping through the stirrup. The boot is especially helpful for riders who have tight heel cords or weak ankle muscles.

Adjustments for Specific Disabilities

The program adjustments and suggestions described in this section are for the balanced forward hunter seat form of horsemanship. Some riding instructors prefer the Western saddle for disabled riders. Although the Western style of riding is not discussed here, we are not trying to indicate that it should not be used.

Some therapeutic riding programs advocate the use of sheepskin and soft pad rather than a saddle to

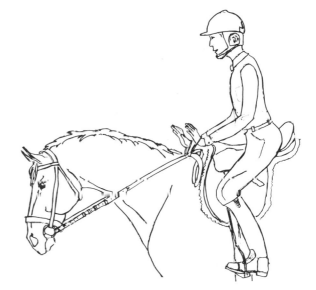

Fig. 7–70. Rider using the Humes Rein. (Courtesy of Mrs. Wallace Winter.)

maximize the walking, motion and warmth generated by the horse. This too provides specific therapeutic advantages for some riders, but will not be discussed in this review.

Abnormal Posture. Therapy for scoliosis, lordosis, and kyphosis is designed primarily to reduce rigidity of the spine, promote correction of the deformity, and

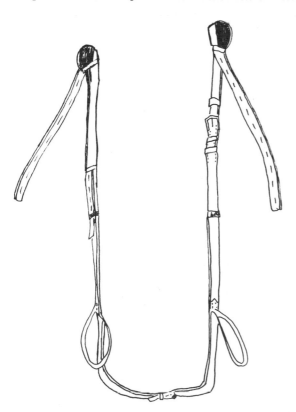

Fig. 7–69. The Humes Rein.

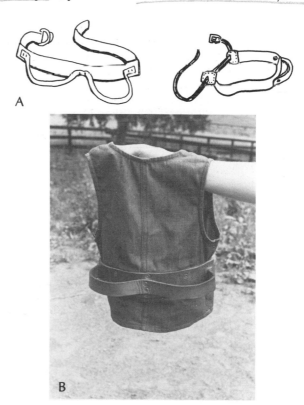

Fig. 7–71. Safety belts.

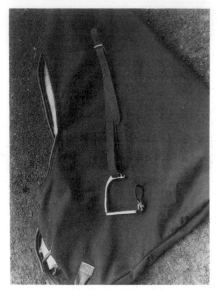

Fig. 7–72. Peacock stirrup.

develop muscle strength. The relaxed spine, as well as movement of the hips, knees, and ankles, is employed as the body's natural shock absorber in riding. The correct riding position facilitates the use of these shock absorbers to their fullest extent. The sitting trot and the canter are particularly useful in promoting purposeful relaxation of the spinal column.

Therapeutic Note: The constant changes in balance reactions created by the moving horse alternately activates and relaxes the spinal extensor muscles. Preriding flexibility and stretching exercises on the mount are also useful for the purpose of strengthening and improving muscle tone of the torso to counteract the effects of bracing.

Riders wearing Milwaukee braces and orthoplast jackets must be observed for possible pressure areas in the pelvic area, and adequate precautions should be taken to avoid fatigue and uncomfortable positions.

Amputations

Unilateral Upper-Extremity. The unilateral upper-extremity amputee can ride either with or without an adapted rein bar or the Humes Rein (Fig. 7–74). No particular problems are associated with this group.

Bilateral Upper-Extremity. In some instances, bilateral upper-limb amputees have been able to ride and control a horse or pony in a slow and gentle walk. However, advanced horseback riding is not usually advisable for this group, because the hook fingers cannot grasp the reins tightly enough to control the sudden movements of the horse's head. These uncontrolled movements may jerk the reins from the terminal device and, possibly, cause the rider to fall off the horse. Modifications to the rein bar may be useful in some situations.

Unilateral Lower-Extremity. The level of amputation will determine the ability to ride in this group of amputees. The below-knee amputee can learn to ride with his prosthesis, since the level of amputation will not interfere with his learning the balanced forward hunter seat. Some riders will use a Devonshire boot for safety reasons. However, the above-knee amputee will lack the necessary leg control for balance. Prior to the fitting of a prosthesis, those with Syme's amputation can ride without any stirrup at all.

Those who wear an above-knee prosthesis may want to use a pelvic band with a double-axis hip joint for flexion, sufficient abduction, and comfortable sitting.[11]

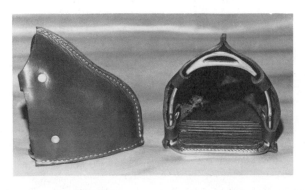

Fig. 7–73. Devonshire boot.

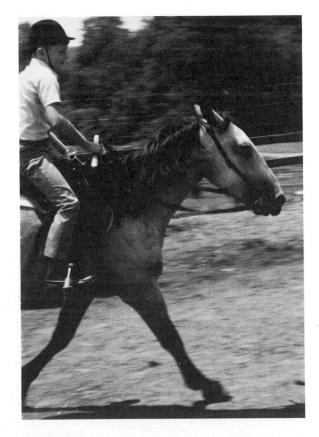

Fig. 7–74. An above-elbow amputee using the adaptive rein bar with the non-affected limb.

Note of Caution: Below-knee amputees with patellar-tendon-bearing prostheses must be watched carefully for chafing and irritation of the skin between the stump and prosthesis.

Bilateral Lower-Extremity. In most cases, the bilateral below-knee amputee can be a successful rider if he has sufficient knee and stump control to maintain a stable seat. Above-knee amputees lack leg control and balance, and this interferes with their ability to control the movements of the horse. "Bucket-type" seats to replace saddles can be designed for riders with short residual limbs.

Therapeutic Note: Teaching amputees to ride offers a particular challenge, since the activity does require movement of the whole body, and the loss of one or more limbs necessitates some adjustment in the conventional equitation position. The complete physical involvement of riding can provide great benefits by offsetting the "dismemberment complex" and eliminating feelings of deprivation and resentment.

Chronic Obstructive Lung Disease. Horseback riding can be successful and rewarding for the asthmatic if the necessary precautions are taken. The instructor should first determine if the individual is allergic to dust or horsehair, since contact with allergens should be eliminated. In some situations, the asthmatic may be instructed to avoid dusty playing fields and riding rings. The second precaution is to avoid undue fatigue and potentially frightening experiences. Asthmatic patients often do not participate in strenuous activity because they fear having an attack. Riding can serve as a progressive developmental activity because it allows time for increased tolerance to exercise as well as to the mental strain involved. The auxiliary breathing muscles can be strengthened by positioning and moving the guiding arm correctly.

Those with cystic fibrosis can also benefit from horseback riding. Exposure to riding definitely aids in developing self-confidence and self-reliance.

Horseback riding does not contribute to diminished endurance levels and early fatigue. For this reason, maximal performance skills are usually possible within a short period of time.

Visual Impairments. Riding can be successful and rewarding for the sightless individual; however, it is important to use a gentle, well-trained horse, maintain close supervision, and give careful directions. The instructor should remember that those with impaired vision usually do not have sound musculature and lag in neuromuscular development. Spatial awareness can be enhanced if the instructor remains in the center of the ring and gives continuous verbal clues to the blind rider. This provides a point of reference which the rider can move toward and away from.

Therapeutic Note: People with impaired vision tend to be more physically tense than sighted persons. It is difficult for them to achieve relaxed, free, and easy movement. The blind rider must develop an awareness of kinesthetic sensations before he can ride in-dependently. A sidewalker is often helpful for the purpose of giving positional sense (touch and verbal) cues. Riding in tandem with a sighted individual is not usually recommended, because this practice hinders the therapeutic objective of riding—to develop self-confidence through improving body control and coordination.

Cardiovascular Disorders. Medical permission must be obtained before enrolling such individuals in a riding program. The strenuousness of riding is determined not by the activity itself but by how hard it is done. Patients whose physical activity is moderately limited may be allowed to ride at a slow walk, and others may be given permission to ride at a sitting trot. The instructor must rely upon the physician's orders and control the level of activity as directed.

Cerebral Palsy. The cerebral palsied rider lacks normal muscular control and balance, and he often has impaired inhibitions, imperfect coordination, and increased reflexes. The teaching program must consist of repetitive movements to improve the whole body image. Riding is an excellent activity for those with good trunk balance, because it requires whole body movement. Coordination can be developed by the maintenance of proper body placement and the learning of repetitive movements, such as posting at the trot. Particular care must be taken in choosing suitable horses and in providing constant supervision.

Riders with spastic diplegia and quadriplegia should benefit from exercises that stress relaxation and postural responses. However, it is important to work slowly and allow the rider to gain confidence before initiating the exercises.

Devonshire boots are especially helpful for riders who have foot and ankle deformities. Adapted reins (Humes or ladder) may be needed for riders who cannot grasp standard ones.

Therapeutic Note: A Western saddle is often recommended for the cerebral palsied rider, because it offers a more secure base. The English Hunter saddle is designed to seat the rider with a remarkable forward incline. This forward seat is often detrimental to the rider because it increases his imperfect coordination. The cerebral palsied rider must have a seat that is centered well back on his buttocks if he is to have functional control of his lower extremities.

The therapeutic effects of riding include neuromuscular stimulation which aids head and trunk control as well as body symmetry and posture. The movement of the horse can replace a lack of normal leg movement in individuals who cannot walk independently. Normal movements of the head and trunk are facilitated by horseback riding. Some instructors prefer to use sheepskin instead of saddles.

Subjective analysis on the effects of therapeutic horseback riding posture and balance in children with spasticity has been debated for a number of years. In a recent study, Bertoti[12] discusses qualitative improvement in muscle tone and balance with this group of riders after participation in a therapeutic horseback riding program. Objective findings were reported after using a postural assessment scale to score alignment and symmetry of five body parts.

Head Trauma. Since head trauma consists of varying types and levels of involvement, each rider will need to be assessed to determine if gross balance deficits or behavioral concerns are disrupting factors. In most cases, the rider will need to be able to follow simple directions (Rancho Level VI) and have some basic processing skills. However, memory problems and delayed response reactions may persist. The instructor may focus attention to certain clinical objectives. For example, the rider can learn to guide his or her mount through obstacle courses while following directional cues to improve attention to task.

Head injuries are the most frequent of all injuries in equestrian sports, so quite naturally caution is of utmost importance in selecting the sport as a rehabilitation tool for someone recovering from a traumatic incident. Wearing of properly fitted headgear is of utmost importance and close supervision is obviously necessary.

Some physicians warn against the risks of repeated trauma to the head. One rule of thumb is that after three severe concussions, the patient should stop riding. However, if he or she is determined to continue, obstacle courses, gymkhana, and timed events should be prohibited.

Additional guidelines are identified in the section on Hemiplegia.

Hemiplegia. In hemiplegia, maximum return of neuromuscular function is the paramount goal. Proper riding position with appropriate placement of the affected extremities aids in muscle reeducation. In some cases, the rein bar may be used as a substitute for the involved arm. It is useful to have the hemiplegic ride with the affected side toward the inside of the arena for most of the lesson. This encourages weight-bearing by the affected leg because of the natural inclination for both horse and rider to lean toward the center of the circle. Also, guiding maneuvers call for the use of extremities on the inside of the circle more frequently than those on the outside; thus they require the hemiplegic to use his involved limbs more often. A hemiplegic can use the ordinary rein on one side and the special rein on the other side.

Hip Joint Disorders. Treatment for Legg-Perthes disease is based on the principle of containment with the head of the femur situated in the acetabulum. The normal riding position assumes this posture with the legs abducted with internal rotation of the hips. For this reason some physicians allow patients time out their abduction orthosis to engage in a therapeutic riding program. However, safety must be emphasized. Unless controlled, the constant bouncing and jostling motion of riding may aggravate the affected area. Horseback riding is a nonweight-bearing activity, but it does not completely unload the pressure on the hip joint. The physician must provide guidance in determining the proper time to initiate the activity. No major problems are anticipated once reossification of the femoral head occurs.

Osteogenesis Imperfecta. Each rider will need to be assessed closely because bone fragility is an obvious need for concern. The biomechanical stress upon the bones of the lower extremities is of concern especially during accelerated movements, i.e. sitting trot. Physicians often do not recommend riding for those with significant short stature, skeletal deformities, and internal fixation pins. Tandem backriding with a qualified instructor or therapist is allowed, in some cases. To provide a safe environment, some instructors limit riding to a slow walk with sidewalkers for security. It should be assumed that not all participants will progress toward independent riding, based on the inherent characteristics of the disease and associated frequent bone fractures.

Overweight and Obesity. Riding is recommended for the overweight individual, because it increases muscle tone and develops greater skill in the use of the body. Most obese riders will need assistance in mounting the horse. Embarrassing situations should be avoided. Many beginners will be unsure of their capabilities and easily frightened by new physical activities.

Paraplegia. Without seat sensation and leg control, the paraplegic will be at a disadvantage. Success in developing a properly balanced seat position depends upon a number of factors, the most important of which are the level of the lesion and possibility of such complications as scoliosis and kyphosis. For example, riders with a lesion lower than T-5 have the extensor muscles in the upper back preserved, and thus they have some potential trunk balance for riding. Many myelomeningocele children with a lesion in the L-4 to L-5 level have motor power present for hip flexion and hip adduction and consequently have good sitting balance. Since the head, trunk, and arms contribute to a properly balanced seat, each individual needs to be carefully evaluated regarding upper-extremity strength and sitting balance, particularly the ability to compensate quickly and accurately in trunk control when trunk balance is upset.

Fleece saddle covers are often recommended for the purpose of preventing pressure sores which develop from lack of seat sensation.

Therapeutic Note: One documented report indicates that riding therapy significantly benefits lateral flexion and trunk rotation through the contact of the rider with the swinging movement of the horse's back if a sheepskin is used instead of a saddle. This form of movement improved righting and balance reactions and strengthened the righting musculature of the trunk in a select group of riders with spina bifida. However, the report suggests that riding therapy is most beneficial for riders with a level of paralysis of L-5 or lower.[13]

Case History: This patient with T-10 myelomeningocele (Fig. 7-75) who required a wheelchair for mobility followed an inpatient treatment program to improve independence and self-care skills. This young girl was insecure and reluctant to engage in new and challenging activities. Horseback riding was recommended to improve body awareness skills and to enhance assertiveness training which carried over into other therapy areas.

The rider demonstrated poor sitting balance affected by weak abdominal and back extensor muscles. However, she had some awareness of joint proprioception in her hips and knees. Other complications included left shoulder mobility restrictions secondary to Springle deformity and bilateral hand weakness. Because of these reasons sidewalker assistance was necessary so she could be positioned securely to enable both hands to be used freely in controlling her mount.

Progressive Muscular Dystrophy. Because of poor body control and balance, horseback riding is not usually recommended for those with progressive muscle disease, unless it is done during the early stages of the disease before the individual becomes a wheelchair user. Riding in tandem with an able-bodied assistant is often encouraged. A Western saddle is recommended for this group of riders.

Therapeutic Note: Muscular dystrophy presents a problem of muscular weakness. Shoulder girdle weakness usually is significant before there is appreciable weakness in the hands and wrists. Weakness of the upper extremities may be present, but trunk muscular function may be spared for an indefinite time. If the

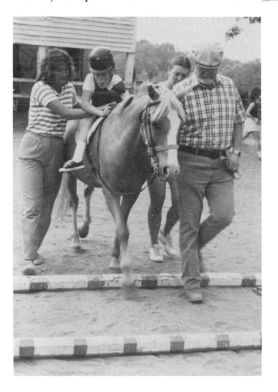

Fig. 7-75. Rider with myelomeningocele requiring sidewalker assistance. Riders who use wheelchairs for mobility find psychologic benefits, as their legs are replaced by the legs of the horse.

rider can fully control his mount, then certain exercises that emphasize halting and turning would exercise the hand, arm, and shoulder muscles. The game "Red Light, Green Light" would be beneficial in such cases.

Quadriplegia. Specially designed saddles with supportive back rests have been used with some low level quadriplegics, but even with this adaptation, considerable assistance must be given by an able-bodied assistant.

Rheumatoid Arthritis. Horseback riding can be a rewarding and relatively successful experience for an individual with rheumatoid arthritis. However, riding is not feasible if the joints are inflamed and range of motion is restricted. A careful evaluation of grip strength and sitting tolerance is required before horseback riding is begun. Careful teaching is necessary to motivate the rider to participate.

Therapeutic Note: For riders with hip involvement, it is possible that riding will stretch tight adductors and maintain range of motion in the hip joint. In any case, riding as a mode of therapy should be geared to the manifestation and extent of disease in each person.

Undernutrition. Rehabilitation of the undernourished patient includes physical exercise, but horseback riding is not recommended until the individual has built up enough endurance and strength to control and master the horse. Sitting posture should be thoroughly evaluated.

Therapeutic Note: The therapist should carefully evaluate each individual when considering the therapeutic appropriateness of riding. The extremely underweight person does not have sufficient fatty tissue to pad the body; as a result, he will not be able to absorb the shock of the horse's movements and will be very uncomfortable.

ICE SKATING

Ice skating, one of the oldest means of locomotion, was first developed by the natives of the prehistoric "pole" villages in the lake regions of the Austrian and Swiss Alps as a means of transportation over the frozen surfaces of the lakes. The first skates used to propel the skater across the ice were made from long bones and long sticks or poles. The oldest bone skate found in Switzerland is believed to be well over 4,000 years old. From the lake regions of the Alps, skating (skidding) migrated to the canals of Holland, the fjords of Scandinavia, and throughout Europe. The oldest skating club in the world was formed in 1742 in Edinburgh, Scotland. Skating was introduced in America by immigrants, and the first American skating club was founded in 1850 in Philadelphia.

Today, ice skaters wear 5½-inch high boots attached to 1¾-inch steel blades of $^5/_{32}$-inch width. Propulsion is achieved by swinging steps from hip to knee to foot with the knee serving as a shock absorber. The skater's task is to cause pressure on the ice by standing in the middle (center) of his blades (Fig. 7–76) with his weight equally distributed. This pressure creates heat, and the skater glides away on the melting ice, using the change in the center of gravity and his muscles to stay in balance and in motion.

Adapted for the Physically Disabled

Ice skating is a sport that can bring great skill and fun to the physically disabled. It was recommended for rehabilitation of various ailments in Austria long before World War II. Due to its close similarity to walking and its demands for the best body position in relation to balance and gravity, skating is a prime instrument in therapeutic recreation programs for physically disabled individuals. With practice, it can be performed by anyone who can stand upright without help. The International Council on Therapeutic Ice Skating (ICOTIS) originated in Charlottesville, Virginia, in July 1974 and was the first known organization associated strictly with therapeutic ice skating. Although it is no longer an operating organization the council was instrumental in building the foundation for using ice skating as a mode of therapy.

Speed skating is a USABA competitive event comprised of 500 and 1,000 meter races. Sighted guides and callers assist the visually impaired skater in negotiating the designated travel route.

Equipment
1. Ice surface: The ice surface, whether it be a frozen pond, tennis court, lake, or an artificial ice rink, should be smooth without cracks, bumps, ruts, or soft spots. An ice rink is preferred to a frozen pond or lake.
2. Ice skates: An ice skate consists of a boot with a mounted steel blade. The skates vary in size, and it is most important, in order to obtain the proper body position and balance, to obtain a properly fitting skate.

Selection: The boot should be sturdy and have strong ankle and arch supports. It must fit the foot (while thin hose are being worn) so that the toes slightly touch the front of the boot and the heel touches the rear. While standing properly on the skates, the skater should feel the blade between the big toe and the second toe in front and in the middle of the heel in the back. The boots should be laced snugly enough to support the ankle but not impair circulation of the foot and leg. The blade must also be sharpened correctly.

Types: The best skate to use is either a figure skate or a hockey skate. At times it is recommended to use a special learning skate, which has a figure-skate-shaped blade without toepicks. Never remove toepicks from a figure skate in order to convert it into a learner's blade, since this will ruin the balance of the blade in relation to the foot.
3. Apparel: Clothing should be loose, leaving room for body movement and yet supply ample warmth.

Falling on the Ice
Many skating instructors advocate, for reasons of safety, that the beginning skater learn to fall correctly. However, in therapeutic ice skating, the instructor must be sensitive to the needs of the skater. One of the main points emphasized by the ICOTIS is that frightening experiences must be eliminated when introducing new physical activities to the disabled. If the skaters are prepared psychologically to fall, then they are likely to fall during the early sessions. Disabled children will sense and overestimate the danger of falling and thus equate the sport with a risky and

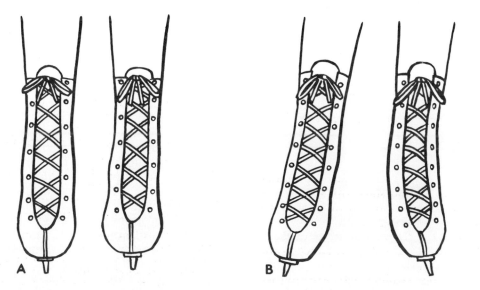

Fig. 7–76. Blade setting. *A,* Correct blade setting with weight equally distributed. *B,* Incorrect blade setting.

threatening experience. Also, since falling usually is an unconscious experience, in most cases a good instructor can provide psychologic help when a first fall occurs. This approach is more logical than overemphasizing the fact that ice skating is a falling experience. Positive aspects rather than negative aspects, of new learning experiences need to be identified.

Immediate success improves self-confidence, and this is why the most critical period in therapeutic ice skating is during the first 5 to 10 minutes on the ice. If the skater has control over his body (using the Oppelt Standard Method of Skating) on an unnatural surface, then in essence he has accomplished a major task.

Technique

How to Ice Skate

The Oppelt Standard Walking Method of Ice Skating is highly recommended because of the simplicity of its teaching method, its effectiveness in teaching groups, and its proven results. It incorporates these principles:

1. Natural positioning (feet slightly apart, turned at a 30-degree angle)
2. Total walking motion (pendulum swing from the hip over the knee to the foot)
3. Change of weight and foot position (lift knee and move toes up and forward; do not forget that feet are turned outward)
4. Use of gravity and pressure (lift off, impact of foot)
5. Edge control (body balanced over the center of blade)
6. Weight transfer (from the right outside to inside edge of the blade while the left foot is in the air; left foot sets down on the outside edge and slowly rolls over to the inside edge while the right foot is in the air)

Many methods of teaching ice skating to the non-disabled can be adapted to the physically disadvantaged, but it must be stressed that each specific handicap must be taken into consideration and that only a highly qualified professional should instruct disabled skaters. Special attention also should be given to physiologic changes such as coldness, joint swelling, skin irritation, blisters, and fatigue. Whenever such changes occur, the proper steps should be taken to eliminate the problem.

The Skating Instructor

Any beginning skater, but especially the disabled one, should get off to a good start with excellent instruction. Never try skating alone for the first time or with the help of a well-meaning friend. Even the best friend does not have the knowledge of a competent skating instructor who is trained to teach ice skating to the physically challenged.

If the instructor is not familiar with working with the disabled, it is advisable for a recreational therapist or someone trained in therapy to assist the instructor. In group instruction, it is recommended to use volunteers who have been trained by qualified skating instructors to help the disabled.

Assistive Devices

Outrigger Skate Aid. This consists of a figure skating blade mounted to a Lofstrand or similar crutch (Fig. 7–77A). Using an outrigger skate increases the base of support for the skater and thus enhances his balance. Force for propulsion is supplied by the upper extremities, which force the edges of the blade into the ice by a rotary motion of the arms, while the lower extremities maintain continuous contact between the blade and the surface of the ice. Hips, knees, and ankles must bend, the toes should point straight ahead, and the knees should bend straight forward—a natural weight-bearing position for many skaters with spastic diplegia. For others, however, propulsion is difficult or even impossible because of equinovarus feet, severe flexion contractures, or both.

Ankle-Foot Orthosis. The vacuum formed, polypropylene ankle-foot orthosis (AFO) (Fig. 7–77B) has been useful to patients with spastic types of cerebral palsy, head injuries, low lumbar level spinal cord injuries, or myelomeningocele, as well as unstable ankles and subtalar joints. The orthosis, which is worn inside the shoe or ice skate, can be fabricated of varying thicknesses of polypropylene, thus altering the rigidity of the orthosis to suit the needs of each individual.

UCB Insert. The University of California at Berkeley (UCB) insert is helpful to patients who are particularly bothered by severely hypermobile, pronated, flat-feet (pes planus) (Fig. 7–77C). This foot orthosis is made by taking a plaster impression of the patient's foot, fabricating a positive impression from the negative, and constructing the foot orthosis over the positive impression. The insert fits in the shoe, and the patient should wear the orthosis when new shoes or ice skates are being fitted.

*Hein-A-Ken Skate Aid.** Development of the skate aid was based on the principle of learning to skate with a chair. The skate aid, however, provides a natural position, ensures proper posture (Fig. 7–78) and even balance, and is more stable than a chair. The device provides physical and psychologic security and is often recommended for skaters who have limitation of the lower extremities.

The skate aid can be used for security or support for skaters who have limited movement, and it is helpful to skaters with neuromuscular disorders, especially those who are unable to achieve reciprocal action of the lower extremities for propulsion over the ice. Actually the device can be used for a number of skaters

*The Hein-A-Ken skate aid also can be used as a walking aid to improve ambulation after an operation has been performed on a lower extremity or after a stroke has occurred. The device, available in two sizes—child and adult—is collapsible and easily transportable. For further information, contact the Hein-A-Ken Corporation, Thief River Falls, Minnesota, 56701.

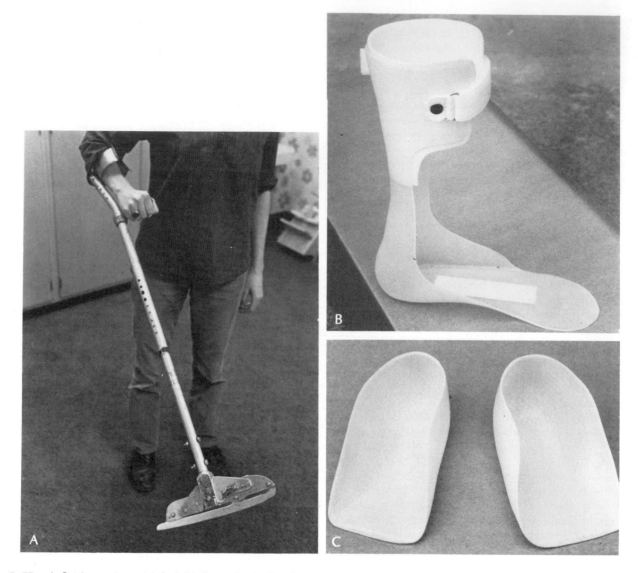

Fig. 7–77.   *A*, Outrigger skate aid. *B*, Ankle-foot orthosis. *C*, UCB insert.

who have difficult coordination because of a physical, mental, or emotional problem.

Nevertheless, do *not* emphasize the skate aid. Emphasize the person's own rehabilitative efforts. Obviously, some skater's achievements will be limited unless the device is used. Remember, however, that normal function is the major goal, even if it is an unattainable ideal. Eliminating the use of the skate aid, therefore, is desirable for some patients.

Wheelchair Runners.* This device was designed by the National Capital Commission of Ottawa. The wheelchair runners (Fig. 7–79) are actually steering skis from a snowmobile which are adaptable (and cost approximately $30.00) for use on wheelchairs.

———

*For further information, contact Director, Parks and Public Activities, National Capital Commission, 48 Rideau, Ottawa-Hull K1N 8K5.

Each winter, the National Capital Commission maintains 5.3 miles on the Rideau Canal for use as a skating rink. As with all its facilities, the Commission encourages use of the Canal Rink by family groups. As a result of this participation by families, the NCC recognized the need to find a means of allowing persons who use a wheelchair to join their families in enjoying this unique leisure time facility. This led to the development of the wheelchair runners.

The runners are fashioned from a pair of steering skis from a ski-doo (Fig. 7–79B). The wheels rest within the channel-like structure of the skis, and this holds the skis at the proper spacing. A horizontal rod passing through the front spring shackle support serves to hold skis in an upright position. A portion of the rear spring shackle support is cut away to allow the wheel of the chair to move farther back. This gives room for the foot boards at the front end to clear the

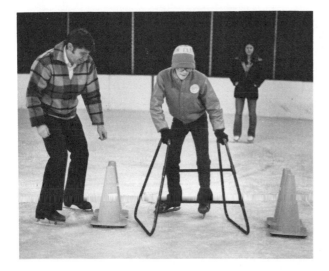

Fig. 7–78. Hein-A-Ken skate aid.

bumpers on the points of the skis. By tightening the turn-buckles on the tie-downs the skis are locked firmly onto the chair.

While intended primarily for use on ice, the runners work reasonably well on roads or sidewalks covered by hard packed snow.

Adjustments for Specific Disabilities

Most disabled persons will be able to skate if they are able to stand upright without help. The most important adjustment is to make sure that the skater stands with his center of gravity exactly above his ankles and hips, having the knees slightly flexed (artificial limbs should have the same Z-effect). If the student is unable to stand properly, he should repeat the following exercise several times before entering the ice surface:

1. Sit on a regular bench with the feet placed flat on the ground.
2. Rise from the bench without using the arms or hands.
3. Sit down slowly.

This exercise will tone the muscles and strengthen them.

Abnormal Posture. Ice skating naturally develops body alignment and musculoskeletal balance. The sport activates the antigravity muscles at the ankle, knee, hip, and back. The erector spinae group, which is attached along the spinal column, is brought into action through posture awareness development. In ice skating, the abdominal muscles are contracting and relaxing, and these work antagonistically in a pair relationship with the erector spinae group to help balance the body segments one over another.

The Milwaukee brace wearer has a distinct advantage in ice skating because the throat mold prevents him from tending to look down at his skates. Also, the brace provides vertical segmental alignment, and

this helps the beginning skater maintain equilibrium much sooner than the average normal skater.

Note: A patient who is being weaned from a Milwaukee brace or orthoplast jacket may participate in both therapeutic and basic figure skating. Special ice skating maneuvers, such as turns, leaps, and controlled landing on impact, should be done only by patients being weaned from the brace, or with special consent from a physician.

Amputations

Unilateral Upper-Extremity. One main objective during prosthetic training for the below-elbow amputee is to develop elbow flexors and extensors and as much supination and pronation of the affected limb as possible. Various exercises such as the backward swizzle can be used to meet these objectives. Steering the body in different directions helps the individual develop bilateral integration skills, because the upper part of his body initiates the change of direction.

Bilateral Upper-Extremity. This group of amputees can adapt to the sport of ice skating without too much difficulty. Power skating for speed has excellent therapeutic merits because the prosthetic limbs are moved in a forceful swing motion to generate forward momentum.

Unilateral Lower-Extremity. Ice skating is a natural sport for this group of amputees. Constant changes that occur in pace and position while ice skating are unanticipated, and thus, prosthetic awareness skills are promoted through unconscious movements. During the forward stroking motion, the skater can analyze his gait by evaluating the length of his stride while skating (Fig. 7–80). For example:

Normal leg—normal stride.

Prosthetic leg—short stride. This may be due to habit or a feeling of instability. The skater might be trying to get back on the normal and more secure leg as quickly as possible.

Ice skating can be used as a therapeutic activity to overcome gait deviations. The skating instructor needs to watch carefully for the "prosthetic limb instability syndrome." It may be caused by one or a number of problems including muscle weakness, anxiety, pain, or faulty alignment of the prosthesis.

Ice skating has additional values for the unilateral lower-extremity amputee:

1. Forward gliding exercises help some amputees overcome abducted gait habits. Many amputees, particularly in the stance phase, have this problem. The usual reason for walking with the abducted gait is to ease discomfort and pain.
2. Ice skating strengthens the quadriceps muscles. Knee flexion and extension power is needed to develop a good gait.

The above-knee amputee will have some problems adjusting to ice skating due to the loss of a knee joint. The loss of a hinge joint means that a major source of stabilization and power is affected, thus causing

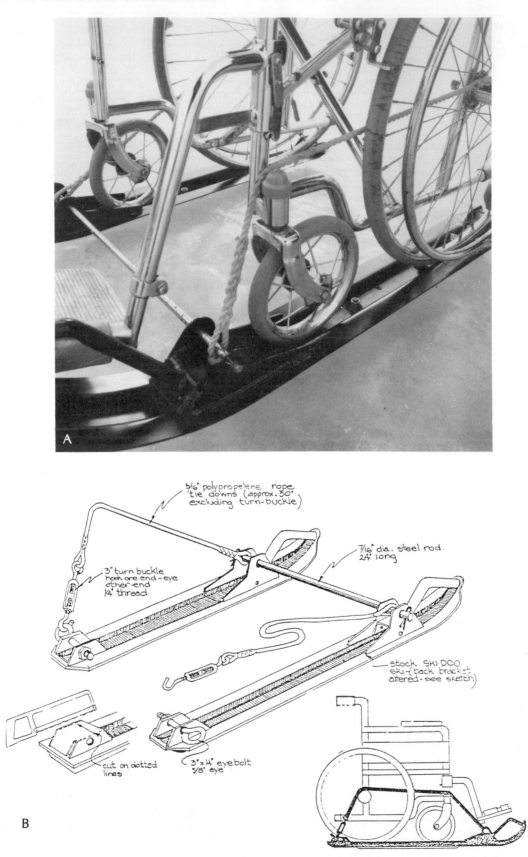

Fig. 7–79.   *A,* Wheelchair runners. An able-bodied skater pushes the wheelchair; however, the disabled person receives the unusual sensation of gliding over a smooth surface. *B,* Specfications for construction of wheelchair runners. (Courtesy of National Capital Commission, Canada.)

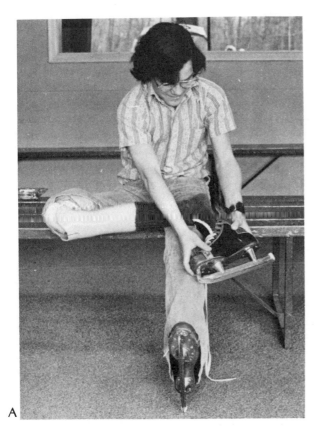
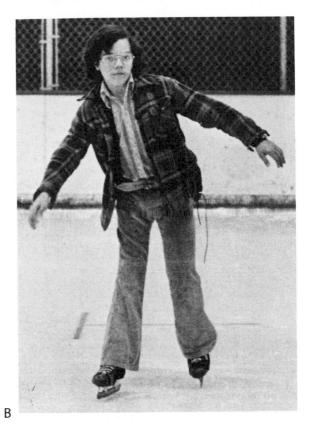

Fig. 7–80. Skater with leg prosthesis. *A,* Position for putting on skates. *B,* Forward stroking motion.

problems with equilibrium reactions on an unnatural surface (ice). Obviously, the main problem deals with lack of stability on the ice. Often, when force is applied to the above-knee artificial limb, the shank will rotate too far backward and cause problems with balance. Learning to use the Oppelt Standard Method of Ice Skating is important. Locking the knee in full extension will enable the amputee to use the scooter exercise as a means of propulsion over the ice.

Bilateral Lower-Extremity. As would be expected, bilateral leg cases pose special problems. Some amputees with 2 good below-knee residual limbs have participated in ice skating with the aid of outriggers (see Fig. 7–77A). Instead of a ski, a blade is mounted at the end of a Lofstrand crutch. Although the sport of ice skating would be challenging to a bilateral lower-extremity amputee, it is unusual to find a bilateral lower-extremity amputee who will use the sport as a recreational outlet.

Chronic Obstructive Lung Disease. Ice skating is an excellent activity for this group. One advantage of skating in an indoor rink is that the air is pure, thus eliminating common irritants to the airway. In addition, the measures aimed at better ventilation can be controlled in an indoor arena that provides a stable temperature. Poor posture and loss of trunk mobility are features commonly associated with individuals who are limited by chronic lung disease. Ice skating

is an excellent activity for improving posture because it exercises the antigravity muscles, particularly through the unconscious contraction and relaxation of the abdominal muscles. Improvements in the capacity for work and the efficiency of breathing patterns are additional therapeutic benefits of ice skating.

Cardiovascular Disorders. Ice skating is a good activity for persons with cardiovascular disorders if it is done regularly and progressively. Most energy expenditure charts indicate that ice skating expends approximately 6.5 cal/min. However, increasing the intensity of skating from a moderate level of exercise intensity to speed skating can result in a high energy expenditure. The American Heart Association indicates that the heart rate can be used to regulate intensity only if both the test and the conditioning activity consist of isotonic exercises that are done in the upright posture and use primarily the large leg muscles. Ice skating fits this description and provides pleasure without causing prolonged discomfort or fatigue.

Therapeutic Note: The heart rate is a good indicator of changes in myocardial and total body oxygen requirements. The skater can be responsible for taking his own pulse during a pause in skating to find the extent of his physiologic stress. Obviously, if ice skating is done for rehabilitative purposes, there should be close medical supervision.

Cerebral Palsy. In some instances, ice skating can be a beneficial and interesting sport for individuals with cerebral palsy. The skating instructor needs to evaluate each case carefully to ascertain the possibility of intellectual retardation and slow motor development. The sport is not recommended for individuals with severe spasticity in the lower extremities or for those with athetosis for whom an abnormal amount of involuntary motion will cause problems with balance.

For those with minimal cerebral palsy (spastic diplegic), ice skating can be used to develop balance awareness and bilateral integration of body sides. Skaters who have good standing balance and reciprocating movements of the legs can use ice skating to develop control of movement through visual and kinesthetic clues. Occasionally, off-the-ice exercises will help a skater who is limited by spasticity in the lower extremities. A physical therapist or physician might recommend that the instructor aid the skater in a series of manual stretching or positional stretching of muscles before and/or during pauses in skating.

Note of Caution: In most cases, a one-to-one ratio is needed when teaching the cerebral palsied. Surgical release of contractures, transplantation of muscles, and foot deformities are common features. A high-topped, well-fitted boot is mandatory, and an ankle stabilizer may be recommended in certain cases. Some cerebral-palsied skaters show hyperkinetic disturbances, most noticeably a distinct inability to relax and perform slow rhythmic movements while learning the Oppelt Standard Method of Ice Skating. However, with medical permission, rapid uncontrolled movement on the ice can be controlled by adding resistance with leaded weight cuffs at the ankle joint, thus allowing the skater to become more kinesthetically aware of his position on the ice.

Hemiplegia. The decision to introduce ice skating to a hemiplegic depends upon a number of factors. The sport involves bilateral integration of body sides; consequently the hemiplegic will be at a distinct disadvantage because of involvement on one side of the body. A high-topped boot and/or ankle stabilizer may be needed, since inversion of the affected foot and instability of the ankle are common problems. The hemiplegic has a natural tendency to do a scooter exercise as a means of propulsion because it uses the motor power of the uninvolved leg more effectively. Another factor that needs to be analyzed is the degree of involvement of the upper extremity. Usually, spasticity in the affected upper limb will cause the wrist and elbow to be held in flexion, a position that causes problems with balance and posture.

From a positive standpoint, ice skating has countless values for the hemiplegic. The sport can develop balance and power in the antigravity muscles of both sides of the body and improve muscle strength, muscle coordination, and endurance. Forward stroking can improve reciprocal movements. Gliding exercises in a straight line have therapeutic value because the skater must maintain both the knee joints and the ankles in functional positions, thus improving joint motion and associated movements of both limbs.

Case History: An 11-year-old, with left spastic hemiparesis wore a polypropylene ankle-foot orthosis to control equinus. His orthopedic surgeon recommended ice skating to help him develop a better body image and bilateral integration skills as he adjusted to his new orthosis (see Fig. 7–78).

The young patient was extremely apprehensive about doing any physical exercise, so it was felt that he should use the Hein-A-Ken skate aid for psychologic reasons. At first he shifted his weight away from his affected side and tended to use the "scooter" exercise for propulsion because it used the motor power in the uninvolved leg more effectively. Also, it was obvious that he was trying to get his weight back on the normal leg as quickly as possible. This caused poor tactile input and resulted in displacement of body segments and disturbed equilibrium of the whole body.

Slowly he began to develop compensatory habits of stroking and gliding with the skate aid; then he was gradually weaned from the device and introduced to elementary stroking and gliding exercises. As his confidence improved, so did his equilibrium reactions. Forward stroking improved his reciprocal movements, and gliding in a straight line helped him maintain both his knee joints and his ankles in functional positions which improved the joint motion and movements of both limbs.

Note of Caution: Some hemiplegics will hold their affected feet in the equinus position. A toe drag results, as it becomes difficult to clear the floor with the toes when the person picks up the hemiplegic foot. The toepicks on a figure skate become hazardous in such situations. In these cases, the instructor should consult with an orthotist or physician concerning the possibility of using an ankle stabilizer to support the foot in a functional position.

Head Trauma. Ice skating is not for everyone, particulary if the patient reacts inconsistently to stimuli. Another concern is the risk of moving on an unnatural surface which could heighten the skater's arousal level and fear responses. This is a concern for even the Rancho Level VII patient who requires minimal supervision for learning and for safety purposes. However, once the recovering head injured patient is oriented to his environment, ice skating can be an excellent rehabilitation medium for increasing tolerance for stress. Also, the skater must elicit judgment in unanticipated circumstances which requires bodily changes for balance and propulsion. Another feature of ice skating is the element of improving cardiovascular fitness. A helmet is often worn for safety reasons. Other considerations are listed under the section on Hemiplegia.

Hip Joint Disorders. Each individual with a hip joint disorder needs to be carefully evaluated in accordance with the degree of involvement and methods of treatment before introducing the sport of ice skating. Obviously, the sport would be contraindicated if a fall on the ice would aggravate the joint disorder. For this reason, two important points need to be considered before ice skating is recommended: (1) roentgenographic findings should show proper healing, and (2) if operative treatment was performed, then the child should have completed the postoperative precautionary period (generally 6 months for Legg-Perthes disease, and 3 months for slipped femoral epiphysis if external pinning was used). If an abduction appliance is the method of treatment for Legg-Perthes disease, then ice skating is not recommended as therapy.

However, late in the rehabilitation period, ice skating could serve a particular purpose. This is contingent on the fact that the individual is on full weight bearing without crutches or containment appliances. Ice skating makes active use of the quadriceps and hamstring muscles, and forward stroking increases range of motion in the lower extremities. The backward swizzle exercise would aid in internal and external rotation of the hips. It would also increase the strength of the adductor muscles of the hip.

Overweight and Obesity. The obese group will generally have problems adjusting to ice skating. Many lack muscle tone and their physical performance is slow because of poor agility, strength, and power. Predominance of weight in the center of body causes a "top heavy syndrome" that makes it difficult for the individual to maintain balance on the blades.

Ice skating is an excellent self-testing medium for individuals on a weight control program. During the early stages, it is important to increase the length of the skating sessions rather than the intensity. The goal is to use up calories; thus ice skating can be used to burn up calories over extended periods of time without becoming fatigued early. Regular exercise is important if physical activity is to be used in conjunction with dietary controls.

Rheumatoid Arthritis. Activities such as ice skating that cause impact to a joint are contraindicated in certain cases of rheumatoid arthritis. Naturally, the severity of the disease must be analyzed before initiating the sport for individuals with joint involvement and limitation of motion. Ice skating should not be allowed during a period when the disease is exacerbated. However, for those with minimal involvement, the sport of ice skating has numerous values. Attention will be directed to a few joints that are often affected.

1. The knee joint is a common area for limitation of motion. Ice skating, during the forward stroking phase, can strengthen the quadriceps muscles. This is important because atrophy of muscles about the knee is common among those with involved knees.
2. The ankle joint and foot need careful attention. Soft-tissue swelling of the ankle is a common problem, as limitation of motion often occurs in dorsiflexion, which is often secondary to tightening of the Achilles tendon. In certain cases a higher boot should be used to provide greater ankle support (provided that there is no swelling of the ankle). This corresponds to the suggestion, made by many physicians, to use a firm, well-fitting shoe for individuals with an involved ankle. A heel wedge or ankle stabilizer may be prescribed in certain cases.

Undernutrition. This group usually needs to be introduced to activities in which they can analyze their self-performance skills. Team games and sports are often contraindicated because the individual must compare his physical attributes (strength, speed) with other team members. During ice skating, the individual can develop neuromuscular coordination and appreciate the value of learning a smooth, efficient pattern of movement. Physiologic advantages of ice skating to the undernourished group include: (1) development of cardiorespiratory endurance and muscular endurance, and (2) increased joint stability through strengthening the ligaments and other connective tissues.

Note of Caution: Ice skating must be started slowly. The main problem with the undernourished group is that their skeletal systems have weak supporting muscles, which causes problems with stability on the ice. A natural tendency to use the inside edges of the blade for support is often due to weakness of the lower extremities and the anti-gravity muscles.

Visual Impairments. Blind people have already adopted the body position needed for navigation on ice. After orientation to the rink while following the word of a person leading him, the blind person can skate well. Championship skaters navigate their bodies the same way as blind people do: heads erect, eyes and ears parallel to the ground. Turns are done by turning the head in the desired direction with the shoulders going along; this turns the hips, and thus the foot will take a curve if not lifted from the ice. Orientation disappears when balance is lost because of a rough surface. The head will move and the eyes and ears will not be parallel to the ice. Blind skaters make excellent ice dancing partners because of their feeling for correct direction change, a feeling essential to pair skaters and dancers.

MARATHON RACING

Marathon racing, a modern road race, was first staged at the revival of the Olympic games at Athens, Greece, in 1896. The race is commensurate with the legendary feat of a Greek soldier who, in 450 B.C., is supposed to have run from Marathon to Athens, a distance of 22 miles, to bring news of his countrymen's victory over the Persians. Except for the Olympic marathon, the most coveted honor in marathon racing is participation in the Boston, Massachusetts Athletic Association race, which has been held annually since 1897.

Adapted for the Physically Disabled

Marathon racing in wheelchairs is a sport in which persons with physical disabilities push their wheelchairs for 26 miles, 385 yards in a race that includes able-bodied runners. Key requirements are: (1) that the athletes *push* their chairs, (2) that the race be a *road* race rather than a track race, (3) that it cover the *full marathon distance* of 26 miles, 385 yards, and (4) that it be *integrated* with able-bodied competitors—it is not a segregated or separate race. For example, the National Wheelchair Marathon is the wheelchair division of the Boston Marathon.

Marathon racing in a wheelchair can be traced back to the 1975 Boston Marathon, when Bob Hall completed the event in 2 hours and 58 minutes. Other road racing in wheelchairs did occur before that time, however. The most significant point in the history of the sport seems to have been the 1977 National Wheelchair Marathon, when 7 athletes entered and completed the Boston Marathon in wheelchairs. This success ignited interest in the sport and wheelchair athletes have been competing in marathons and other road races in increasing numbers.

The uniqueness of the sport is magnified by its technological sophistication, its capacity for integration into mainstream sporting events and its development of a competitive series with thousands of dollars in funding. Of special interest is the racing athlete who devotes countless hours to following a rigorous training schedule. This, coupled with the intense physical effort and tactical strategy that is involved during competitive races makes it one of the premier wheelchair athletic events.

It has been reported that the average racer has to perform up to 10,000 strokes during the marathon, and the impulse applied to the rims during each stroke is critical in chair speed.[14] Marathoning for 26 miles is an ambitious feat, sometimes heightened by the speed and challenges imposed by a fellow competitor. To master the effects of "togetherness," racing leaders often cooperate in a so-called "drafting alliance." That is, one racer takes the lead while the others follow behind to obtain a drafting effect. Racers take turns moving from the pack to the point position until the final 200 meters or so. At this time intensity of effort breaks open with each racer sprinting toward the finish line.

Like endurance runners, long distance wheelchair racers need to maintain a rigid training schedule and work on aerobic conditioning to tax the cardiorespiratory system. Wheelchair propulsion exercise needs to be of a sustained nature to reach 70 to 85% of the maximum heart rate. This includes using sprint intervals (gradually increasing distance over time with shorter rest periods) combined with propulsive efforts over 400 and 800 meter distances. Work output is increased and fitness level enhanced by challenging efforts to propel over uneven terrain such as up steep slopes and hills. Top wheelchair racers push 80 to 100 miles per week to attain high standards and peak performance levels.

Rules/Regulations

Long distance wheelchair racing is administered by a committee within the athletics governing body of the NWAA. The wheelchair must be NWAA approved; hand driven without use of gears, chains, and other mechanical devices. Use of pushing cuffs or protective gloves are recommended to protect the hands and wrists from chafing. It should be pointed out that pushing is done with the heel of the hand. Seat belts are discouraged because it is safer to fall free of the chair in case of an accident. Head starts of 5 to 15 minutes before the open class is frequently allowed. This avoids any congestion that might occur between the able-bodied runner and the wheelchair racer.

Technique and Adjustment for Specific Disabilities

The technique chosen to propel the wheelchair depends on several factors: the most important of which is the level of spinal lesion and the classification of the athlete which determines the strength of muscles used to apply force to the rims. Another important factor is the strength of the wrist and handgrip. The traditional technique consists of simply grasping the rims at the top and pushing down and forward until the arm is extended close to the bottom of the rims (Fig. 7–81). However, this technique is not as useful for the quadriplegic classes because they do not have the wrist and finger flexors for a strong handgrip on the rims. Many quadriplegics have used the traditional technique in their races, but it has been less effective for them because they are unable to grasp the rims firmly. Most of these athletes have relied on palm pressure assisted by shoulder depression to apply force for propulsion against the rims. However, even palm pressure requires strong wrist flexors to pull the hands inward toward the wheels, and most quadriplegics do not have strong wrist flexion.

A new technique of wheelchair racing, developed especially for quadriplegics, has overcome the need for strong wrist flexors or a strong handgrip in racing. This new backhanded style (Fig. 7–82) has been adopted by many top quadriplegic racers, and is successful due to the use of alternative muscle groups which are more powerful than those used in the traditional style. Instead of gripping the rims in the traditional way at the top of the stroke, the athlete uses the back of the hand on the rim, and may even contact the rim before the top. The hand is protected by a racing glove which is further reinforced with a thick rubber pad on the back, to prevent injury to the back of the hand which has no extra padding or fat for protection. The hand is then drawn up and over the top of the wheel, and down the front of the rim to the bottom—all with the back of the hand in contact

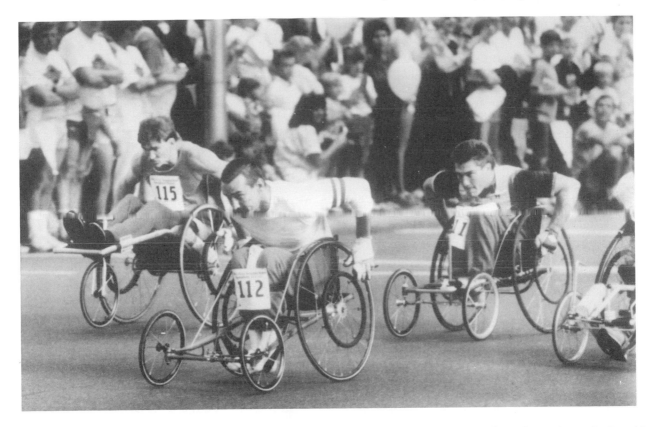

Fig. 7–81.   Wheelchair marathon racer using traditional stroke technique necessitating strong wrist and finger flexors for application of force production. (Courtesy of Sports 'N Spokes.)

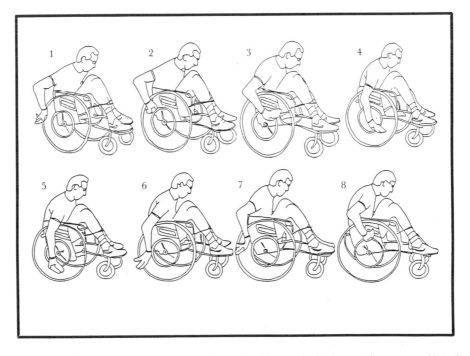

Fig. 7–82.   Wheelchair Racing Backhand Technique, an alternative method for quadriplegic marathon racers. Note that the rims do not have to be grasped and ungrasped for each stroke. (Reprinted wth permission from Palaestra magazine.)

with the wheel. The stroke is similar to the traditional technique in that much of the force is produced by the forceful elbow extension, shoulder flexion, and shoulder adduction during the downstroke. The major differences lie in the addition of the movements of wrist extension, supination and shoulder lateral rotation to the power phase of the stroke.

The movement of wrist extension is generally quite strong in 1B quadriplegics, while the wrist flexion and finger flexion is often weak. By turning the hand over, the athlete has substantially increased his potential for force by using his well-developed wrist extensors to provide much of the power for pressure against the rim for the stroke. The isometric wrist extension at initial contact with the rim provides the friction necessary for the athlete to apply force to the rims, while the final concentric wrist extension provides additional propulsion to the chair. Another positive aspect of the backhanded technique for quadriplegics is the recruitment of additional muscle groups which are often stronger in quadriplegics, including the wrist extensors, supinators and lateral shoulder rotators. These muscles are more active during the downward part of the stroke, providing additional force to the rim and increasing propulsive force.

The technique chosen by all wheelchair marathon racers above Class I (quadriplegics) is the traditional technique, in which the rims are grasped by the thumb and fingers, and the forces transmitted to the rims by the hands in a natural position of mid-pronation. Since all of these athletes have good control over their hand muscles, most feel it is more effective to apply forces to the rims using this grasping technique. Those athletes with lower spinal lesions can also use trunk flexion during the propulsive phase to increase the forces applied to the rims.

Some of the disadvantages associated with the traditional technique include: the time it takes to grasp and let go of the wheel for each stroke, and the difficulties of applying force to the rim near the end of the stroke (bottom of the rim). At this point, the hand and wrist are fully flexed and adducted, so the wrist and finger flexors are in too shortened a position to apply strong forces to the rim, so the forces diminish greatly. These are disadvantages only if the force per unit time is small—in the top paraplegic athletes and amputees who are extremely strong in the arms and shoulders the impulse is so large in a short period of time that these disadvantages are negligible.

POCKET BILLIARDS (POOL)

England, France, Ireland, Spain, Germany, Italy, and China—each has claimed to have originated billiards, and if Shakespeare is accurate, the game was played in the shadow of the pyramids before the Christian era began. Whatever its origin, billiards won popularity in the courts of Europe after 1400 and was played with regal enthusiasm by Louis XI, Louis XVI,

and Charles IX of France, as well as by Mary, Queen of Scots, and James I of England.

Pocket billiards, usually called *pool*, is played on a table that has 6 pockets, or openings, into which 15 object balls (numbered 1 through 15) are hit. Play begins in most pocket billiard games with the 15 object balls being racked at the foot end of the table with the ball that is at the apex of the triangle resting on the foot spot. See Figure 7–83 for positions of balls when racking and spotting. There are many different games of pocket billiards, and each has variations.

Adapted for the Physically Disabled

Billiards has been a popular recreation in hospitals for many years. As a result of the promotional efforts of billiards manufacturers, this sport grew tremendously during the 1960s. Various kinds of assistive devices have been designed recently for the physically

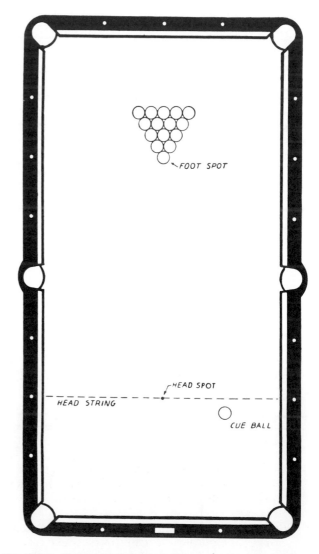

Fig. 7–83. Table with balls in position for basic pocket billiards. (Courtesy of the Billiard Congress of America.)

disabled; as a result, participation has been made possible for many more persons.

Pocket billiards is a quiet game of low intensity with little movement. However, the sport is a good tension reliever and in many cases promotes social benefits for patients undergoing active treatment in a hospital. It is also a popular alternative for individuals who have orthopedic conditions and are unable to engage in active exercise. The billiard table is a ready made support system. For example, crutch users can often shift their body weight from their crutches to the table when resting or maneuvering about for shots.

Snooker, a form of pocket billiards played with 21 object balls and a cue ball, is played at the Stoke Mandeville Games for Paraplegics in England, but it is not an event at the National Wheelchair Games.

Equipment

The following equipment is needed:
1. Table (Fig. 7–83): Regulation pocket billiard tables are either 4 feet by 8 feet or 4½ feet by 9 feet.
2. Billiard Balls: Pocket billiard balls weigh between 5½ and 6 ounces and are 2¼ inches in diameter.
3. Cue Stick: Custom sticks are often handmade of exotic woods, and the weight, length, and balance are suited to the player (Fig. 7–84). Pocket and carom cues can weigh from 14 to 22 ounces, snooker cues from 12 to 19.
4. Tips (Fig. 7–84): Leather tips should be properly crowned, resilient yet firm, and slightly "roughed." A crown (1) is necessary for the fullest possible contact on the cue ball.

    The shoulder (1B) of the tip is a ⅛-inch surface flush with the sides of the cue. Tips are glued to the flat base (1C) at the end of the ferrule (1D), which is a plastic or fiber shock absorber glued to the end of the shaft (2), which is glued at the 4 "points" to the butt (4).

    A 2-piece custom cue is fastened by means of a metal screw at the joint (3).
5. Rack: This is the triangular wooden or plastic frame into which the balls are grouped for beginning the play. Balls are racked on the foot spot for the start of most pocket billiard games.

Techniques and Rules

How to Play

Ambulatory Players
1. Gripping the cue: The cue stick is gripped lightly with the thumb and first 3 fingers. This gives a spring action to the stroke and permits better control. A tight grip tends to decrease the action of the ball.
2. Stance: The player should face in the direction of the shot, and the cue arm should move freely. He should lean forward at the hips, with his body weight distributed evenly on both feet. He

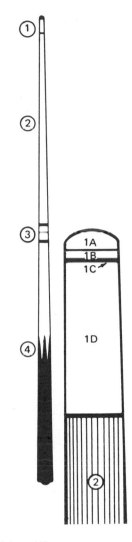

Fig. 7–84. Cue stick and tip.

should place the left arm (reverse directions for left handers) as far forward on the table as possible. The right forearm should be as vertical as possible. The head is over the cue in the line of aim.
3. Bridge: The bridge is made by making a fist with the left hand. It is rested on the table, palm side down, from 6 to 8 inches behind the cue ball. A circle is formed with the index finger and thumb, into which the cue is inserted; the index finger pulls firmly against the cue. The heel of the hand is placed firmly on the table, and the last 3 fingers are spread outward. The bridge should be firm so that the cue will not wobble. Other types of bridges are used when the cue ball is against the cushion or when the player must reach over an object ball.
4. Aim: The objective is to hit the cue ball in such a way that it in turn knocks an object ball into a pocket. To do this, an imaginary line from the object ball to the pocket is sighted; the cue ball

is aimed at the point on the object ball that lies on the imaginary sight line.

5. How to hit the cue ball: The tip of the cue is chalked before any shot is attempted. The best way to hit the cue ball is to feel that the cue stick is moving right through it; that is, by following through about 12 inches or so. The cue ball can be made to behave in different ways by hitting it at different points: it will "follow" the object ball after being hit above center; it will "draw" after a hit below center; "English" is caused by hits to left or right of center. But for best results on most shots, the cue stick should be held level and should hit the cue ball in the center (Fig. 7–85).

BASIC STROKES.* Perfect Rolling: A cue ball skids for a short distance when it is struck by the cue tip. If it is struck slightly above center (six-tenths of its height), the entire circumference of the ball will come in contact with the covering of the table in the shortest possible time—that's perfect rolling.

Follow Ball: A ball struck about two-thirds of its height will rotate forward around the horizontal axis more times than in normal rotation (imperfect rotation). When it strikes another ball, it tends to follow it.

Draw Ball: As shown in Figure 7–86, a ball struck below center revolves with a backward motion which catches the felt and causes the cue ball to draw, or move backwards after striking object ball or cushion.

WHERE TO STRIKE THE CUE BALL

C Center Ball: With cue level, stroke through the cue ball. The ball rebounds in direct line with point of aim.

RE Right English: The cue ball spins to the left (counterclockwise) and curves right. It rebounds from cushion or ball to the right, and throws object ball to the left.

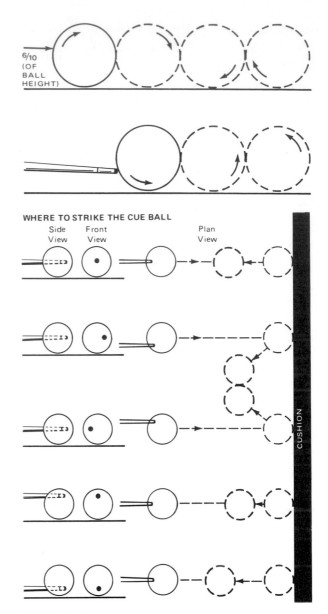

Fig. 7–86.   Ball maneuvers.

LE Left English: Cue ball spins to the right and curves left. It rebounds from cushion or ball to left, and throws object ball to the right.

F Follow: Cue ball rebounds from cushion or ball in direct line of aim, but for a shorter distance.

D Draw: A snappy wrist action and followthrough returns the ball in direct line of aim.

Hitting the Object Ball: In pocket billiards, the eyes should be on the object ball when the cue ball is struck. The point of aim on an object ball can be determined by drawing a line from the center of the pocket which bisects the object ball. Where the line extends through the object ball is the point of aim.

Wheelchair Players. The fundamentals will be the same as those for ambulatory players except that the section on stance is inapplicable. Range of motion will

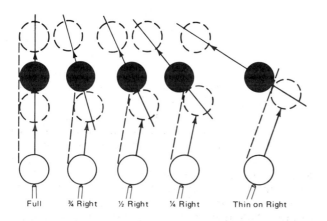

Fig. 7–85.   Aiming a cue ball.

*Reprinted with permission from FALK SPORT FACTS newsletter, The Falk Corporation, Box 492, Milwaukee, Wisconsin 53201.

be restricted, since the wheelchair player will be unable to bend forward over the cue to line up the cue ball with an object ball.

General Rules

Basic pocket billiards is often played with the rule that a player forfeits one ball (in addition to those pocketed on a foul stroke) for the following fouls: failure to comply with break-shot requirements; scratching (pocketing the cue ball) or forcing the cue ball off the table; shooting while balls are in motion; failure (after break shot) to pocket a ball, cause an object ball to hit a cushion, or cause the cue ball to hit a cushion after hitting an object ball; striking the cue ball twice on same stroke; touching the cue ball or object balls with anything other than a legal stroke with the cue.

Spotting balls: Balls pocketed illegally are "spotted," or placed, on the long string (an imaginary line running from the foot spot to the center of the foot rail). Balls are spotted in numerical order; for example, if the 1- and 3-balls are illegally pocketed, the 1-ball is placed on the foot spot and the 3-ball is frozen behind it on the string (placed so close that it touches the next ball). If the foot spot is occupied, the spotted balls are placed on the long string as close as possible to the spot, still in numerical order. If an object ball or the cue ball is resting on the long string, it is never moved to make way for a ball to be spotted. Spotted balls are placed either in front of or behind such object balls on the long string (Fig. 7–87).

If the long string is totally occupied, the balls to be spotted are placed in front of the foot spot as close as possible to it.

If the cue ball rests on the long string, thus interfering with the placement of an object ball, the object ball is placed either in front of or behind the cue ball, so close that it touches the cue ball (which means frozen to the cue ball).

Jumped balls: If one or more object balls jump the table, they must be spotted. If the player contacts a legal object ball first and then causes one or more object balls to jump the table, he continues play and is credited with any object balls pocketed on the stroke. If he fails to count, it is a miss and ends his inning.

If the cue ball jumps the table, it is an error and it ends the player's inning. Balls pocketed on such a

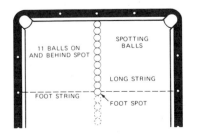

Fig. 7–87. Spotting balls.

stroke are spotted. The incoming player proceeds with the cue ball in hand and places it at a point behind the head string.

Balls within head string: In rotation, if a legal object ball lies between the head string and the head of the table, and the striker has the cue ball in hand, the legal object ball is placed on the foot spot.

Loss of game: After a player has pocketed all the balls in his numerical group, he tries to pocket the 8-ball, specifying into which pocket he will try to shoot it. If shooting directly at the 8-ball (that is, not banking the shot), the player must either pocket the 8-ball or cause the 8-ball or the cue ball to contact a cushion.

If the player, shooting directly at the 8-ball, fails to cause the cue ball to go to a cushion after hitting the 8-ball, or if the 8-ball fails to contact a cushion, he loses the game. If the 8-ball is pocketed on the break, it is a loss of game for the breaker. If banking the 8-ball, the player must hit the 8-ball. If a player accidentally pockets the 8-ball before he pockets all the balls of his numerical group, he loses the game.

When playing for the 8-ball, the player must hit that ball first. If he pockets the 8-ball on a combination, he loses the game. If he fails to hit the 8-ball on bank, he loses the game.

Since a player is required to call his shot when playing for the 8-ball, he loses the game if the 8-ball drops into any pocket other than the one he designated on the call.

Official Billiard Rules

Rotation (Fig. 7–88). Rotation pocket billiards is played with a cue ball and 15 object balls, numbered from 1 to 15. The object balls are racked in a triangle at the foot spot. The 1-ball is at the apex of the triangle of the foot spot; the 2-ball is at the left apex of the triangle; the 3-ball is at the right apex; the other balls are placed at random.

BREAK. Order of play may be determined by lagging or lot. The player making the first, or break, shot has the cue ball in hand. The opening player is compelled to make the 1-ball the first object ball. If he fails to contact the 1-ball first on the break shot, it is an error and ends his inning. Any balls pocketed on the shot are spotted. A player beginning his inning accepts the balls in position. The 1-ball is the first object.

SCORING. The player or side who first scores 61 points wins the game. The score for a ball is the same as its number. The 1-ball is the first object ball until it is legally pocketed. Then the 2-ball becomes the legal object ball; then the 3-ball; then the 4-ball, etc. The cue ball must strike the legal object ball before touching another ball; failure is a miss and ends the inning. Balls pocketed on an illegal contact are spotted.

If a player makes a legal contact on the object ball, he is entitled to all balls pocketed on that stroke, whether or not he pocketed the legal object ball. For example, if a player contacted the 1-ball, which failed to fall into a pocket, but pocketed the 15-ball or some other ball as the result of a combination or a carom, he is entitled to the ball or balls. The lowest numbered ball on the table is the object ball.

POCKETING CUE BALL. If the cue ball is pocketed, it is a scratch and ends the inning. Balls pocketed on the stroke are spotted.

EIGHT BALL, OR STRIPES AND SOLIDS (Fig. 7–88). The game is played with a cue ball and 15 object balls numbered from 1 to 15. Balls are racked at the foot spot, with the 8-ball in the center of the triangle.

One player or side must pocket the solid-colored balls which are numbered from 1 to 7; the other player must pocket the striped balls which are numbered from 9 to 15. The opponent pockets the group of balls not selected by the player with the original choice; for example, if the player with the first choice chooses to pocket balls from 1 to 7, the opponent must pocket balls from 9 to 15. Choice of stripes or solids is made by the first player to pocket a ball legally. The player who has pocketed all of his numerical group shoots at the 8-ball; the player who legally pockets the 8-ball wins the game. (See earlier section on loss of game.)

BREAK: Order of play can be determined by lagging or lot. The starting player is not compelled to make a choice on the opening shot, nor must he call his shot on the break. If the opening player pockets a ball on the break, the group from which that ball comes shall be the object group for that player or his side. If one ball from each group is pocketed the opening player must then declare his group before shooting again. If the breaker fails to pocket a ball on the break, the incoming player accepts the ball in position and can shoot at any ball. No determination of object balls is made until a ball is legally pocketed.

SCORING: The striker is entitled to all balls legally pocketed, unless he pockets a ball belonging to his opponent, in which case the opponent is credited with that ball. If a player pockets only an opponent's ball and none of his own group, it is a miss. If the shooter strikes one of his opponent's group or the 8-ball with the cue ball before it strikes his own object ball, the shot is not legal and any of his own group pocketed on the shot must be spotted; an opponent's ball pocketed on this shot shall remain pocketed.

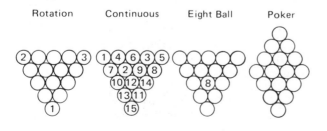

Fig. 7–88. Ball set-ups.

Special Billiard Games

Spot Billiards. Before the game starts, a numbered ball is placed directly in front of each pocket (pocket spot). The cue ball is placed in the middle of the table, and from there, the opening shot of the game is placed. This game was originally designed for cerebral-palsied players, because a slight touch is enough to pocket the object ball. The first player shoots until he fails to pocket an object ball. In case of a scratch shot (pocketing the cue ball), the following player can place the cue ball anywhere on the table. If a player scratches and also pockets an object ball, then the following player must return the object ball to the table and place it at a pocket spot of his choice. If a player pockets all 6 balls on the opening round, then the following player or players must match this feat to gain a tie or draw. The player who pockets the last object ball, provided that it is not a scratch shot, is declared the winner.

Rattlesnake. The "rattlesnake trap" (one of the 6 pockets) is chosen by the players before the game starts. Players proceed by attempting to pocket 14 object balls in any of the 6 pockets, including the rattlesnake trap. The object of the game is to "catch" (pocket) the "rattlesnake" (last remaining object ball on the table) in the "trap." It is a foul to: scratch the cue ball when attempting to pocket the rattlesnake; fail to hit the "rattlesnake" with the cue ball; pocket the "rattlesnake" in a pocket other than the "trap." A foul can be ruled loss of game or removal from game (if more than 2 players are competing).

Golf Pocket. A single object ball is assigned to each player. The object is to play "6 holes" in the fewest number of strokes. Players must bank the object ball off the foot cushion of the first stroke into hole number one—all succeeding shots may be banks or straight-ins. On each succeeding hole, players start by spotting the object ball on the foot spot with the cue ball left where it came to rest.

Break-Plus-One. This game was originally designed for the blind. Fifteen object balls are racked in a triangle at the foot spot. The first player breaks, and if a ball is pocketed (excluding the cue ball) then the player continues to shoot until he fails to pocket an object ball. If a numbered ball is not pocketed on the break, then the player is awarded another opportunity (bonus) to pocket the scattered object balls. The player shoots until he fails to pocket a ball. He then tabulates the number of object balls pocketed. The second player follows the same sequence, and high score wins. A player must forfeit a bonus shot in case of a scratch. The maximum score is 15; however, different score variations can be used such as playing in a series of frames similar to bowling. This game allows the blind to play without interference from hitting an opponent's ball. A sighted coach should aid the player in lining up shots.

Dutch. To start this game, the balls are racked at the foot spot. By choice, a player breaks. Two points are awarded for any striped ball pocketed, one point for any solid ball pocketed. Any ball that is pocketed is returned to the table at the *Dutch Line* (an imaginary line running from the foot spot to the center of the foot rail). As such, there are always 15 balls on the table. A bonus shot is allowed after a numbered ball is pocketed. In case of a scratch shot, the following player can return the cue ball to *any place* on the table. No score is awarded if a numbered ball is pocketed along with the cue ball; nor is a bonus shot awarded to the player.

The first player to score 25 points wins the game. Another alternative is to set a time limit, such as letting the high score at the end of 15 minutes win the game. Any number of players can play.

Assistive Devices

Because of the rapid rise in popularity of billiards, a number of assistive devices have been designed within the last few years. Many of the adapted devices discussed here can be made in an orthotics, a prosthetics, or a carpenter's shop. Scrap wood or metal can be used.

Adapted Bridge. The adapted bridge device is helpful and often necessary for the individual with cerebral palsy, muscular dystrophy, amputations, or other severely limiting upper-extremity problems. It is inexpensive and easy to make and is similar to a regular pool bridge. The holes in the bridge steady the cue in a particular shooting position for players with limited muscle control or ability (Fig. 7–89).

The materials required for the bridge are: a piece of ¼- or ⅜-inch plywood, approximately 4 inches by 6 inches; an old cue or a 36-inch long piece of ⅜-inch dowel; and a 5-inch strip of moleskin, light leather, or felt.

With a hand or coping saw, cut the plywood into the shape of a half circle. Smooth the edges with sandpaper. With a ¾-inch bit, drill 3 holes in the half circle. Two of the holes are placed ¾ inch from the flat bottom of the half circle and ¼ inch from the outer edge. The other hole is placed in the middle of the board with its outer edge ¼ inch from the top.

A hole for the handle is drilled in the middle of the half circle with its outer edge ¼ inch from the bottom of the board. This hole should provide a snug fit for the handle which is then glued or wedged in.

Sand any rough edges and paint. When the paint is dry, glue the moleskin, leather, or felt on the bottom of the cue rest to protect the playing surface of the pool table.

Swivel Cue Holder. The swivel cue holder illustrated is slightly more stable and somewhat more permanent than the adapted bridge, since it is made of steel (Fig. 7–90). It is a one-handed bridge which has been of great benefit both to amputees and to other patients whose upper-extremity involvement leaves them with only one functional hand.

The materials required to make the holder are: Two pieces of stock steel, 7½ inches by 1 inch by ⅛ inch; an eyebolt with a ¾ inch opening; 2 washers and one nut to fit the eyebolt.

Bend the stock steel into half circles that will fit together as shown. It may be necessary to trim one leg so that the pieces fit properly. Weld or braze the two pieces together, and drill a hole through the junction that is large enough to accommodate the eyebolt.

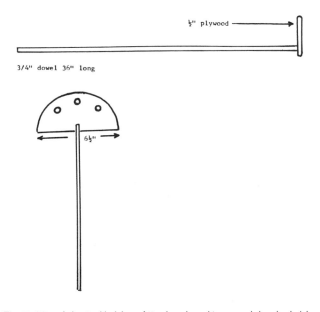

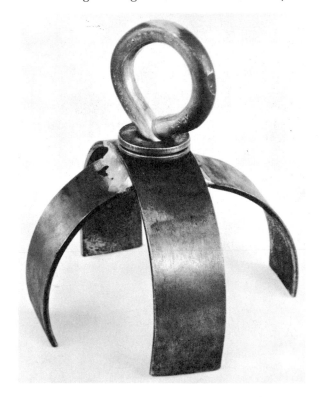

Fig. 7–89. Adapted bridge. Attach a dowel to a semicircular bridge with glue or nails. Cover the bottom of the bridge with felt or moleskin.

Fig. 7–90. Swivel cue holder. Courtesy of David Field.

File the joint to a smooth finish and paint. Pass the eyebolt through the washers and the hole; put on the nut and tighten it until there is a little play or swivel in the eyebolt. Make a mark on the bolt right below the nut. Disassemble, and saw the eyebolt at this point. Coat the eyebolt and nut with oil, and reassemble.

The eyebolt should swivel easily, but it should not slip from side to side. When it functions satisfactorily, set the nut by using a punch on the cut end of the eyebolt to expand the threads so that the nut will not work loose.

To protect the surface of the pool table, the four legs of the rest should be covered with moleskin or other soft material.

Wheeled Cue Rest. This simple device was designed and used by an older amputee, who suggested its use for children. Although the designer had parts of his aid machined and used machined ball-bearing wheels, simple wheels and axles and a block of oak are sufficient for training patients to shoot pool (Fig. 7–91).

The materials required are: an oak or other hard wood block, approximately ¾ inch by 1⅝ inches by 2⅜ inches; 2 model car axles; 4 model car wheels to fit the axles; 2 strips of 12-gauge aluminum, 2½ inches by ¾ inch; three ¹/₁₆-inch stove bolts and nuts; and a pool cue.

Drill two holes through the block of wood to hold the axles. These holes should be no more than ⅛ inch from the bottom edge of the block and approximately ⅝ or ¾ inch from its ends. Drill holes through the centers of both metal strips ⅛ inch from each end; drill holes to fasten the aluminum strips to block as shown.

Attach the metal strips to the block with bolts. Drill a ⅛-inch hole no more than 3 to 4 inches from the tip end of the cue. Align the metal strips on each side of the cue. Put the stove bolt through one strip of metal, through the cue, and then through the other strip of metal. Tighten the nut on the bolt. Clip off the excess bolt. Place the axles through the bottom holes and put on the wheels, checking to see that they are free wheeling and level.

Mobile bridges with larger wheels are also available from distributors.

Uni-que* ("Hot Shot"). The aluminum spring-loaded cue, known as the Uni-que, was designed by

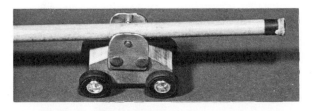

Fig. 7–91. Wheeled cue rest.

*This item can be purchased from Flaghouse Inc., 150 No. MacQuesten Pkwy., Mt. Vernon, NY 10550.

For additional information including warranties against manufacturing defects and workmanship write to Clyde Fox, 11107 Duller Ave., Northridge, CA 91326

a quadriplegic (Fig. 7–92). Power is generated from the thumb to a lever which then activates a spring-loaded shaft toward the ball. The spring-loaded extension shaft is loaded, depending on the impact needed for a particular shot. It is pushed in slightly for a soft shot and completely for a crisp, hard shot. The cue can be "reloaded" by pushing the tip against any stable object (floor, table, etc.).

Control Cuff Billiard Cue. Quadriplegics (C-5 and below) who have the major muscles of the rotator cuff with accompanying elbow flexion have successfully used an adapted device called a control cuff cue. The cuff (Fig. 7–93) which is made of Velcro material is screwed into the shaft of a regular cue stick. The palm of the hand is fixed to the shaft of the cue by the overlapping strap. Functionally, this maintains the hand in a stable position and compensates for lost finger strength and dexterity.

Adjustments for Specific Disabilities

Amputations

Unilateral Upper-Extremity. The adapted bridge and wheeled cue rest is particularly helpful to the postoperative amputee as a substitute for the missing bridge hand. The instructor should encourage the amputee to use the artificial limb as a functional hand; immediately after the prosthesis is properly fitted, the hook fingers can provide a firm bridge for the cue stick.

Bilateral Upper-Extremity. Before the fitting of the prostheses, billiards will be impossible for most above-elbow amputees. Adaptations to the butt of the cue can be made to accommodate the hook fingers, and the wheeled cue rest has been used successfully in some cases. Participation in billiards can assist in teaching control and use of the artificial limbs during the prosthetic training period. Bilateral shoulder disarticulation patients may lack sufficient energy to control assistive devices.

Unilateral Lower-Extremity. In most instances, prior to application of the prosthesis, the individual will be ambulatory with crutches, and standing balance will be precarious to play from the upright position. Under these circumstances, participation from a wheelchair is encouraged. No major problems should be encountered after the individual has learned to balance himself on his prosthesis.

Bilateral Lower-Extremity. Participation from wheelchairs is recommended for the immediate postoperative amputee. Participation in billiards is encouraged during the prosthetic training period to practice balance skills. The pool table is an excellent standing assist for this group of amputees, and billiards may be the first recreational activity that is recommended after fitting of the prosthesis. Those with two good below-knee residual limbs will be able to master the fundamentals without difficulty. However, special attention may be required for some above-knee amputees who are unable to distribute their weight

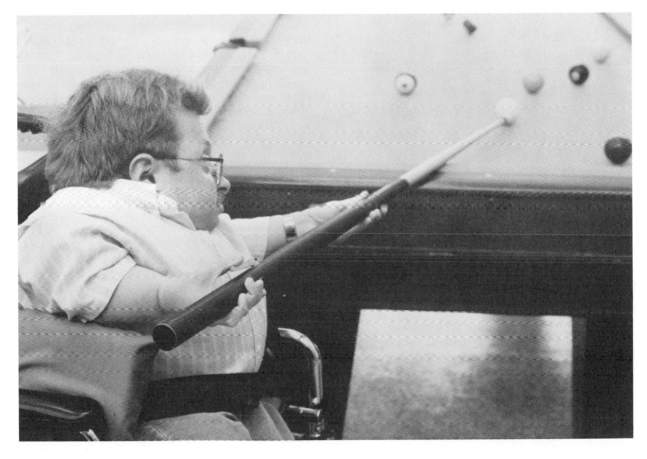

Fig. 7–92. Player with osteogenesis imperfecta using the Uni-Que.

evenly on both feet. The amputee will usually make his own adjustments and overcome this problem through practice.

Therapeutic Note: The use of adapted equipment can be either beneficial or detrimental to the amputee. With the amputee who has recently lost his arm, adapted devices are a definite advantage in that they allow him to participate actively during the healing and fitting process; they are detrimental if they are

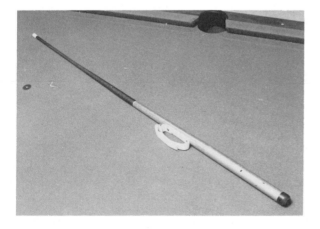

Fig. 7–93. Control cuff billiard cue.

depended upon in place of the prosthesis. The therapist who allows the upper-extremity amputee to continue using an adapted device after he has received his prosthesis and training is misinterpreting the purpose of these devices.

Chronic Obstructive Lung Disease. Individuals with chronic lung disease need to participate in physical activities that are within their capacity. Success in the performance of lighter forms of recreational games, such as billiards, develops self-confidence and leads to a lifelong hobby. Some players will lack strength and endurance; however, these problems are minimal and should not interfere with learning pocket billiard skills.

Hospitalized patients with CF undergoing prolonged I.V. therapy and using an intravenous system such as a heparin lock can play billiards without difficulty (Fig. 7–94).

Visual Impairments. It is usually difficult for the sightless individual to play regular pocket billiards. Modified games that keep the object balls near the pockets can be introduced. Beginners should learn to play the game called break-plus-one.

Special mini-beepers attached to the pockets are commercially available that provide for auditory tracking. Also, billiard guides made of plastic are

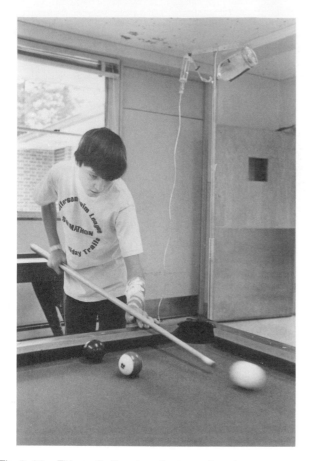

Fig. 7–94.   This cystic fibrosis patient was placed on a demanding 10-day course of I.V. therapy. Billiards was chosen as a therapeutic modality to permit the patient to be physically mobile and to reconstruct his body image and social role. The affected limb receiving I.V. infusion was mobilized as a bridge hand and extra I.V. tubing was used to increase range of motion.

available that provide an identification point for the cue ball and bridge for the cue stick.

Cardiovascular Disorders. Pocket billiards is an excellent activity for those with cardiac disturbances because the individual effort is under the direction of the performer himself. The game is often used to hasten the convalescent period with postoperative cardiac patients by allowing them to play from an upright position for short periods of time. Improvement of general physical and heart-muscle strength is an important therapeutic goal when using billiards as a graded exercise.

Cerebral Palsy. Program adjustments will depend upon the level of disability. An adapted cue stick and bridge are recommended for those limited by extraneous movements. An assistant may need to help the player line up shots, place the adapted bridge in correct alignment with the cue ball and/or hold the shaft of the cue stick steady. Less severely involved cerebral palsied children and adults, such as those with spastic diplegia, can play billiards without assistive devices.

Many beginners tend to "top" the cue ball because they follow through poorly on their strokes. Modified games, such as spot billiards, should be encouraged for beginners so that success is immediate. "Hand" pool is another alternative for players who lack purposeful control of their upper-limbs.

Head Trauma. The ability to play billiards will depend upon the behavioral and cognitive capacity of the patient. Careful monitoring of rules may be necessary so there is not an overload of information to process. Spot billiards is recommended for beginners. Some recovering patients who have trouble manipulating a cue stick can play "hand" games while rolling the cue ball at numbered balls. Certain assistive devices may be necessary.

Therapeutic Note: Billiards is a safe game that fosters processing of basic input. It is an excellent rehabilitation activity because it can be used to develop memory, sequencing, and concept formation. In addition, it is often played in a relaxed environment (tandem or group) which can be used to facilitate social interaction.

Hemiplegia. Before a program of billiards is initiated for the hemiplegic, his personal limitations and abilities should be clearly understood. Those with severe contractures of the affected limb can use the mobile or swivel cue holder to compensate for the loss of the bridge hand. Some players may be able to use the affected hand as a bridge for the cue stick; however, movement must be slow in the beginning to avoid an improper follow-through with the cue. The Uni-que can be helpful in some instances.

Hip Joint Disorders. Depending upon medical orders, players can participate in billiards from a wheelchair or in some cases a bed if traction is used. The instructor should reinforce treatment and discourage the individual from bearing weight on the involved side. During the acute stage, children with Legg-Perthes disease have difficulty adjusting to their wheelchair existence or when using crutches, and often attempt to stand and bear weight on the unaffected side when reaching to hit the cue ball. After the disease is arrested and muscular re-education is nearly complete, participation need be limited only by the structural limitations of the individual. Standing tolerance must be carefully evaluated during the early stages of ambulation.

Players wearing abduction appliances are encouraged to play billiards because the game is so safe. Also, the table can support segments of the body when the player has insufficient standing tolerance and balance skills. This support system is also helpful for postoperative patients using crutches.

Osteogenesis Imperfecta. Depending upon the degree of mobility limitations, most players can play billiards or modifications of the game. The wheelchair player will often need to use the Uni-que (Fig. 7–92) or Wheeled Cue Rest due to restrictions in trunk mobility and short stature. Most ambulatory players without decreased range of motion and contractures can play the game without adapted equipment.

Overweight and Obesity. Many overweight persons become proficient billiard players. Billiards, however, is not a vigorous game and does not contribute significantly to a program of weight reduction.

Therapeutic Note: The therapeutic benefits of billiards are generally psycho-social in nature, assuming that the actvity is not physically challenging. The overweight participant is not at a disadvantage because of the fine motor dexterity required for skill development and success.

Paraplegia. Involvement of both lower limbs will not interfere with learning the fundamentals of billiards from a wheelchair. In some situations, the adapted bridge can be used to compensate for weakness of the arm and shoulder musculature and range of motion restrictions. The use of adapted equipment should be kept to a minimum, since active bimanual upper-extremity exercise is the primary therapeutic value of the game.

Progressive Muscular Disorders. Certain assistive devices can be used to help patients. A short, lightweight cue stick can be substituted for a regular cue if the individual is capable of playing from a standing position. Since muscle function is limited, the participant will have difficulty hitting the cue ball at an object ball accurately. The wheelchair-bound player may need to use the wheeled cue rest to compensate for upper-arm and shoulder-girdle weakness. In addition, the ball bearing feeder (see adapted table tennis) or deltoid sling can be used to promote broader and freer movements of the affected limbs. Even individuals with severe involvement who are required to use assistive devices can gain some degree of proficiency in billiards. Competition must be controlled to avoid frustration.

Frequently, however, an able-bodied assistant will need to help stabilize the cue stick, including the Unique, to give the player a secure base of support. For the severely involved player, an assistant will also need to help line up shots.

Quadriplegia. The individual with severe involvement in all 4 extremities will have difficulty participating in billiards. Modified games, such as spot billiards, that provide for instant success should be encouraged whenever possible or as a lead-up to more advanced games. Early fatigue must be avoided. Some quadriplegics (C-5 and below) have used the control cuff cue, Uni-que and mobile cue with varying degrees of success.

Rheumatoid Arthritis. Those with severe involvement of the interphalangeal joints will have difficulty forming a bridge circle with the index finger and thumb; consequently, they will need to use an open bridge hand or the mobile cue rest, Uni-que, or adapted bridge. As participation becomes more active, joint range of motion is increased, and motor function

is improved. In such cases adapted equipment should be kept to a minimum.

Abnormal Posture. There are usually no contraindications for participation in billiards for ambulatory patients with spinal deformities. The ambulatory player in a Milwaukee brace or postoperative cast will find little anatomic restriction, although some players will be unable to lean forward comfortably at the hips to sight the cue ball.

Undernutrition. The major physical characteristics of undernutrition—muscular weakness, poor coordination, and low vitality—will not interfere with learning pocket billiard skills, since the game is not strenuous. Poor forearm and upper-arm strength will hinder some players in executing a smooth, straight follow-through with the cue. Lack of muscle control will also interfere with developing a stable bridge. In some situations, a lightweight cue stick can be used to compensate for lack of strength.

Therapeutic Note: Adapted devices should not be encouraged. The underweight individual needs to be shown that his condition does not necessarily interfere with learning successful motor skills.

TARGET SPORTS/GAMES

There are many target throwing activities that can be included in general and therapeutic recreation programs including disc sports, darts, and horseshoes to name a few. The popularity of these activities are related, in part, to the affordable price range of equipment, and the adaptability such as using variations in distance throwing to various disability groupings. It is impossible to review many target sports/games due to space limitations. However, two will be discussed; precision javelin, known mostly as a competitive sport event, and blowdarts, a new recreational outlet for the severely involved participant.

PRECISION JAVELIN

The spear has played an important part in history from earliest times. Javelin throwing can be traced to primitive man's use of the spear for hunting and fighting. Precision was acquired by primitive men, since they depended upon a sharp eye to kill animals for survival. The spear was the chief weapon used in the battles of ancient Asia and Europe. The Swedes and Finns were the first to introduce the javelin throw to modern athletic programs.

The javelin is essentially a long spear with a sharp metal tip. The object of the sport is to throw the javelin from behind a restraining line to a ground target made of circular rings (Fig. 7–95). Each competitor throws 6 times, and the best 5 scores count.

Adapted for the Physically Disabled

Precision javelin for the disabled was a popular competitive NWAA event for a number of years until

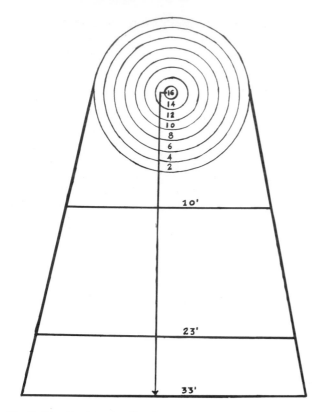

Fig. 7–95.   Precision javelin court.

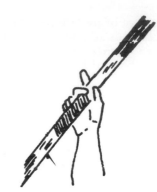

Fig. 7–96.   Finnish hold.

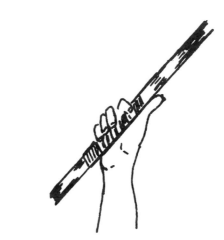

Fig. 7–97.   American hold.

it was phased out after 1972. Precision javelin eliminates the running approach and throwing for distance which characterize the regular javelin throw seen in track and field events. The sport is very adaptable. For example, mainstream instruction to include precision javelin would fulfill certain needs for a mobility impaired student in a regular physical education unit that includes track and field.

Equipment
The following equipment is needed:
1. Javelin: The official javelin for precision throwing is the international ladies' javelin. The javelin is made of wood with a point of solid metal and is between 7 feet 2⅝ inches and 7 feet 6½ inches in length and weighs at least 1 pound 5¼ ounces.

Throwing Technique
The type of grip that an individual selects will depend upon the length and strength of his fingers, the size of the javelin shaft, and personal preference. Two methods of holding the javelin are:

The Finnish hold (Fig. 7–96): The thrower grasps the javelin at the rear of the binding so that his second finger encircles the shaft and barely touches the extended thumb. The first finger is approximately in line with the wrist and curls slightly around the shaft. The Finnish hold finds ready acceptance among throwers, since the shaft lies in the natural cradle of the palm of the hand, giving a feeling of security.

The American hold (Fig. 7–97): This hold is somewhat different, since the javelin is held with three fingers encircling the whipcord with the thumb resting lightly along the shaft. The difference between this hold and the Finnish style is that the pull is exerted by the first finger with the American hold.

Throwing Distances
From end line to center of circle:
Severely involved—10 feet
Ladies—23 feet
Men—33 feet

Adjustments for Specific Disabilities
Almost everyone can gain a satisfactory degree of proficiency in the sport of precision javelin. Discussion will be limited to the wheelchair participant who has a moderate or severe disability, since the sport was originally intended for this group.

Cerebral Palsy. The Class IV athlete (moderate to severe diplegia), and above athlete with good hand function and normal strength can usually learn to throw the javelin. Naturally, those with exaggerated stretch reflex movements will have difficulty in learning the fundamentals of the javelin throw. The major problem will be their inability to develop a smooth release. Most players with spasticity and athetosis will have a poorly timed, jerky release movement which will cause the javelin to be released improperly. Since the javelin throw is primarily a single-response activity, active physical training may improve body mechanics and muscular control. However, some patients with moderate to great limitation of activity will be unable to adjust to the sport, regardless of the amount of training.

Paraplegia. Most paraplegics can become proficient javelin throwers (Fig. 7–98). This is particularly true for those with very low lesions because the abdominal and back muscles are spared. Those with a high lesion (between T 2 and T 7) will have a balance problem when shifting their body weight in the wheelchair during the forward thrust motion. With sufficient practice, the paraplegic should produce accurate precision scores. Two positions for throwing are possible: (1) the wheelchair is placed at a 90-degree angle to the target for participants with good sitting balance; or (2) the wheelchair faces the target for participants with poor sitting balance.

Quadriplegia. Depending upon the level of involvement, the quadriplegic can either use the forward or backward method of throwing the javelin. The instructor should introduce both methods and choose the type which is most suitable. Various assistive devices can enable the quadriplegic to throw backward,

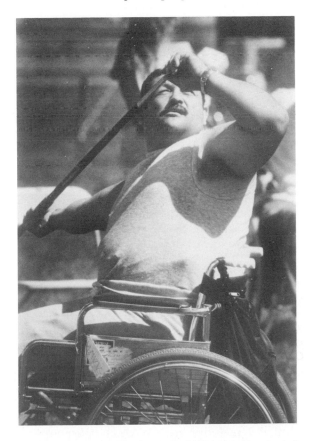

Fig. 7–98. Javelin thrower demonstrating position technique. (Courtesy of Paralyzed Veterans of America.)

thereby allowing him to utilize his remaining upper-arm muscles. This is particularly the case with athletes at the C-6 level of functioning in which no triceps function can assist in the forward throwing motion.

Program Notes
The target has 8 concentric circular rings, each 8 inches wide. The target may consist of tubular rings flush to the ground, or painted lines on a cloth laid and fixed on the ground, or some similar device.

The center rings will count 16 points; each ring away from it, 2 points less than the previous ring.

The competitor will throw 6 times at a distance of 33 feet from the throwing line to the center of the middle ring. (Note: In ladies' competition, the distance will be 23 feet.) The best 5 scores will count.

All throws will conform to legal javelin throws. Each javelin will be removed from the target before the next one is thrown.

In the event of any tie, the higher rank should be awarded to the competitor with the most center rings scored, and followed by the most of the next higher rings scored, etc.

BLOWDARTS
The use of a blowgun to propel darts at a target has been used for centuries as a primitive means of hunting. The concept of using a blowgun as a recreational activity for disabled persons who have little or no use of their arms and hands was developed by Andrew I. Batavia, J.D., M.S., Program Director for Health Services Research at the National Rehabilitation Hospital in Washington, DC (Figs. 7–99 and 7–100).

Equipment*
There are three basic pieces of equipment needed to conduct the activity of blowdarts; a blowgun, blowdarts, and a target. The blowgun is a metal cylinder with a rubber or plastic mouthpiece into which the participant blows. The blowdarts are darts that are specially designed to be propelled from the blowgun. The target is basically the same as the target used in the game of darts. For use in institutions, velcro-tipped blowdarts and targets are suggested to minimize safety concerns.

Therapeutic Implications
The therapeutic benefits of blowdarts as an activity for disabled persons have not yet been empirically tested. However, there are strong reasons to believe that blowdarts has therapeutic value in terms of increasing respiratory strength and capacity. Disabled persons who have tried the activity report that it appears to be a valuable respiratory exercise. Further, blowdarts is one of the few respiratory exercises available for severely disabled persons (high level quad-

*For price list and order form, write AIB Unlimited, Inc., P.O. Box 3635, Boynton Beach, FL 33424

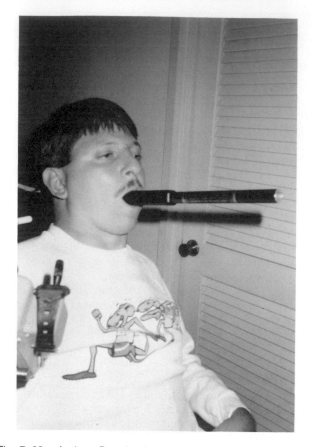

Fig. 7–99. Andrew Batavia, the developer of blowdarts demonstrates the activity. Directions for person with limited or no use of arms and hands: An able-bodied person loads the blowgun. The shooter places his lips and teeth around the mouthpiece, and bites gently on the shaft. Using head and neck, aim carefully at the target, breathe in around the mouthpiece, and exhale sharply into mouthpiece to shoot the dart.

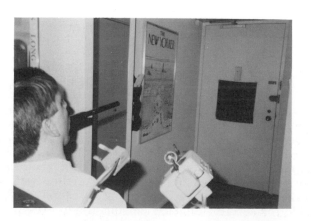

Fig. 7–100. Blowdart target range. Even with velcro blowdarts, it is important to aim and play with care.

riplegics and advanced muscular dystrophy). It would also benefit patients with chronic obstructive pulmonary disease. Finally, blowdarts appears to be an attractive social activity, therefore well-suited for use in therapeutic recreation.

Further Information

For further information on blowdarts, please contact:

Andrew I. Batavia
700 7th Street S.W. #813
Washington, DC 20024
(202) 863-2783

QUAD RUGBY

The game of muderball, now known as quad rugby was started in 1976 by a group of Canadian quadriplegics. The sport slowly gained popularity in the United States headed by the efforts of Brad Mikkelson who formed the first team with support from the Disabled Student Services at the University of North Dakota. The year 1982 marked for showcasing the sport of quad rugby competition in the United States with an exhibition game at the National Wheelchair Games. It was also the same year for the first International Quad Rugby Tournament which was held at the University of North Dakota.

The game can be aggressive, and for this reason provides a physical challenge to many quadriplegics (Fig. 7–101). In addition, it is a promising team sport that provides an alternative to playing wheelchair basketball.

Equipment

Quad rugby is played on a regulation basketball court with two restricted zones marked at each end with cones (Fig. 7–102). The official game ball is a regulation-weight volleyball.

Techniques and Rules

Each team is comprised of four quadriplegics who attempt to control a volleyball from player to player, similar to basketball. Strategy for scoring points entails breaking a line of defense to cross the opponent's goal line with the ball. Like hockey, a player who commits defensive penalties and other violations such as holding and pushing must sit out time in the penalty box.

A zone defense can be used to control the offensive threat of the opposing team. Strategic positioning to take advantage of the player's mobility and height is used to control specific zones. For example, a chaser must be quick and strong enough to apply constant pressure to the offensive ball handler in the front court area (Fig. 7–102).

There is a team balance rule based on an eight point system. This includes the NWAA classification system (with adjustments for trunk stability): Class 1A = one point, Class 1B = two points, Class 1C = three points.

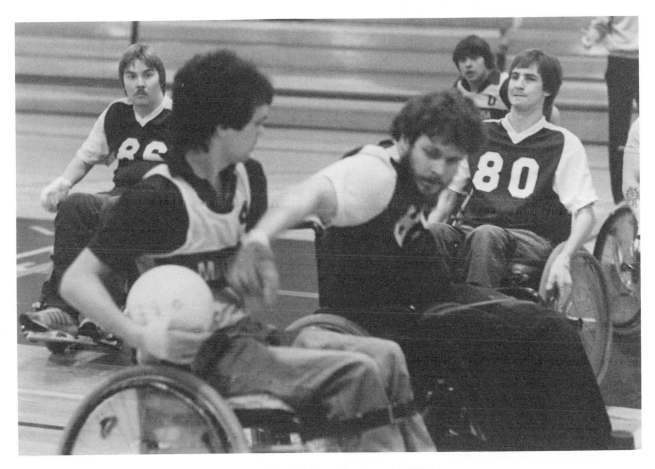

Fig. 7–101.   Quad rugby action between Manitoba and North Dakota. (Courtesy of USQRA.)

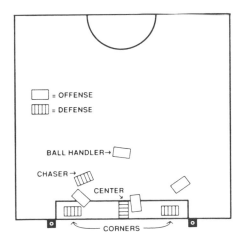

Fig. 7–102.   Typical zone defense that is used in quad rugby. By permission of Sports 'N Spokes, Copyright 1988. Paralyzed Veterans of America.

For more information on the game of quad rugby including specific rules, readers are encouraged to write to the USQRA, 2418 West Fall Creek Court, Grand Forks, ND 58201 Attention: Brad Mikkelson.

SKIING

Skiing is a way of moving over snow wearing a pair of long, flat runners attached to the shoes or boots. It was first developed as a method of transportation in regions with heavy snowfall. Skiing as a sport originated in Norway and Sweden in the early 1800s, and immigrants from these countries introduced the sport to the United States in the mid-1800s. The Federation Internationale de Ski (FIS) was founded by representatives of 26 countries in 1924.

Handicaps in skiing are not unique to those with physical, sensory, or mental disabilities. Every person who attempts to ski is somewhat handicapped and thus requires special equipment to compensate. Ski boots provide support for inadequate ankle stability, and skis compensate for inadequate length of the feet. Everyone to a degree is handicapped when learning to ski. Additional aids or teaching methods may be necessary for amputees or skiers limited by cerebral palsy to help them overcome their limitations and ski successfully.

Downhill Skiing for the Physically Disabled

Early attempts at disabled skiing can be traced to the immediate post World War II era in Europe. In 1968, at Arapahoe Basin, Colorado, a program was put into use for teaching three-track skiing to those with lower-extremity amputations. In 1970, the program moved to Winter Park, Colorado under the direction of George Engle of Winter Park Ski School. Winter Park's program has expanded greatly in the past 20 years and now works in conjunction with the Denver Children's Hospital. The program for disabled skiers, now under the direction of Hal O'Leary, offers qualified instruction to hundreds of disabled individuals weekly. National Handicapped Sports (NHS) is the leading organization for disabled skiing in the United States. The major governing body of competitive racing which includes stand-up and sit ski athletes comprising the United States Disabled Ski Team (USDST) is the United States Ski Association (USSA).

To the individual who is blind, deaf, and amputee, mentally retarded, or affected by cerebral palsy, skiing can provide an opportunity to participate successfully in a rewarding recreational sport. The provision of the opportunity for these individuals to move with speed and grace is unique to skiing. Initiation of enough force to provide speed is very difficult for an amputee or the cerebral palsied; however, in skiing, gravitational pull provides the force and allows the experience of fast, free movement.

United States Disabled Ski Team

Disabled ski racers from all over the nation compete in a number of regional events for an opportunity to qualify for national competition. Sanctioned by the USSA, skiers who qualify for the Nationals must do so at two different regional race sites. Qualifying times are based on winning efforts from the previous national championships. The World Disabled Alpine Ski Championships, an F.I.S. sanctioned event, is the world's most challenging ski event for disabled skiers. Athletes compete in four race events: Slalom, Giant Slalom, Super-G, and Downhill. Affiliated organizations include NHS, United States Olympic Committee, and the USSA.*

Goals

In developing goals of skiing for the disabled, **safety** must be the first item considered. With care, skiing can be a safe, enjoyable experience for the disabled. Concerns for safety must start with the assurance that equipment fits properly and is adjusted appropriately for each skier. This includes boots, bindings, skis, ski clothing and adapted equipment. Safety also includes

*Handicapped Sport Report, vol. 8, no. 1, Winter edition 1988–89, NHSRA, Washington, DC

instruction in proper chairlift embarkment and disembarkment. Depending upon the skier's movement potential and skiing ability, the chair lift may need to be slowed down or stopped for him to get on and off it safely. Lift operators and ski patrol should be made aware of what assistance the disabled will need prior to the day they ski.

Another goal of a skiing program is to learn to ski. Obviously, learning to ski is important in meeting the other goals, however it can receive less emphasis until the individual decides that he wants to learn to ski properly.

Ski instruction should be provided by qualified, knowledgeable instructors who have a good understanding of the principle of skiing and various methods of instruction. They must also have a basic understanding of the individual's limitations and specific needs. The NHS has a certification program for instructors wanting to teach adaptive ski techniques.

Three-Track Skiing

The history of three-track skiing dates back to the early 1940s in European countries especially in Austria, Germany, and Switzerland. It was not until the late 1950s that three-track skiing became popular in the United States, and it has now grown considerably.

Three-track skiing is the use of one ski, along with two outriggers to help provide balance. Lower extremity amputees have had the greatest success with this method of skiing, but it may also be used by individuals such as post-polio persons who have generalized weakness in one lower extremity.

Essentially, the three-track skier must learn to ski by the principles of the Professional Ski Instructors Association American Teaching Methods (ATM) with the exception of stemming skills. Space does not permit elaboration on instruction in three-track skiing, however important guidelines to follow are:

1. Establish a good rapport with the student.
2. Watch for fatigue. This can be lessened by preconditioning the leg and arms, eliminating excess standing, and avoiding skiing in windy conditions.
3. Care properly for the hands and stump. The hands are under constant pressure, which causes poor circulation and excess cold. Better quality mittens usually will keep the hands warmer. The stump should be protected by a protector made of either leather or light, molded plastic. This, in addition to a wool residual limb sock, should provide adequate protection, but due to the possibility of poor circulation to the residual limb, extra precautionary checks are advisable.
4. Build confidence by starting beginning skiers on a flat surface. Work first on walking with the ski, falling, and getting up. Then work on straight running.

5. Instruct the skiers in how to use the brakes on the tail of the outriggers for initial speed control and stopping.
6. Teach the steering actions required by the foot and knee to make desired turns.
7. Teach down unweighting.
8. Explain the proper chairlift procedure prior to first attempt.
9. Build rhythm with small deflections and encourage smooth technique by teaching turn anticipation.

Three-track skiers can develop into beautiful skiers under any conditions. Their skiing style must be aggressive and strong, but, most importantly, dynamic. There is nothing static about the fluid, rhythmic form that their skiing presents.

Case History: A.P. at the age of 5, had a below-knee amputation following an auto accident. As a 12-year-old, she attempted to ski while wearing her prosthesis and had little success. Being from a skiing family, she felt frustrated about her inability to ski and participate in family outings. This, as well as her difficulty walking in the snow, made her dislike the winter months.

She attempted three-track skiing at the age of 15 in the adaptive ski program at the Kluge Children's Rehabilitation Center, Charlottesville, Virginia. On her first day, she was able to handle the beginner slope quite well and ride the chairlifts. She progressed to the point of riding all the chairlifts and skiing all the intermediate trails by the end of her second day of skiing (Fig. 7–103).

Case History: A.H., a former certified ski instructor and member of the University of Colorado ski team, is again an enthusiastic skier (Fig. 7–104). In 1969, at the age of 23, as a member of the U.S. Marine Corps, A.H. was cut down by an explosive device that blew off both his legs above the knee and half the fingers and palms of both hands. A.H. came through his rehabilitation quite well. Upon his return home he renewed his interest in personal physical fitness. Although his competitive interests never waned it was now harder for him to find outlets. However, he participated in sailing, weight lifting, and fitness, and then, he finally renewed his interest in skiing. Upon the urging of friends, A.H. once again attempted the sport he had loved before. Through trial and error and finding a way with skis and outriggers (four-tracking), A.H. has gained enough proficiency to compete nationally in races for the handicapped.

Four Track Skiing

Four track skiing is used by people with a variety of disabilities including double A/K amputees, spina bifida, stroke and paraplegia. An individual with two legs and arms, natural or prosthetic, who is capable of standing independently or with the aid of outrigger could use this method (Fig. 7–104).

Four trackers may use one of three body positions (normal, jacknife, or leaning back for skiers who rely on leg braces for stability and who often need a ski bra or other device for ski tip stabilization).

Different holds and assists can be used by the instructor, but will not be discussed in this report. The main concern is to gradually decrease physical sup-

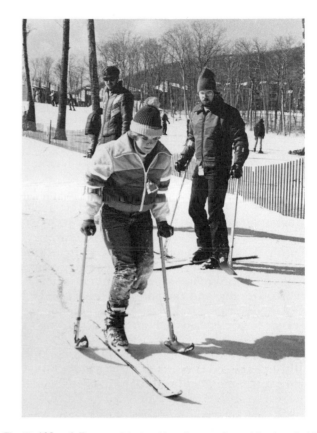

Fig. 7–103.   A.P. was able to ski well enough to ride the chairlift and successfully ski down the beginner's hill on her first attempt at three-track skiing.

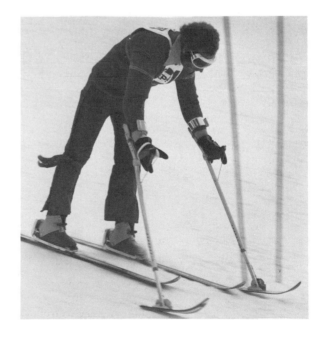

Fig. 7–104.   A.H., a double-amputee, is obviously about to 4-track quite effectively. (Courtesy of Bill Stieler.)

port as the skier gains independent control in maintaining stability and a good body position.

Skiing for Neurologically Impaired

The ability to move with speed and grace is impossible for many of those with a neurologic impairment, but with low level myelomeningocele individuals may indeed be able to enjoy the sport of skiing, as may those with spinal cord injuries, multiple sclerosis, and mild cases of cerebral palsy. These people may need to use adapted equipment, such as the ski bra, and/or outrigger, to be successful. The assistance of an able-bodied person may also be necessary to allow the person to experience skiing. The ability to become independent as a skier varies for each person (Fig. 7–105). Potential for movement often varies like the severity of the disability, that is, some are more severe than others, but desire and determination also contribute to becoming an independent skier. Each skier is different, and this must be considered when a teaching approach is developed. Equipment and its use must be prescribed and adapted according to individual needs.

In general, the beginner skier with cerebral palsy should not use ski poles, and short skis (130 to 150 cm) are recommended for those who have lower limb

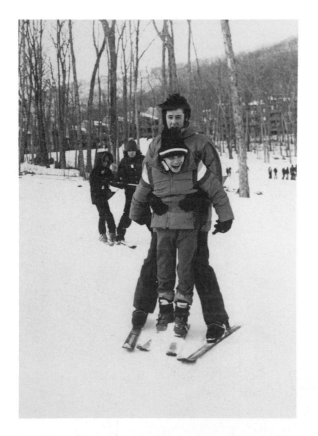

Fig. 7–105. In the foreground, an adolescent with CP experiences the freedom of moving rapidly. In the background, a skier with CP (spastic diplegia) skis in tandem with a volunteer using the ski pole method.

impairment. Longer skis can be used as the student progresses.* Since involvement is often asymmetrical, the skier will have difficulty turning to the more involved side. When selecting progression skills, the instructor should know that a wedge often increases spasticity, as does traversing. Ski poles can be introduced if the skier has good hand function as often seen with the skier with spastic diplegia.

The social and emotional implications of skiing for these skiers is of primary importance. The interaction with others in an exhilarating outdoor sport provides a great boost in self-esteem. The more severely involved may never be able to ski independently, however with assistance, they too can experience the thrill of skiing. The enjoyment derived from skiing is tremendous but its benefits also include physical exercise. Often, those with neurologic impairments and cerebral palsy exercise less than others because it is difficult and awkward for them to do so. Skiing enables them to find an enjoyable, graceful means of exercise.

Assistive Devices

The following equipment is needed for adaptive skiing:

1. Outriggers (Flipski†): Shown in Figure 7–106, these are used primarily by individuals who need assistance in balance. They are not used as a steering device, but may be used for initial braking by the beginning skier. The device may be used by amputees, people with one strong leg and one weak leg or people whose legs are both mildly involved. The skier must have the strength and coordination to handle the outriggers, thus eliminating those with upper extremity spasticity or weakness. Flipskis can also be used as crutches when necessary.

2. Canting Wedge: This is a polypropylene wedge that is installed between the boot and the ski to adjust the lateral tilt of the boot on the ski. This is often used by three-track skiers who have difficulty turning on their outside edge.

3. Ski-bra‡ (Fig. 7–107): This device stabilizes the skis by temporarily securing their tips. It stabilizes the base of support and thus improves the balance of individuals with insufficient strength or control of their lower extremities. The Ski-bra may work well for skiers with CP including those with hemiparesis.

4. Ski Pole: Ski poles can be used in the traditional manner, or they can be used as an assistive device for skiers with more severe handicaps. If the skier and instructor stand side by side and grasp the ski pole horizontally between them, the instructor can apply forward pressure with the pole to help the skier keep his weight forward

*NHS, Adaptive Skiing Technique (Manual), Orangevale, CA
†PSI, 141 Jonathon Blvd., N. Chaska, MN 55318
‡Multi-Leisure Products, 11952 Vose, N. Hollywood, CA 91605

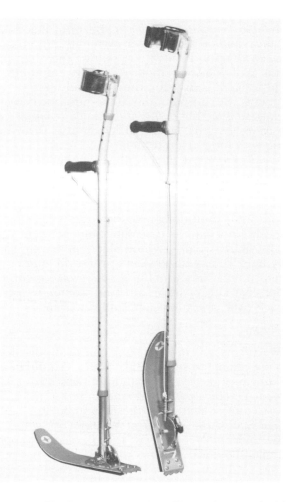

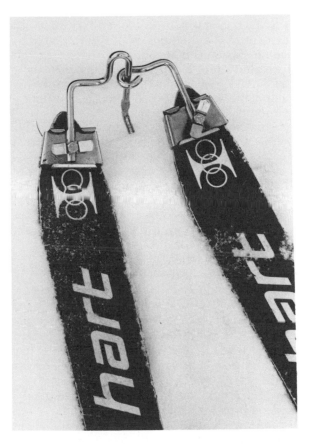

Fig. 7–107.   A Ski-bra in use.

Fig. 7–106.   The Flipski in 2 positions. The outrigger on the left is in the skiing position; the one on the right can be used as a crutch. (Courtesy of Paul's Sports, Inc.)

on the skis. The pole can also help the instructor assist the skier in other ways. The instructor should always grasp the basket end of the pole and have his inside arm over the skier's with the palm up. This can help skiers gain confidence and aid them to shift their weight and control turns and speed.

5. Rod: A 15-foot pole may also be used by 2 instructors and one skier to provide the same assistance as a ski pole.
6. Toe Bar: The toe bar mounts under the toe binding and enables skiers without lateral control (those with cerebral palsy and neurological impairments) to keep their feet apart. The bar is connected with ball joints to allow for sufficient independent leg action both forward and backward and up and down. It is often used in conjunction with the Ski-bra, providing a stable brace.
7. AT-Ski-TD:† The All Terrain Ski Terminal Device is a ½ in. diameter fitting that fits into a

† Write to Therapeutic Recreation Systems, 1280 28th St., Suite 3, Boulder, CO 80303-1797 for information.

standard prosthetic wrist. Safety features include a quick disconnect pole and "flex away" joint allowing the pole to pivot during a fall.
8. Hosmer Ski Hand: This ski-pole prosthesis is made of silicon rubber and is shaped to resemble a closed hand (Fig. 7–108). The ski pole is inserted into a hole in the center of the hand.

Adjustments for Specific Types of Disabilities

Below-Knee Amputations. It may be stated with a reasonable degree of confidence that a unilateral below-knee amputee can usually ski satisfactorily with two skis and an unmodified prosthesis. The commonly

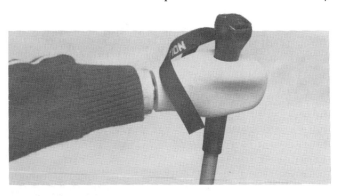

Fig. 7–108.   Hosmer Ski-Hand. Courtesy of Hosmer Dorrance Corp., 561 Division St., P.O. Box 37, Campbell, CA 95008.

used SACH foot will function satisfactorily without adjustment of the bindings or of the foot itself. Two difficulties have been encountered: (1) In extremely cold weather there has been a tendency for the glue of the SACH foot to loosen; (2) The prosthesis will not stand the strain imposed upon it by skiing over large moguls or small jumps.

Residual limb circulation may pose a problem; however, this problem can be prevented with insulated protectors (which can be made from leather at small cost by a prosthetist or leather worker).

The methodology for teaching below-knee amputees wearing one or two prostheses is the same as that for teaching normal skiers; however, the following guidelines are necessary for satisfactory progress:

1. Adapting the prosthesis.
2. Conditioning the muscles.

Preconditioning of the leg and knee muscles is extremely important because the hips and knees are used extensively in total body motion, leverage, edge setting and release, and weight transfer. Because of lack of use, these muscles deteriorate in both strength and tonus. Several exercises will develop the extensor, flexor, abductor, and adductor muscles. The use of both isometrics and isotonic exercises on a regular basis will decrease the time needed to gain good control of the prosthesis and, therefore, the ski. A below-knee amputee who can walk upstairs using alternate steps will be able to adequately control the muscles used in skiing.

Upper-Extremity Amputations. In most instances the power in the prosthesis is not sufficient to permit a ski pole, however it is fixed, to be used in a normal manner. A firm attachment between the terminal device and the pole may possibly create an unnecessary hazard. The amputee can nevertheless become proficient without poles, and he can eventually learn to rise after a fall without needing to use poles. The AT-Ski-TD or Hosmer Ski Hand are viable alternatives for the absent pole hand.

When unilateral upper-extremity amputees have started skiing with two poles, they have used the pole on the involved side essentially as a balance aid. However, most of these skiers prefer to use a single pole.

The unilateral upper-extremity amputee can use his prosthesis for balance, but he must protect the residual limb and provide warmth to prevent circulatory difficulties.

Amputations Following Malignancy. These individuals can ski successfully provided that there is no evidence of local recurrence in the residual limb and that no bony metastases are present. Where bony metastases are present, with possible increase in the danger of fracture, skiing is generally contraindicated.

In weighing the dangers of skiing, the psychologic benefits of not being considered an invalid and the opportunity to live a more nearly normal life, regardless of life expectancy, must be considered.

Multiple Amputation Problems. Bilateral below-knee amputees and bilateral upper-extremity amputees can be given an opportunity to try skiing using their prostheses. With bilateral upper-extremity amputees, the main problem is in using the tows and lifts.

Patients with amputations at the hip-disarticulation level, as well as those with above-knee residual limbs of various lengths, have participated in three-track skiing with little or no difficulty.

Visually Impaired. The NHS recommends teaching the ATM to visually impaired skiers, and readers are encouraged to read other sources for progression levels of this method. Various assists or holds are used initially and continuous verbal contact is necessary to keep the blind skier at ease. Once independent skiing is achieved, partially sighted skiers generally follow the guide. Totally blind skiers prefer the guide to be behind them. This way the guide's voice is directed to the skier and provides a better position to call out obstacles and assist in establishing rhythm.

Sit Skiing

Sit skiing is a term used by persons with disabilities who are unable to stand while skiing. Candidates for sit skiing include persons with multiple sclerosis, CVA (stroke), cerebral palsy and spinal cord injuries. The first attempt at skiing for the non-ambulatory in the United States was in 1977 at Winter Park where the Norwegian "pulk" was used. It was a sled designed to be pulled behind a cross country skier. In 1978, the Arroya sled was designed by Peter Axelson which opened up the world of downhill sit skiing for paraplegics.

Typically, the beginner sit skier is tethered by an able bodied instructor who skis behind the sled to assist in maintaining control (Fig. 7–109). The tetherer must demonstrate the ability to ski under control while being ready to assist the sit skier at all times (assist in turns, obstacle avoidance, etc.). The sit skier, in turn, must ski under good control and speed in most snow conditions. This is done by shifting body weight and using modified ski poles. Eventually many sit skiers can learn to control the sled safely without

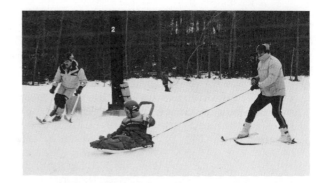

Fig. 7–109. Sit skiier and tetherer demonstrating speed control during downhill ski run.

the need for a tethering assistant. National Handicapped Sports has a certification examination and issues a card certifying the skier's qualifications without the aid of a tetherer. Evaluation criteria includes control of speed, turning skills, rolls, and basic skiing skills. Many ski areas now have guidelines for use of sit skiers. This includes skiing procedures, chairlift operations, and safety precautions.

Skill level development depends upon a number of factors, most noticeably good sitting balance and upper body strength. Surprisingly, some low level quadriplegics have achieved levels of proficiency in a sit ski device. Most sit skis have straps to support the upper trunk to assist the quadriplegic in maintaining good sitting balance. Other accessories include knee and waist straps that are used for stabilization purposes, and a padded back support and waterproof nylon cover for the legs.

The rapid growth in skiing the past 10 years has led to further improvements in re-designed devices to aid the disabled downhill skier. Most notably, the Mono-ski has been designed that allows even greater maneuverability and control for the agile paraplegic. The skier utilizes a Mono-ski with the aid of short outriggers adjusted to the person's sitting height. The Mono-ski is, from a technical point of view, a dynamic skiing orthosis. This device is complete with customized hydraulic shock absorbers, cams and artificial linkages to assist the skier in shock absorption on the slopes. Equally as important, the Mono-ski allows the skier to have control of the skis edges, thus greatly improving turning and control. The custom fitting of a Mono-ski depends upon the person's functional ability and body size. The skier is capable of riding the chairlift safely, however, adjustments may be necessary depending upon the height of the chairlift and depth of the snow. These devices have further improved the skiing options available to disabled skiers (Fig. 7–110).

Safety is a major concern for individuals learning to Mono-ski. Due to the potential speed factor and the fact the person is rigidly fixed to the Mono-ski, the skier must take safety precautions to protect himself/herself from injury. Safety precautions include seat padding, warm clothing that will not bunch up or wrinkle in the seating area, warm boots, goggles and a helmet. Additionally, the skier should learn to appropriately fall. It is suggested to ball up and try to slide following a fall. Certainly, do not try to use the outrigger to brake the fall.

Mono-ski competition is slowly maturing as equipment technology, technique and training improves. Competition for mono-skiing is divided into three categories by classification. The system based on tested ability includes:

    LW-10 class—higher level disabled skier who
        generally has less balance and control.
    LW-11 and LW-12—competitors who have increasingly better physical ability.[15]

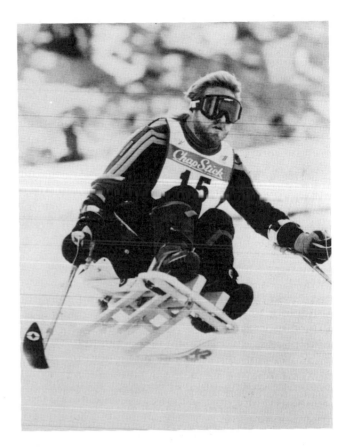

Fig. 7–110. Dan Ansley of Chula Vista, CA using Unique-1, a high performance mono-ski. (Courtesy of Enabling Technologies, 2411 N. Federal Blvd., Denver, CO 80211.)

Cross Country Skiing

Cross country skiing is one of the fastest growing outdoor sports. The sport involves either following prearranged tracks or making your own tracks through unbroken snow, up hill and down, across a serene and snow laden landscape, whether on a secluded mountain or a city golf course. Cross country skiing began more than 1,500 years ago in Scandinavia. The sport as it is adapted for the handicapped originated in 1955, in Norway. Today, Norway's unique Beitostolen Health Sports Center, one of the world's outstanding facilities, promotes ski touring (and other sports) as a means of rehabilitation. The annual Knights' Race has been held there every year since 1964, and it provided the inspiration for the Ski for Light program in the United States.

Recently the NHS and the USSA have made significant committments to building a solid, ongoing nordic program. The United States Disabled Nordic Ski Team consisting primarily of amputees and visually impaired skiers is now gaining international recognition as evident with medal winning performances in the Winter Games for the Disabled. This increased excellence in cross country racing should propel the United States further with feeder programs to the USDST from the NHS and United States Association of Blind Athletes. Nordic sit skiing is dominated by the Norwegians and Swiss. However, the United States is presently laying the foundation for future growth and development through year round training programs.

Cross country skiing builds endurance and muscle strength, especially in the legs. For this reason, the sport is becoming popular with individuals recovering from cardiovascular impairments and persons following rehabilitation programs after reconstructive surgery of a lower extremity. Since both arms and legs are actively involved in cross country skiing, it exercises a greater percentage of the body's major muscles than running does. The sport is not expensive in comparison with downhill skiing; it is self-regulated in terms of energy output; and it provides the participant with a safe lifetime sport. Cross country skiing conditions the whole body, develops one's sense of balance and rhythm, and seldom leads to injuries.

Organized cross country skiing for the blind is becoming popular in America. Further information here is limited to that group. Cross country skiing for the blind is not much different than it is for sighted persons except that a sighted guide skis alongside the blind skier giving verbal instructions and noting terrain. Skiing in previously prepared tracks provides the blind skier with a sense of security. The 2 sets of parallel ski tracks are a little wider and deeper than ordinary tracks and about 3 to 3½ feet apart, from center to center. Normally, the sighted skier skis in the left tracks and his blind partner in the right tracks (Fig. 7–111). Skiing on a prepared track is helpful, because the guide can be aware of the distance to curves and hills and also of the length of the hills. For instance, the sighted guide might say, "15 yards to a 30-yard-long uphill."

As skiers and guides work together on skiing techniques, many strong friendships develop. When skiing with a competent instructor or friend, the blind skier is quite safe and, in fact, usually indistinguishable from a sighted skier.

WATER SPORTS

Water sports for disabled persons including scuba diving, water skiing, canoeing, kayaking, and other forms of boating are becoming popular recreational outlets. With the advent of outdoor adventure programs in the last 10 years, water sports has opened up an assortment of new "high risk" challenges. More recently, triathlon competitions have emerged which include high level proficiency skills in rowing and swimming combined with wheelchair propulsion skills. This adds another dimension to the ever growing field of water sports.

This section will focus attention to only two water sports (sculling and water skiing) which will give the reader some indication of what the participant may

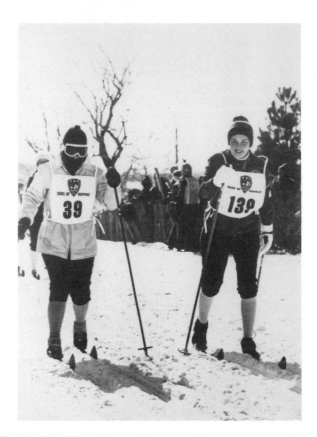

Fig. 7–111. Blind skier and sighted guide during annual Ski for Light International program of cross country skiing. (Courtesy of Ski for Light.)

expect from each. Readers are encouraged to read other sources of information for a broader overview of the subject.

PARA- AND QUAD-SCULLING

Single hull sculls are unique exercise and recreational vehicles because of their lightness and potential for speed. The scull's lightness allows a small amount of effort to generate movement. At the same time, maximal exertion and large amounts of effort can be employed to produce fast movement through space. This range of useful effort can accommodate a wide continuum of disability levels making it a potential rehabilitation, exercise and recreational vehicle for paraplegic and quadriplegic individuals.

Single hull sculls are unstable and require good balance. The catamaran-type single scull that is currently on the market offers the best design. The craft is lightweight (60 pounds), virtually impossible to tip over, and very easy to adapt for the handicapped.

The major adaptation needed to permit the paraplegic and quadriplegic to scull involves mounting a stationary seat in place of the regular sliding seat (Fig. 7–112). A piece of ½-inch plywood is bolted to the underside of the metal tubes connecting the hulls. A commercial plastic seat covered with foam on the

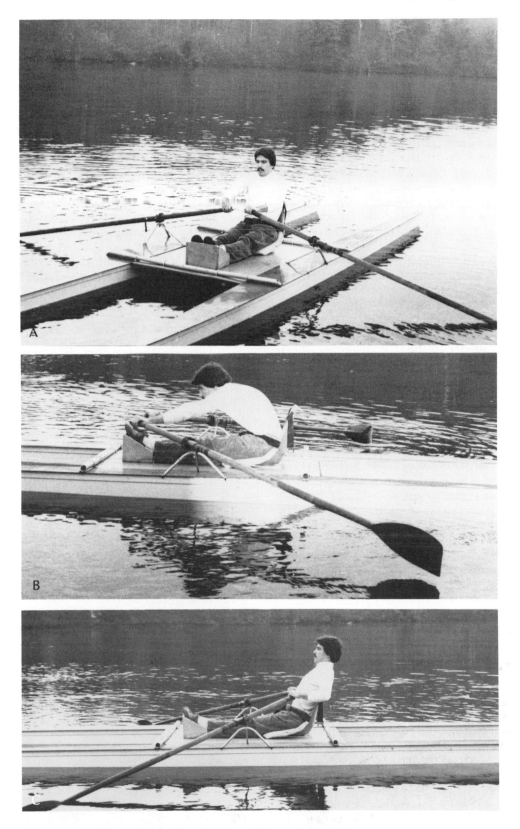

Fig. 7–112. Range of movement skills used in sculling. Note the stationary seat.

lower seat area is then mounted on the plywood. Seat belts are mounted at hip and chest levels to give support when needed. The seat should be positioned where it will produce the most effective stroke action, and therefore it should be adjustable for different limb lengths and ranges of motion.

The oars, which normally rotate in the oar locks for feathering, are secured with a bolt in the early stages of sculling and they are kept bolted for quadriplegics with poor hand strength. Securing the oars in this way reduces the complexity of the task and enables the individual to concentrate on generating the correct pattern of movement. Quadriplegics who lack the hand strength to grip the oars require an additional support system. Gloves with Velcro straps can be used to secure their hands to the oars.

An adjustable foot positioning box is placed in front of the seat. The box secures the feet and aids in maintaining an upright posture which allows for a maximal range of motion during the sculling process. Some paraplegics do not find the box useful and remove it, resting their feet directly on the deck.

A person can transfer to the craft from his wheelchair in several ways. The easiest transfer is performed by sliding the craft onto a beach or low, grassy banked area along the body of water. Paraplegics with good transfer skills can transfer themselves to the deck and into the seat. Paraplegics and quadriplegics who need assistance can be transferred easily to the seat due to the space available immediately behind the seat. If a shore docking is not possible, a special dock can be constructed or adaptations made to an existing dock to permit safe transfers.

The potential for range of motions and muscle group involvement is considerable (Fig. 7–112B & C). The individual can use a pushing or a pulling motion or both and involve a large number of upper body muscles. Done repeatedly, sculling has the potential to produce changes in both strength and cardiovascular fitness.

WATER SKIING

Water skiing is a dynamic and challenging sport that is gaining popularity among the disabled population. The sport is relatively new, especially the sit-down version which will be discussed in this section. In tracing historical roots, Norway was using specialized equipment for skiers in the 1960s. Introduction to training courses for disabled skiers were first held in Great Britain in 1979 and 1980. More recently, research efforts and product designs in the United States were done at California State University in Chico, where Ability First Program was funded by a grant from the Department of Education, Rehabilitation Services Administration. Recently the American Water Ski Association (AWSA)* has acknowl-

*AWSA, P.O. Box 190, Winter Haven, FL 33882

edged water skiing for the disabled by establishing a committee within its organization to promote the sport.

There are some basic requirements to the sport. The skiers should be able to swim and tolerate cold water. The spinal cord injured skier lacks sensation in the lower extremities and will be unable to sense cold water (although muscle spasms may occur as a warning signal). A spinal cord injury impairs both heat production and heat loss, and for this reason a wet suit is recommended. Good upper-body strength is important and most paraplegics have little trouble learning the skills. The values of developing and maintaining organic strength and vigor are incalculable to the disabled individual's mental and physical well being. Adapted equipment can be used for skiers with limited functional skills. For example, some quadriplegics with lesions at C-5 and below have been able to master the sport with ski gloves and velcro straps attached to the handlebars.

Equipment
Emphasis will be placed on the Kan-Ski (Fig. 7–113) since it is the standard ski for disabled skiers. It was designed by Royce Andes, a former national barefoot competitor, and now a C-4 quadriplegic. In addition to the spinal cord injured, the Kan-Ski has been used successfully by skiers with a number of other disabilities including bilateral lower-extremity amputees, cerebral palsy, and spina bifida to name a few. Two models will be discussed.

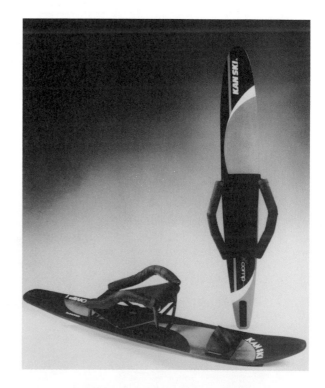

Fig. 7–113.   Kan Ski water ski. (Courtesy of Kan Ski, 2704 Hwy. 99, Biggs, CA 96917.)

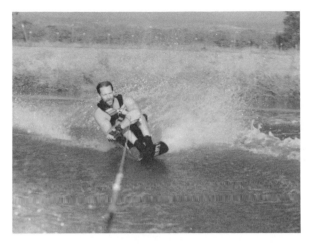

Fig. 7–114. Water skier demonstrating tilting forces for speed control. (Courtesy of Kan Ski.)

Beginner-Quad Ski: This ski is 16 in. wide with a flat bottom design for stability. It includes a slot in the board nose for the tow line which provides for easier and straighter starts. For skiers who are unable to grasp the ski handle, the rope may be attached directly to the ski. When this is done, the rope must be attached to the boat using a "quick release," enabling the rope to be disengaged by an observer if the skier falls.

Recreation–Competitive Ski. This ski has a 13 in. bottom for easier maneuverability. It has a high seat cage design and moderate rocker shape (front and back with double wing fin that adds stability).

Initiation to the ski is done first on dry land, then in shallow water. This is to allow the instructor to be in close proximity during the early training period. It also enables the beginning skier to overcome any fear as expectations of the unknown.

While submerged in the water, most disabled skiers can eventually learn to board the Kan-Ski independently. To start, the skier positions his feet in the bindings and bends slightly forward while holding onto the ski handle. Once out of the water, steering is done by leaning in the desired direction. After sufficient practice, the skier can exaggerate tilting force from side to side to increase the ski's turning speed (Fig. 7–114). A quick release rope which releases a ski line under tension from the boat may be used as a safety precaution.

REFERENCES

1. Parks, B.: Wheelchair Tennis is Here to Stay. Sports 'N Spokes, 6: May, 1980, p. 24.
2. Cowart, J.: Guidelines for Adaptations. IRUC Briefings, 2:12, 1977.
3. The World Book Encyclopedia. Field Enterprises Educational Corporation, 1970.
4. Marksmanship for young shooters. Washington, D.C.: AAHPER, 1960.
5. Harper, J.: Guts, grit and guns. Guns and Ammo, 14 (5): May 1970.
6. Bear, F.: *The Archer's Bible*, Garden City, N.Y., Doubleday and Company, 1968.
7. Hyman, D.: Programs for the handicapped. JOHPER, 40 (4): 1969.
8. Kay, H., et al.: A bowling device for bilateral arm amputees Inter-Clinic Information Bulletin, 9 (7); April, 1970
9. Bauer, J.: Riding for Rehabilitation. Toronto, Ontario, Canadian Stage and Arts.
10. McCowan, L.: It is Ability That Counts (A Training Manual on Therapeutic Riding for the Handicapped). Olivet, Michigan, The Olivet College Press.
11. Kegal, B.: Sports and Recreation for Those with Lower Limb Amputation or Impairment. J Res Develop, Clinical Supplement No. 1, Wash., D.C. 1985, pg. 25.
12. Bertoli, O.: Effect of Therapeutic Horseback Riding on Posture in Children with Cerebral Palsy. Physical Therapy, 68:1505–1512, 1988.
13. Van Vliet, A. and de Ross, Y.: Indications and Contraindications for Therapeutic Horseriding in Patient with Spina Bifida. Proc. from 3rd Int. Conf. on Riding for the Disabled. 1979, pp. 4–5.
14. Alexander, M.: Aspects of Performance in Wheelchair Marathon Racing. CAHPER Journal—Jan, Feb., 1989. pgs. 26–32.
15. Crase, N.: Winter Heat. Sports 'N Spokes, Vol. 15, No. 1, 1989, pgs. 9–14.

BIBLIOGRAPHY

Axelson, P.: Sit Skiing. Sports 'N Spokes. Jan.–Feb. Pg. 28–33, 1984.
Axelson, P.: Hitting the Slopes, Sports 'N Spokes. Nov.–Dec. Pg. 22–34, 1984.
Freeman, G.: Hippotherapy/Therapeutic Horseback Riding Clinical Mgmt. in Physical Therapy. Vol. 4, No. 3, pg. 20–26.
Mood, D., Musker, F., and Armbruster, D.: *Sports and Recreational Activities for Men and Women.* St. Louis, C.V. Mosby, 1983.
NHSRA, Sit Ski Qualification Exam Manual, Orangedale, CA, 99662.
NAGA, Amputee Golfer Magazine, Challenge Publications, Macomb, IL 1989.
Paciorek, M. and Jones, J.: Sports and Recreation for the Disabled: A Resource Manual, Indianapolis, IN, Benchmark Press, Inc., 1989.
Parker B.: How to: Wheelchair Tennis, Part 2: Mobility and Ground Strokes. Sports 'N Spokes, Nov.–Dec. pgs. 29–31, 1980.
USTA, Tennis Programs for the Disabled, Princeton, N.J.
Mission Bay Aquatic Center, Waterskiing for the Physically Disabled, San Diego, CA.

8 *Aquatics*

Swimming has been viewed by many as one of the most beneficial mediums of exercise. It provides an opportunity to improve such physiologic components as cardiovascular strength and endurance and general muscular strength and endurance. Swimming exercises the entire body without putting extreme amounts of stress or tension on the specific body parts. The body moves through a relaxing environment in which circulation, respiration, muscle endurance, and body secretions are elevated slightly to become more efficient in maintaining general body fitness.

THERAPEUTIC EFFECTS OF AQUATICS

The therapeutic effects of swimming benefit many domains of the child's total development. The physiologic aspect of aquatic exercise is extremely beneficial. The positive effects of whole body immersion in warm water (88° to 96° F) are one of the greatest benefits of pool therapy. The temperature of the water can help increase circulation and aid in the healing process for those with temporary orthopedic problems. The warmth of the water also aids relaxation of muscles and encourages further exploration of movement in the water. This relaxation can help in gaining normal postural tone to encourage more efficient movement. The increasing ability to relax, along with the reduction of gravitational pull increases the mobility and movement potential of a variety of physically handicapped individuals. Buoyancy, a physical property of water, is described in the Archimedes' Principle: "When a body is wholly or partially immersed in a fluid at rest, it experiences an upward thrust equal to the weight of the fluid displaced."[1] The property of buoyancy can work in numerous ways in assisting movement for the physically disabled. The lessened gravitational pull provides less resistance to total body movement.

DEVELOPMENTAL OBJECTIVES IN PROGRAM PLANNING

Earlier in this text, the Developmental Objectives of Physical Education (see Chap. 1) were cited as guidelines to implementation of a program. The objectives fall under 5 categories: (1) organic, (2) neuromuscular, (3) interpretive, (4) social, and (5) emotional. The potential of aquatics to meet each type of objective will be reviewed here.

The organic objective refers to development of specific goals aimed at increasing the functioning of the systems in the body. This includes such goals as increasing cardiovascular endurance through sustained exercise or increasing flexibility in joint range of motion through active and assistive stretching. Muscle strength and endurance are also components of the organic objective and they both can be geared either toward particular muscle groups or toward general body fitness. An important function of the organic objective is that increased activity increases circulation, and this aids in the healing process by preventing stasis. This is particularly evident in temporary orthopedic problems such as Legg-Perthes disease or in most postoperative patients. By aiding in the healing process, swimming helps return the patients to the regular, independent mobility to which they are accustomed.

The neuromuscular objective is based on increasing opportunities for perceptual-motor development. Attainment of skill in various sports activities requires specific perceptual-motor development in areas such as hand-eye coordination and eye-foot coordination. The aquatic domain offers numerous possibilities for increasing proficiency in many of the perceptual-motor deficiencies that often prevail in the physically disabled. It provides an additional medium in which specific input may be channeled to overcome an existing deficit. The patient can receive positive input in development of locomotor skills, such as hopping, skipping, jumping, galloping, and running. The water, in some cases, provides a supportive base in addition to slight resistance, which slows down the sequential movement to permit a more effective teaching situation. Hopping, for example, is often difficult for individuals with mild ataxia; however, it is possible within the pool environment.

Non-locomotor skills, such as bending or twisting, are incorporated nicely into the aquatic program. They can be used as forms of exercise or even more beneficially as methods to aid in water adjustment. Movements such as these add extra dimensions to otherwise less interesting games, plus are beneficial in developing balance.

The opportunities for increased stimulation of hand-eye coordination and game-type skills (i.e., catching, throwing, striking, etc.) are innumerable in the swimming pool. Sponges provide excellent soft, lightweight objects that can be used for such motor development. The sponges also aid in the water adjustment process.

The interpretive objective is a comprehensive category that emphasizes self or body awareness. Understanding movement potential and capabilities is a primary segment of the interpretive objective. Aquatics presents the individual with a multidimensional medium in which to explore, discover, and experience new movement capabilities. Space perception, body-object perception, and body awareness activities integrate nicely into water exploration. Hula hoops, tubes, balls, and kick boards are examples of objects that help the swimmer increase awareness of himself in relation to objects surrounding him. The interpretive objective also helps individuals gain awareness of their own bodily functions in physical activity. This is especially evident in individuals who have newly acquired handicapping conditions (such as spinal cord injury, stroke, and traumatic amputation). The aquatic environment enables such persons to gain a better understanding of how body positioning and movement capabilities inter-relate for efficient body propulsion.

The social objective of physical activity is appreciated in many forms of recreation. Interacting with other people to form better communication skills is beneficial for the disabled. The development of positive personality traits often needs to be emphasized by instructors. Swimming is beneficial to social development in that it is often a group activity (Fig. 8–1). Obviously this can boost the self-concept. The confidence of an individual in his ability to make social contacts can be increased. Another important factor which swimming presents is that it encourages constructive use of leisure time.

The final developmental objective is the emotional benefit that swimming can provide. Gaining a healthy response to physical activity is beneficial for all people. Outlets for suitable physical interaction are often limited for disabled persons, but enjoyment and the feeling of success are tremendously important to them, so successful opportunities for these things should be incorporated into every session of aquatics.

The physically disabled person may be able to leave all the assistive devices necessary for ambulation (i.e., wheelchair, crutches, braces) in the locker room and move himself independently in the water. This can provide a tremendous boost to his psychologic state. The fact that swimming is somewhat a "risk" sport, in which not everyone is capable, makes successful participation even more gratifying.

PLANNING AN ADAPTED AQUATICS PROGRAM

The implementation of an adapted aquatics program justifies looking directly at the interrelationship between all of the developmental objectives. However, the emphasis placed on each objective must be

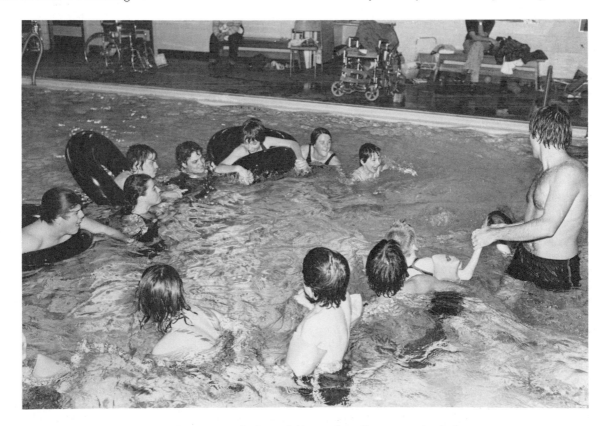

Fig. 8–1. Group games provide an excellent opportunity for social interaction with peers and volunteers.

weighed in relation to its total benefit for each person. For instance, if a child needs to concentrate on the organic objective (development of strength and endurance), but is not maintaining enough motivation to continue, emphasis must be placed on the emotional objective to improve the enjoyment.

Developmental objectives must essentially be given second priority in planning an aquatic program. *Safety* must be the most important objective. Concentration on learning safety skills and an awareness of pool rules and regulations should be integrated into every program of aquatics. The rules should be interpreted to each group of swimmers at the level of their intelligence. Consistency in explaining and enforcing the rules is requisite in adapted aquatic programs. Safety decisions must be firm, quick, and consistent. The safety rules also apply to the instructors and teacher's aides who handle disabled persons in and around the pool. A more detailed description of specific handling techniques is given later in the chapter.

A safe but enjoyable swimming environment is essential. Disabled individuals often need to be motivated to achieve their utmost in a learning situation. By making the learning situation more enjoyable, the swimmers maintain a higher level of motivation. Making the swimming pool enjoyable must also be a main priority in organizing a program. Safety must be the top priority, but if the swimmers do not benefit from the emotional objective, then further learning is impossible.

Learning specific swimming skills and stroke techniques must be the last of the high priorities in developing goals for an adapted program. Although skills are the means by which the objectives are developed, the importance of learning to swim must be secondary to a safe, enjoyable experience.

IMPLEMENTING AN ADAPTED AQUATICS PROGRAM

Implementation of adapted aquatic programs often requires more than an understanding of the potential benefits of the program for the disabled. The American Red Cross can provide much necessary program information. They have training programs (American Red Cross Adapted Aquatics course) taught by certified personnel to help people gain an awareness of the needs of physically challenged individuals. This section emphasizes elements that are critical in implementing a program.

It is important to evaluate how many people potentially would benefit from a program, the resource help (professionals and paraprofessionals) that would be available to provide instruction for the program, and the financial obligations that would have to be met if a program were initiated. A survey is the most widely used method of identifying critical elements. Contacting the community through a mailed survey can identify some areas of concern in planning. How-

ever, in large communities this can be expensive and the ratio of replies to inquiries may be significantly low. Surveying local organizations to find the number of potential participants may be a more effective method of collecting needed information. Community health agencies and school districts can provide information on the number of available participants. Social service agencies can also provide detailed information to benefit the cause. Such service agencies as child development centers, hospitals, and parks and recreation departments may also be of assistance. Close communication with service agencies can consolidate the essential ingredients in forming the necessary plans. It is beneficial to find out not only how many persons are aided by or associated with the organizations contacted, but also the levels to disability, age, and social ability of the potential participants, as well as their experience with previously existing programs.

Upon gaining enough information to substantiate the need for a program of this kind, it is helpful to establish a committee to secure community interest in the project. Educating the entire community about the need for such a program may be made simpler by gaining support from local agencies or prominent community members. Their support is needed before attempting to gain the support of an entire community. Educators, physicians, social workers, clergy, and service organization leaders can be influential in gaining the needed support.

The groundwork done to establish the need for the program and the supportive community members and agencies will help in locating adequate facilities for the program. Obviously, a swimming program cannot function without adequate facilities. Accessibility of the pool is beneficial but not essential. Most local communities have facilities that are adequate for the summer months but often inadequate during the winter. Considerations in selecting a pool include its availability for disabled people (i.e., proximity and hours when usable). Other important considerations are pool temperature and depth. It is beneficial to have water temperatures of about 85° to 95° F in order to allow enjoyable participation early in the session. This temperature is also more beneficial for specific disabilities as will be discussed later in the chapter. Pool depth is important because many swimmers may never reach the stage of being independent and comfortable when swimming in deep water. Their fear of failure is an even bigger obstacle in this situation. Accessibility of dressing rooms, bathrooms, and locker rooms also needs to be considered.

Local school districts, area colleges, recreation centers, and even motels and hotels may have suitable facilities available for use. It is essential for the sponsoring committee to take full responsibility for the program and prove that it can operate independently of the organization whose facilities are to be used, if need be (this would include responsibility for insurance, liability of lifeguards, equipment, and supervision).

Volunteer and instructor training are essential ingredients in developing a successful adapted aquatics program. The topics discussed in training should include motivational techniques, handling of the disabled, background material on their special needs, safety equipment and its use, beginning swimming skills, and cardiopulmonary resuscitation. It is vital that an understanding of the handicapped and their needs be made apparent prior to the program. The participants, in most cases, do not want sympathy, but only understanding. Providing films, slides, and published information prior to the program may also help educate the instructors. It is their understanding and assistance that make a program successful. Encourage the staff to keep daily records of the progress of each of their students, because this will make them more perceptive to gains in proficiency. This record should also indicate emotional characteristics of the swimmer on each day.

A frequent concern is the adequate student-to-instructor ratio. Obviously, one-to-one instruction is the ideal situation. With the severely disabled (physically, sensory, and mentally), it is often necessary to have the ratio remain one-to-one in the beginning of the program. This ratio is quite variable according to pool size, number of participants, swimming ability of each, medical indications, and other specific variations. Safety is the prime consideration and must remain so when assigning student-teacher ratios.

A vital aspect of an adapted aquatic program is the use of special equipment and flotation devices. This cannot be overlooked if a successful program is to be implemented. Further information is presented later in the chapter.

IMPLICATIONS OF SPECIFIC DISABILITIES FOR AQUATICS

Cerebral Palsy

The person with cerebral palsy has great difficulty developing normal movement patterns. This is because of abnormal muscle tonus which results from insult to the brain in the developmental period. This hypertonus affects the development of normal movement and causes inappropriate compensatory action that further impedes development. The most important elements in working with cerebral palsied persons in the water are: (1) establishment of safe breath control procedures; and (2) maintenance of more normal postural tone. The person with cerebral palsy can experience movement with more freedom while in the swimming environment, because the buoyancy decreases the gravitational pull and allows for a greater range of movement. Usually it is best to encourage swimming in the horizontal plane, because it is the area of greatest mobility. The swimming environment

can be used to aid in the development of motor skills and achieve independent mobility.

Establishing more normal postural tone in the cerebral palsied is essential if they are to achieve effective movement. Therapeutically warm water temperatures (approximately 85° to 95° F) can help reduce the amount of muscle activity physiologically. This can contribute to a more normal postural tone. The warmth of the water helps the person relax, thus decreasing muscle hypertonus that is due to anxiety. This relaxation is necessary before any attempts are made at stroke technique or movement exploration in the water.

The cerebral palsied person has a tremendous fear of falling when in an unfamiliar environment. This is due, in part, to a lack of balance capabilities resulting from the brain lesion, but this fear must be overcome to help achieve the necessary relaxation. Providing a calm environment with little extraneous noise (splashing, yelling, intruding audience) can help ease the sense of fear so often present. Instilling confidence and trust between pupil and instructor is essential in helping the pupil to relax. Background music also helps create a relaxing atmosphere in which to learn to swim. Entering the water needs to be a safe and calm experience for those with cerebral palsy.

This fear of falling is usually exaggerated in the pool because of the effects of buoyancy, along with fear of the water. The person with ataxic elements of cerebral palsy experiences problems in balance while walking. These problems worsen in the pool because of the lack of gravitational pull and limited balance reactions.

Special Considerations. Cerebral palsied individuals are often multiply handicapped. Additional problems need to be understood and planned for when developing a program. A communication system may need to be developed to insure adequate understanding between student and instructor. For instance, a special cue may be needed to signal "I'm tired," or "I want up," and these cues should be worked out well in advance of the time they are initially needed. However, every effort to understand the speech of the cerebral palsied helps them maintain a better self-image.

The medical history of the swimmer should be understood by the instructor. This is especially relevant when seizure activity can be prevented with prescribed medications. Included in the medical history must be medications received, allergies, medical persons to contact in emergencies, movement contraindications, and other specific problems associated with each person.

Handling Techniques. Helping the person maintain symmetric segmental alignment will assist in achieving better muscle tonus. Thus, the instructor should attempt to keep the head, neck, trunk, and pelvis in a symmetric, proportional alignment. The most important consideration is control of the swimmer's head. If adequate head control is not possible for the swimmer, then the instructor must provide support with his hands. Included in head control is control of jaw and mouth closure. Those who are incapable of jaw closure can be assisted if an index and middle finger are placed around their chin with the thumb on the outer border of the jaw and chin. Often the person with cerebral palsy will have enough head control and mouth closure to be independent of support. However, there is a possibility of occasional thrusts of the extensor muscles of the neck that can submerge the head if not controlled. It is important to encourage the swimmer to maintain his head in the neutral position, neither flexed nor extended. This is often overlooked by attempting to teach the backfloat, which entails extension of the neck and back. This is contraindicated for those with cerebral palsy if extension of the head increases extensor tone throughout the back as is often the case. The increased extensor tone virtually eliminates any possibility of relaxation, thus making independent floating impossible. Because of this tendency, good floating technique is difficult for the cerebral palsied, and additional flotation devices are often necessary.

The most desirable teaching position is from behind the swimmer, with the hands placed in the axillary area and the forearms held in underneath the swimmer's head (Fig. 8–2). This position is best for three reasons: (1) the potential for controlling the head and neck area is better, and this obviously improves safety; (2) the potential movement of the arms is not obstructed as it is when support is from the side; and (3) constant eye contact is possible to ensure security. Another way for the instructor to increase the swimmer's feeling of security is to provide his shoulder as a resting place for the swimmer's head. This maintains

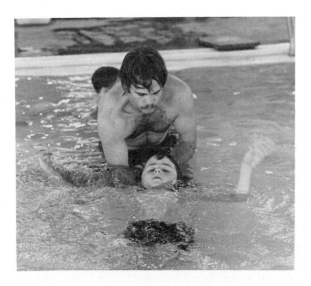

Fig. 8–2. Proper teaching position for students needing minimal assistance with head control. The head should be flexed slightly.

close contact, and the shoulder can help maintain proper positioning of the head. An additional benefit of this teaching position is the ability it provides to create a "drafting effect," which will assist the swimmer. This can be done while walking slowly ahead of the swimmer without touching him. The swimmer's self-concept can be promoted greatly by this, because it shows him his potential for independent swimming. However, it must be used with discretion, depending upon the individual situation.

The instructor's position for a swimmer in the prone position also needs to be at the head. This is also essential for the previously listed reasons. It must be remembered that extension of the head may increase extensor tonus throughout the back, so swimming in the prone position needs to be limited until the face can be, at least periodically, submerged with the head maintained in a neutral position. The possibility of holding the person prone with his head extended completely out of the water should be avoided at all times.

Preferred Strokes for Cerebral Palsy. Movement potential for the cerebral palsied is usually greatest in the horizontal plane. Thus, strokes that are more efficient, and more beneficial, are those that require only horizontal-type movements. These include finning, sculling, elementary backstroke, and breast stroke. One essential element in each of these strokes is that each movement requires an identical bilateral movement. This is easier to comprehend perceptually than are reciprocal and/or unilateral motions such as those of the crawl stroke or sidestroke. Encouragement should be given to achieve maximal range of movement with each stroke. Often, attempting to slow down the stroke can result in a more efficient power phase for propulsion.

The kicks for each of these strokes may make achievement of efficient propulsion difficult. It is felt that limited kicking, if any, helps gain the more effective stroke. Kicking is a fun way to move and explore in the water and should be a part of the learning process. However, most often it does interfere with attaining good arm function because integration of both is extremely difficult. Attempting the flutterkick is contraindicated for the cerebral palsied, particularly those with spastic diplegia. This kick requires reciprocal flexion and extension of the hips, and this may increase the muscle tonus in the extensor muscle groups of the hips, trunk, and back. It also encourages internal rotation at the hips which leads to the "scissoring" gait pattern (a common characteristic of persons with spasticity). Essentially, the flutterkick produces a log-rolling motion of the entire body and increases muscle tonus, neither of which effect is beneficial for the circumstances. A "frog-type" kick with bilateral abduction may be used in place of the flutterkick. The standard whip kick may be attempted by those with mild cerebral palsy.

Integration of body movements is the essential area of concentration in swimming for the cerebral palsied. Achieving more functional use of the involved extremities necessitates good integration of movement capabilities. Thus, strengthening a particular muscle group through swimming is not beneficial. Harmonious functioning of both sides of the body is the goal of these specific strokes, and this is achieved most easily through reduction of muscle tonus and integration of bilateral strokes in the horizontal plane.

The use of flotation devices is often necessary for the cerebral palsied to achieve independence in the water. We feel that, in many cases, inflatable arm supports (i.e., Water wings, Floaties, etc.) are viable and effective. They work well on individuals who have adequate head control and can possibly be independent in the water. These devices work well because they allow for full range of movement and work effectively in both the prone and supine positions. Also, swimmers can be weaned from them gradually, because they can be inflated to lesser degrees as tolerated. However, they are *not* to be considered a life jacket, and constant supervision is still necessary. The standard Personal Flotation Device (PFD), or life-preserver, works well with those needing support of the head and neck. This device, however, restricts swimming to the supine or backstroke position. The Delta Swim System is a viable alternative and is adaptable to meet multiple needs in the course of therapy (refer to section on Equipment). A Danmar head float may be recommended, and is especially useful when the swimmer is placed in the vertical position.

Tire inner tubes can be used effectively by those with more severe involvement. Motorcycle inner tubes are best because their smaller size and bulk result in a better fit. The tubes are good because they move the shoulder and elbows forward, out of the spastic abduction position, thus making handling of balls and toys more possible. The inner tubes also must be considered only as aids to movement and *not* as life preservers.

The USCPAA allows the use of flotation devices in competition, but only by Class I and Class II athletes.

Inner tubes are not allowed.

Myelomeningocele

The child with myelomeningocele presents an entirely different picture than children with other physical handicaps. These children usually have multiple problems that require attention when planning a swimming program. The problems often include mental retardation, short attention span, obesity, social immaturity, emotional lability, multiple perceptual deficits, bowel and bladder incontinence, and scoliosis, as well as little or no use of the lower extremities. Each of these problems requires special attention in program planning. However, swimming provides these children with a vast amount of benefits that cannot be attained collectively in any other single activity.

Problems and Implications with Myelomeningocele. Many children fall into the range of mild mental retardation. This necessitates clear, concise teaching methods that are consistent from day to day. Demonstrations usually gain the child's understanding. Repetition is usually critical to insure that comprehension takes place. Often, a child will appear to not have difficulties understanding directions in an attempt to prove his abilities. They often attempt to manipulate situations with excess verbiage in order to cover difficulties in comprehension. Their short attention span often adds to problems in communication.

Perceptual deficiencies also vary from child to child. However, a majority of those with myelomeningocele demonstrate figure-ground problems, laterality and directionality deficits, hand-eye difficulties, and poor body awareness, as well as poor motor planning skills. Many opportunities for perceptual input should be incorporated into the aquatic program. Body awareness skills using hoops, rings, and balls can provide positive input. Helping the children gain an understanding of left, right, over, under, around, and through are indispensable benefits for them.

The social immaturity of children with myelomeningocele may also be the result of the difficulty they have in playing peer related activities at an early age. They can be highly verbal, yet unable to provide actions commensurate with their verbal ability. Encouragement of appropriate social skills is important for any child, but it is particularly so for those with myelomeningocele.

Swimming provides strenuous, whole-body activities that improve general body fitness. Swimming also may help in increasing circulation to aid in the prevention of decubitus ulcers (pressure sores), and it may actually aid in the healing process of previously developed ulcers. The increase in circulation also aids in the function of exocrine glands and the regeneration of tissue. Encouragement to increase upper-extremity strength and endurance is valuable in promoting independence in daily living skills. Whole-body activity also may limit contractures of the lower extremities.

The inadequate lower-extremity function of myelomeningocele children may present a few problems other than lack of kicking ability. These children often exhibit a great imbalance between upper-body weight and lower-body weight. This makes it difficult or impossible for them to right themselves in the water once they have achieved the backfloat. A large fear obviously develops because of their difficulty in this skill. However, they can learn to perform this movement quite well once they have thoroughly adjusted to the water. Another associated problem is the danger of fracturing or scraping the lower extremities when around or in the pool. Due to the common inability to stand and walk, the bones of the legs do not maintain suitable levels of minerals, causing the bones to fracture easily. The lack of sensation in the lower extremities makes it critical for the instructor, as well as the student, to be cautious when using transfer techniques. Socks can be worn to help avoid unnecessary scratches or scrapes on the feet from abrasive surfaces. This should be a portion of the care in prevention of decubitus ulcers. The instructor also needs to be aware of the method of elimination from bowel and bladder (refer to section on users of treatment devices).

Teaching Progression and Stroke Analysis. Emotional maturity with myelomeningocele people is decisively important to the rate of progress in learning swimming skills. The initial steps most easily accommodated to by children are: (1) being held in the upright position, face to face with the instructor. In this position, water adjustment is a more secure experience for the individual, and support from the instructor is readily available; (2) developing prone skills to an extent that ensures breath control and adaptation to the water environment; (3) gaining understanding of supine skills such as backfloat and sculling. Skills in the supine position are often frightening because of the difficulty the nonambulatory child with myelomeningocele has in righting himself. These steps are adaptable to each individual, and no approach should be considered rigid.

Once independence in the water is gained, any stroke that is productive should be encouraged. However, strokes that require bilateral mirroring of the stroke are usually easier to comprehend, thus learned more easily. These strokes include elementary backstroke, breast stroke, sculling and finning. Progression to more difficult strokes is indicated when appropriate. If kicking is a viable alternative, the flutterkick is probably the only kick possible due to neurologic impairment. The instructor needs to analyze the available movement and prescribe the appropriate kick accordingly.

Spinal Cord Injuries

Swimming can be used effectively to increase upper-extremity strength and endurance. The individual with a spinal cord injury relies, to a great extent, on the strength of his arms to successfully perform all the activities of daily life. Swimming can be used as an adjunct to weight lifting to gain the necessary strength. The rehabilitative process after a spinal cord injury stresses independence in daily living skills, and upper-extremity strength is the primary force through which goals are accomplished. Contractures of the joints may also be relieved by swimming. Whole-body activities out of the wheelchair are one of the best therapies available, and swimming is the finest example of such. Obesity often hinders independence, and the energy expended in endurance swimming ranks high among all sporting activities.

For the spinal cord injured, when anesthetic skin is present, the development of decubitus ulcers is a constant concern. Because circulation is poor in the affected extremities, an increase in circulation to the whole body is valuable. Swimming increases circulation and relieves the constant pressure on the areas that are susceptible to skin breakdown.

Excelling in any activity helps those with spinal cord injuries develop constructive goals to increase their self-esteem. Swimming provides an outlet in which the assistive devices (braces or crutches) and wheelchairs can be left behind and physical activity tremendously enjoyed. Competitive swimming is available through the National Wheelchair Athletic Association on the state, national, and even international levels. Goals may be set and accomplished through participation in such competitive situations.

Paraplegia. Paraplegics can be taught stroke mechanics in essentially normal teaching situations. They can learn almost any stroke successfully. Strokes that require kicking to be a large propulsive force (e.g., breaststroke, sidestroke, butterfly) are often more difficult but still beneficial for the swimmer.

A common problem for paraplegic swimmers is overcoming the drag effect produced by nonfunctioning legs. This problem is accentuated in swimmers who have spasms in their lower extremities. One method that helps to reduce drag is the use of slightly inflated arm floaties around the knees. This is not recommended for those training for NWAA Games, because flotation devices are not allowed in the competition except with Class IA swimmers.

Swimming also provides a risk of injury to those with little or no sensation and function in the legs. Scrapes and scratches can be a problem because of the chance of poor healing and resulting pressure sores. Socks (even sweatpants) can be worn to limit the possibility of such a problem. Most paraplegics are capable of moving independently from the wheelchair to the deck and back; however, the instructor should check for abrasive surfaces around the pool and take appropriate protective measures.

An additional element to be understood and dealt with is incontinence of bowel and bladder. This is not always present, but if it is, appropriate precautions should be taken. If an external catheter is worn by a male, the device can be easily removed for swimming. Every effort to void (by Credé's method) should be made prior to entering the pool. An internal catheter worn by a female can be either disconnected at the collection device and the tubing clamped shut or emptied entirely and attached underneath the swimsuit. Bowel management is usually under control, however accidents can take place; and if they do, action should be swift with little embarrassment to the person.

Quadriplegia. The quadriplegic may also experience tremendous enjoyment and success from swimming. Stroke technique is more limited, however, due to limited movement potential. Essentially, the functional movement present should be evaluated and a stroke devised to accommodate that movement. Through experience, it has been found that bilateral strokes (breast stroke, inverted backstroke and elementary backstroke) provide the best method of movement for quadriplegics. An out-of-water recovery stroke often is effective to help improve shoulder position and increase arm speed for the power phase of the stroke.

The precautions discussed in the section on paraplegia also apply to the quadriplegic. Additional items to be cautious of are the breathing potential of the individual and his breath control. Many quadriplegics lose function of the musculature that assists in the breathing process, thus making inhalation of water more problematic. They also may have difficulty rotating their bodies or lifting their heads to take a breath. Warning signals may be necessary in the early stages of learning to swim after a spinal cord injury. Thus, strokes performed from the supine position are usually more successful initially since breathing is easier from that position. Use of the Delta Swim System is often indicated to aid in progressive swimming development.

An additional element present in many cases is the psychologic effect of swimming after the accident. Many quadriplegic patients acquire their disabilities in swimming-related accidents. The emotional component of fear plus the realization of the inability to move at will can both be accentuated on the first return to the pool after the injury. Support needs to be provided by the instructor and trust developed to help insure a more safe, enjoyable experience upon the first attempt.

Muscular Dystrophy and Muscular Atrophies

The child with muscular dystrophy is continually faced with obstacles to the achievement of functional movement. As the disease progresses, the potential for movement decreases. The major obstacle to movement is the pull of gravity, which must be overcome to an extent that allows a body part to move. Success in active games and sports gradually becomes more and more limited. Swimming, however, provides a medium in which independent movement is made possible for a much longer period of time. This movement is possible without the braces, chairs, and other devices that are otherwise needed, and this gives patients tremendous emotional benefits. Aquatics can benefit the person with muscular dystrophy in each of the developmental objectives.

Specific Benefits and Implications. Moderate exercise and activity may be beneficial to those with muscular dystrophy. It is hoped that exercise will maintain enough active strength in the unaffected muscle groups to prolong daily living skills and independence. Many people with muscular dystrophy are capable of swimming short distances independently. Swimming may also be beneficial in decreasing flexion

contractures. Active exercise out of the seated position may reduce the possibility of developing these contractures thus increasing range of motion and flexibility (Fig. 8–3). Cardiopulmonary strength and endurance are other facets of the organic objective that can be incorporated successfully into swimming programs for those with muscular dystrophies. Breathing exercises and breath control are a vital part of swimming for anyone but they are even more important for those with muscular dystrophy.

The neuromuscular objective includes integration of body parts through performance of a variety of motor skills. Swimming can be the medium in which to concentrate on the development of such perceptual-motor skills. It is often possible to practice such nonlocomotor skills as bending, twisting, swaying, and reaching from a standing position in the water. Locomotor skills are also possible in the water for a greater length of time than they are out of the water. Many times, standing and walking are still possible without braces in the pool, and this gives great satisfaction.

Swimming also helps those with muscular dystrophy develop body awareness. They realize and understand the limitations imposed on them by their disease, but must learn to compensate in various ways in order to continue to enjoy swimming. Appreciation of participation is also an element. Movement exploration can be incorporated into a swimming program more easily and with more movement than it can into a gymnasium program.

The physical benefits attributable to swimming should not overshadow the tremendous social and emotional benefits it also provides to those with muscular dystrophy. Swimming is a great outlet because it provides the possibility of success in a "risk" sport. Gaining proficiency in swimming makes people feel they are competing adequately with a potentially fearful environment; thus, swimming improves their self-esteem. Swimming also provides an excellent opportunity for group interaction with able-bodied classmates and friends.

Precautions in Programming. A major contraindication for the swimmer with muscular dystrophy is over-fatigue while swimming, although frequent rest periods may be a sufficient guard against this danger. Excessive chilling can also be harmful. People with muscular dystrophy may be more susceptible to pulmonary infections, which can be difficult for them to overcome since they are generally inactive and have low cardiopulmonary fitness. Warm air and water are often sufficient precautions, however drying off quickly and putting on warm clothing is necessary in many instances.

Transferring nonambulatory patients from their wheelchairs to the pool must be done carefully, because the musculature of the shoulder area is often weak in the later stages of the disease. The techniques to be used are outlined later in this chapter.

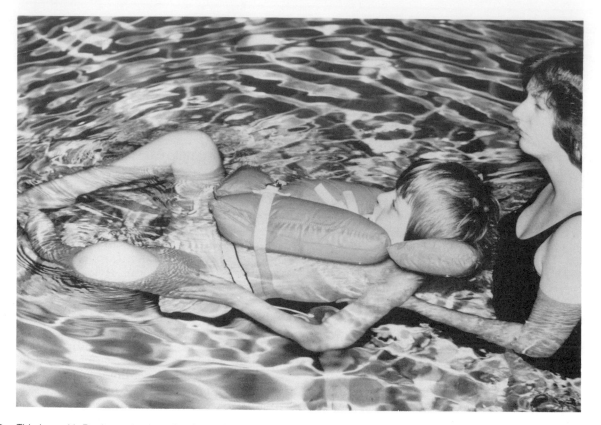

Fig. 8–3. This boy with Duchenne's muscular dystrophy enjoys swimming. Note the hip and knee flexion contractures and the equinovarus deformity of his feet.

Stroke Technique. The elementary backstroke (also finning and sculling) is generally the best stroke for those with muscular dystrophy to learn. It is recommended for the carry over effect it has throughout the disease. It is important to evaluate the swimmer's functional ability at regular intervals in order to maintain for him the most effective technique. A dolphin kick and/or flutterkick may be integrated into the stroke. When arm movement no longer provides efficient propulsion, kicking by flexing the leg at the knee (in supine position) will help the person move in a feet-first manner.

Abnormal Curvatures of the Spine

Swimming provides for those with abnormal curvatures of the spine a therapeutic form of exercise not possible in any other activity. It enables them to actively exercise the antigravity muscles when the body is in the horizontal plane. General body fitness is important for those with abnormally curved spinal columns who are undergoing treatment with exercise and an orthotic appliance. Swimming out of the brace can activate major muscle systems to help improve muscle tone and strengthen key postural muscles.

Scoliosis. The objectives of corrective exercise for scoliosis are to increase trunk flexibility, strengthen the postural muscles to improve general posture, pull the body into general alignment, and improve breath-ing muscles. These elements can be incorporated into the swimming program.

Almost any swimming strokes will help achieve these goals. However, the side stroke is probably the best stroke for aiding in correction of the spinal deformity. It is best to teach the person to do the stroke with the concave portion of his primary curve down in the water. This is the side opposite the thoracic pad on the Milwaukee brace or other prescribed device. With this side down, the person gets the maximal stretching effect in the propulsion and glide phases of the stroke. The back crawl start may also be beneficial in maximizing spinal flexibility.

Bilateral strokes, such as the breast stroke and elementary backstroke are beneficial in maintaining strength on both sides. However, any stroke will aid in the correction of the spinal deformity.

Kyphosis. Major objectives of treatment are to stretch the internal rotators of the shoulder, stretch the scapular abductors, and strengthen the external rotators of the shoulder and the scapular abductors. Specific strokes that may be beneficial are the inverted breast stroke, the elementary backstroke, and the back crawl.

Again, any stroke, other than the butterfly stroke, is beneficial and encouraged. The crawl stroke may be performed if an attempt is made to maintain a flat body position with the head slightly up and the recovery stroke low to keep from aggravating the deformity by strengthening the internal rotation of the shoulder.

Lordosis. Any swimming stroke will aid general body fitness for those with a lordotic problem. Kicking can be made more beneficial by stretching the hip flexors and lumbar extensors. This may be done using a scissors kick practiced on both sides. Another good practice is to place a kickboard under the lower back and keep the back flat on the kickboard while kicking.

General Implications. Swimming is beneficial not only in achieving organic developmental objectives, but also in achieving social and emotional benefits. The swimmer is able to remove the brace to swim and not consider that time out of the brace. This is due to the benefits that swimming offers.

Amputee Swimming

The person with an incomplete extremity (or extremities) is able to swim successfully with the appropriate stroke technique or adapted devices. The instructor must look at the functional capabilities of the individual and choose the most effective stroke. Independence through movement is a goal for which amputees continually strive, and swimming supports this goal. Recent amputees commonly experience balance problems in their first swimming experience, because of the effects of buoyancy.

Upper-Extremity Involvement
1. Partial amputation. Perform arm action to the extent of movement. A finning action may be possible with a partial arm amputation.
2. Complete bilateral. Concentrate on kick for propulsion. The whip kick and scissors kick are the most suitable.
3. Complete unilateral. The side stroke is preferred, with the usable arm down. A slightly deeper arm pull aids propulsion. Oftentimes, flippers or a similar adapted device can add surface area to aid in propulsion.

Lower-Extremity Involvement
1. Partial amputation. Perform leg action to the extent of movement or substitute a flutter kick.
2. Complete bilateral. Concentrate on arm action and the glide portions of strokes. Encourage lower body movement if possible.
3. Complete unilateral. Teach correct use of usable leg. A flutterkick will help overcome directional control, as will a stronger pull with the opposite arm.

A common problem with bilateral lower-extremity amputees is surface diving. They are often too buoyant without their legs, the greatest negative factor in floating, and have difficulty diving beneath the surface.

Some amputees prefer not to become involved with a swimming program in a group situation, because they fear teasing about the residual limb. The instruc-

tor should be aware of potential problems and handle the situation prior to any inconvenience.

Visual Impairments

The visually impaired person can enjoy physical activity as much as sighted persons. However, successful participation in many activities requires special equipment containing electronic auditory cues or the presence of sighted guides who provide the necessary cues. Swimming presents an alternative, because the blind swimmer can swim freely in most situations with little adapted equipment. Swimming also provides a great opportunity for physical development and general fitness.

When introducing a blind person to a new environment he should be given the opportunity to explore and discover the surroundings. A tour with a sighted person helps him acquaint himself with the pool and the equipment in the area. Tactile and auditory cues help him distinguish necessary characteristics. The exploration should include the entire deck, the locker rooms, the pool, and the equipment around the pool area (ladders, diving boards). It is important to minimize extraneous noise and hazards in the area, particularly if their placement is temporary. When "surveying" the area, the sighted guide should offer the preferred elbow to be used as a contact point. Rarely will a blind person want to be guided by another's hand. Be cautious of the tone of voice used while speaking to the blind. The guide should not feel uncomfortable asking the blind person questions about the area they are touring and he should emphasize the importance of total understanding. Many blind individuals prefer not to accept assistance, but would rather explore the area independently. Simply ask the person whether he would like assistance or not.

Teaching Recommendations. Obviously, the totally blind individual must rely on auditory, tactile, kinesthetic and proprioceptive sensory input. Visual cues from the teacher are thus eliminated, and verbal cues from the teacher indicated. Verbal cues must be clear, concise, and detailed. The explanation is reinforced with appropriate tactile input by placing the person's body in the desired position. Guiding the person's hand and arm or having him maintain contact during the demonstration will help him gain understanding. It is helpful initially to avoid totally submerging the ears until orientation to the surroundings is complete (Fig. 8–4).

The instructor should time his voice to coincide with the time at which the swimmer's ear is out of the water. Swimming should not be learned with the head always out of the water, even for the blind person. Concentration on kinesthetic perception will help the blind swimmer swim straight. Lanes can be marked off if necessary.

Special Aids. Various devices have been used by blind swimmers once they have established competent

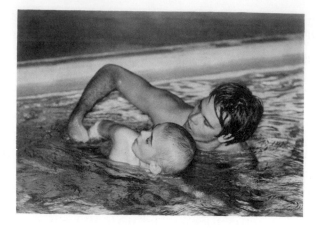

Fig. 8–4. Tactile, as well as verbal, input helps a blind swimmer to understand the proper movement.

swimming ability. These devices, such as "tapping poles" operated by a sighted person, provide cues as to direction in the pool and distance from the wall. Metronomes have been used to provide auditory cues to a blind swimmer doing laps. However, this may not be desired by all those who swim laps.

Seizure Disorders

A person with a known seizure disorder may actively participate in swimming. Safety must be the prime concern, and the lifeguard should be notified before the child enters the pool. A one-to-one student to instructor ratio is advisable, if possible, for those with more severe seizure disorders.

If a major motor seizure happens in the pool, the correct procedure is simply to maintain the head above the water (with the head tilted back to insure a clear airway) and allow the seizure to take place. Perhaps a blanket can be spread under the person or two people can support the entire body. It is not indicated to attempt to remove the person from the pool immediately because of the risk of injury. When the seizure has ended, authorized personnel should be contacted and the person allowed to rest in a warm, dry area.

Springboard diving is usually contraindicated for those with seizure disorders because of the risk of a seizure while on the ladder or board. Diving from the deck is a suitable skill to develop.

Swimming can provide a tremendous outlet and opportunity for general physical conditioning for those with a seizure disorder. The social and emotional objectives should be primary considerations in many cases.

Chronic Obstructive Lung Disease

Asthma. Swimming has been considered for many years to be an outstanding form of exercise for the asthmatic. A study by Fitch and Morton, in 1971, showed submaximal aerobic exercise to be more favorable than running or cycling. Exercise induced asthma was observed in 72.5% of those participating in the running test, and 65% of those in the cycling test, but in only 35% of those in the swimming test. These significant findings accentuate the importance of swimming as a form of aerobic fitness for asthmatics. The American Academy of Pediatrics recommended that children with asthma participate in physical education and sports.[3] Every effort should be made to ensure that restrictions set by school districts on the activity of asthmatic children are minimized. Breathing humidified air is helpful for asthmatics and this often aids controlled respiration.

Asthmatics may have to limit their participation in stressful active exercise. The need for athletic involvement and development of skills make swimming an excellent outlet. It is important to ensure that appropriate medical personnel are aware of the swimming program. According to the treatment plan of the physician, the necessary medication must be available. The arrangements must be made prior to a bronchospasm attack.

Cystic Fibrosis. Children with cystic fibrosis also have a need for expression through physical activity. Oftentimes limited in full-activity sports, their total involvement in any physical activity is important. The swimming environment can provide them with many social contacts as well as physical benefits. Accumulated secretions in the bronchial tree may be relieved by physical activity.

A problem that commonly develops in those with cystic fibrosis is chest deformity and kyphosis. As discussed earlier, swimming can help inhibit the development of kyphosis. The most important considerations, however, for those with cystic fibrosis are psychologic. Gaining the most out of life and fulfilling aspirations to normal group interaction are the most important reasons to participate in a recreational pursuit such as swimming, from which great enjoyment and satisfaction may be derived.

Temporary Orthopedic Impairments

Swimming is a tremendous therapeutic medium for rehabilitation of an orthopedic impairment. In most cases, immobilization of a joint area and its surrounding muscle groups causes deficits in passive and active ranges of motion, as well as muscular atrophy. The swimming environment can be an asset to rehabilitation by concentrating on these two areas. The instructor should work in conjunction with the physical therapist and/or physician in charge to provide the best possible therapeutic program for the individual.

The increase in circulation to the area often helps to remove swelling and speed the healing process. This increase in circulation occurs as a result of general swimming activity or intense work of the affected area. An increase in general muscle strength and endurance can help return the body to a more normal level of function, which is vital for independence upon return to normal living. Active exercises can be de-

---

signed for specific muscle groups. Suggestions should be shared with appropriate medical personnel prior to initiation. These can help increase muscle tone and joint range of motion.

Precautions need to be taken in transferring persons with orthopedic impairments to and from the pool. Assistance for each impairment should be under the direction of a medical team.

Juvenile Rheumatoid Arthritis (JRA)

Physical activity for those with JRA is often limited to mild forms of games and sports in order to prevent undue stress on joints affected by the disease. Swimming, however, can help increase muscle strength and joint range of motion, and submergence in therapeutically warm water often provides welcome relief for the joints during an active inflammation of the disease.

JRA can cause greatly varied degrees of limitation of movement in different persons. Particular swimming strokes should be recommended according to the amount of active movement available. Often, the range of motion in the horizontal position with the aid of buoyancy may be greater than when assessed in a gravitational position.

Success in activities is important to the arthritic and must be considered when planning a program. Stressful situations must be avoided. The important rules to follow are: (1) consult with the appropriate medical team (i.e., physician, therapist); (2) provide frequent rest periods; (3) avoid exercising to the point of fatigue; and (4) work within limitations of range of motion.

Arthritis aquatic programs are carried out jointly by local YMCAs and Arthritis Foundation chapters in most localities. Both organizations arrange for training of instructors and oversee the classes held in YMCA pools. It is possible for staff who are not from a YMCA aquatic facility to receive training.[4]

Osteogenesis Imperfecta

Depending upon the type of swim therapy (postsurgical treatment for gradual weight bearing or general mobilization exercise) the following guidelines should prove helpful.

Gentle, active movements of the legs should be encouraged. This can be done from the vertical position in deep water with the feet clearing the floor of the pool while the instructor gives support to the swimmer's waist. With some swimmers, as further weight-bearing is allowed, activity is carried out in progressively shallow water. Movements can include flexion/extension, abduction, adduction of the hips with the knees straight, and hip and knee flexion. These movements can also be performed in supine position while the child is supported by the instructor's hands lightly held under the waist. The child's head rests gently on the instructor's shoulders. In both vertical and horizontal positions active arm movements can be encouraged. Some swimmers will be independent in performing the range of motion exercises while using flotation devices.

Many persons with OI become independent swimmers and the water provides a support system for an unstable bone structure.

EQUIPMENT

Various equipment has been designed to make the swimming experience more valuable and successful for disabled individuals. Standard safety equipment can be used to encourage therapeutic gains as well as to provide needed flotation. Personal flotation devices (PFD) can be used in the standard position or various other ways to help provide support.

Arm floaties can be used independently of PFDs or in addition to them. They also can be used on legs as well as arms. It must be remembered that these devices are inflatable and not life preservers but support devices that help promote independence.

Transferring Devices For Pool Entry. Various devices have been designed that assist in lifting a person to and from the pool. No method is set for transporting people to the pool; each case must be evaluated individually. If the person is capable and prefers independent water entry, encourage it.

Swimming Aids. Swim mitts and paddles aid in movement by increasing surface area for water resistance. They are especially useful with the hemiplegic and the amputee. The greater resistance caused by the additional surface area is also beneficial in muscle strength development.

Masks, snorkels, and goggles may also be used. Safety requirements should be followed when underwater equipment is used.

Kickboards can be used in a variety of ways and their use by the disabled population should be encouraged. They can be valuable teaching aids for amputees, blind swimmers, those with temporary orthopedic impairments, and those with chronic lung disease.

Games and Toys. Games are an important aspect of enjoyable aquatic experiences for the disabled. Many skills can be taught effectively in the aquatic environment. The skills that can be emphasized include: (1) perceptual motor skills, (2) academic skills, (3) fundamental motor skills, (4) movement exploration experience, and (5) basic swimming skills. These skills can be woven successfully into the teaching environment by an innovative instructor.

The use of games as a teaching tool is beneficial. Games can provide important psychologic advantages that make a child more able to learn. These advantages include increasing the motivation of the student to the point of optimum learning.

The student and instructor both can relax and this helps ease the pressure on developing and improving skill techniques. By helping the student lose awareness of particular fears, games often make the student learn skills unconsciously. A pleasant atmosphere can allow for less pressure, and the desire to learn can be improved.

Delta Swim System. This system (Fig. 8–5) is designed to allow the swimmer to float in either prone or supine positions. Depending upon each individual situation, any combination of parts can be added or removed to facilitate the desired position in the water. The system is useful for swimmers who lack mobility skills, or have difficulty synchronizing body parts for propulsion. The sectional flotational device allows for freedom of extremity movement, and aids handling skills if the instructor is engaged in specific hydrotherapy exercises with a patient.

Creative Games. The movement education approach can be incorporated successfully into an aquatic program. This approach encourages independent decision-making and creative play. The children experience success readily, and hopefully, their fear of failure is eliminated. This is especially useful for children with low self-esteem. Creative play allows the students to be the major decision-makers in how the game is played. The instructor's job is to guide the students or encourage them to be creative within the boundaries of safety. These noncompetitive games encourage continuous activity among all the students.

Competitive games can also be used appropriately to help skill development. Some students respond favorably to competition and enjoy the opportunity to win or lose. The emphasis on winning must be held in the proper perspective by all children. Children with low self-esteem may not thrive on competition, and efforts must be made to encourage their participation to the limits of their abilities. Tag games and relays are competitive games in which all students can participate.

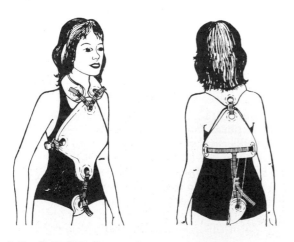

Fig. 8–5.   Delta Swim System. Courtesy of Danmark Products, Inc., 2390 Winewood Ave., Ann Arbor, MI 43103. Readers are encouraged to write to Danmark for further information.

Game Equipment. The great thing about aquatics and equipment for the pool is that almost everything can be used. Leftover and inexpensive equipment often works best in a pool, provided that a little imagination goes along with it. Objects that sink can be used for retrieval games, while floating objects have many uses.

Equipment that helps the beginning swimmer adjust to the water includes: sponges, wash cloths, squeeze water bottles, pots, pans, old milk jugs, blow tubes, straws, plastic buckets, and the child's favorite plastic game or toy.

Equipment that can be incorporated into games is uncountable. Examples include: plastic balls, wiffle balls, balloons, deck tennis rings, Hula hoops, kickboards, cones, Nerf balls, golf balls, plastic flowers, basketballs, beach balls, etc.

Perceptual-motor skills and academic skills can be improved with equipment that incorporates shapes, textures, color, and sounds. Such equipment may include multicolored hats, sponges in shapes or that are numbered, squeeze toys, hoops, rings, and ropes. Ropes can be used to make many shapes and sizes.

Evaluation. An important part of any game and activity are the teacher's evaluation of the effectiveness of the game. The teacher must determine whether the game he presented met the students' needs. These needs include physical, social, and emotional needs. Success needs to be built-in to the games, however, the games also need to present new and different experiences and challenges.

CONTRAINDICATIONS FOR SWIMMING

In developing an adapted aquatics program, the supervisor must be aware of certain conditions that make swimming unadvisable. A medical consultant should be available if questions arise. When no such consultant is available and a medical question remains unanswered, abstention from the activity is recommended. Medical approval should be indicated prior to the beginning of the program, however, a general contraindication list for swimming includes:

1. Infectious diseases in the active stage, i.e., the person still has an elevated temperature.
2. Chronic ear infections.
3. Chronic sinusitis.
4. Allergies to chlorine or water.
5. Skin conditions such as eczema.
6. Open wounds and sores such as draining decubitus ulcers (see note below).
7. Osteomyelitis in the active stage (see note below).
8. Acute episodes of rheumatoid arthritis.
9. Venereal diseases.
10. Severe cardiac conditions.

Note: Barrier protection with a WaterGard product (refer to later section) is possible for patients with I.V. therapy skin openings and open lesions. However, there are concerns for every case and a physician will need to make the final decision regarding permission to swim.

LIFTS AND TRANSFERS

The most important aspect in transferring a person into the pool is insuring the safety of all who are involved. All too often, inappropriate techniques are used that frighten the swimmers and put them at a risk of unnecessary injury. The following steps are helpful:

1. Safety first! Employ all possible help when lifting a person. Depending on the person's size, two adults are usually adequate.
2. Make certain that the brakes on the wheelchair are locked. If additional people are available, have someone hold the wheelchair in addition to locking the brakes.
3. Lifters should use good body mechanics when lifting. The distance the person is lifted should be as small as possible.
4. Lifters should lift the person in unison, with one person giving directions.
5. Explain to the person prior to lifting him the plans of the lift to the deck.
6. The swimmer should be lifted from the chair to the deck, then from the deck to the pool. The deck should be non-abrasive. If the deck is abrasive, use a towel or blanket to pad the surface.
7. Insure that a helper is available to support the person on the deck if necessary.
8. Always have a helper in the pool to help the swimmer into the water.
9. If the swimmer is independent in transferring to the deck of the pool safely, provide a safe environment and promote his independence but be available to assist when necessary.
10. When a lifting procedure is not possible, ramps can be used to transport the person into the water in a wheelchair.
11. Make sure the wheelchair has the wheels locked, is positioned as close to the pool as possible and has towels covering the seat.

2-Man Lifts

1. The 2 lifters grasp opposing wrists with 2 arms under the thigh area and 2 arms in the mid-back region.
2. Lifters can grasp with one hand under the axillary area and one hand under the thigh. With one person on each side of the swimmer, lift together.
3. With a lifter on each side, grasp the swimmer's wrist, palms down, with the forearm under the axillary area and the other hand under the thigh.
4. One lifter can grasp both legs under the thigh and the other can place both his hands either in the axillary area or in front of the swimmer with his arms around the chest.

4-Man Lifts

All of the previous lifts can be done by 4 people, having one person grasp each extremity.

Large Towel or Blanket Lift

Slip a blanket behind the person and completely underneath his body (from shoulders to knees). The blanket should be rolled up from the sides so that it can be grasped securely. Lift in unison from the chair to the deck. This can also be used from the deck into the water (Fig. 8–6). An ideal aspect of this lift is that the blanket can be positioned in the water for the return lift to the deck. Either 2 or 4 people can lift in this manner. If needed, a person may maintain proper head position of the person in the towel (Example, a person with muscular dystrophy or cerebral palsy may lack appropriate head control).

A hydraulic pool lift is a useful piece of equipment that can be installed on the pool deck to assist with the transfer of a swimmer to and from the water. The lift eliminates physical strain and can be used to transfer swimmers who lack mobility and/or who are heavy.

Aquatic programs offer tremendous benefits that may not be achieved through any other single medium. Swimming is not only a beneficial exercise for the physically challenged, but more importantly, it

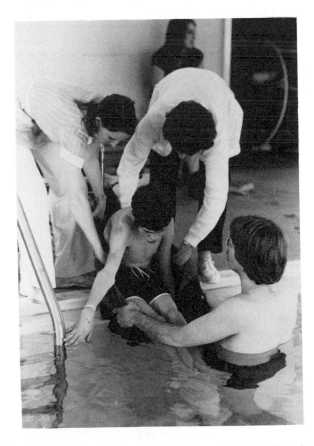

Fig. 8–6. This young man with athetoid cerebral palsy is assisted to the deck by means of the blanket lift.

provides a lifetime recreational and leisure time out-let.

ADAPTED COMPETITIVE SWIMMING

The Adapted Swimming Committee of United States Swimming, Inc. (USS) advocates assistance including rule modifications for swimmers who are physically disabled. For example, a blind swimmer can participate in (USS) sanctioned meets. A coach can use a "tap pole" to make contact with the swimmer's head or shoulder to indicate when to make a flip turn, or to provide a warning that the pool edge is within reach. Many other considerations that would enable disabled swimmers to compete with their non-disabled peers are fully discussed in the Handbook for Adapted Competitive Swimming published by USS.*

SPECIAL CONSIDERATIONS FOR USERS OF TREATMENT DEVICES

The rehabilitation process often focuses on physical restoration, and water therapy is frequently referred to as hydrotherapy, or in some circles as aquatic therapy. Physicians recognize the health and rehabilitation benefits of hydrotherapy as a specific treatment medium especially in clinical and rehabilitation agencies where an interdisciplinary team provides early and aggressive treatment strategies.

This section focuses attention to patients who require certain temporary or permanent devices for personal care or treatment. Many of these patients will demonstrate obvious concerns as to being candidates for an aquatic program. So many factors are involved in any one condition, that it is impossible to discuss the many variables that might influence each case. It is hoped that certain conclusions can be made to the indications, complications, and other considerations entering into the selection process. It is not unusual for swimming instructors, and in some instances therapists, to be unfamiliar with the use and management of these devices in a pool setting. The following information will point out practical guidelines for including users of treatment devices in swimming and/or hydrotherapy programs.

Butterfly Infusion Needle, Angiocath, Heparin Lock Needle (Fig. 8–7)

Reason for Usage. These medical devices are used for inserting fluids utilizing a needle into the desired vein. Intravenous medication and fluid administration provides a quick and accurate method of supplying medication and the replacement of fluids.

Population. These medical devices are used with individuals requiring rapid infusion of medication or fluid replacement, the most common being those treated with antibiotics (cystic fibrosis, osteomyelitis).

---

*U.S. Swimming Inc., 1750 E. Boulder St., Colorado Springs, CO 80909

Adaptive Apparatus. WaterGard, manufactured by CABA Medical Products, Inc. (Fig. 8–7). Also, a latex surgeon's glove with the fingers cut off can be secured over the heparin lock. A second glove can be added over the first layer to give added protection. Careful taping of the glove is required to provide waterproof covering.

Implications and Precautions. Although usage of the WaterGard device should provide adequate protection against water penetration to the intravenous site, it is important that care still be implemented. Patients should feel comfortable continuing their daily swimming exercise regimen, although sustained pressure or contact to the intravenous site should be avoided as displacement of the needle is possible. However, normal swimming strokes are permissible as long as the WaterGard device is correctly worn. During application, it is important to squeeze all the air out of the bag, otherwise the unit will float.

Arm Cast (Below or Above Elbow) and Leg Cast

Reason for Usage. Arm and leg casts promote fixed healing of bone matter.

Population. These medical devices are used with persons with post-fracture orthopedic impairments.

Adaptive Apparatus. WaterGard device (Fig. 8–7).

Implications and Precautions. The individual's limb mobility will be limited by the size and location of the cast. The affected arm or leg can be used with the WaterGard device when correctly worn; however, physician approval should be granted before exercise procedures are undertaken in the pool.

Ostomy Collection Device (Fig. 8–8)

Reason for Usage. Ostomies are essentially artificial openings from the inside to the outside of the body, the purpose being to eliminate waste matter. The three most common types of ostomies are colostomy, ileostomy, and ureterostomy. The colostomy opens into the colon, an ileostomy opens into the ileum, and the ureterostomy opens into the ureters. The difference between the colostomy and ileostomy is the type of fecal waste that is discharged through the artificial opening or stoma. The ureterostomy discharges urine.

Population. This surgery is performed for a number of reasons, including bladder or bowel damage or obstructions. This procedure can be permanent or temporary in nature, depending on the extent of damage or defect.

Adaptive Apparatus. Urinary diversion pouch, fecal stoma bag.

Implications and Precautions. Individuals with ostomy collection devices certainly can participate successfully in swimming, although it is important that the appliance seal is water tight. If the individual chooses to wear a belt with the pouch or bag, the belt should be made of rubber since elastic cloth belts have a tendency to lose their elasticity when wet. Females

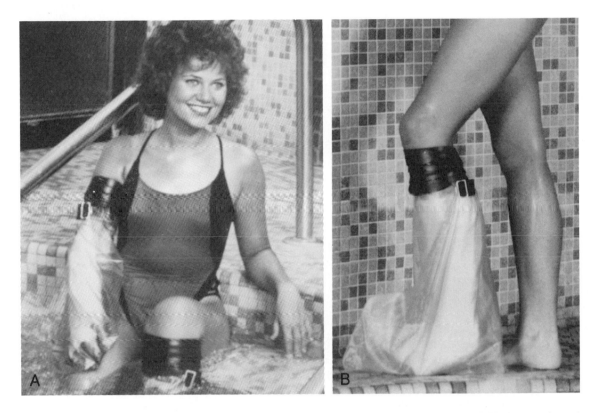

Fig. 8–7. The WaterGard can be used to protect arm and leg casts from direct exposure to water. In addition, many therapists are now using WaterGard to cover sutures before they are completely healed for quicker access to water rehabilitation programs. (Courtesy of CABA Medical Products, Ltd., Medical Arts Center, Suite 101, 35 W. Clay, Muskegan, MI 49440.) Readers are encouraged to write CABA for further information, or call 1-800-777-3500.

can successfully wear the device using a suit with a skirt while males are able to conceal the device by wearing boxer shorts. It is advisable that the collection device be emptied before any swimming participation. Although vigorous physical activity should be avoided, persons wearing these devices should feel free to participate in normal swimming activity.

Nagogastric Feeding Tube (N.G. Tube) (Fig. 8–9), Gastrosomy Tube, (G. Tube) (Fig. 8–9).

Reason for Usage. The nasogastric feeding tube is inserted into the stomach via the nose for the purpose

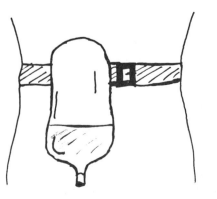

Fig. 8–8. Urinary diversion pouch. The pouch can be worn with a belt and concealed under the bathing suit.

of instilling food and/or fluids. The gastrosomy tube is surgically inserted through the abdominal wall and into the stomach with the objective of giving the patient liquid nutrients.

Population. The nasogastric tube is used for the purpose of feeding and as a route for medication when the patient is unable to take oral nourishment. These feeding problems could be the result of an injury, developmental delay, or a health impairment. The implementation of the nasogastric tube is commonly found in newborn infants who have problems with sucking and swallowing. Gastrosomy tube implementation is commonly seen in long-term rehabilitation patients who have suffered a head injury or who have complete obstruction of the esophagus due to tumor or scar tissue contractures.

Implications and Precautions. There is no reason why persons with nasogastric and gastrosomy tubes should not receive hydrotherapy. However, possible displacement of the nasogastric tube from the stomach can take place if adequate care is not provided. Coughing can be a factor in tube displacement; therefore, the therapist should ensure that no amount of water enters the nostrils. Since nasogastric tube placement is usually a temporary measure, breath control procedures should be postponed until the nasogastric tube has been permanently removed from the patient.

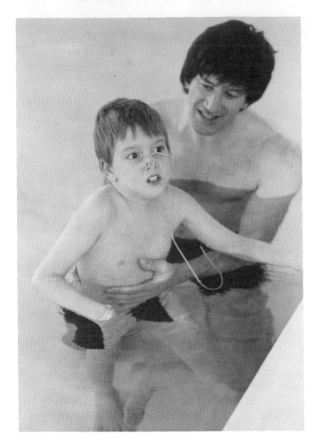

Fig. 8–9. This 10-year-old male, who sustained a closed head injury, is equipped with a nasogastric tube and is primarily working on leg strengthening and ambulation skills in the swimming pool.

Fig. 8–10. This 18-year-old male with a diagnosis of a closed injury is fitted with a gastrosomy tube which has been clamped and tucked under his trunks.

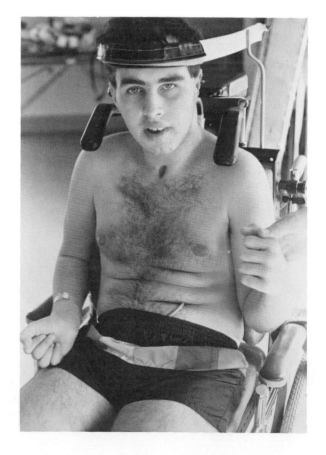

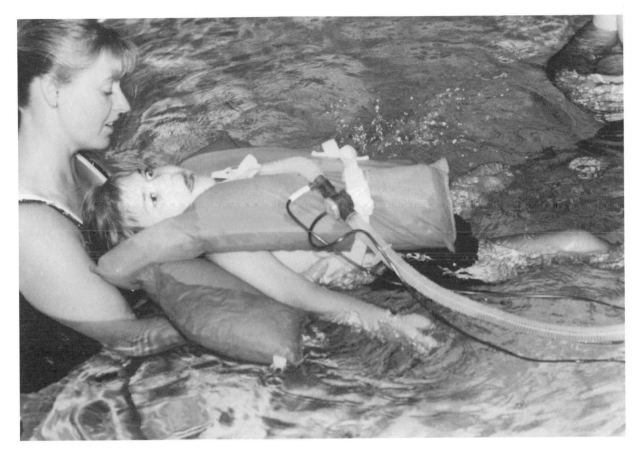

Fig. 8–11. A ventilator patient afflicted by myasthenia gravis. This 6-year-old male, although needing continuous respiratory support from a ventilator, was able to engage in hydrotherapy (note tubing extending from tracheal site). Active range of motion exercises to maintain strength, flexibility, and endurance were performed in calm water.

Exercise and strokes done primarily from the supine position can be performed successfully by the patient wearing the nasogastrc tube; of course, adequate support from the therapist or instructor is an absolute ncccssity from a safety standpoint. "Stoppers" or "plugs" can be placed in a N.G. or G. tube to ensure that entrance of water does not occur. In addition, to maximize protection, a rubber band or clamp can be placed at the end of the gastrosomy tube and tucked under the swimming trunks (Fig. 8–10).

A patient wearing a gastrosomy tube can undertake most types of exercises in the pool, care being given that the tube is not pulled which may create discomfort for the patient.

Tracheostomy Device (Fig. 8–11)

Reason for Usage. A tracheostomy is an incision into the trachea and the placement of the tracheostomy tube below the larynx so as to produce and maintain an open airway.

Population. These medical devices are used with individuals who have damage to the trachea which has resulted in a restriction of the airway. Initial rehabilitation for head-injured patients usually involves tracheostomy care.

Implications and Precautions. A therapist working with a patient who has a tracheostomy device should take care that water does not enter the air passageway by way of the stoma. Therefore, extra support for the patient is required when he or she is placed in the supine or vertical position. It is essential that the patient's neck is above the surface of the water. Therefore, the positioning of the patient in the prone position is not recommended.

Extra support from the therapist and a personal flotation device are required to keep the stoma site above the surface of the water. However, qualified personnel, such as a nurse familiar with tracheostomy suctioning procedures, should be close at hand in the event that water enters the swimmer's air passageway. This safeguard is crucial, particularly for patients who have no cough reflex.

Halo-Cervical Orthosis (Halo Vest)

Reason for Usage. These medical devices stabilize injured spinal columns by immobilizing the head and cervical spine.

Population. These devices are used with individuals who have injuries to the C1–T1 cervical segments of the spinal column.

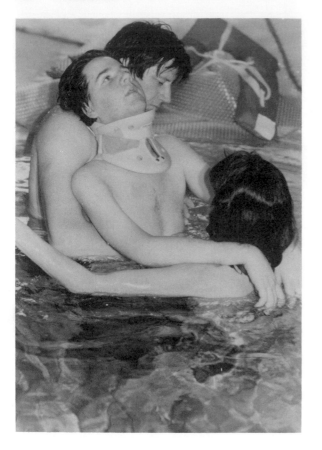

Fig. 8–12. This 18-year-old male who sustained a closed head and spinal cord injury is being given range of motion exercises by two therapists. In this instance, the Philadelphia collar facilitates the desired head position.

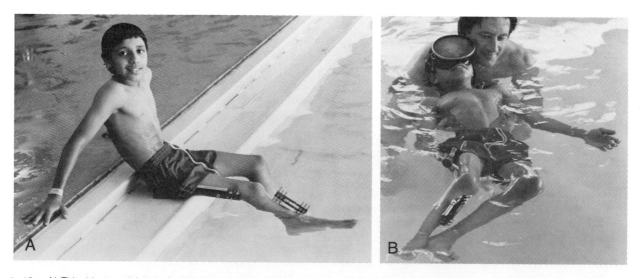

Fig. 8–13. A) This 11-year-old male is seen with the dynamic axial fixator device for limb lengthening of both his femur and tibia. Wearing this device as opposed to a cast, allows the patient to participate in hydrotherapy. B) This patient fitted with the dynamic fixator device can actively range his affected extremity in the water, and also perform functional swimming skills.

Implications and Precautions. Although some high-level spinal cord injured patients do participate in hydrotherapy, it is recommended that patients not participate while wearing a halo vest due to possible cervical instability. In addition, skin breakdown is a problematic complication when the halo lining of the jacket is allowed to get wet, as adequate drying of device proves difficult. However, after the halo vest is removed and physician approval has been obtained, these spinal cord injury patients benefit from hydrotherapy.

Philadelphia Collar (Fig. 8–12)

Reason for Usage. The collar prevents flexion, extension or hyperextension of the cervical column and reduces lateral flexion and rotation. In addition, the device reminds patients to curb head and neck movement.

Population. The Philadelphia collar (Fig. 8–12) is used for individuals who require mechanical restraint/support of the cervical column.

Implications. The Philadelphia collar is a useful support item made out of resilient polyethylene which is durable in water. However, it is recommended that the patient requiring cervical neck support change into a dry collar after the completion of the hydrotherapy session. Skin breakdown may result from the wearing of a wet or partially wet collar.

Dynamic Axial Fixator (Fig. 8–13)

Population and Reason for Usage. This versatile orthopaedic instrument can be used for a number of different surgical procedures, including the repair of open and closed fractures, the fixing of diaphyseal osteotomies in arthrodesis of joints and limb lengthening.

The implementation of the Dynamic Axial Fixator in the lower extremities allows the patient to partially bear weight and exercise the affected extremity immediately after surgery. Exercising the limb will decrease muscle atrophy and curtail conditions of osteoporosis which might occur had the affected limb been immobilized in a cast. Thus the patient is more responsible and productive in terms of improving his own physical prognosis. Unlike the Dynamic Axial Fixator, the cast prevents access to the affected site consequently inhibiting the patient's progress.

Implications and Precautions. A patient wearing a Dynamic Axial Fixator device can take advantage of swimming as an invaluable exercise medium, provided suitable precautions are made to ensure that the skin at the pin sites is kept clean and infection free. Problems in relation to the pin sites should be immediately referred to the patient's physician. Patients should also exercise care in transferring from the pool deck into the water and seek the therapist's assistance if necessary. Once in the pool, individuals can perform active range of motion in an attempt to increase blood flow to the weakened site and to maintain flexibility, strength, and endurance in the affected limb. Movement in the water will also have a natural cleansing effect on the skin surrounding the fixation pin sites.

REFERENCES

1. Bolton, E., and Goodwin, D.: An Introduction to Pool Exercises. Phys Ther, 58:1978.
2. Fitch, K.D., and Morton, A.R.: Specificity of exercise in exercise-induced asthma. Br Med J, 4:577, 1971.
3. American Academy of Pediatrics: The asthmatic child and his participation in sports and physical education. Pediatrics, 45:150, 1970.
4. McDuffie, M., and Boutaugh, M.: Pool Exercise Programs for People with Arthritis. Clin. Rheumatol. in Practice, July-Aug., 168–169, 1985.

ADDITIONAL REFERENCES

Adamo, P.: A Guide to Pediatric Tracheostomy Care. Springfield, Charles C Thomas, 1981.

Aquatics for Special Populations. Champaign, IL, Human Kinetics Publishers, Inc., 1987.

Atlas of Orthotics. Biomechanical Principles and Applications. American Academy of Orthopaedic Surgeons. 2nd Ed. St. Louis, The C.V. Mosby Co., 1985.

Auxter, D.: Physical fitness and adapted physical education. Exceptional Education Quarterly, 3 (1):54–63, 1982.

Campion, M.R.: Hydrotherapy in Pediatrics. Rockville, MD, Aspen Publications, 1985.

De Bari, A.: (Dept. of Orthopaedic Surgery, School of Medicine, University of Virginia). Private Correspondence, 1988.

De Bastiani, G., Aldegheri, R., and Renzi-Brivio, L.: The treatment of fractures with a Dynamic Axial Fixator. J Bone Joint Surg, 66-B:538–545, 1984.

De Bastiani, G., Aldegheri, Renzi-Brivio, L., et al.: Limb lengthening by Callus Distraction (Callotasis). J Pediatr Orthoped, 7 (2):129–134, 1987.

Elkington H.: Swimming—A Handbook for Teachers. Cambridge, Cambridge University Press, 1978.

Hollister Incorporated: Managing a Urostomy . . . So It Doesn't Manage You. Chicago, Hollister Inc., 1974.

Siegel, R., and Papush, H.: The A.B.C. of Ileostomy. Miami Beach, Harriett Papush Custom Service, Inc., 1970.

Sorensen, K.C., and Luckman, J.: Basic Nursing. A Psychophysiologic Approach. Philadelphia, W.B. Saunders Co., 1978.

The International Directory of Recreation—Oriented Assistive Device Sources. Marina del Ray, CA, Lifeboat Press, 1986.

Urinary Ostomies. A Guidebook for Patients. Los Angeles, United Ostomy Association, Inc., 1978.

Wang, G.W.: (Dept. of Orthopaedic Surgery, School of Medicine, University of Virginia). Private correspondence, 1988.

8 *Low Organization Games*

Low organization games are those requiring little organization, few rules, little equipment, and limited activity. Since there are many types of disabled individuals with varied interests and different needs, a program of low organization games includes a wide variety of activities. Regardless of the extent of physical or mental involvement, most individuals need social stimulation and interaction with others, especially their own peers. This section on low organization games is designed primarily for those whose physical and/or mental disabilities restrict the type and range of movements that can be used.

SUGGESTIONS FOR SPECIFIC DISABILITIES

In order to aid the more severely involved individual, the instructor must become acquainted with some general leadership suggestions for specific disabilities.

Mental Retardation

Persons with mental retardation have short attention spans and most have problems with coordination, balance, agility, directionality, laterality, strength, body awareness, and self-image. In many situations, these problems are the result of inactivity and lack of opportunity to participate in group activities. Mentally retarded children are often overprotected and discouraged from exploring the world; consequently, they have fewer opportunities to learn. Research clearly indicates that, with training and practice, people with mental retardation can develop skills in physical fitness and motor abilities.

Leadership Suggestions
1. Groups of 5 or 6 are generally best to work with, particularly during the early phases of the program.
2. Groups should be organized by developmental abilities and chronologic age.
3. Play and activity periods should be frequent, but relatively short. Play periods should not last more than 30 minutes.
4. A variety of activities should be introduced in order to hold the attention of the child.
5. Instructions should be brief.
6. Demonstrations should accompany instructions.
7. Pictures, stories, colorful equipment, and visual aids will stimulate the program.
8. Physical activities should be coordinated with art and music activities.

9. Names for the games or activities should be attractive.
10. Games and activities should be taught with overlearning to reinforce the person's learning process. Overlearning is necessary to improve the persons retention of the skill.
11. It is important to remember making the activity age appropriate. The activity should also be functional or able to be utilized by the person in a community living situation. Help the student learn a skill that he/she can continue to use outside the particular school or rehabilitation area. This is of particular importance with the mentally retarded pupil.

Visual Impairments

Impaired vision or blindness is always a handicap, but if newly acquired, the patient requires much help and understanding. He will need to relearn some things or make adjustments in doing them. Familiarity with location of materials will be necessary.

Leadership Suggestions
1. Activities that will not neglect the totally blind in favor of the partially seeing child should be selected.
2. Circle and line formations are effective in keeping the group together.
3. Counting and clapping help keep blind people in touch with each other.
4. The leader should indicate where he is at all times and he should inform the group what the others are doing.
5. Rattles and bells should be placed inside balls to help the blind follow their movement.
6. A totally blind person should be paired with a partially sighted one, if possible.
7. Balls for the partially sighted should be soft, larger than normal, and painted white or brightly colored.
8. The leader's voice should be loud enough to be heard by everyone.
9. Music and rhythmic sounds are highly motivating. Rhythmic activities and simple dances are recommended.
10. Activities that are complex (contain many steps) should be broken down into the simple components before being taught to the visually impaired person.

Auditory Impairments

Impaired hearing or deafness, especially if newly acquired, requires many adjustments. Warmth and understanding can be communicated by actions and facial expressions as well as by speaking and writing. One main concern is that the deaf person may have difficulty in understanding complex rules and strategies for games, especially during large group encounters.

Leadership Suggestions

1. Speak moderately and at a normal pace to improve the possibility of lip reading. Do *not* speak slowly as this will confuse the person.
2. Gestures, sign language, and demonstrations should be used when giving instructions. Face the group at all times.
3. If possible, have a hearing partner pair up with the hearing impaired person to facilitate communication.
4. Use signs, overheads or other written forms of communication to assist the learner.
5. If outside, do not have the hearing impaired person looking into the sun for instructions.

Immobilized Patient (Activity Suggestions from a Bed)

The psychologic impact of an illness or accident serious enough to warrant hospitalization with confinement to bed is often of enormous consequence to the victim. The physical and mental condition of the patient often limits the type and range of movements; therefore, activities may be limited because of: (1) the physical incapacity of the patient; (2) the contraindications for movement due to injury, medical, or surgical conditions; (3) the immobility of the patient due to traction, casts, braces, catheters, or various other medical equipment; or (4) the mental ability of the patient.

The use of low organization games presents the therapist with opportunities for motivation and psychologic encouragement which often stimulate the patient to better efforts.

Leadership Suggestions

1. Children may experience discomfort when sitting in bed as a result of exaggerated joint and muscle pressure; therefore, short but frequent play periods should be provided for such children.
2. Large and light, or improvised, balls should be used in place of regulation balls.
3. A balloon is useful for volleyball and toss games for children in bed because it moves and falls slowly.
4. Court dimensions should be smaller than those for regulation courts, and the equipment should be lighter.
5. Physical limitations may be handled by pairing players so that each does one part of a skill and together they accomplish the entire act.

6. The program leader should consider the physician's recommendations and any contraindications for activity.

ADAPTING GAMES AND ACTIVITIES

To achieve the desired results, it is important to create a framework from which a low organization game can be analyzed. Prior to the actual adaptation of games and activities, the program leader has the responsibility of assessing 4 important factors relative to the participants in question. These factors are:

1. Physical abilities
2. Mode of transportation (independent walker, wheelchair-user, etc.)
3. Ocular functioning and communicative ability
4. Intellectual level

After the initial assessment, the choice of game components can be investigated. Game components include the number of players on a team, the equipment to be used, the organizational framework (circle, straight line, triangle, etc.) of the playing area, and rules and purpose of play. The purpose of playing a low organization game is not always to play to win. For example, a game can be designed to promote independent locomotor skills or to elicit cooperative play attitudes.

There are literally hundreds of games that can be adapted for physically disabled children. As indicated previously, the program leader, in many cases, has the responsibility of selecting games based upon the needs of each participant. For this reason it is important to review and analyze the general qualities inherent in each game situation (Table 9-1).

To categorize each game in some logical sequence for quick reference is useful. An inspection of the following strategies can give the reader an idea on how such reference material can be readily used (Table 9-2). Hopefully this information will encourage readers to explore additional literature on the subject.

Target Badminton

The game consists entirely of serving, which allows the player who is limited in mobility skills to compete on an equal basis with a normal or less involved player. All game skills are performed from a stationary position, and the game is based on offensive performance ability. No defensive maneuvers are utilized. For this reason, players who are confined to stretchers, crutches, standing platforms, and wheelchairs can play and stay within a margin of safety. Movement patterns are basically of a single response (flexion-extension) nature and in one plane.

Target badminton can be played indoors or out, in singles or doubles matches. Two archery target faces are used, each one placed in an opposite court approximately 10 feet from the net. No boundary or court lines are required (Fig. 9-1).

Table 9–1. Factors to Consider When Selecting Games

Time—Approximate duration of the game.

Min. # of Participants—*Minimum* number of participants needed for the game.

Equipment—Special equipment used in the game.

Warm Up—A good game to begin a session with, ice breaker.

Active—A high-paced game; may become aggressive. Monitor closely.

Passive—A game offering a calming effect and/or requiring minimal physical movement.

Trust—A game requiring and/or developing trust.

Team Development—A game that tends to develop teamwork or sense of community.

Problem Solving—Usually an initiative game requiring the group to work together to solve a problem.

Strategy—A game requiring individual or group strategy to overcome the challenge.

Leadership—A game requiring and/or developing leadership.

Self-Confidence—While most of the initiatives/games are structured to enhance self-confidence, these games specifically focus on self-confidence.

Quick Thinking—A game that requires and/or develops quick thinking.

Hand/Eye Coordination—A game that requires and/or develops hand/eye coordination.

Balance/Coordination—A game that requires and/or develops balance and coordination.

From Initiatives and Games for Recreation, Leisure, and Therapy. Courtesy of Douglas Bowne, Bureau of Health and Recreation Services, Division For Youth, 84 Holland Avenue, Albany, NY 12208.

Play

The badminton net is usually lowered to equalize competition and provide opportunities for early success. Two shuttlecocks are given to each player. Players alternate serves, each attempting to stroke the shuttle over the net so that it lands on the target face. Each server has two opportunities to strike the shuttle over the net. If, on the second attempt (contact with racket must be made for legal serve), the server fails to hit the shuttle over the net, then one point is deducted (individual or team) from the score. A deduction is made only for points already accumulated. No deduction is made from an individual or a team with no earned points. The opposing player or team serves after a deduction in score has been made.

The scoring system is based on the same values used for archery: gold, 9; red, 7; blue, 5; black, 3; white, 1. Score is counted after each serve for any part of the shuttle (cork or feathers) touching the colored score zones.

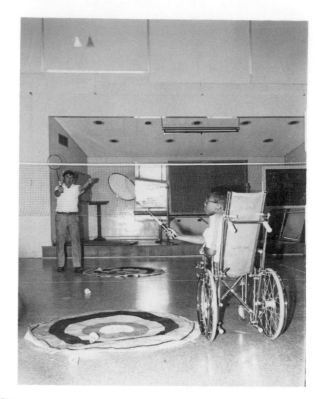

Fig. 9–1. Target badminton game.

The game is won by the first player or team to score 50 points (or a score of another total depending upon agreement of the players).

Modified Serve. Serving skills can be adapted for players who cannot use the conventional serving technique. With the player holding the racquet at shoulder level, an assistant places the shuttle (feathers down) on the racquet face (Fig. 9–2). By holding onto the handle with either one or two hands, the player extends the arms upward, thrusting the shuttle over the net.

Target Tennis

A vigorous game for 2 or 4 wheelchair-bound or ambulatory players.

Equipment
The following equipment is needed:
1. Target screen (Fig. 9–3). The screen should be permanently attached to a base approximately 4 inches from the ground. It is easily movable with four 1½-inch rubber casters attached to the base. It has a frame 2 by 4 inches with a ⅜-inch rim of pine plywood. Ten-inch diameter open spaces are spaced equally on a net, wire, or similar backdrop.
2. Target tennis court (Fig. 9–4): The target tennis screen should be placed near a wall or a canvas backdrop. The side and end zones should be marked with white tape.

Table 9–2.

Initiative or Game	Text/pg. #	R.L.T.	Time	Min. # of Participants	Activity Level	Equipment	Warm-Up	Active	Passive	Trust	Team Develop.	Problem Solving	Strategy	Leadership	Self-Confidence	Quick Thinking	Hand/Eye Coordination	Balance and Coordination	Remarks
A What	MNG 73	L	10	6	Lo	Objects	X		X							X	X		Humorous
All Aboard	SB 106	T	10	6	Med		X			X	X	X	X	X	X				
Almost Infinite Circle	SB 131	L	10+	2	Lo	See Remarks			X		X	X	X			X			2' Piece Rope/Person
Amoeba Race	NG 159	R	15	6	Med	Rope		X		X	X	X	X	X					
Balance Broom Relay	CC 18	R	10+	2	Hi	2 Brooms		X									X	X	Humorous
Bola	NG 49	R	10	8	Hi	Schmerltz		X								X		X	Jump Rope
Bone Game	NG 79	L	20	6	Lo	4 Bones			X				X	X					Bones can be matches/sticks
Bloop	SB 49	R	15+	6	Hi	Beach Ball	X	X					X			X	X	X	
Bottoms Up	SB 159	R	5+	2	Med		X		X				X		X		X	X	
Chute Volley	MNG 173	R	15+	8+	Med	Parachutes/Balls		X					X			X	X	X	Pitch and Catch
Circle the Circle	SB 60	R/L	10	6	Med	Hula Hoops	X	X					X			X		X	Group Against Time—Team Against Team
Commons (Snap)	MNG 25	R/L	10	2	Lo			X								X			
Data Processing	MNG 139		5	4	Lo		X		X			X							Used to Form Into Teams
Diminishing Load	SB 138	T	15	6	Hi			X		X	X	X	X	X		X		X	

*Initiatives and Games Reference Chart. Courtesy of D. Bowne.
Key: R = Recreation oriented game/activity
    L = Leisure oriented game/activity
    T = Therapeutic oriented game/activity

3. Badminton or tennis racquets.
4. Tennis balls.

Play
Serve. The player must position himself behind the end zone line. He then tosses the ball into the air and strikes it with an overhand stroke so that it will bounce on the floor (Fig. 9–5).

Scoring a Point. To score a point, the player serves the ball so that it bounces once on the floor (midway between the player and the screen) and then goes through one of the five open spaces in the target screen. A bonus serve is allowed for every point scored. No point is scored if the ball bounces two or more times on the floor. Modifications in scoring are allowed for the player using an adapted racquet.

Rules
1. A referee is chosen to be responsible for keeping score, retrieving dead balls, and keeping official time.
2. Each player receives 2 balls and chooses his racquet.
3. A flip of a coin decides which player serves first.
4. Each player must stay in his half zone of the court and behind the end zone.
5. Player 1 attempts to score by serving the ball.
6. After the referee has ruled Player 1's ball "dead," Player 2 takes his turn.
7. Players alternate serves until the 4 balls are ruled "dead." This completes a round.
8. Play continues for 15 minutes. The player with the highest score at the end of that time is the winner.
9. In case of a tie, play continues as before until the deciding point is scored.

Re-serve
1. After a player scores a point, he is awarded another serve.

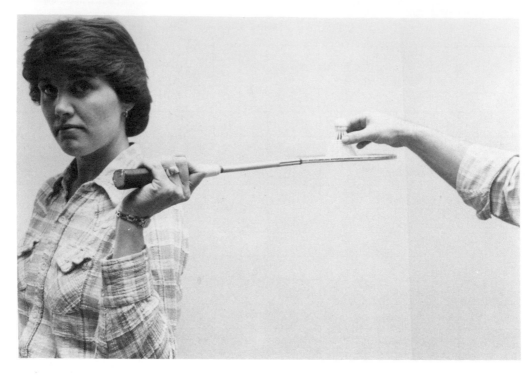

Fig. 9–2.   Modified serving technique.

2. If the player misses the ball when attempting to serve, he is allowed to continue until he strikes the ball.
3. If the ball hits the target screen and rebounds to the server, the player must remain behind the end zone line; however, it is permissible to cross over the end zone line with the racquet and retrieve a ball in the playing court. The player cannot cross the end zone line and retrieve a ball with his hands or feet. The server is not allowed to cross into his opponent's court to retrieve the ball. If the player is confined to a wheelchair, a re-serve is allowed if the ball is "trapped" or "stopped dead" by the player's racquet. The referee hands the ball to the server, and play continues.

Loss of Serve. If a player serves and the ball "stops dead" in the restricted zone (Fig. 9–4), he loses one serve on the next round.

Organizing the Instruction
Stress body control and form. Speed and power are not essential game skills in target tennis.
1. Grip: The player should use a firm grip on the racquet handle. A loose grip will cause the rac-

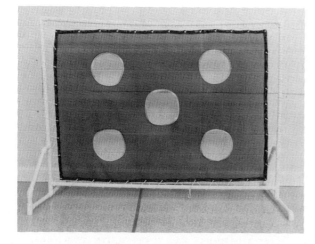

Fig. 9–3.   Target screen.

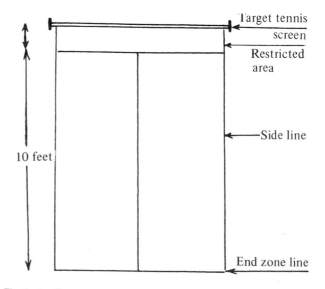

Fig. 9–4.   Target tennis court.

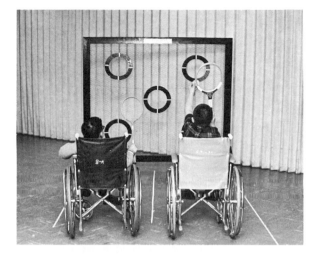

Fig. 9–5. Overhead serve.

quet head to tilt when hitting the ball. If the ball is constantly hit to the left or right of the intended flight, the problem is usually a loose grip.

2. Positioning of feet (ambulatory players): Standing tolerance must be thoroughly evaluated. The stance that is used will depend upon the involvement in the lower limbs. Usually, for the right handed player, both feet are pointed toward the screen, with the left foot slightly forward.

3. Forehand stroke: This is the fundamental stroke in target tennis. The ball should be stroked at about eye level with the wrist held firm as the ball makes contact with the racquet. Body weight is shifted to the front foot as the racquet hits the ball. The instructor should understand that shifting of body weight is not essential when completing the forehand stroke motion. This is particularly true for ambulatory players with involvement in their lower extremities.

Assistive Devices

Underhand Control Racquet. The severely handicapped individual with weak upper-extremities can play the game with the aid of an adapted racquet (Fig. 9–6). The racquet was originally designed for players with muscular dystrophy; however, other patients handicapped by weakness in their arms and shoulder girdle can use the device.

The adaptations can be made to a regular aluminum badminton racquet. The palmar support section, located next to the racquet face, includes a swivel and an adjustment to allow for different hand sizes. The forearm control cuff is located next to the handle. The cuffs can be made from $1/16$-inch stainless steel with Velcro straps.

Use of Racquet

1. The racquet is firmly strapped around the player's serving arm.
2. The player is moved to a position near the target screen. In some instances, the player will have

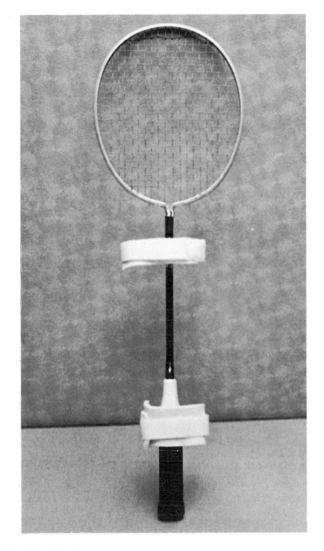

Fig. 9–6. Underhand control racquet.

enough strength to play from behind the end zone line. The therapist should determine the best playing position.

3. The player leans over the side of the wheelchair in position to serve the ball. Ambulatory players stand.

4. The referee (kneeling or standing) bounces the ball once close to the face of the racquet, and the player uses a pendulum motion to hit the ball toward the target screen.

Scoring. The player using the underhand control racquet can score a point by hitting the ball through a hole, either on the bounce or in the air.

Ball Suspension Table Tennis

This game is designed for players who have severe mobility and balance problems, such as players that need a motorized chair. One physical requirement is that the server must have some active arm extension with accompanying shoulder rotation to play successfully. The game is also designed to allow play with an able-bodied opponent. *The disabled player does all the serving.* This occurs after each "dead ball" situation thereby eliminating rallies between opponents.

Play

A suspended ball is hung above head level by cord or yarn with a loop at the end for ball placement. The wheelchair player is positioned slightly off center of the suspended ball so the serving hand is in line with the ball. With the paddle above shoulder level, the ball is struck by a forehand motion, releasing it from the suspended line (Fig. 9–7). The ball is hit so it bounces over the net as in regular table tennis and returned by the opponent. (The net can be lowered depending upon the serving ability to the disabled player.) Points are awarded as follows:

1. If the disabled server fails to strike the ball so it bounces over the net, then the receiver scores the point. No infraction is called if on the striking motion the ball is missed or fails to release from the loop on contact.

2. If the receiver fails to return the ball over the net, then the server scores a point. Another alternative is to award 2 points depending upon player skill levels, etc.

Play stops (dead ball) and the ball returned to the suspended loop after every serve and return action. The first player to score 15 points wins the game.

Miniature T-Tether Ball

A moderately active tabletop game for 2 to 4 players.

Equipment

1. Paddles: Regular Table Tennis paddles are used.
2. Miniature T-tether ball table (Fig. 9–8). The pole, 30 inches in length, is made from a ⅜-inch dowel. The base of the pole is whittled so that it will fit snugly into a ½-inch hole bored through the center of a 2-inch block. The ball is fastened by a length of strong cord to a small staple on screw eye in the top of the pole. The ball should hang 6 inches below the T-peg.

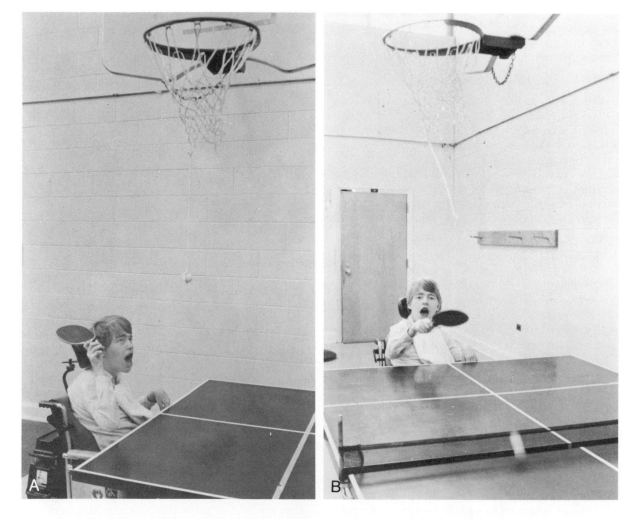

Fig. 9–7. *A.* Player in position to strike suspended ball. *B.* Contact-made, with successful serve over the net.

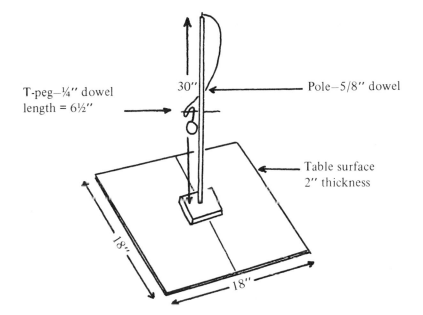

Fig. 9–8. Miniature T-tether ball table.

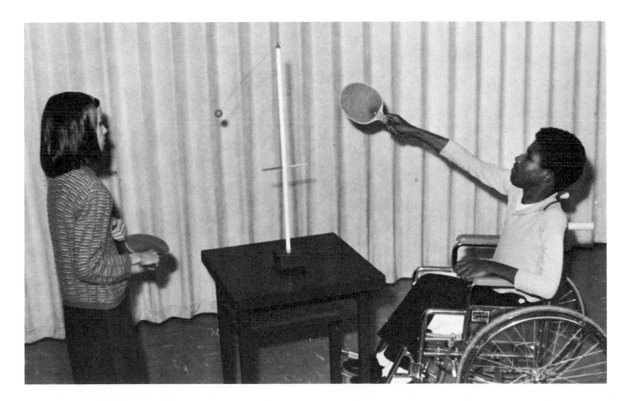

Fig. 9–9. T-tether ball match involving girl with anorexia nervosa and boy with progressive muscle disease.

The T-peg should fit into a hole drilled through the pole 17 inches from the top of the pole. One side of the peg should be painted red and the other side yellow.

The rubber ball which is attached to the cord should be approximately the size of a golf ball.

Play

Each player must face his opponent (Fig. 9–9). The ends of the T-peg must point toward the players. The server starts the game by tossing the ball in the air and striking it in any direction around the pole. His opponent then attempts to return the ball. The players alternate hitting the ball in an attempt to wind the string and ball around the T-peg on the opponent's side of the table. A hit is legal if the paddle hits either the ball or the string.

Rules

Singles (2 Players)
1. Players alternate hits.
2. A ball that had stopped swinging is a "dead" ball. Play is resumed with a serve by the player who is next in turn to hit the ball.
3. Each player must keep his paddle on his side of the court. It is illegal to cross the center line to hit the ball.

Doubles (4 Players)
1. Teammates are stationed on the same side of the table.
2. Rules for singles play also apply to doubles play.

Scoring
1. The first player to win 5 points, or the first team to win 10, wins the game.
2. If a player hits the ball or string twice in succession, then his opponent scores a point. Players must alternate hits.
3. If a player hits any part of the tether ball pole, including the T-peg, with his paddle, then his opponent scores a point.
4. A point is scored if a player hits the ball so that the string wraps around the T-peg on his opponent's side of the table (Fig. 9–10).

Special Rule: A point cannot be scored on a direct serve. The ball must be returned by the opponent to the server before point action can start.

Organizing the Instruction

Development of hand-eye coordination is the primary game value. Proper timing is required to hit the moving ball at the T-peg; this basic game skill can be learned through practice. The ball will not move on a fixed pathway; however, the player can learn to shift the blade of the paddle to control the movement of the ball toward the T-peg.

Development. Hand-eye coordination, directionality, ocular pursuit, upper-extremity strength and body awareness are developed by this game.

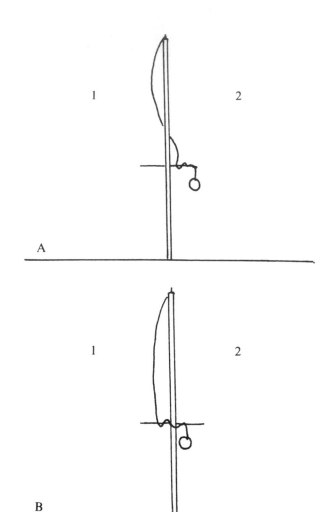

Fig. 9–10. Scoring in T-tether ball. *A*, Point for Player 1. Ball rests on T-peg of Player 2. *B*, Point for Player 1. No change in scoring if cord is partially wrapped on opposite side. The position of the ball itself determines the score.

GAMES WITH LIMITED EQUIPMENT

Hoop-Scotch

Equipment: 8 hoops.

Setup: Place hoops in hoop-scotch formation (Fig. 9–11).

Procedure 1: Child is asked to jump or hop forward in the hoops. Start with one foot in each of the double hoops, then hop on one foot to the single hoop, then one foot in each of the double hoops, and finish by hopping on one foot in the last two hoops.

Procedure 2: The child starts with single hoop and hops in the other direction.

Procedure 3: Same as #1, except the child jumps or hops backward.

Development. Hoop-scotch develops balance, agility, and coordination.

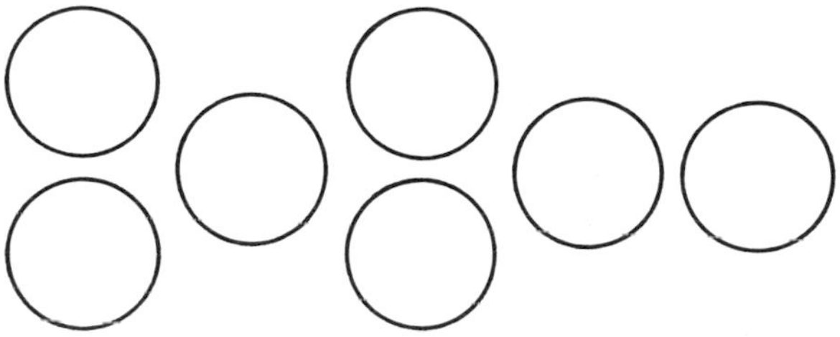

Fig. 9–11. Hoop-scotch formation.

Hoop-Around

Equipment: 10 or 26 hoops, construction paper, marking pen, masking tape, flash cards, or spelling list.

Setup: Print numbers 1 to 10 or letters A to Z on construction paper. Place hoops in 2 straight lines (Figs. 9–12 and 9–13). Tape a piece of the construction paper to the floor inside of each hoop.

Procedure 1: The instructor holds up flash cards for mathematics, and the child hops or jumps to the center of the appropriate hoop. This game can be used for addition, subtraction, division, and multiplication.

Procedure 2: The instructor reads out a word, and the child hops to the proper blocks in sequence to spell out the word.

Development. Hoop-around develops balance, agility, and coordination, in addition to academic skills.

Obstacle Course

Equipment: Tables, chairs, desks, mats, balance beam, or other large objects.

Setup: Place objects about room or outside.

Procedure: The child, in following a course laid out and demonstrated, climbs over, crawls under, jumps, and hops about the various obstacles placed about the room or play area.

Development. This game develops balance, agility, coordination, directionality, and body awareness.

Follow the Pattern

Equipment: Chairs, striped cones or playground markers, Indian clubs, colorful small objects, and masking tape.

Setup: Start game with chairs or other markers spaced about 3 feet apart (Fig. 9–14). Different patterns can be made by changing the arrangement of the equipment.

Procedure 1: Child moves in and around chairs first forward and then backward.

Procedure 2: Progress to smaller objects as child is able to move about large objects in different patterns.

Development. This game develops directionality, laterality, agility, balance, and coordination.

Follow the Ball

Equipment: String or light rope, various sizes of "whiffle balls" or balls made of plastic or soft rubber, 2 standards or poles, paddle.

Setup: Tie string or light rope between 2 poles, trees, or standards. Tie another piece of string to a large ball, and attach it to the string between the poles.

Procedure 1: Swing the ball in various directions. The child must keep his head still and just follow the movement with his eyes.

Procedure 2: Swing ball, and have the child try to hit it with a wooden paddle.

Development. This game develops hand-eye coordination and ocular pursuit.

Body Parts

Equipment: Mats or small throw rugs, phonograph records (if desired).

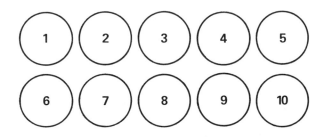

Fig. 9–12. Hoop-around formation for arithmetic game.

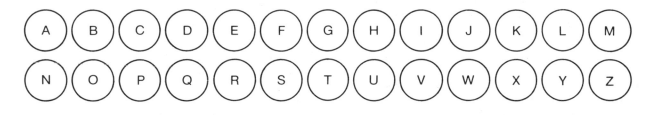

Fig. 9–13. Hoop-around formation for spelling game.

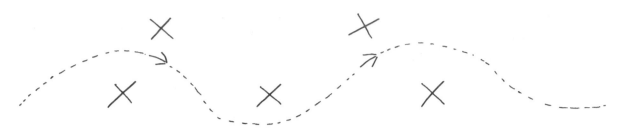

Fig. 9–14.   Follow the pattern. The child moves around the objects (X-marks) as indicated by the dotted line.

Setup: Children lie on mats or rugs or stand. Music is played quietly in the background, or a record about the identification of body parts is played. A record is not needed, as the instructor can call out the names of various parts.

Procedure 1: Instructor asks the children to touch all the major body parts: nose, head, knee, and so forth.

Procedure 2: If the child has no difficulty in identifying the body parts, the instructor asks him to touch his nose with the left hand, to touch the right knee with the left hand, and so forth.

Development. This game develops body awareness, laterality, and directionality.

Yarn Ball Games

Equipment: A yarn ball is made of wool yarn of various colors wound together. It is soft and will not injure students if they are hit directly. They can be purchased commercially and are especially good for play in limited spaces and with fearful children.

Setup: The yarn ball can be used for most ball games, such as relays, volleyball activities, catching and throwing, tossing into boxes or bags, bowling activities, dodgeball, and hit the opponent.

Procedures: Follow the basic rules of the game chosen. The instructor can modify any number of games for use with the yarn ball.

Development. Yarn ball games develop coordination, agility, balance, flexibility, body awareness, directionality, and laterality.

Bean Bags

Equipment: Bean bags can be made from any material and filled with small stones or beans. Boxes, empty coffee cans, or similar objects can be used for targets.

Setup: For games of toss, place boxes ranging from large to small at various distances from a throwing line. A variety of cans may also be used.

Procedure: Toss the bean bags at targets or objects. The distance from objects and targets depends on the age and throwing ability of the individuals and the size of the room. Points can be awarded for each hit or for each bag going into the target.

Development. Bean bag games develop coordination, agility, and hand-eye coordination.

Ropes

Equipment: Ropes of various lengths.

Procedure 1: Balance-walk along rope laid on floor.

Procedure 2: Stand facing rope on floor; jump over and jump back.

Procedure 3: Stand facing 2 to 5 ropes on the floor; jump forward into the spaces between them; then jump backward.

Procedure 4: Jump over ropes held at various heights.

Procedure 5: The instructor swings a rope with a weight on its end in a circle close to the ground; students jump over as rope passes.

Procedure 6: The child holds rope in his hands. He walks as rope is brought over head.

Procedure 7: The child holds rope in his hands. He skips as rope is brought over head.

Procedure 8: The child holds rope in his hands. He moves forward or backward as rope is brought over head.

Development. Rope games develop agility, coordination, balance, strength, and body awareness.

GAMES WITH NO EQUIPMENT

I Say Stoop

Basic Skill: Bending.

Space: Classroom or playground.

Description: Leader stands in front of the group and gives commands. When he commands, "I say stoop," all players stoop; when he commands, "I say stand," all stand. Players should not follow instructions unless the leader says, "I say." Anyone making a mistake is eliminated.

Animal Trap

Basic Skill: Running.

Space: Playground.

Description: Half of the pupils join hands and form a circle, and the other half stay outside the circle. The players outside decide what animal they want to pretend to be. At the teacher's signal, the "animals" run in and out of the "trap." When the teacher claps his hands, the trap is closed. All animals caught inside the trap join the circle. After all the animals have been caught, the players change positions and start a new game.

I'm Tall, I'm Small

Basic Skill: Walking.

Space: Playground or multipurpose room.

Description: One child stands in the center of a circle with his eyes closed. Other players walk slowly around in a circle and sing:

I'm tall, I'm very small.
I'm small, I'm very tall.
Sometimes I'm tall.
Sometimes I'm small.
Guess what I am now.

As the children walk and sing, they stretch or stoop according to the words. When the singing is over, the teacher signals the players to assume a stooping or stretching position. The child in the center tries to guess which position they have taken. If he guesses correctly, he stays in the circle; if incorrectly, a new player is chosen to stand in the circle.

Hopping Relay

Basic Skills: Hopping, skipping.

Space: Playground.

Description: The players line up in single file in 2 lines. On signal, the first in each line hops on one foot to the turning line and returns hopping on the other foot. The turning point should be approximately 30 feet away. The team whose last player finishes first is the winner.

Variation 1: Same as above, except the players skip.

Variation 2: Same as above, except the players skip rope.

Crows and Cranes

Basic Skills: Listening, running.

Space: Playground or gymnasium (2 goals, 50 feet apart).

Description: Children are divided into 2 groups, the "crows" and the "cranes." The groups line up and face each other in the center of the playing area about 5 feet apart. The leader calls out either "crows" or "cranes" using a prolonged "K-r-r-r-r" sound at the start of either word to mask the one he will call. If "crows" is the call, the "crows" chase the "cranes" to the goal. If "cranes" is the call, the "cranes" chase the "crows." Any child caught before he reaches his goal goes over to the other side. The team having the most players when the game ends is the winner.

Beefsteak

Basic Skills: Listening, running.

Space: Playground or gymnasium.

Description: The players stand in a single line along the starting line; one child is chosen to be "it" and stands on the finish line, which is 20 to 25 feet away from the starting line, with his back to the others. "It" counts aloud to 10 and then calls "Beefsteak," and turns around to face the other players. As "it" is counting, the others are running forward trying to cross the finish line. Any player caught stepping or running after "Beefsteak" is called is sent back to the starting line. The first player over the finish line becomes "it."

Chain Tag

Basic Skills: Running, evading.

Space: Playground or gymnasium.

Description: Players are scattered over the playing area. One player who is "it" attempts to tag another. Any player tagged must join hands with "it," and the two attempt to tag someone else. As players are tagged, they join hands with the player who tagged him. Only players on the end of the line may tag others. No player may be tagged while the line is broken. Players may not break through the line but are allowed to go under it. Last player tagged is the winner.

Partner Tag

Basic skill: Running.

Space: Outdoors or gymnasium.

Description: One child is chosen to be "it" and another to be the "chaser." Other children select partners and link elbows. The "chaser" tries to tag "it" who may run anywhere in the play area. Whenever "it" links elbows with a player, he is safe. The partner at the opposite side where "it" linked on becomes the new "it." If the "chaser" tags "it" they change positions, and the game continues.

Caterpillar Race

Basic Skills: Coordination, bending.

Space: Any smooth area.

Description: Two teams line up single file behind a common starting line. Each child bends forward and grasps the ankles of the child in front of him. At a starting signal, the teams move forward as best they can, continuing to hold ankles. The first child may use his hands in any manner to help his team. The first team to have all its members cross the distance line, which is 60 feet away, wins. If the line breaks, it must join again before it proceeds.

BEAN BAG ACTIVITIES

Bean bags are good implements for mentally retarded children because they stop where they land after being thrown, they do not bounce away like balls, and they tend to wrap themselves around the hand when being caught. Retarded children are more successful in catching them than balls because they do not need to be quite as accurate in the skill. Bean bags also lend themselves to creative activity, and the children can make up their own games.

Suggested Activities

The following suggestions for activities with bean bags are not to be regarded as comprehensive, and the ingenious instructor will adapt, modify, and invent other activities.

1. Freely throwing the bean bag in the air and catching it with both hands.
2. Freely throwing the bean bag in the air and catching it with one hand.
3. Freely throwing the bean bag from one hand to the other overhead.
4. Freely throwing the bean bag into the air and jumping to catch it with 2 hands; with one hand.
5. Throwing the bean bag into the air and clapping the hands (turning about, touching the ground, and so forth) before catching it.
6. Walking freely about the area and throwing the bean bag in the air and catching it with both hands; with either hand.
7. Running freely around the area and throwing the bean bag in the air and catching it with both hands; with either hand.
8. Throwing the bean bag from behind the back and over the shoulder and catching it in front of the body (either side).
9. Throwing the bean bag from behind the body and under the opposite arm and catching it in front of the body (either side).
10. Standing with the bean bag at arm's length in front of the body; dropping it and trying to catch it with the same hand before it hits the ground (either hand).
11. Standing and throwing the bean bag for distance. No specific method of throwing.
12. Throwing the bean bag for distance with an underarm throw; an overarm throw.
13. Free walking with the bean bag balanced on the head.
14. Balance walking on beams, logs, or along a paint line with the bean bag on the head.
15. Balance walking along a beam, tossing the bean bag in the air and catching it.
16. Balance walking along a beam bending down and passing the bean bag under the beam.
17. Standing with the bean bag balanced on one foot and kicking the bean bag for distance; for accuracy.
18. Standing with the bean bag balanced on one foot, hopping about trying to keep the bean bag on the foot.
19. With bean bag gripped between the heels, jumping up and kicking the bean bag up behind to be caught in the hands.
20. Standing astride the bean bag on the floor and jumping to click the heels above the bean bag.
21. Lying on the floor on the back, picking up the bean bag between the feet and raising overhead to place it on the floor above the head (vice versa).
22. Throwing and catching bean bag with a partner.
23. Exchange catching with a partner (both players have a bean bag).
24. Throwing through a hoop held by partner.
25. Juggling with 2 bean bags.

PARACHUTE ACTIVITIES

The possibilities of physical education activities using parachutes are numerous. Not only do they provide an excellent opportunity for strengthening arm and shoulder girdle muscles but they are also lots of fun for the child.

Area: Playground or gymnasium.

Players: The number is limited only by the size of the chute to the number that can group around its perimeter.

Equipment: Parachute.

Formation: Circle.

Age Group: Any age group.

Starting Position: All activities begin with the parachute deflated and flat on the floor. Students form a circle around the outside of the parachute and grasp the edge with both hands.

Suggested Activities

1. Inflate parachute by raising arms over head and then pulling the chute down; repeat.
2. Inflate parachute; students holding on to edge walk under and back before parachute comes down; repeat.
3. Merry-Go-Round: Inflate chute; hold with right hand and raise left hand; walk 8 steps with right hand raised. Hold with left hand; go in opposite direction.
4. Outside Mushroom: Raise chute and sit down outside parachute; keep hold with both hands. Deflate; repeat.
5. Inside Mushroom: Inflate chute and pull chute with both hands over head and down behind the back; sit down inside chute. Deflate; repeat.
6. Partners Change: Give every student a number. Children inflate chute; instructor calls number, and students with numbers called exchange places, running under raised parachute. Deflate; repeat, calling different numbers.
7. Ball Control: Place a rubber ball or volleyball in center of deflated parachute. Divide students into 4 teams grouped around chute. Inflate chute; when pulling chute down, each team tries to get the ball to roll down to their team. Repeat entire action.
8. Ball Flip: Divide group into 2 teams by counting off 1, 2, 1, 2 for middle and upper elementary grades and by assigning names of animals, such as bears and tigers, or cartoon characters for primary grades. Team members alternate positions around the parachute. Place 2 balls (volleyball and soccer ball) in the chute, which is held in a stretched position. Each team is given 10 points at the start of the game. At a signal, teams attempt to flip the other team's ball out of the

chute by vigorously moving their arms up and down. Points are lost every time a team's ball is flipped out. The team first to lose all its points loses the game. As soon as a ball is flipped out, the instructor throws it back in the chute.

9. Group Exercises: The parachute can be used to facilitate physical fitness by including its use in group exercises. An example would be to have all the students raise the parachute up and quickly return it to the floor, then have all the students (still holding the parachute) do push-ups until the parachute is laying on the ground. Another example would be to do group sit-ups, while sitting and holding the parachute (underhand grip), all pupils do sit-ups simultaneously. Yet another exercise would be to get all the students to pull the parachute towards their chin or knees etc. to build strength through isometric type exercises. This creates a motivating environment to exercise.

ADDITIONAL GAMES

Balloon Battle

Equipment: 2 or 3 balloons.

Setup: Players are divided into 2 teams. Each team forms 2 ranks, facing the opposite team. The players line up, one behind the other, with about 2 feet of space between the ranks and the teams. The players may stand or sit.

Procedure: The leader tosses up 2 or 3 balloons between the teams. The players bat the balloons, trying to make them go over the heads of the opposing team. One point is scored for the team batting the balloon over the opposing team. If a balloon goes out at either end, it does not score but is tossed in again by the leader, and the game continues.

Animal Blindman's Bluff

Equipment: Blindfold and broomstick.

Setup: The players form a circle. One player is blindfolded and takes his position in the center of the circle.

Procedure: The players in the circle grasp hands and move around the blindfolded player until he taps the floor with the broomstick. The "blind man" then points the broomstick at some player and commands him to make a noise like a cat, dog, duck, or other animal. From this, the blind man tried to guess the name of the player. If he succeeds, they exchange places. If he fails, the game is repeated with the same blind man.

Hot Potato

Equipment: A bean bag or a balloon. The balloon travels more slowly and gives the one who is "it" more time to accomplish his objective.

Setup: The players form a circle with one person who is "it" in the center.

Procedure: The players in the circle throw the balloon to one another, trying not to hold it long enough to be tagged by the player in the middle. The player who is caught with the balloon takes the place in the center of the circle and becomes "it."

Take Away

Equipment: 10 to 20 small and interesting objects, a table, and chairs.

Setup: The objects are placed on the table, around which the players sit.

Procedure: The players study the objects. Then one player leaves the room while another is chosen to take an object from the table and hold it out of sight. The first player returns and guesses what is missing.

Cat and Rat

Equipment: 2 bean bags or balls.

Setup: Players form a tight circle.

Procedure: One bag or ball is designated the "cat," and the other the "rat." The "cat" is given to a player in one part of the circle and the "rat" to a player in another section. At the signal "go" the bags are passed to the right, with the "cat" trying to overtake the "rat." The person who is caught with both bags at the same time becomes the "cheese" and leaves the circle. The game is continued.

The game may be varied by having the leader give the command to "change" and the bags then move in the opposite direction. The changes may come close together or far apart.

Wonder Ball

Equipment: Rubber ball.

Setup: The group forms a circle.

Procedure: The players sing as the ball is passed around the circle:

"The wonder ball goes round and round.
To pass it quickly you are bound.
If you're the one to hold it last,
Why then for you the game is past,
and you are O-U-T."

The player holding the ball as O-U-T is being sung has a point scored against him.

Balloon Keep Up

Equipment: Inflated balloons.

Setup: The players form a circle.

Procedure: Players tap the balloon lightly, trying to keep it within the circle. A point is scored by the person last touching the balloon if it either hits the floor or goes out of the circle. The player with the lowest number of points wins. Two balloons in the circle make an interesting addition.

Balloon Volleyball

Equipment: 2 balloons and a net about 6 feet high, or lower, stretched across the playing area.

Setup: The players are divided into 2 equal teams, each confined to one half of the playing area.

Procedure: One balloon is given to each team, and on the signal from the leader, it is butted across the net. The object of the game is to make the balloon touch the floor on the opposite side. The game is continuous. There are only 2 rules: (1) the balloon must be butted, not thrown, and (2) it must go over the net in order to score. Each time the balloon touches the floor one point is scored.

Saucer Toss (Fig. 9–15)

Purpose. Helps improve or maintain range of motion and strength.

Appropriate For. Those with full or limited range of motion and good or fair strength.
Both sexes.
All grade levels.
Sitting or standing position.

Activity

1. Draw 5 lines on the ground, making them 12 feet long and 3 feet apart. (Use rope if playing on the grass.)
2. Label the lines 1, 3, 5, 7, 9.
3. Label the spaces between the lines 2, 4, 6, 8, 10.
4. Draw a starting line.

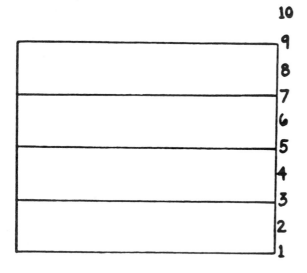

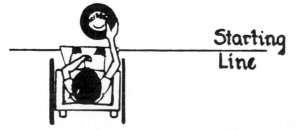

Fig. 9–15. Saucer Toss. (Courtesy Muscular Dystrophy Association.)

5. Position player in front of starting line.
6. Player throws saucer and receives score indicated by the number on line or area where saucer lands.
7. Players are given alternate turns.
8. Each player receives 3 throws.
9. Winner is player who scores the most points.

Time. About 30 minutes.

Variation. Vary the distance between the starting line and line 1, depending on the ability of the players.

Equipment. Saucers (pie tins, frisbees, etc.), chalk or rope.

Arm Ball (Fig. 9–16)

Purpose. Helps improve or maintain range of motion.

Appropriate For. Those with full or limited range of motion and good or fair strength.
Both sexes.
Individual (two or more).
Sitting and standing position, or lying on chest.
All grade levels.

Activity

1. Construct a wooden box 2 ft. by 8 ft. Divide it in the middle with a "bridge" that has an opening in the center. Place a tone bell in the middle of each side. (See diagram.)
2. Position the two players (A & B) next to the box, one at each side.
3. Each player attempts to roll a ping pong ball through the opening in the bridge and ring the tone bell on the other side.
4. Each player begins with 6 ping pong balls.
5. A player scores one point each time he makes a "ring."
6. When game ends, player with the most points is the winner.

Variation. Score ½ point for getting ball through opening, and 2 points for "ring."

Time. About 20–30 minutes.

Equipment: Wooden box, bridge, 2 tone bells, 12 ping pong balls.

Ramp Ball (Fig. 9–17)

Purpose. Helps improve or maintain range of motion and strength.

Appropriate For. Those with full or limited range of motion and poor as well as better strength.
Both sexes.
All grade levels.
Sitting or standing position.

Activity

1. Place "Porta-Pit" ramp in center of room.
2. Place an extension ladder at start of ramp incline (see diagram).

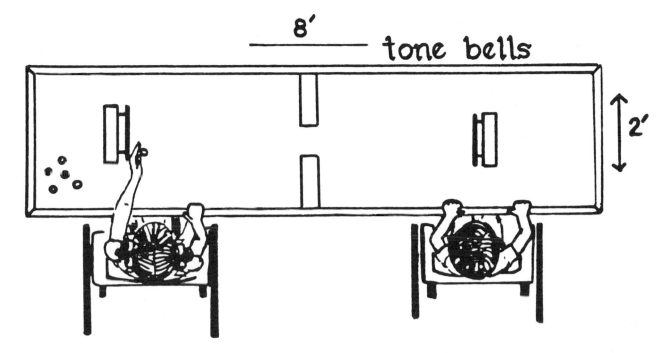

Fig. 9–16. Arm Ball. (Courtesy Muscular Dystrophy Association.)

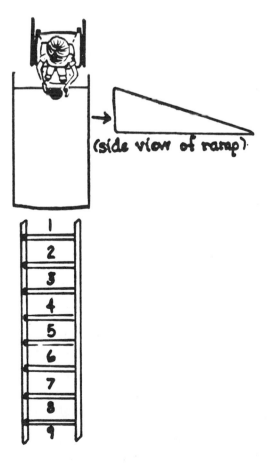

Fig. 9–17. Ramp Ball. (Courtesy Muscular Dystrophy Association.)

Table 9–3. Classification

Class I-A	For quadriplegics, who are so severely disabled that a push is required for mobility.
Class I-B	For quadriplegics, who are so severely disabled that an electric wheelchair is necessary for mobility.
Class II	For quadriplegics, who are severely limited in their upper extremities and push with their feet.
Class III	For quadriplegics, who are able to manipulate a wheelchair with their arms, but limited in their effectiveness and control because of spasticity and functioning levels.
Class IV	For individuals using a wheelchair, who have good control of their upper body.
Class V	For individuals who are severely limited in mobility on their feet, and who use assistance devices.
Class VI	For individuals who are involved to such a degree that they are unable to run or jump freely, but still have good mobility.
Class VII	For individuals who are hemiplegic or only have one limb involved, who are very mildly involved, so as to be able to throw, run or jump with little difficulty.
Class VIII-A	Individuals with no vision or those who have so little vision that it would not be an advantage over someone with no vision at all.
Class VIII-B	Individuals with partial vision; enough so as to be an advantage over totally blind participants.

In classifying people, some participants may fit into one class for most events, but in a different class for some events. This is permissible so long as it is indicated ahead of time on the Entry Form.

3. Number the spaces between the rungs of the ladder (see diagram).
4. Position player at starting line.
5. Player rolls or throws ball down ramp trying to get it to land in a space between rungs of the ladder.
6. Each player receives 3 turns.
7. His total score is the sum of the points indicated by the numbered space in which the ball lands. The ball has to remain in a space to be counted.

Time. About 20 minutes.

Variation. Vary the type and size of ball. Vary the number of turns. Vary the distance between the ladder and rungs. Divide players into teams.

Equipment. Porta-Pit ramp, extension ladder, tennis ball.

COMPETITIVE GAMES

Competitive game situations for the physically disabled can take the form of an Olympic-style format. Classification levels (Table 9–3) can focus on functional ability levels similar to other national sport associations. However, the events are less traditional than those designed for other competitive arenas (NWAA, USCPAA), but yet provide the participant an opportunity to be challenged regardless of his limitations.

Listed below is a sample of the organization structure of the Oregon Games for the Physically Limited

which emphasizes the uniqueness of the competition and event designs.

Manual Wheelchair Obstacle Course Demo (Code: WOCD)

Competition/Demonstration Event

Classes. IV (people who use manual *w/c* and have very good upper body strength)

Description. (See diagram), athletes go from the start line, 10 feet to seven traffic cones spaced 32″ apart. After slaloming the cones, go 5 feet, cross line, turn left and go around the left side of a hula hoop. Go clock-wise, 270 degrees around the hula hoop, 15 feet to a wheelchair ramp, over the ramp, five feet to a 4-foot-square, 4-inch-high platform. Move the wheelchair straight up onto the platform. Pivot-turn, left, 90 degrees (in place) and *back* off the platform. Continue backing until in line with the last leg of the course. Back-turn so as to line up with that last leg and go forward 8 feet to another wheelchair ramp. Go over the ramp and go 5 feet to a 5′ × 10′ obstacle frame made up of 2″ × 4″ lumber. After crossing the frame on the 10′ axis, go 7 feet to the finish. Fastest time wins.

Equipment: Seven traffic cones, one hula hoop, two wheelchair ramps, one 4′ square and 4″ high platform, one 5′ × 10′ obstacle frame, one stopwatch. *Note: make sure the ramps are wide enough to accommodate a standard wheelchair wheel-span. Spotters should be ready to prevent wheelchairs from tipping as athletes negotiate the course—*

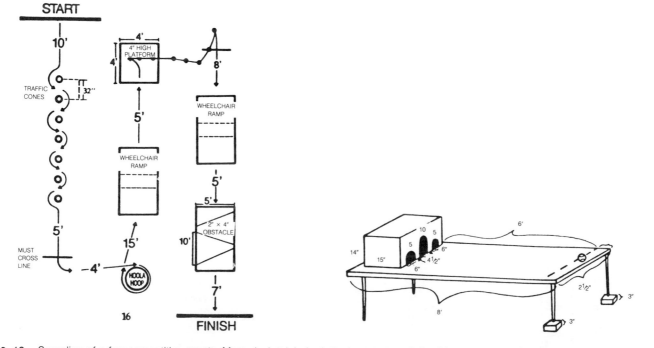

Fig. 9–18. Sampling of a few competitive events. Manual wheelchair obstacle course and tilt table target ball. (Courtesy of Oregon Games for the Physically Limited, Inc. This non-profit corporation is responsible for coordinating local, regional, and statewide recreation and sports programs in the state of Oregon. For further information, write P.O. Box 665, Salem, OR 97308.)

especially at the obstacle frame where a forward tip could occur.

Tilt-Table Target Ball (Code: TTTB)

Classes: Open to all classes

Description. Five tennis balls are released, one at a time, from behind the foul-line, toward the target box which has three holes (see diagram). Scoring: Center hole = 10 pts. side hole = 5 pt. each, miss box = 0 pt. One point will be awarded for each ball that comes to rest against the box and does not enter a scoring hole.

Equipment. An 8' × 2½" folding table is raised 3 inches (double 2 × 4" blocks under legs) at the foul line end, one 14 × 15 × 21" plywood box—with scoring numbers, five tennis balls.

Wheelchair Rope Pull (Code: WCRP)

Classes: III, IV, VIII-A, VIII-B

Description. Each end of the rope is secured so the rope is tight and 30" high. The course is 20' long. The participant uses hands only and pulls self along while in the chair. This is a timed event. Fastest time wins. The longest distance after 90 seconds will determine the winner.

Equipment. One 30' × ½" rope, knotted every 8", 2 securing posts, one stopwatch.

BIBLIOGRAPHY

Clifton, M.: A developmental approach to perceptual motor experiences. JOHPER, *41*:34, 1970.

Cratty, B.J.: *Developmental Sequences of Perceptual Motor Tasks.* Freeport, LI, NY, Educational Activities, 1967.

Cratty, B. and Breen, J.: *Educational Games for Physically Handicapped Children,* Denver, Lowe Pub. Co., 1973.

Herkowitz, J.: A perceptual motor training program to improve the gross motor abilities of preschoolers. JOHPER, *41*:38, 1970.

Kephart, N.C.: *The Slow Learner in the Classroom.* Columbus, Ohio, Charles E. Merrill, 1960.

Muscular Dystrophy Association, This is Patient Service, New York, NY 10019, Spring, 1979.

New York State Division for Youth, Initiatives and Games for Recreation, Leisure, and Therapy, 1986.

Oregon Games for the Physically Limited, 1988 Rule Book, Salem, OR.

Radler, D.H., and Kephart, N.C.: *Success Through Play.* New York, Harper & Row, 1960.

Smith, H.M.: Implications for movement education experiences drawn from perceptual-motor research. JOHPER, *41*:30, 1970.

Appendix A

Therapeutic Exercises

Therapeutic exercises are divided into the following classifications:

1. Passive exercises: Exercises that cannot be accomplished by the patient but must be done entirely by the instructor or therapist.
2. Active assistive exercises: Exercises that are accomplished in part by the patient with the assistance of the instructor or therapist.
3. Active exercises: Exercises that are accomplished by the patient against gravity without assistance.
4. Resistive exercises: Exercises that are accomplished against gravity by the patient with some additional form of resistance such as weights, springs, or manual resistance.

The person under treatment may be able to accomplish resistive exercises for some parts of his body, but may need assistance in performing passive exercises for other parts. It is important to evaluate each patient and to plan a firm and sound exercise program based on his own needs and abilities.

It is important to keep accurate records on the status of the patient in a therapeutic exercise program. This information should include the amount and type of exercise, the number of repetitions, the times per day, the amount of resistance used (if any), and the condition of the patient after completing a specific routine.

The exercises on the following pages are active exercises, with the exception of certain resistive exercises. However, the exercises given here are not to be interpreted as the only ones to be used for a particular disability. All 4 classifications of exercises can be appropriate for use, depending on the condition of the patient and his medical treatment.

The therapist or instructor must remember to treat the whole individual and not just the joint or area involved. For example, if the patient has a condition affecting his knee, the hip and ankle on the involved side should also be treated, as well as the general condition of the entire body.

EXERCISES FOR THE UPPER BACK

1. a. Prone position
   b. Arms at sides
   c. Elbows straight
   d. Palms of hands upward
   e. Pull scapulae together
   f. Do not move shoulders
   g. Hold
   h. Return to starting position
2. a. Prone position
   b. Arms at sides
   c. Elbows straight
   d. Palms of hands upward
   e. Raise arms to 45 degree angle
   f. Do not move shoulders
   g. Hold
   h. Return to starting position
3. a. Prone position
   b. Place hands in the small of the back
   c. Palms of hands upward
   d. Raise elbows and shoulders
   e. Do not move head
   f. Hold
   g. Return to starting position
4. a. Prone position
   b. Arms at sides
   c. Elbows straight
   d. Raise head, shoulders, and chest
   e. Hold
   f. Return to starting position
5. a. Prone position
   b. Arms at shoulder level, at a right angle to the body
   c. Elbows straight
   d. Palms of hands facing downward
   e. Raise arms
   f. Hold
   g. Return to starting position
6. a. Prone position
   b. Arms at 45 degree angle to body
   c. Elbows straight
   d. Palms of hands facing downward
   e. Raise arms
   f. Hold
   g. Return to starting position
7. a. Prone position
   b. Forehead resting on table, mat, or support

   c. Arms extended overhead
   d. Elbows straight
   e. Palms of hands facing downward
   f. Raise arms
   g. Hold
   h. Return to starting position

8. a. Sit on stool
   b. Back flat against a wall
   c. Arms at shoulder level (abducted)
   d. Elbows flexed to 90 degrees
   e. Backs of hands against wall
   f. Slowly raise arms upward and outward
   g. Keep backs of hands against wall
   h. Stretch to maximum
   i. Hold
   j. Return to starting position

*9. a. Stand facing wall pulleys; grasp handles
   b. Arms at shoulder level (abducted)
   c. Elbows flexed to 90 degrees
   d. Palms of hands facing downward
   e. Pull elbows backward, moving weights
   f. Keep arms and elbows flexed
   g. Hold
   h. Return to starting position

*10. a. Stand facing wall pulleys; grasp handles
   b. Arms at shoulder level (abducted)
   c. Elbows straight, palms of hands facing downward
   d. Pull arms backward, moving weights
   e. Arms remain at shoulder level
   f. Hold
   g. Return to starting position

*11. a. Stand facing wall pulleys; grasp handles
   b. Arms straight overhead
   c. Elbows straight
   d. Raise arms upward and backward, moving weights
   e. Keep chest up
   f. Hold
   g. Return to starting position

12. a. Sit on stool
   b. Back flat against wall
   c. Arms at shoulder level
   d. Elbows straight, back of hands against wall
   e. Keep hands against wall
   f. Move arms upward overhead and touch hands
   g. Hold
   h. Return to starting position

*13. a. Stand facing wall pulleys; grasp handles
   b. Arms at shoulder level
   c. Elbows straight, palms of hands facing downward
   d. Pull arms downward to sides and then backward, moving weights
   e. Keep chest up
   f. Hold

*Weights can be used.

   g. Return to starting position

14. a. Sit on stool
   b. Place fingers against back of neck
   c. Elbows forward, level with shoulders
   d. Head up
   e. Pull elbows backward
   f. Hold
   g. Return to starting position

15. a. Sit on stool
   b. Place fingers against back of neck
   c. Elbows forward, level with shoulders
   d. Head up
   e. Therapist places foot on stool behind patient
   f. Therapist grasps elbows and pulls gently backward
   g. Hold
   h. Return to starting position

16. a. Sit on stool
   b. Arms extended overhead
   c. Head up
   d. Pull arms upward and backward
   e. Hold
   f. Return to starting position

17. a. Sit on stool
   b. Arms extended overhead
   c. Head up
   d. Therapist places foot on stool behind patient
   e. Therapist grasps elbows and pulls gently backward
   f. Hold
   g. Return to starting position

EXERCISES FOR THE LOWER BACK

18. a. Supine position
   b. Knees flexed, feet flat on floor
   c. Roll pelvis backward
   d. Try to force lower back flat against floor
   e. Contract abdominal muscles
   f. Hold
   g. Return to starting position

19. a. Supine position
   b. Knees bent, feet flat on floor
   c. Roll pelvis backward
   d. Try to force lower back flat against floor
   e. Contract abdominal muscles
   f. Lift head and shoulders upward, touch knees with fingertips
   g. Hold
   h. Return to starting position

20. a. Supine position
   b. Knees bent, feet flat on floor
   c. Roll pelvis backward
   d. Try to force lower back against floor
   e. Contract abdominal muscles
   f. Slide one leg down until it is out straight on floor
   g. Lift leg, keeping it straight, upward to 90 degrees if possible

   h. Bend knee toward 90 degrees, straighten knee, and lower leg back to floor
   i. Slide leg upward until knee is bent and foot flat on floor
   j. Repeat exercise on opposite leg
   k. Remember to keep pelvis tilted backward

21. a. Supine position
   b. Legs out straight
   c. Bend one knee to 90 degrees
   d. Grasp with hands, pull knee to chest
   e. Hold
   f. Return to starting position
   g. Repeat on other leg

22. a. Supine position
   b. Legs out straight
   c. Bend both knees to 90 degrees
   d. Grasp with hands; pull knees to chest
   e. Hold
   f. Return to starting position

23. a. Stand with back against wall
   b. Heels 4 inches from wall
   c. Head, shoulders, and hips are against wall
   d. Roll pelvis upward, pull in abdomen
   e. Try to force lower back against the wall
   f. Hold
   g. Return to starting position

24. a. Repeat first 5 steps of above exercise
   b. Raise heels, bend knees, slowly squat as far as possible
   c. Hold
   d. Slowly rise from squat, keeping back flat against wall
   e. Return to starting position

25. a. Sit on stool with back against wall
   b. Slowly bend forward at the hips
   c. Bend forward as far as possible
   d. Hold
   e. Slowly straighten up until lower back, shoulders, and head touch wall
   f. Relax
   g. Return to starting position

26. a. Prone position
   b. Arms at sides
   c. Knees straight
   d. Raise one leg slowly as far as possible
   e. Hold
   f. Lower slowly
   g. Repeat with other leg
   h. Return to starting position

27. a. Prone position
   b. Arms at sides
   c. Knees straight
   d. Raise both legs together as far as possible
   e. Hold
   f. Lower slowly
   g. Return to starting position

28. a. Prone position
   b. Arms extended overhead
   c. Elbows straight
   d. Slowly lift one arm as high as possible
   e. Hold
   f. Lower slowly
   g. Repeat with other arm
   h. Return to starting position

29. a. Prone position
   b. Arms extended overhead
   c. Elbows straight
   d. Slowly lift both arms as high as possible
   e. Hold
   f. Lower slowly
   g. Return to starting position

30. a. Prone position
   b. Arms extended overhead
   c. Elbows straight
   d. Legs straight
   e. Slowly lift an arm and leg on the same side of the body as high as possible
   f. Hold
   g. Do not roll body away from side that is being exercised
   h. Lower slowly
   i. Return to starting position
   j. Repeat with other side

31. a. Prone position
   b. Arms extended overhead
   c. Elbows straight
   d. Legs straight
   e. Slowly lift right arm and left leg as high as possible
   f. Hold
   g. Return to starting position
   h. Repeat with other arm and leg

EXERCISES FOR ABDOMINAL MUSCLES

32. a. Supine position
   b. Knees flexed, feet flat on floor
   c. Arms extended overhead
   d. Slowly raise arms forward toward knees
   e. With chin to chest, raise the upper body approximately 45 degrees
   f. Hold
   g. Lower slowly
   h. Return to starting position

33. a. Supine position
   b. Knees flexed, feet flat on floor
   c. Arms folded across chest
   d. Contract abdominal muscles
   e. Slowly raise the upper body to a semisitting position
   f. Hold at approximately a 45 degree angle
   g. Lower slowly
   h. Return to starting position
   i. Repeat exercise with 3- to 5-lb. weight on chest

34. a. Supine position
   b. Knees flexed, feet flat on floor
   c. Hands clasped behind head

d. Elbows back
e. Contract abdominal muscles
f. Slowly raise the upper body to a semisitting position
g. Hold at approximately a 45 degree angle
h. Lower slowly
i. Return to starting position
35. a. Supine position
b. Knees flexed, feet flat under bottom rung of stall bars or being held flat by therapist
c. Hands clasped behind head
d. Elbows back
e. Slowly raise head and shoulders until they are 6 inches off floor
f. Hold
g. Lower slowly
h. Return to starting position
36. a. Supine position
b. Knees flexed, feet flat under bottom rung of stall bars or being held flat by therapist
c. Hands clasped behind head
d. Elbows back
e. Slowly raise head and shoulders off floor
f. Rotate upper part of body to left while rising
g. Hold
h. De-rotate
i. Lower slowly
j. Return to starting position
k. Repeat exercise, rotating to right
37. a. Supine position
b. Legs extended, knees straight
c. Arms down at sides
d. Raise head and shoulders and rotate upper body to right
e. Touch right foot with left hand
f. De-rotate
g. Lower slowly
h. Return to starting position
i. Repeat exercise rotating to left and touching left leg with right arm
38. a. Supine position
b. Legs extended, knees straight
c. Arms down at sides
d. Raise head and shoulders and rotate upper body to left
e. Touch left foot with right hand
f. De-rotate
g. Lower slowly
h. Return to starting position
i. Repeat exercise rotating to right and touching right leg with left arm
39. a. Supine position
b. Legs extended, knees straight
c. Hands clasped behind head
d. Slowly raise both feet about 6 inches off floor keeping knees straight
e. Hold
f. Lower slowly
g. Return to starting position

40. a. Supine position
b. Legs extended, knees straight
c. Hands clasped behind head
d. Slowly raise both feet about 6 inches off floor
e. Keep knees straight
f. Slowly spread legs
g. Hold apart to a count of 5
h. Return legs together
i. Lower slowly
j. Return to starting position
41. a. Supine position
b. Arms extended sideward (abducted) at shoulder level
c. Legs extended vertically, feet toward ceiling
d. Knees straight and legs together
e. Slowly move legs to left side and lower to floor
f. Legs should be at 90 degree angle during exercise, arms on mat
g. Slowly lift legs
h. Return to starting position
i. Repeat to opposite side
42. a. Supine position
b. Arms at sides
c. Legs extended about 6 to 12 inches apart, knees straight
d. Lift left arm and shoulder at the same time
e. Lift right leg upward, keeping it straight
f. Rotate upper part of body to the right
g. Reach with left hand to right leg
h. Touch outside of right knee
i. Hold
j. De-rotate—lower arm and leg
k. Lower slowly
l. Return to starting position
m. Repeat exercise rotating to left and using right arm and left leg

EXERCISES FOR THE HIP

43. a. Supine position
b. Legs extended, knees straight
c. Slowly raise left leg as high as possible
d. Hold
e. Lower slowly
f. Return to starting position
g. Repeat with right leg
44. a. Supine position
b. Legs extended, knees straight
c. Slowly raise left leg
d. Slowly flex left knee to approximately a 90 degree angle
e. Straighten knee slowly
f. Lower slowly
g. Return to starting position
h. Repeat with right leg
45. a. Supine position
b. Legs extended, knees straight
c. Slowly raise left leg

    d. Bend knee and bring to chest
    e. Straighten left leg slowly
    f. Lower slowly
    g. Return to starting position
    h. Repeat with right leg
46. a. Supine position
    b. Legs extended, knees straight
    c. Move (abduct) left leg slowly as far as possible to the side
    d. Point toes toward ceiling, knees straight
    e. Hold (abducted)
    f. Slowly return to starting position
    g. Repeat with right leg
47. a. Supine position
    b. Legs extended and internally rotated
    c. Keep knees straight
    d. Move (abduct) left leg slowly to the side as far as possible
    e. Keep leg internally rotated
    f. Slowly return to starting position
    g. Repeat with right leg
48. a. Supine position
    b. Legs extended, knees straight
    c. Flex left hip and knee
    d. Grasp left knee with both hands
    e. Pull knee toward chest slowly
    f. Release and slowly straighten left leg
    g. Lower slowly
    h. Return to starting position
    i. Repeat with right leg
49. a. Supine position
    b. Legs extended, knees straight
    c. Contract gluteal (buttocks) muscle
    d. Hold
    e. Relax
50. a. Lie on left side
    b. Flex knee of left leg slightly
    c. Keep knee of right leg straight
    d. Raise (abduct) right leg as far as possible
    e. Hold
    f. Return slowly to starting position
    g. Repeat exercise on other side
51. a. Lie on left side
    b. Flex knee of left leg slightly
    c. Internally rotate right leg, keep knee straight
    d. Flex right leg slightly at hip
    e. Raise right leg slowly as far as possible
    f. Keep leg internally rotated
    g. Hold
    h. Lower slowly
    i. Return to starting position
    j. Repeat exercise on other side
52. a. Prone position
    b. Legs extended
    c. Keep knees straight
    d. Raise (extend) one leg as far as possible
    e. Hold
    f. Lower slowly
    g. Return to starting position

    h. Repeat exercise with other leg
53. a. Prone position
    b. Legs extended
    c. Flex knee of one leg to 90 degree angle
    d. Keep other knee straight
    e. Raise (extend) flexed knee as far as possible
    f. Hold
    g. Lower slowly
    h. Return to starting position
    i. Repeat exercise with other leg
54. a. Sit on table with legs over the edge
    b. Knees flexed to approximately 90 degree angle
    c. Do not lean backward; hold edge of table with hands
    d. Raise (flex) one knee toward chest
    e. Hold
    f. Lower slowly
    g. Return to starting position
    h. Repeat exercise with other leg
55. a. Sit on table with legs over edge
    b. Knees flexed to approximately 90 degree angle
    c. Do not lean backward; hold edge of table with hands
    d. Raise (flex) knee slightly; externally rotate and slightly abduct leg; raise heel toward opposite knee
    e. Hold
    f. Lower slowly
    g. Return to starting position
    h. Repeat exercise with other leg
56. a. Supine position on table
    b. Left leg over front of table, knee flexed to 90 degree angle
    c. Right leg flexed at hip and knee, foot flat on table
    d. Rotate left ankle inwardly (external rotation of hip)
    e. Hold
    f. Return slowly to starting position
    g. Repeat exercise with other leg
57. a. Supine position on table
    b. Left leg over front of table, knee flexed to 90 degree angle
    c. Right leg flexed at hip and knee, foot flat on table
    d. Rotate left ankle outwardly (internal rotation of hip)
    e. Hold
    f. Return slowly to starting position
    g. Repeat exercise with other leg
58. a. Stand between 2 chairs, hands on backs of chairs for support
    b. Elevate one foot slightly off floor
    c. Full weight on other leg, keep knee straight
    d. Swing leg with pendulum motion
    e. Return to starting position
    f. Repeat exercise with other leg

59. a. Stand facing table, hands on table for support
    b. Elevate one foot slightly off floor
    c. Full weight on other leg, keep knee straight
    d. Move leg with sideward motion (abduct)
    e. Return to starting position
    f. Repeat exercise with other leg
60. a. Stand with feet 12 inches apart
    b. Elevate left foot slightly off floor
    c. Full weight on right leg, keep knee straight
    d. Internally and externally rotate left leg
    e. Return to starting position
    f. Repeat exercise with right leg
61. a. Stand facing up stairway
    b. Step up one step with one leg
    c. Bring other leg up to the same step
    d. Repeat all the way to top
62. a. Stand facing down stairway
    b. Step down one step with one leg
    c. Bring other leg down to the same step
    d. Repeat all the way down
63. a. Stand facing stairs
    b. Go up and down normally

EXERCISES FOR THE KNEE

64. a. Supine position
    b. Legs extended
    c. Place small rolled towel under one knee
    d. Tighten thigh musculature and raise heel
    e. Push back of knee against towel
    f. Hold for count of 5
    g. Return to starting position
65. a. Supine position
    b. Legs extended
    c. Tighten thigh musculature
    d. Lift one leg 6 inches; keep knee straight
    e. Hold
    f. Lower slowly
    g. Return to starting position
66. a. Supine position
    b. Legs extended
    c. Tighten thigh musculature
    d. Lift one leg; keep knee straight
    e. Try to lift leg to right angle with table
    f. Flex knee slowly; then extend
    g. Lower leg to starting position
67. a. Sit on edge of table
    b. Posterior thigh supported
    c. Slowly flex knee
    d. Flex knee to maximum
    e. Extend knee
    f. Repeat
68. a. Sit with body erect
    b. Legs extended, knees straight
    c. Reach forward and touch toes with fingers
    d. Return to starting position
69. a. Prone position
    b. Legs extended

c. Slowly flex knee
d. Bring heel toward buttocks
e. Hold at maximum flexion
f. Extend slowly until knee is straight
70. a. Prone position
    b. Legs extended
    c. Loop rolled sheet around ankle
    d. Grasp both ends of sheet
    e. Flex knee to maximum without aid
    f. Flex knee further by pulling sheet
    g. Slowly extend knee to starting position
71. a. Prone position
    b. Legs extended
    c. Flex knee by rotating lower leg outwardly
    d. Flex knee to maximum; hold
    e. Extend knee to starting position
72. a. Prone position
    b. Legs extended
    c. Flex knee by rotating lower leg inwardly
    d. Flex knee to maximum; hold
    e. Extend knee to starting position
73. a. Stand facing stall bars
    b. Place both feet on lower rungs
    c. Spread feet about 12 inches apart
    d. Hold onto stall bars with hands at shoulder height
    e. Slowly lower body for knee flex
    f. Slowly raise body for knee extension
74. a. Stand
    b. Slowly flex knees by squatting
    c. Keep heels on floor
    d. Squat to maximum
    e. Return to standing position slowly
75.   Ride stationary bicycle
76. a. Supine position
    b. Lift legs to a 60 to 90 degree angle with hips
    c. Place hands under hips for support
    d. Pedal as if riding bicycle
    e. Return to starting position
*77. a. Sit on table
    b. Body erect, hands grasping front of table
    c. Small rolled towel under uninvolved knee
    d. Small stool supporting involved leg when knee is flexed to 90 degrees or maximum
    e. Fasten foot boot, or other weight device securely on uninvolved leg
    f. Determine maximum amount of weight that can be lifted with uninvolved knee (this is to be used as a guide for the involved knee)
    g. Knee must come to full extension
    h. Must complete 10 repetitions of heaviest weight
    i. Leg must not swing pendulum fashion; patient must lift weights
78. a. Sit on table
    b. Body erect, hands grasping front of table
    c. Small rolled towel under knee

*testing exercise

d. Small stool supporting foot when knee is flexed to 90 degrees or maximum
e. Fasten foot boot, or other weight device securely on foot
f. Attach light weight (1¼ to 2½ lbs.)
g. Extend knee, hold for count of 3, and then lower; repeat 10 times
h. Continue to add weights; extend knee, hold for count of 3, and then lower; repeat 10 times with full extension, if possible, of knee until patient reaches maximum without pain
i. Next treatment session: take 50% of heaviest weight lifted (example: 50% of 10 lbs. = 5 lbs.)
j. Start with 5 lbs.: proceed as outlined in step g.
k. Next step: lift 75% of the maximum load on involved side (example: 7½ × 10 repetitions)
l. Final step: 100% (10 lbs. × 10 repetitions)

79. a. Sit on table
b. Body erect, hands grasping front of table
c. Small rolled towel under involved knee
d. Knee flexed 10 to 20 degrees, foot resting on stool
e. Attach foot boot with 50% of maximum weight (see Exercise 78)
f. Extend knee to lift weight through this short range of motion (to increase strength of vastus medialis for full extension)
g. Hold at full extension to count of 5; repeat 10 times
h. Continue with weighted boot; hold knee in full extension for longer periods; first 5 seconds then 10 seconds

80. a. Sit in rocking chair
b. Flex involved knee as much as possible
c. Flex uninvolved knee to approximately a 90 degree angle
d. Rock slowly; try to obtain more flexion of involved knee

EXERCISES FOR THE ANKLE AND FOOT

81. a. Sitting, prone, or supine position
b. Foot in neutral position
c. Dorsiflex (pull up) foot as far as possible
d. Hold
e. Plantar flex (push down) foot as far as possible
f. Hold
g. Return to starting position

82. a. Sitting, prone, or supine position
b. Foot in neutral position
c. Dorsiflex foot and invert (pull medially) as far as possible
d. Hold
e. Do not rotate hip or upper leg
f. Return to starting position

83. a. Sitting, prone, or supine position
b. Foot in neutral position
c. Plantar flex foot and invert (pull medially) as far as possible
d. Hold
e. Do not rotate hip or upper leg
f. Return to starting position

84. a. Sitting, prone, or supine position
b. Foot in neutral position
c. Plantar flex foot and evert (pull laterally) as far as possible
d. Hold
e. Do not rotate hip or upper leg
f. Return to starting position

85. a. Sitting, prone, or supine position
b. Foot in neutral position
c. Flex toes as far as possible
d. Do not plantar flex foot or ankle
e. Hold
f. Return to starting position
g. Extend toes as far as possible
h. Do not dorsiflex foot or ankle
i. Hold
j. Return to starting position

86. a. Sitting or supine position
b. Foot in neutral position
c. Instructor or therapist takes patient's heel in palm of hand
d. Instructor's or therapist's fingers are across heel near insertion of "Achilles tendon"
e. Upper part of instructor's or therapist's hand, wrist, and forearm is placed against sole of foot
f. Opposite hand is placed on anterior surface of knee to keep knee straight
g. Instructor or therapist slowly pushes toes, foot, and ankle into dorsiflexion by moving hand and forearm toward the knee
h. Hold at maximum stretch
i. Release slowly
j. Return to starting position

87. a. Stand
b. Feet parallel, 4 to 6 inches apart
c. Knees slightly flexed
d. Raise heel from floor into plantar flexion
e. Hold
f. Lower slowly
g. Return to starting position

88. a. Stand
b. Feet parallel, 4 to 6 inches apart
c. Knees slightly flexed
d. Raise heel from floor into plantar flexion
e. Swing heel outward
f. Hold
g. Swing inward
h. Return to starting position slowly

89. a. Stand, facing a wall about arm's length away
b. Feet parallel, 6 to 12 inches apart
c. Place toes and upper part of foot on book or piece of wood

    d. Heel of foot on floor
    e. Knees straight
    f. Hands against wall
    g. Keep body erect, buttocks in line with upper body
    h. Slowly lean forward toward wall
    i. Hold at maximum stretch
    j. Return to starting position slowly

90. a. Stand
    b. Feet parallel, 6 to 12 inches apart
    c. Walk on toes
    d. Hold
    e. Return to starting position

91. a. Stand
    b. Feet parallel, 6 to 12 inches apart
    c. Walk on heels
    d. Hold
    e. Return to starting position

92. a. Sit on stool
    b. Towel on floor
    c. Feet parallel, 6 to 12 inches part
    d. Flex toes and try to grasp towel
    e. Extend toes to release towel
    f. Return to starting position

93. a. Sit on stool
    b. Towel on floor, marbles on towel
    c. Flex toes, try to pick up marbles and move to another part of the towel; extend toes to release marbles
    d. Return to starting position; repeat

94. a. Stand
    b. Feet parallel, 6 to 12 inches apart
    c. Place weight on outer surfaces of feet by inverting feet
    d. Walk on outer surfaces of feet
    e. Return to starting position

95. a. Stand
    b. Feet parallel, 6 to 12 inches apart
    c. Place weight on inner surface of feet by everting feet
    d. Walk on inner surface of feet
    e. Return to starting position

EXERCISES FOR THE FINGERS

96. a. Sit at table
    b. Palm flat on table
    c. Spread fingers apart
    d. Raise (extend) fingers from table one by one
    e. Return to starting position

97. a. Sit at table
    b. Back (dorsal surface) of hand on table
    c. Fingers extended
    d. Flex fingers one by one at metacarpophalangeal joints
    e. Keep interphalangeal joints extended
    f. Hold
    g. Return to starting position

98. a. Sit at table
    b. Back (dorsal surface) of hand on table
    c. Fingers extended
    d. Flex distal and then middle interphalangeal joints
    e. Do not flex metacarpophalangeal joints
    f. Hold
    g. Return to starting position

99. a. Sit at table
    b. Palm (volar surface) of hand on table
    c. Fingers extended
    d. Slowly spread (abduct) fingers as far as possible
    e. Hold
    f. Slowly bring fingers together (abduct) and squeeze
    g. Hold
    h. Do not lift fingers from table
    i. Relax
    j. Return to starting position

100. a. Sit at table
    b. Palm (volar surface) of hand on table
    c. Flex fingers slightly
    d. Slowly extend proximal phalanges
    e. Keep fingers slightly flexed
    f. Hold
    g. Return to starting position

101. a. Sit at table
    b. Back (dorsal surface) of hand on table
    c. Flex distal and then proximal phalanx of thumb
    d. Pull thumb across into palm of hand
    e. Hold
    f. Return to starting position

102. a. Sit at table
    b. Palm (volar surface) of hand on table
    c. Extend thumb as far as possible
    d. Hold
    e. Return to starting position

103. a. Sit at table
    b. Palm (volar surface) of hand on table
    c. Extend fingers and thumb
    d. Keeping fingers and thumb extended
    e. Bringing fifth finger and thumb together
    f. Touch tip of fifth finger and tip of thumb together
    g. Hold
    h. Return to starting position

104. Squeeze small piece of sponge or small rubber ball

105. Pick up coins and buttons of assorted sizes

106. Crumple sheet of newspaper into small ball with one hand

107. a. Gently pull fifth finger outward
    b. Flex metacarpophalangeal joint

108. a. Gently pull fifth finger outward
    b. Flex middle interphalangeal joint
    c. Repeat with other fingers

109. a. Gently pull fifth finger outward
    b. Flex distal interphalangeal joint

c. Repeat with the other fingers
110. a. Hand pronated, fingers slightly flexed
  b. Place other hand on top, fingers over metacarpophalangeal joint
  c. Slowly flex fingers
  d. Exert pressure with cupped hand
  e. Hold
  f. Return to starting position

EXERCISES FOR THE WRIST

111. a. Sit
  b. Hand in relaxed position
  c. Make a fist (flex fingers and thumb) as tight as possible
  d. Hold
  e. Extend and spread (abduct) fingers and thumb as far as possible
  f. Hold
  g. Return to starting position
112. a. Sit at table
  b. Forearm resting on table
  c. Hand midway between supination and pronation
  d. Flex wrist and raise (elevate) side of hand off table
  e. Hold
  f. Return to starting position
113. a. Sit at table
  b. Forearm resting on table
  c. Hand fully supinated
  d. Slide wrist toward fifth finger
  e. Keep hand flat on table
  f. Hold
  g. Return to starting position
114. a. Sit at table
  b. Forearm resting on table
  c. Flex wrist as far as possible
  d. Hold
  e. Return to starting position
115. a. Stand facing a table
  b. Hand palm down, forearm, and elbow resting on table
  c. Back (dorsal surface) of other hand on table
  d. Slowly raise elbow and forearm upward from table
  e. Hold
  f. Return slowly to starting position
116. a. Grasp door knob
  b. Turn right
  c. Hold
  d. Turn left
  e. Hold
  f. Return to starting position
117. a. Stand facing wall
  b. Arm extended at shoulder level, elbow slightly flexed
  c. Place palm against wall
  d. Extend fingers and point them upward
  e. Keep hand against wall; slowly slide arm downward
  f. Do not lift hand away from wall
  g. Do not bend knees
  h. Hold at maximum stretch
  i. Return to starting position

EXERCISES FOR THE ELBOW

118. a. Sit or stand
  b. Arm at side, forearm supinated
  c. Elbow extended
  d. Flex elbow
  e. Bring fingertips to shoulder
  f. Hold
  g. Extend elbow to maximum
  h. Hold
  i. Return to starting position
119. a. Sit or stand
  b. Forearm pronated
  c. Elbow flexed to 90 degree angle, resting on hip
  d. Slowly turn forearm and hand until palm is up (supinated)
  e. Hold
  f. Slowly return to starting position
120. a. Stand facing a bar at shoulder height
  b. Grasp bar
  c. Try to flex elbow (isometric)
  d. Hold
  e. Try to extend elbow (isometric)
  f. Hold
  g. Return to starting position
121. a. Sit at table
  b. Forearm resting on table
  c. Grasp a 12- to 18-inch rod or pole at one end
  d. Slowly pronate as far as possible
  e. Hold
  f. Slowly supinate as far as possible
  g. Hold
  h. Return to starting position
122. a. Sit facing mirror
  b. Rod or pole resting on thighs
  c. Grasp rod or pole with both hands
  d. Raise (flex) arms to shoulder level
  e. Hold
  f. Flex elbows; bring rod or pole to nose
  g. Hold
  h. Extend elbows
  i. Hold
  j. Return to starting position
123. a. Sit facing mirror
  b. Arm at side
  c. Flex elbow bringing fingers to shoulder
  d. Hold
  e. Lift arm over head, elbow extended
  f. Hold
  g. Flex elbow, bring fingers to shoulder

h. Hold
i. Lower (adduct) arm to 90 degrees
j. Extend elbow
k. Hold
l. Return to starting position
124. a. Stand facing a wall about arm's length away
b. Feet parallel
c. Place palms on wall, fingers extended and pointing inward
d. Keep heels on floor and body erect
e. Slowly flex elbows
f. Move body toward wall
g. Hold
h. Extend elbows and push body away from wall
i. Return to starting position

EXERCISES FOR THE SHOULDER

125. a. Stand alongside table or chair
b. Bend over at the waist
c. Place uninvolved hand on table or chair for support
d. Arm on involved side hangs loose
e. Slowly swing arm forward and backward (pendulum action)
f. Stop swinging slowly
g. Slowly swing arm across body and then back (pendulum action)
h. Stop slowly
i. Slowly make circles left and then right
j. Stop swinging slowly
k. Return to starting position
126. a. Stand or sit facing a mirror
b. Arms at sides
c. Raise (elevate) shoulders (shrugging motion)
d. Hold
e. Lower
f. Pull shoulders forward
g. Pull shoulders backward
h. Return to starting position
127. a. Stand facing wall
b. Arms at side
c. Place fingers on wall at hip level
d. Slowly move fingers with elbow straight, up wall
e. Flex shoulder as far as possible
f. Hold
g. Return to starting position slowly
128. a. Sit facing mirror
b. Wand resting on thighs
c. Grasp wand with both hands, shoulder width apart
d. Keep elbows straight
e. Slowly flex shoulders
f. Bring wand up over head
g. Do not arch back
h. Hold
i. Return slowly to starting position

j. Do exercise without wand
129. a. Sit facing mirror
b. Arm at side, elbow straight
c. Slowly raise (abduct) arm as far as possible to the side
d. Keep palm down
e. Do not lean in opposite direction
f. Hold at maximum
g. Lower slowly to starting position
130. a. Sit facing mirror
b. Arm at side, elbow straight
c. Slowly raise (flex) arm as high as possible toward the front
d. Palm down
e. Hold
f. Do not lean backward
g. Lower slowly to starting position
131. a. Sit facing mirror
b. Wand resting on thighs
c. Grasp wand with both hands shoulder width
d. Keep elbows straight
e. Raise wand toward mirror to shoulder level
f. Hold
g. Pull wand to left as far as possible
h. Hold; return to front
i. Pull wand to right as far as possible
j. Hold; return to front
k. Lower slowly to starting position
l. Do exercise without wand
132. a. Sit on stool
b. Back against wall
c. Raise (abduct) arms to shoulder height at sides
d. Flex elbows to a 90 degree angle on shoulder-height plane
e. Palms facing downward
f. Slowly lift hands—try to touch wall with backs (dorsal surfaces) of hands; hold
g. Keep shoulders and elbows at 90 degree angles during motion
h. Slowly lower hands and try to touch wall with palms (volar) of hands; hold
i. Keep shoulders and elbows at 90 degree angles during motion
j. Slowly return hands to shoulder height
k. Return to starting point
133. a. Standing or supine position
b. Fingers interlaced behind neck
c. Elbows are forward
d. Pull elbows back
e. Hold
f. Return to starting position
134. a. Stand facing chair
b. Grasp top of chair, palm up
c. Elbow at waist level
d. Slowly turn body away from chair
e. Elbow remains at waist level
f. Hold maximum stretch
g. Return slowly to face chair

   h. Return to starting position
135. a. Stand facing mirror
   b. Place hands in small of back
   c. Grasp wand, cane, or pole
   d. Keep body erect
   e. Try to lift wand, cane, or pole upward
   f. Hold at maximum stretch
   g. Return to starting position
136. a. Sit on stool
   b. Pulley with rope through it attached overhead on door, ceiling, or extension of metal
   c. Elbows straight, shoulders flexed
   d. Body erect
   e. Grasp one end of rope with each hand
   f. Pull rope down into extension
   g. Opposite will go into flexion
   h. Hold at maximum pull
   i. Pull from flexion into extension
   j. Hold at full extension
   k. Repeat, alternating from flexion to extension
   l. Return to starting position
137. a. Sit on stool
   b. Use pulley as in 136 b above
   c. Shoulders abducted to a 90 degree angle, elbows straight
   d. Grasp ends of rope one end in each hand
   e. Pull one arm down in shoulder adduction
   f. Other arm will go into shoulder abduction
   g. Hold in full abduction
   h. Reverse procedure, pull arm that is abducted into adduction
   i. Hold
   j. Repeat
   k. Return to starting position
138. a. Sit on stool
   b. Bend slightly at waist
   c. Arms at sides, elbows straight
   d. Swing arms forward and upward (flexion)
   e. Then downward and backward (extension)
   f. Repeat
   g. Return to starting position

EXERCISES FOR HEAD AND NECK

139. a. Sit facing mirror
   b. Body erect
   c. Pull chin down and slightly back, but not down on chest
   d. Slowly rotate head to right
   e. Hold
   f. Rotate back to midpoint
   g. Slowly rotate head to left
   h. Hold
   i. Rotate back to midpoint
   j. Return to starting position
140. a. Sit facing mirror
   b. Body erect
   c. Pull chin down and slightly back, but not down on chest

   d. Slowly tilt head toward right shoulder
   e. Hold
   f. Do not rotate head or raise (elevate) shoulder
   g. Return to midpoint
   h. Repeat on left side
   i. Hold
   j. Return to midpoint
   k. Return to starting position
141. a. Sit on bench facing stall bars or wall
   b. Arms flexed to shoulder level, elbows straight, palms on walls or bars
   c. Chin tucked in
   d. Instructor or therapist places hand behind patient's head
   e. Patient presses head backward
   f. Instructor or therapist gives resistance
   g. Hold
   h. Relax
   i. Return to starting position

EXERCISES FOR DEEP BREATHING

142. a. Supine position
   b. Hips and knees flexed
   c. Feet flat on floor
   d. Inhale through nose to maximum
   e. Hold briefly
   f. Exhale through mouth with hissing sound
   g. Repeat
143. a. Supine position
   b. Hips and knees flexed
   c. Feet flat on floor
   d. Place one hand on upper chest
   e. Place other hand on abdomen
   f. Inhale through nose and try to elevate the chest only
   g. Hold briefly
   h. Exhale through mouth with hissing sound
   i. Abdomen should remain fairly still during exercise
   j. Repeat
144. a. Supine position
   b. Hips and knees flexed
   c. Feet flat on floor
   d. Place one hand on each side of ribs
   e. Inhale through nose; try to elevate chest only
   f. Hold briefly
   g. Exhale through mouth with hissing sound
   h. Push hands together during expiration
   i. Abdomen should remain fairly still during exercise
   j. Repeat
145. a. Supine position
   b. Hips and knees flexed
   c. Feet flat on floor
   d. Place folded towel around chest
   e. Cross arms across chest
   f. Grasp ends of towel
   g. Inhale through nose; try to elevate chest only

h. Hold briefly
i. Exhale through mouth with hissing sound
j. Pull towel tight during expiration
k. Repeat
146. a. Sit in chair
   b. Arms relaxed at sides
   c. Slowly flex at waist
   d. Exhale through mouth as you flex body toward floor
   e. Hold briefly at maximum position
   f. Slowly sit up
   g. Inhale through nose
   h. Hold at sitting position
   i. Repeat

EXERCISES FOR THE SPINAL ORTHOSIS USER

The following exercises are designed to improve the strength of the muscles of the torso to counteract the effects of bracing and to activate the abnormal curvature of the spine. These exercises are not to correct the spinal curve, but to maintain strength and flexibility in the spine.

147. *Pelvic Tilt.*
   a. Lie in supine position, knees bent, feet flat on floor
   b. Tighten abdominal muscles, pinch the buttocks muscles together, tilt pelvis to force the small of the back against the floor. (Do not hold breath.)
   c. Hold for a count of 5
   d. Return to starting position
   e. Variations on the pelvic tilt can be done while lying, standing, walking, and in or out of the brace

The following exercises are done daily out of the brace:

148. *Sit-ups.* To strengthen and/or maintain good abdominal muscles
   a. Lie in supine position, knees bent, feet flat on floor
   b. Do the pelvic tilt
   c. Keep the pelvic tilt, roll upward starting with the head, lifting shoulders and head only; hold for a few seconds, making the abdominal muscles very tight
   d. Return to the starting position, maintaining the pelvic tilt
   e. Do 10 consecutive times. Do 5 times diagonally to each side, turning in the spine

149. a. Lie in supine position
   b. Put arms around the knees, pull them to the chest, then touch forehead to knees
   c. Hold for several seconds
   d. Do 2 times

150. *Push-ups.* To strengthen and/or maintain shoulder and upper back muscles
   a. Kneeling on hands and knees, arms out from body at shoulder level with the elbows straight
   b. Do the pelvic tilt
   c. Keeping the head level with shoulders, lower the body to the floor (touch nose to floor) by bending elbows. Keep pelvic tilt
   d. Straighten elbows and return to starting position
   e. Do 10 times

151. *Hamstring Stretching* (only if tight)
   a. Supine position with knees straight
   b. Raise one leg at a time with knee straight until "pull" is felt behind thigh and knee. Keep the opposite leg flat on the floor
   c. Return to starting position

152. *Hyperextension.* To strengthen scapula and upper back, reduce round shoulders
   a. Lie in prone position with arms by the sides of body
   b. Do pelvic tilt
   c. Squeeze shoulder blades together
   d. Lift the shoulders, upper chest, and legs off the floor
   e. Keep the head level with shoulders and maintain the pelvic tilt. Hold for 5 seconds
   f. Return to starting position
   g. Do 5 times with arms at sides, 5 times in "Superman" position with arms extended in front of body

153. a. Lie in supine position
   b. Put arms around knees, pull them to chest, then touch forehead to knees
   c. Hold for several seconds
   d. Do 2 times

154. a. Sit in Indian style position
   b. Reach one arm over head, and lean sideways
   c. Put both hands on the floor on one side while rotating the spine
   d. Keep hips on the floor
   e. Do 5 times to each side

155. *Deep Breathing.* Refer to Exercise #142.

Appendix B

General Exercises for Physical Reconditioning

The exercises listed in this appendix were selected to provide instructors and therapists with some basic physical reconditioning activities. This is not to imply that these are the only useful and valuable exercises. There are many others that can be utilized to supplement the exercises listed in this appendix.

Listed under each physical reconditioning exercise are the primary and secondary sites of development in the body. The authors wish to point out that some of the muscles in the primary and secondary sites listed will act as prime movers, synergists, or muscles of fixation. These specific muscles may perform all or one of the above actions during the exercises.

A discussion of the kinesiologic activity of a specific muscle or muscle group is not the intent of the authors. Rather, our intent is to give the instructor or therapist a general overview. If the instructor or therapist is interested in specific muscle activity, a good anatomy or kinesiology book is recommended.

All physical reconditioning exercises can be divided into four types: strength, flexibility, endurance, and cardiovascular.

The instructor or therapist must constantly keep in mind the disease, medical problem, or condition of the person with whom he is working. The mental, as well as the physical, status of the person must also be considered before any exercises are initiated. Many of the reconditioning exercises may only develop one aspect of strength, flexibility, endurance, or cardiovascular activity. Other exercises based on factors of repetitions and periods of time may develop 2 or more aspects of strength, flexibility, endurance, or cardiovascular changes.

All physical reconditioning exercises should be initiated slowly. Give a few specific exercises and a set number of repetitions for each exercise. Do not leave these matters up to the individual. The exercises and repetitions should be increased as the individual gains in one or all of the factors of strength, flexibility, endurance and/or cardiovascular activity. Do not overwork the individual. Overwork may cause a relapse or slow the healing process. A well-planned and gradually increased physical reconditioning program is the safest.

1. Push-ups from kneeling position
   a. Lower arm
   b. Upper arm
   c. Shoulder
   d. Shoulder girdle
   e. Anterior chest
   f. Upper back
   g. Lower back
   h. Abdominals
2. Push-ups
   a. Lower arm
   b. Upper arm
   c. Shoulder
   d. Shoulder girdle
   e. Anterior chest
   f. Upper back
   g. Lower back
   h. Abdominals
3. Pull-ups—overhead grip, feet on floor
   a. Fingers
   b. Hand
   c. Wrist
   d. Lower arm
   e. Upper arm
   f. Shoulder
   g. Shoulder girdle
   h. Anterior chest
   i. Upper back
   j. Abdominals
4. Pull-ups—overhead grip, feet off floor
   a. Fingers
   b. Hand
   c. Wrist
   d. Lower arm
   e. Upper arm
   f. Shoulder
   g. Shoulder girdle
   h. Anterior chest
   i. Upper back
   j. Lower back
   k. Abdominals
5. Pull-ups—underhand grip, feet on floor
   a. Fingers
   b. Hand

c. Wrist
d. Lower arm
e. Upper arm
f. Shoulder
g. Shoulder girdle
h. Anterior chest
i. Upper back
j. Lower back
k. Abdominals

6. Pull-ups—underhand grip, feet off floor
   a. Fingers
   b. Hand
   c. Wrist
   d. Lower arm
   e. Upper arm
   f. Shoulder
   g. Shoulder girdle
   h. Anterior chest
   i. Upper back
   j. Lower back
   k. Abdominals

7. Moving forward and backward on horizontal ladder from arm hanging position
   a. Fingers
   b. Hand
   c. Wrist
   d. Lower arm
   e. Upper arm
   f. Shoulder
   g. Shoulder girdle
   h. Anterior chest
   i. Upper back
   j. Lower back

8. Hanging tolerance from overhead bar
   a. Fingers
   b. Hand
   c. Wrist
   d. Lower arm
   e. Upper arm
   f. Shoulder
   g. Shoulder girdle
   h. Upper back
   i. Anterior chest
   j. Abdominals

9. Arm support with forward and backward movement on parallel bars
   a. Fingers
   b. Hand
   c. Wrist
   d. Lower arm
   e. Upper arm
   f. Shoulder
   g. Shoulder girdle
   h. Anterior chest
   i. Upper back
   j. Lower back
   k. Abdominals

10. Medicine ball activities
    a. Fingers

b. Hand
c. Wrist
d. Lower arm
e. Upper arm
f. Anterior chest
g. Upper back
h. Shoulder
i. Shoulder girdle

11. Sit-ups—knees and hips flexed
    a. Neck
    b. Abdominals
    c. Anterior chest
    d. Hip
    e. Anterior hip

12. Sit-ups—knees straight
    a. Neck
    b. Abdominals
    c. Anterior chest
    d. Hip

13. Straight leg raises
    a. Knee
    b. Hip
    c. Abdominals
    d. Anterior thigh
    e. Anterior calf

14. "Jumping Jacks" (side straddle hop)
    a. Shoulder
    b. Shoulder girdle
    c. Anterior chest
    d. Upper back
    e. Midback
    f. Abdominals
    g. Hip
    h. Knee
    i. Ankle
    j. Foot

15. Trunk bending: forward, sideways, and backward
    a. Neck
    b. Anterior chest
    c. Upper back
    d. Midback
    e. Lower back
    f. Abdominals
    g. Anterior thigh
    h. Posterior thigh
    i. Hip

16. Toe touching—sitting
    a. Upper back
    b. Anterior chest
    c. Shoulder
    d. Shoulder girdle
    e. Lower back
    f. Abdominals
    g. Hip

17. Toe touching—standing
    a. Upper back
    b. Midback
    c. Lower back

    d. Anterior chest
    e. Shoulder
    f. Shoulder girdle
    g. Hip
    h. Abdominals
18. Squat thrust
    a. Anterior thighs
    b. Hip
    c. Upper back
    d. Lower back
    e. Hand
    f. Wrist
    g. Lower arm
    h. Upper arm
    i. Shoulder
    j. Shoulder girdle
    k. Anterior chest
    l. Abdominals
    m. Posterior thighs
    n. Calf
    o. Ankle
    p. Foot
19. Trunk twister
    a. Hip
    b. Abdominals
    c. Upper back
    d. Lower back
    e. Anterior chest
20. "V" seat
    a. Knee

    b. Hip
    c. Abdominals
    d. Lower back
    e. Upper back
    f. Anterior chest
    g. Posterior thigh
    h. Anterior thigh
21. Standing run
    a. Foot
    b. Ankle
    c. Calf
    d. Knee
    e. Hip
    f. Anterior thigh
    g. Posterior thigh
22. Rope climbing (legs wrapped around ropes)
    a. Fingers
    b. Hand
    c. Wrist
    d. Lower arm
    e. Upper arm
    f. Anterior chest
    g. Shoulder
    h. Shoulder girdle
    i. Upper back
    j. Lower back
    k. Abdominals
    l. Hip
    m. Anterior thigh
    n. Posterior thigh

Appendix C

Weight Training and General Conditioning

Use of the proper weight is the most important factor in weight training. The proper weight should be selected for each exercise with consideration given to the strength of the muscles utilized. The following procedures comprise the best approach to successful weight training.

1. Start with a weight that can be lifted or moved through a given motion for 10 repetitions, with the proper form and without strain.
2. Try to increase the number of repetitions done each day with proper form and without strain.
3. When 15 repetitions are accomplished using proper form without strain, increase the weight by 5 pounds.
4. With the increased weight, begin a new series with 10 repetitions and follow steps 1 through 3 again.
5. Some exercises will be easier to do than others; keep accurate records of the weight used and number of repetitions done for each exercise.

GENERAL WEIGHT TRAINING EXERCISES

1. Two arm curl
   a. Stand, body erect, feet about 12 inches apart
   b. Arms at sides
   c. Grasp bar with undergrip, palms up, shoulder width apart
   d. Keep elbows at hips
   e. Slowly lift weights by flexing elbow
   f. Bring weights toward shoulders
   g. Hold
   h. Do assigned number of repetitions
   i. Lower to starting position; straighten elbows completely
2. Two arm press
   a. Stand, feet about 12 inches apart
   b. Bar on floor in front of feet
   c. Bend knees; grasp bar with overgrip, knuckles up, shoulder width apart
   d. Bring bar and weights to chest in one clear motion by flexing elbows and straightening knees
   e. Hold weight at chest level
   f. Slowly push bar and weights overhead

g. Hold; lower slowly to chest
   h. Repeat overhead
   i. When assigned repetitions are completed, return to chest, then lower to starting position
3. Two arm reverse curl
   a. Stand, body erect, feet about 12 inches apart
   b. Arms at sides
   c. Grasp bar with overgrip, knuckles up, hands about 6 inches apart
   d. Bar at thigh level
   e. Extend wrist to maximum
   f. Flex elbows, lifting bar to chest
   g. Keep elbows close to hips
   h. Hold bar at chest level
   i. Lower bar to thighs; hold
   j. Repeat lift to chest; do assigned number of repetitions
   k. Return to starting position
4. Supine press
   a. Supine position
   b. Shoulders comfortable on floor or bench
   c. Bar and weights are resting behind head
   d. Grasp bar
   e. Lift slightly to be sure bar is balanced
   f. Lift bar upward; straighten elbows; arms should be perpendicular to the floor
   g. Slowly lower bar and weights to chest
   h. Slowly push bar and weights upward until elbows are straight
   i. Be sure arms are perpendicular to floor
   j. Repeat number of assigned repetitions
   k. Return to starting position
5. Rise on toes
   a. Stand, body erect, heels together, toes turned out
   b. Place bar behind the neck
   c. Grasp bar with hands at shoulder width or beyond
   d. Slowly raise up on toes as high as possible
   e. Hold
   f. Lower slowly
   g. Repeat until assigned number of repetitions are completed

h. Return to starting position
6. Sit-ups
   a. Supine position
   b. Feet slightly higher than head if inclined board is available
   c. If board is not available, use mat or lie on floor
   d. Therapist should hold ankles
   e. Place bar and weights behind neck, grasp bar at shoulder width
   f. Slowly come to a sitting position
   g. Hold
   h. Return to full supine position
   i. Repeat assigned number of repetitions
   j. Return to starting position
7. Rowing
   a. Stand, feet 12 inches apart
   b. Bar and weights resting on floor approximately 12 to 18 inches in front of feet
   c. Flex trunk at waist
   d. Arms hanging straight down
   e. Grasp bar with overgrip
   f. Keep elbows straight after grasping bar
   g. Flex elbows bringing bar and weights to chest
   h. Hold
   i. Lower to straight elbow position
   j. Repeat to complete number of assigned repetitions
   k. Return to starting position
8. Quadriceps lift
   See therapeutic exercises 77, 78, and 79.
9. Forward raise
   a. Stand, feet 12 inches apart
   b. Bar with weight in middle
   c. Grasp bar with overgrip, knuckles up, hands shoulder width apart
   d. Bar at thigh level
   e. Lift bar and weights forward and overhead
   f. Keep elbows extended
   g. Lower weights with elbows extended
   h. Return bar to thigh level
   i. Repeat to complete number of assigned repetitions
10. Shoulder shrugging
   a. Stand, feet 12 inches apart
   b. Arms at sides
   c. Grasp bar with overgrip, knuckles up, hands shoulder width apart
   d. Bar at thigh level
   e. Elbows extended
   f. Shrug shoulders
   g. Lower shoulders to starting position
   h. Repeat to complete number of assigned repetitions
11. Upright rowing
   a. Stand, feet 12 inches apart
   b. Arms at sides
   c. Grasp bar with overgrip, knuckles up

d. Hands are placed in the center of the bar about 6 inches apart
e. Keep elbows extended
f. Bar and weights at thigh level
g. Flex elbows; bring bar and weights upward to chin (elbows should go up and out to shoulder level when lifting)
h. Hold
i. Lower to straight elbow position
j. Repeat to complete number of assigned repetitions
12. Regular dead lift
   a. Stand, feet 12 inches apart
   b. Bar and weights on floor, feet under barbell
   c. Arms at sides
   d. Flex hips and knees
   e. Grasp bar with overgrip, knuckles up, shoulder width apart
   f. Knees flexed as far as possible
   g. Back flat, head up
   h. Slowly straighten knees until body is straight
   i. Bar and weights at thigh level, elbows extended
   j. Flex knees; keep back straight; return weights to floor
   k. Repeat to complete number of assigned repetitions
13. Straddle lift
   a. Stand; feet straddling bar on floor
   b. Feet flat on floor, one foot slightly forward of the other
   c. Knees flexed, back straight
   d. Grasp bar, front hand overgrip, knuckles upward, rear hand undergrip, palm up
   e. Slowly stand upright by straightening knees
   f. Bring bar and weights upward between legs
   g. Keep back straight, head up
   h. Flex knees; keep back straight and return to starting position
   i. Repeat to complete number of assigned repetitions
14. Straight arm pullovers
   a. Supine, hips and knees straight
   b. Arms extended overhead, shoulder width apart
   c. Grasp bar, palms up
   d. Bar resting on floor behind head
   e. Keep elbows extended and slowly raise bar above chest
   f. Hold
   g. Return bar slowly to the floor behind the head
   h. Repeat to complete number of assigned repetitions
15. Triceps press (supine)
   a. Supine, hips and knees straight
   b. Arms are straight, elbows extended up toward ceiling

c. Bar is placed in hands
d. Grasp bar with overgrip, knuckles up
e. Hands 3 to 6 inches apart
f. Lower bar to the bridge of the nose
g. Keep elbows pointed toward the ceiling
h. Slowly straighten the elbows, keeping the upper arms vertical
i. Repeat to complete number of assigned repetitions

(Caution: weight must be controlled so it does not drop on the face.)

16. Triceps press (standing)
    a. Stand, feet 12 inches apart
    b. Hold bar above head
    c. Arms straight, elbows extended
    d. Bar grasped with overgrip
    e. Slowly lower the bar behind the head
    f. Keep elbows pointed toward the ceiling
    g. Try to keep the forearms vertical
    h. With the elbows pointed toward the ceiling, extend the arms slowly until weight is directly overhead
    i. Repeat to complete number of assigned repetitions

17. Back lift
    a. Stand, feet 12 inches apart
    b. Arms at sides
    c. Bar is resting behind heels
    d. Flex hips and knees
    e. Grasp bar with overgrip
    f. Knees bent, back straight, head up
    g. Slowly come to a standing position
    h. Hold
    i. Slowly return weight to floor by flexing knees
    j. Repeat to complete number of assigned repetitions

18. Lateral raise (standing)
    a. Stand, feet 12 inches apart
    b. Arms at sides, elbows straight
    c. Grasp dumbbell in each hand with overgrip
    d. Palms facing thighs
    e. Slowly raise dumbbells to shoulder level
    f. Keep elbows extended
    g. Hold
    h. Slowly lower dumbbells to starting position
    i. Repeat to complete number of assigned repetitions

19. Forward raise
    a. Stand, feet 12 inches apart
    b. Arms at sides, elbows straight
    c. Grasp dumbbells in each hand with overgrip
    d. Dumbbells rest across the thighs
    e. Slowly raise dumbbells directly overhead
    f. Keep the elbows straight
    g. Hold
    h. Lower dumbbells to starting position
    i. Repeat to complete number of assigned repetitions

20. Alternate curl
    a. Stand, feet 12 inches apart
    b. Arms at sides, elbows straight
    c. Grasp dumbbells in each hand with overgrip
    d. Palms facing thighs, arms straight
    e. Slowly flex right elbow and supinate hand; bring dumbbell to right shoulder
    f. Keep right upper arm close to body
    g. Slowly extend right elbow and pronate hand, returning dumbbell to starting position
    h. As the right dumbbell is being lowered, left dumbbell begins curl
    i. Continue alternating dumbbells in rhythm
    j. Repeat to complete number of assigned repetitions

WEIGHT (RESISTANCE) TRAINING SYSTEMS

Comprehensive exercise systems (single and multi-units) with variable resistance loads that provide wheelchair users (manual and motorized) with easy access are commercially available (Fig. C–1). Many of the systems are designed to simulate a wheelchair push motion, overhead press/pulldown, rowing, etc. Padded wrist cuffs and other restraining aids are available for hand-impaired individuals.

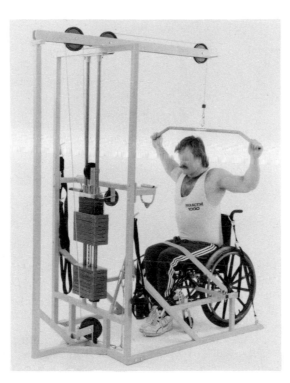

Fig. C–1.   Repetitive action against submaximal resistance while using multi-exercise unit. (Courtesy of ParaMed Exercise Equipment, Inc., P.O. Box 7304, Jackson, MS 39212.)

Appendix D

Crutches

MEASURING FOR CRUTCHES

a. Patient should be in a supine position
b. Use a steel tape
c. Measure from under arm to a point 6 inches in front and to the side of the foot
d. Space between the axillary bar (top of crutch) and the axilla should be 1 to 2 inches or about 2 or 3 fingers
e. Stand patient up against wall or supportive device
f. The elbow should be flexed in a 25 to 30 degree angle when the hand is on the handgrip
g. Patient should not lean on axillary bar at any time, either resting or moving

TYPES OF CRUTCH GAITS

1. Four-point gait
   a. Advance left crutch
   b. Advance right foot
   c. Advance right crutch
   d. Advance left foot

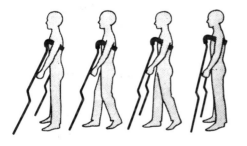

2. Two-point gait
   a. Advance left crutch and right foot simultaneously
   b. Advance right crutch and left foot simultaneously

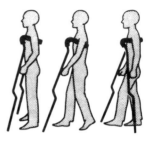

3. Three-point gait
   a. Advance both crutches and the involved leg together (the physician will specify if the involved leg should bear weight or not)
   b. Advance uninvolved lower extremity in between or in front of crutches
4. Drag-to gait
   a. Place both crutches in front of body
   b. Lean into crutches
   c. Drag body in between crutches
5. Swing-to gait
   a. Place both crutches in front of body
   b. Lean into crutches, lifting body off floor by extending elbows
   c. Advance feet in between crutches
   d. Keep shoulder back
   e. Move crutches slightly forward when feet strike

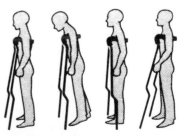

6. Swing-through gait
   a. Place both crutches in front of body
   b. Lift body off floor by extending elbows
   c. Move hips forward with a jerking motion
   d. Advance feet to a position slightly in front of crutches

---

*Illustrations reproduced from the crutch training manual of Lumex Inc., Bay Shore, N.J.

e. Move crutches slightly forward as feet strike

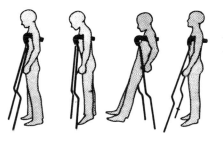

STAIRS

1. Ascending stairs
    a. Stand facing steps
    b. Crutches close to bottom step

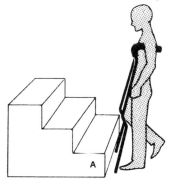

c. Extend elbows
d. Step up on first step with stronger leg
e. Balance on step

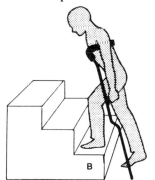

f. Bring both crutches and weaker leg up on first step

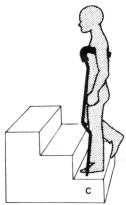

g. Continue to top of steps
h. Crutches are used the same way when ascending a curb
i. If handrail is present, place both crutches under the arm opposite handrail
j. Use handrail as crutch

2. Descending stairs
    a. Stand with crutches facing steps
    b. Stronger leg is placed close to edge of step

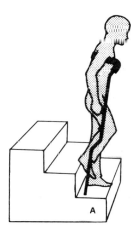

c. Place both crutches and weaker leg on next step
d. Bend knee of stronger leg for balance

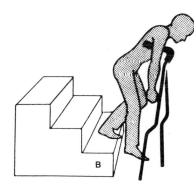

e. Balance on crutches on step
f. Bring stronger leg down to step

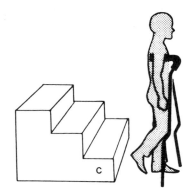

g. Continue to bottom of steps

h. Crutches are used the same way when descending a curb

i. If handrail is present, place both crutches under arm opposite handrail and use handrail as crutch

Appendix E

Balance Beam Exercises

Two heights are used as a standard reference: the low beam is 3 to 7 inches high, and the high beam 15 to 24 inches high. Variations in height can be made to adjust to individual problems. It is advisable to start at the lower level and then progress to the higher level.

Adhering to the following procedures will provide uniformity of exercising or testing:

1. Remove shoes and stockings. If this is impractical, then sneakers or tennis shoes should be worn.
2. Always approach the beam with the dominant foot.
3. Walk the beam slowly.
4. Use a heel-to-toe gait.
5. Place the whole foot straight on the beam.
6. Keep the head up, and do not watch feet.
7. Arms may be used to adjust center of gravity when starting to walk the beam or when performing dynamic balance exercises.
8. Student should focus his eyes on a given area when performing all exercises unless otherwise stated.

STATIONARY (STATIC BALANCE) EXERCISES

The following exercises are done with the arms extended sideward (abducted) at shoulder level and the weight on the balls of the feet.

1. a. Stand on beam
   b. Feet sideward, side by side
   c. Time number of seconds balance is maintained
2. a. Stand on beam
   b. Feet in heel-to-toe position
   c. Eyes closed
   d. Time number of seconds balance is maintained
3. a. Stand on beam
   b. Feet in heel-to-toe position
   c. Raise left foot, stand on right
   d. Time number of seconds balance is maintained
4. a. Stand on beam
   b. Feet in heel-to-toe position

   c. Raise right foot, stand on left
   d. Time number of seconds balance is maintained
5. a. Stand on beam
   b. Feet in heel-to-toe position
   c. Keep back straight
   d. Take left foot off beam and let foot hang to left side
   e. Bend right knee as far as possible
   f. Hold
   g. Straighten right knee
   h. Return to starting position
   i. Repeat on right side
6. a. Stand on beam
   b. Feet sideward, side by side
   c. Keep back straight
   d. Bend both knees as far as possible
   e. Hold
   f. Return to starting position
7. a. Stand on beam
   b. Feet sideward, feet apart 4 to 6 inches
   c. Keep back straight
   d. Bend both knees as far as possible
   e. Hold
   f. Return to starting position
8. a. Stand on beam
   b. Feet in heel-to-toe position
   c. Stand on left foot and raise right knee toward chest
   d. Keep back straight
   e. Hold
   f. Return to starting position
   g. Repeat on opposite side

MOVEMENT (DYNAMIC BALANCE) EXERCISES

The following exercises are done with the arms extended sideward (abducted) at shoulder level and weight on the balls of the feet.

1. a. Stand on beam
   b. Feet in heel-to-toe position
   c. Slowly walk forward
   d. Arms held sideward
   e. Use heel-to-toe gait
2. a. Stand on beam

    b. Feet in heel-to-toe position
    c. Slowly walk backward
    d. Arms held sideward
    e. Use heel-to-toe gait
3. a. Stand on beam
    b. Feet in heel-to-toe position
    c. Hands on hips
    d. Slowly walk forward
    e. Use heel-to-toe gait
    f. Repeat, walking backward, toe-to-heel gait
4. a. Stand on beam
    b. Feet in heel-to-toe position
    c. Arms folded across the chest
    d. Slowly walk forward
    e. Use heel-to-toe gait
    f. Repeat, walking backward, toe-to-heel gait
5. a. Stand on beam
    b. Feet in heel-to-toe position
    c. Arms at sides
    d. Place chalkboard eraser on top of head
    e. Slowly walk forward
    f. Use heel-to-toe gait
    g. Repeat, walking backward, toe-to-heel gait
6. a. Stand on beam
    b. Feet in heel-to-toe position
    c. Place chalkboard eraser in middle of beam
    d. Slowly walk forward
    e. Use heel-to-toe gait
    f. Pick up eraser
    g. Continue to end of beam
7. a. Stand on beam
    b. Feet in heel-to-toe position
    c. Place chalkboard eraser in middle of beam
    d. Slowly walk forward
    e. Use heel-to-toe gait
    f. Pick up eraser

    g. Turn
    h. Return to starting position
8. a. Stand on beam
    b. Feet in heel-to-toe position
    c. Slowly walk forward
    d. Stop in center of beam
    e. Bend one knee; place one foot off to side
    f. Hold
    g. Straighten knee
    h. Continue walking to end of beam
    i. Repeat, bending opposite leg
9. a. Stand on beam
    b. Feet in heel-to-toe position
    c. Slowly walk forward
    d. Keep right foot always in front of left
    e. Repeat, keeping opposite foot in front
10. a. Stand on beam
    b. Feet in heel-to-toe position
    c. Slowly walk backward
    d. Keep right foot always in front of left
    e. Repeat, keeping opposite foot in front
11. a. Stand on beam
    b. Feet in heel-to-toe position
    c. Slowly walk forward
    d. Use heel-to-toe gait
    e. Walk to middle of beam
    f. Balance on one foot
    g. Turn (half circle) on this foot
    h. Walk to end of beam
    i. Repeat, on opposite foot
12. a. Stand on beam
    b. Feet in heel-to-toe position
    c. Balance chalkboard eraser on head
    d. Slowly walk forward
    e. Use heel-to-toe gait
    f. Repeat, walking backward, using toe-to-heel gait

Appendix F

Rehabilitation Calisthenics

MODIFIED CARLSON FATIGUE-CURVE TEST

This test was modified from the Carlson Fatigue-Curve Test by substituting rhythmic calisthenics performed at different levels of exercise intensity for spot running. The test may be used to evaluate the physical work capacity that an individual has at different levels of exercise intensity. The pulse rate is used as a parameter to indicate physical work capacity and physical fitness. The pulse rate response to a given work load is dependent on many factors, among which are body position, age, time of day, and emotions. Thus, it is important to administer the test while the subject is in a room that is free from noise and congestion. The test should be administered at the same time every day, preferably early in the morning. The test is easy to administer and provides objective evidence of physical performance under stress. Another advantage is that the test can be used in a home exercise program or at school as part of an adapted physical education program.

Administration of Test

1. The test can be administered only after written permission is given by a physician. The subject rests in the supine position for a period of 5 minutes. The resting pulse (radial or apical) is taken for one full minute after this period of rest.
2. The subject completes the exercise protocol. Six exercises are chosen from the Montefiore Cardiac Fitness Program (Fig. F–1). The pulse is recorded immediately after exercise and known as the *exercise pulse*. The selection of exercises depends upon the condition of the subject and the amount of stress that is recommended by the physician. For convenience, the following classification of intensity is suggested:

Classification of Intensity	Heart Rate
Very light to light	80–99
Moderate	100–119
Heavy to unduly heavy	120–179
Exhaustive	180

The subject should start at a low energy cost level, and carry out 6 exercises (to caloric levels

of 2.5 calories per minute). Depending on his tolerance for exercise, the subject can slowly follow a graded exercise protocol by deleting the less strenuous exercises after every 4-day interval and adding others that expend higher levels of energy. It is suggested that the subject perform a series of exercises for a minimum of 4 days before increasing the intensity and duration. The number of exercises can be increased from 6 to 10 after the subject has advanced to the "heavy" range of exercise intensity.

3. The pulse is taken at 2, 4, and 6 minutes after exercise and, when plotted on a graph, is known as the *general fatigue curve* or post-exercise pulse (Fig. F–2). The recovery pulse, the last pulse rate that is documented, is taken 6 minutes after exercise.

In summary, the pulse is recorded 5 times during the test:

1. After the initial 5 minute rest period.
2. Immediately after exercise (taken for 15 seconds and multiplied by 4).
3. At 2, 4, and 6 minutes after exercise.

   The pulse should be taken for one full minute, except immediately after exercise as noted above. This permits greater accuracy when the cardiac rhythm is irregular.
4. The physical conditioning exercises program should continue on a daily basis until the subject is allowed full, unsupervised activity or until the physician issues other instructions.

Variables Used in Appraising Physical Work Capacity

1. The pulse rate count 6 minutes after exercise (*recovery pulse*) should correspond approximately to the count immediately before exercise (resting pulse). (Give or take 5 pulse counts, higher or lower.)

   Example 1: resting pulse = 96; recovery pulse = 98.

   The resting-recovery pulse rate variable would be satisfactory.

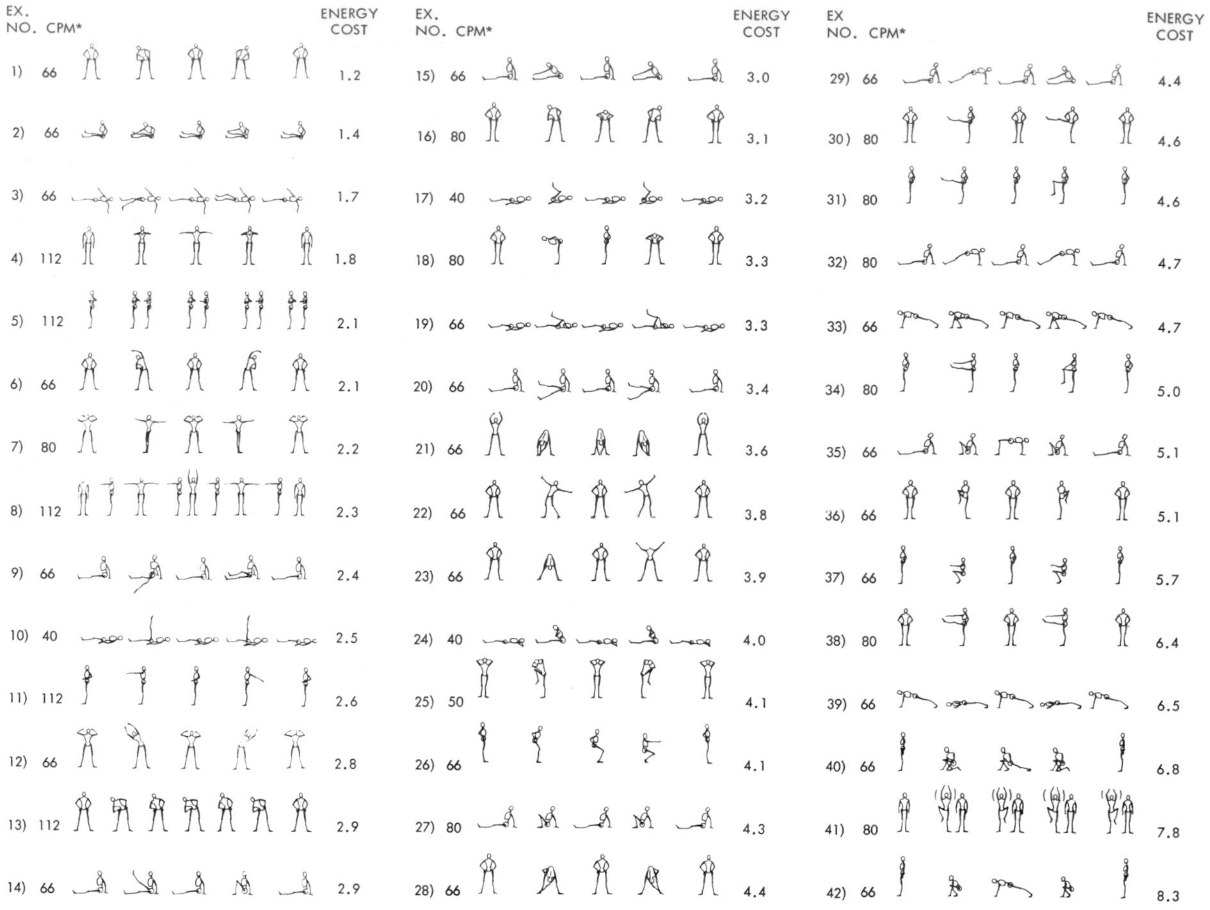

EX. NO.	CPM*	ENERGY COST	EX. NO.	CPM*	ENERGY COST	EX. NO.	CPM*	ENERGY COST
1)	66	1.2	15)	66	3.0	29)	66	4.4
2)	66	1.4	16)	80	3.1	30)	80	4.6
3)	66	1.7	17)	40	3.2	31)	80	4.6
4)	112	1.8	18)	80	3.3	32)	80	4.7
5)	112	2.1	19)	66	3.3	33)	66	4.7
6)	66	2.1	20)	66	3.4	34)	80	5.0
7)	80	2.2	21)	66	3.6	35)	66	5.1
8)	112	2.3	22)	66	3.8	36)	66	5.1
9)	66	2.4	23)	66	3.9	37)	66	5.7
10)	40	2.5	24)	40	4.0	38)	80	6.4
11)	112	2.6	25)	50	4.1	39)	66	6.5
12)	66	2.8	26)	66	4.1	40)	66	6.8
13)	112	2.9	27)	80	4.3	41)	80	7.8
14)	66	2.9	28)	66	4.4	42)	66	8.3

Fig. F–1.   Exercise instructions given to cardiac rehabilitation patients at Montefiore Hospital. Energy cost means the number of calories of energy needed to perform the particular exercise continuously for a minute. CPM means counts per minute. The CPM divided by four tells how many times the entire sequence is carried out in one minute. (From Weiss, R.A., and Karpovich, P.V.: Energy cost of exercise for convalescents. Arch Phys Med Rehabil, 28:447, 1947.)

Example 2: resting pulse = 80; recovery pulse = 88.
The resting-recovery pulse rate variable would be unsatisfactory.

If the work has been severe, no appreciable decrement in recovery pulse rate ensues. The recovery pulse rate comes down faster if the individual is more physically fit.

2. Alarming irregularities in the pulse rate are a contraindication to further exercise. If the work has been exhausting, an inverse recovery with an increase of pulse rate will occur. The general fatigue curve or post-exercise curve variable is unsatisfactory if there is a 5 pulse count increase between pulse recording intervals (activity; 2 minutes after; 2 to 4 minutes after; 4 to 6 minutes after exercise).

Example 1: Resting = 84
Activity = 105
Two minute interval = 90
Four minute interval = 84
Recovery = 84

General fatigue curve would be satisfactory.

Example 2: Resting = 80
Activity = 110
Two minute interval = 116
Four minute interval = 104
Recovery = 110

General fatigue curve variable would be unsatisfactory. The same holds true for the resting recovery variable.

If both variables are satisfactory, the test is scored SATISFACTORY.
If one variable is satisfactory and the other unsatisfactory, the test is scored FAIR.
If both variables are unsatisfactory, the test is scored UNSATISFACTORY.

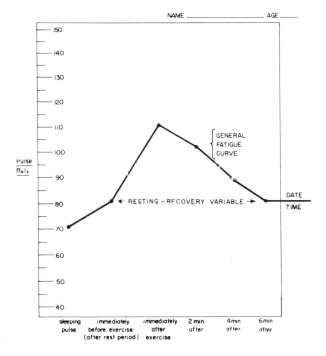

Fig. F–2. Modified Carlson Fatigue-Curve Chart.

Progressive Work Load with Aerobic Components

After the target heart rate has been determined, exercise(s) with an aerobic component such as bench steps, spot running, and brisk walking can be interspersed with the rehabilitation calisthenics. Aerobic exercises can be performed for any specified time, provided that the target heart rate is not exceeded. (Take carotid pulse for 15 seconds and multiply by 4.) The pulse can be taken during a pause in the exercise protocol. Another alternative is to use opto-electronic pulse detection with a wristwatch style digital pulse monitor. Body composition, cardiovascular efficiency, and endurance are enhanced by endurance activities that expend large amounts of energy. The aerobic component program can be used to increase the intensity and total amount of energy expended for any one session. It is recommended to work at lower intensities (rehabilitation calisthenics), especially at the beginning of a program, and then gradually increase the amount of work that is done within the same time period by interspersing aerobic components.

Appendix G

Sports Associations for Disabled Persons*

American Athletic Association of the Deaf
1134 Davenport Drive
Burton, MI 48529

United States Cerebral Palsy Athletic Association
34518 Warren Road, Suite 264
Westland, MI 48185

National Wheelchair Athletic Association†
1604 East Pikes Peak Avenue
Colorado Springs, CO 80909

United States Association for Blind Athletes
33 N. Institute Street
Brown Hall, Suite 015
Colorado Springs, CO 80903

United States Amputee Athletic Association
P.O. Box 210709
Nashville, TN 37221

United States Les Autres Sports Association
1101 Port Oak Blvd.
Suite 9-486
Houston, TX 77056

International Sports Organization for the Disabled
Idrottens Hus
S-123-87 Farsta
Sweden

National Handicapped Sports
1145 Nineteenth Street, Suite 717
Washington, D.C. 20036

---

* This is only a partial listing. Readers are encouraged to read the resource manual, *Sports and Recreation for the Disabled* (Benchmark Press) for a comprehensive review of national and international sports organizations.

† The governing body for Archery Sports Section, U.S. Wheelchair Weightlifting Federation, Physically Challenged Swimmers of America, Wheelchair Athletics of America (track and field), National Wheelchair Shooting Federation, and American Wheelchair Table Tennis Association.

Index

Page numbers in *italics* indicate figures; those followed by "t" indicate tables; those followed by "n" indicate notes.